D1441143

(continued on back)

**RADON
AND ITS DECAY
PRODUCTS
IN INDOOR AIR**

RADON AND ITS DECAY PRODUCTS IN INDOOR AIR

Edited by

WILLIAM W. NAZAROFF
California Institute of Technology
Pasadena, California
and
Lawrence Berkeley Laboratory
University of California
Berkeley, California

and

ANTHONY V. NERO, JR.
Lawrence Berkeley Laboratory
University of California
Berkeley, California

A WILEY-INTERSCIENCE PUBLICATION
JOHN WILEY & SONS
New York • Chichester • Brisbane • Toronto • Singapore

363.179
R1312

Copyright © 1988 by John Wiley & Sons, Inc.

All rights reserved. Published simultaneously in Canada.

Reproduction or translation of any part of this work
beyond that permitted by Section 107 or 108 of the
1976 United States Copyright Act without the permission
of the copyright owner is unlawful. Requests for
permission or further information should be addressed to
the Permissions Department, John Wiley & Sons, Inc.

Library of Congress Cataloging in Publication Data:

Radon and its decay products in indoor air / edited by William W.
  Nazaroff and Anthony V. Nero, Jr.
      p.   cm.

    "A Wiley-Interscience publication."
    Includes bibliographies and index.
    ISBN 0-471-62810-7 :

    1. Radon--Toxicology. 2. Radon--Isotopes--Toxicology. 3. Air-
-Pollution, Indoor--Hygienic aspects. 4. Radon--Environmental
aspects. 5. Housing and health. I. Nazaroff, W. W. II. Nero,
Anthony V.
RA1247.R33R32 1988
363.1′79--dc19   87-18915
                                                           CIP

Printed in the United States of America

10 9 8 7 6 5 4 3 2 1

CONTRIBUTORS

F. T. CROSS, Biology and Chemistry Department, Pacific Northwest Laboratory, Richland, Washington

SUZANNE M. DOYLE, Indoor Environment Program, Lawrence Berkeley Laboratory, University of California, Berkeley, California

ANTHONY C. JAMES, Radiological Measurement Department, National Radiological Protection Board, Chilton, Didcot, Oxfordshire, England

NIELS JONASSEN, Laboratory of Applied Physics I, Technical University of Denmark, Lyngby, Denmark

ATIKA KHAN, Department of Chemical Engineering and Applied Chemistry, University of Toronto, Toronto, Ontario, Canada

EARL O. KNUTSON, Aerosol Studies Division, Environmental Measurements Laboratory, U.S. Department of Energy, New York, New York

HELEN M. Y. LEUNG, Department of Chemical Engineering and Applied Chemistry, University of Toronto, Toronto, Ontario, Canada

J. P. MCLAUGHLIN, Physics Department, University College, Dublin, Ireland

BARBARA A. MOED, Indoor Environment Program, Lawrence Berkeley Laboratory, University of California, Berkeley, California

WILLIAM W. NAZAROFF, Environmental Engineering Science, California Institute of Technology, Pasadena, California and Indoor Environment Program, Lawrence Berkeley Laboratory, University of California, Berkeley, California

ANTHONY V. NERO, JR., Indoor Environment Program, Lawrence Berkeley Laboratory, University of California, Berkeley, California

COLIN R. PHILLIPS, Department of Chemical Engineering and Applied Chemistry, University of Toronto, Toronto, Ontario, Canada

ARTHUR G. SCOTT, American Atcon/Arthur Scott and Associates, Mississauga, Ontario, Canada

RICHARD G. SEXTRO, Indoor Environment Program, Lawrence Berkeley Laboratory, University of California, Berkeley, California

F. STEINHÄUSLER, Institut für Allgemeine Biologie, Biochemie und Biophysik, Universität Salzburg, Salzburg, Austria

ERLING STRANDEN, National Institute of Radiation Hygiene, Østerås, Norway

v

University Libraries
Carnegie Mellon University
Pittsburgh, Pennsylvania 15213

Environmental Science and Technology

The Environmental Science and Technology Series of Monographs, Textbooks, and Advances is devoted to the study of the quality of the environment and to the technology of its conservation. Environmental science therefore relates to the chemical, physical, and biological changes in the environment through contamination or modification, to the physical nature and biological behavior of air, water, soil, food, and waste as they are affected by man's agricultural, industrial, and social activites, and to the application of science and technology to the control and improvement of environmental quality.

The deterioration of environmental quality, which began when man first collected into villages and utilized fire, has existed as a serious problem under the ever-increasing impacts of exponentially increasing population and of industrializing society. Environmental contamination of air, water, soil, and food has become a threat to the continued existence of many plant and animal communities of the ecosystem and may ultimately threaten the very survival of the human race.

It seems clear that if we are to preserve for future generations some semblance of the biological order of the world of the past and hope to improve on the deteriorating standards of urban public health, environmental science and technology must quickly come to play a dominant role in designing our social and industrial structure for tomorrow. Scientifically rigorous criteria of environmental quality must be developed. Based in part on these criteria, realistic standards must be established and our technological progress must be tailored to meet them. It is obvious that civilization will continue to require increasing amounts of fuel, transportation, industrial chemicals, fertilizers, pesticides, and countless other products; and that it will continue to produce waste products of all descriptions. What is urgently needed is a total systems approach to modern civilization through which the pooled talents of scientists and engineers, in cooperation with social scientists and the medical profession, can be focused on the development of order and equilibrium in the presently disparate segments of the human environment. Most of the skills and tools that are needed are already in existence. We surely have a right to hope a technology that has created such manifold environment problems is also capable of solving them. It is our hope that this Series in Environmental Sciences and Technology will not only serve to make this challenge more explicit to the established professionals, but that it also will help to stimulate the student toward the career opportunities in this vital area.

ROBERT L. METCALF
WERNER STUMM

∎∎∎∎∎ PREFACE

In recent years, society's perception of the importance of indoor radon has altered drastically. Until the late 1970s, it was thought that elevated indoor radon concentrations were largely an isolated concern associated with the inadvertent presence of certain industrial and mining residues in or near buildings. Subsequent events—notably the observations around 1980 in Sweden, Canada, and the United States of a high incidence of ordinary houses with elevated radon levels—forced a major revision of that view within the scientific community. It is now widely understood that the most important component of radiation exposure to the public is due to the inhalation of radon decay products indoors. Even more significant is that the estimated level of health risk associated with average indoor radon levels is much higher than those due to other environmental carcinogens. Furthermore, and perhaps most importantly, radon concentrations ten or even a hundred or more times the average are observed with startling frequency, even in buildings that are otherwise quite ordinary. Long-term exposure to these higher concentrations leads to individual risks of lung cancer that are so high as to be unacceptable by almost any standard.

With its emergence as a major environmental concern, indoor radon has drawn considerable attention. Public awareness of the problem is keen in several European countries and Canada. In the United States, the discovery in 1984–85 of extraordinarily high radon levels in ordinary homes in Eastern Pennsylvania drew the problem to the attention of the public, legislators, and governmental agencies. From an element residing in an obscure corner of the periodic table, and of concern only to health physicists, radon has been propelled into a topic of front-page news and dinner-time discussion. Several scientific meetings are held to discuss new results each year. A new industry has even been created to diagnose and correct excessive indoor concentrations.

Consequently, considerable resources are being devoted to a wide range of activities aimed, ultimately, at limiting human exposures to radon decay products. As yet, however, a very small fraction of the necessary work has been completed. For ongoing efforts to be effective requires thorough understanding of an issue that is broadly interdisciplinary. Although there is a large and growing literature, there are too few works that provide insightful analysis of important aspects of the indoor radon problem, and none that do so comprehensively.

This book is designed to address that deficiency. As a whole, the volume is structured to examine the current state of knowledge of all major aspects of the indoor radon problem. Each chapter is in the nature of a review article, providing a critical synthesis of its topic with sufficient detail to be accessible to those who are technically trained but lack prior direct experience.

The core of the book is divided into four major sections. The first is concerned with the generation and migration of radon in source materials, and its entry into buildings. In the second section, the physical and chemical behavior of radon and radon decay products in indoor air are addressed. In the third section, evidence is discussed pertaining to the health effects and risk of exposure to radon decay products. The final section deals with both strategic and tactical aspects of controlling exposures. The book's core is framed by an overview chapter, which is a comprehensive introduction to the present state of knowledge, and by an appendix that provides a summary of measurement techniques and instrumentation.

In addition to its direct importance as a health hazard, indoor radon is exemplary of the broader issue of indoor air quality. Studies of radon can have important implications for studies of other indoor pollutants, and vice versa. On the one hand, the fairly detailed studies of the behavior of other airborne pollutants—including combustion emissions and organic chemicals—in the outdoor atmosphere and, increasingly, in the indoor environment provide a model approach and, in some cases, results that apply directly to the understanding of radon. On the other hand, the study of radon's behavior in the indoor environment per se, being somewhat more fully developed than the study of the behavior of other species in this setting, can produce generally useful information on the dynamics of indoor atmospheres. Similarly, policy approaches developed for indoor radon can help in dealing with other pollutants. An additional important aspect of radon is that it represents a relatively simple carcinogenic agent when compared, for example, with tobacco smoke. Consequently, our understanding of carcinogenesis may be advanced by focusing efforts on radon as a model agent. Thus, careful consideration and a reasoned response to the problem of indoor radon should take account of results from related studies. Conversely, efforts to gain further understanding of the nature of indoor radon could provide benefits beyond those that are immediately perceived.

WILLIAM W. NAZAROFF
ANTHONY V. NERO, JR.

Pasadena, California
Berkeley, California
April 1987

◼◼◼ ACKNOWLEDGMENTS

We are grateful for the efforts of the following scientists in reviewing chapters of this book: R. C. Bruno, R. Collé, R. Cuddihy, P. K. Hopke, H. M. Sachs, R. G. Sextro, A. B. Tanner, and M. E. Wrenn. Ultimate responsibility for the contents lies, of course, with the chapter authors and with the editors. Additionally, W.W.N. wishes to thank his wife, Ingrid, for her patience and support during the book's preparation.

CONTENTS

PART ONE: SOURCES AND TRANSPORT PROCESSES

2. Soil as a Source of Indoor Radon: Generation, Migration, and Entry   57

*William W. Nazaroff, Barbara A. Moed, and
Richard G. Sextro*

PART TWO: CHARACTERISTICS AND BEHAVIOR OF RADON DECAY PRODUCTS

5. Modeling Indoor Concentrations of Radon's Decay Products

Earl O. Knutson

PART THREE: THE BASIS FOR HEALTH CONCERNS

7. Lung Dosimetry   259

Anthony C. James

**RADON
AND ITS DECAY
PRODUCTS
IN INDOOR AIR**

1

Radon and Its Decay Products in Indoor Air: An Overview

ANTHONY V. NERO, Jr.

Indoor Environment Program, Lawrence Berkeley Laboratory, University of California, Berkeley, California

1 INTRODUCTION

The radiation dose from inhaled decay products of ^{222}Rn is the dominant component of natural radiation exposures of the general population. Monitoring in various countries yields average residential ^{222}Rn concentrations ranging from 10 to 100 Bq/m^3 (0.3–3 pCi/L; see Section 8.1 on quantities and units). For a country such as the United States, with an average of about 40 Bq/m^3, the average lifetime risk of lung cancer caused by exposure to radon decay products is estimated to be about 0.3%, causing on the order of 10,000 cases of lung cancer annually among the U.S. population of 235 million. As illustrated in Figure 1.1—showing data from the United States—this average risk is more significant than that received on the average from all other natural radiation sources or from medical exposures. And the radon dose exceeds by a factor of 10 to 100 the average doses from nuclear power or weapons testing.

Moreover, in any country indoor levels a factor of 10 or more higher than the average sometimes occur. In fact, it is the common experience of the radon research community that ^{222}Rn concentrations in the range of 200–2000 Bq/m^3 are found with startling frequency. And although the lung cancer risk associated even with an ordinary concentration such as 40 Bq/m^3 is very large compared with many environmental insults of concern, living for prolonged periods at concentrations above 200 Bq/m^3 leads to estimated individual lifetime risks exceeding 1%. The highest values found—more than 2000 Bq/m^3—have risks even larger than those from cigarette smoking. However, unlike smokers, those living in unusually high radon concentration are rarely aware of the large risks they may thereby be suffering.

The principal basis for present concern about exposures to radon's decay products is the experience with lung cancer incidence among underground miners. High fatality rates observed among miners as early as the sixteenth century were only

1

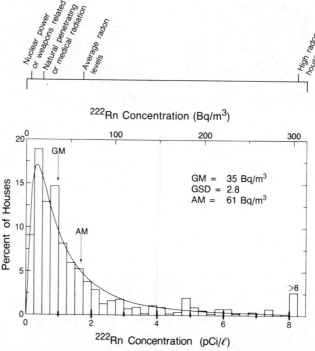

Figure 1.1. Probability distribution of ^{222}Rn in U.S. homes. These data result from direct aggregation of 19 sets of data, totaling 552 homes, from the United States. The smooth curve is a lognormal function with the indicated parameters. The upper scale indicates approximately the relative effective doses from radon and other sources of radiation exposure. From Ref. 10.

later ascribed to lung cancer. And it was only after recognition in the 1950s that excessive lung cancer rates were occurring among uranium miners in the United States and elsewhere that examination of exposure history versus incidence indicated a relationship between added risk of lung cancer and exposures to ^{222}Rn decay products. Broadly speaking, results from a number of studies conducted among various miner groups, uranium or otherwise, have shown roughly consistent results. In the meantime, substantial efforts have been devoted to lowering exposure rates below occupational limits that—although much lower than earlier conditions—still entail a significant risk and, indeed, one that is larger than the risk associated with most occupational standards. The experience gained in the uranium mines provided, not only information on health risks, but also the initial tools for understanding the occurrence, behavior, and control of radon and its decay products in the more general environment. The various isotopes of radon—^{222}Rn is the most important—are present to a greater or lesser degree in all environmental media—air, water, and soil—and arise naturally from the radioactive decay of radium, whose isotopes are members of the decay series originating with uranium and thorium, primordial constituents of the earth's crust.

The initial focus of environmental studies, however, was still exposures resulting from industrial processes—primarily the mining and milling of uranium—that increased the accessibility of radon to the outdoor atmosphere or to indoor environments. A principal example has been high ^{222}Rn concentrations inside homes and other buildings in the vicinity of Grand Junction, Colorado, that were built on or with radium-rich tailings from uranium milling. Another case, in Canada, is that of the communities of Port Hope, Uranium City, Elliot Lake, and Bancroft, where remedial action programs were undertaken because of the possibility that indoor concentrations were unusually high owing to local mining, milling or refining activities. A comparable example is observation of higher-than-average indoor concentrations in homes built on lands in Florida that have been disturbed as the result of phosphate ore mining. These ores typically have elevated concentrations of the uranium series, and resulting waste products have high concentrations of radium. Although exposure limits were set by the United States and Canada for each of these cases (cf. Chapter 12), it is now clear that the concentrations found in these communities—although higher than average—are no higher than those occurring in other buildings due merely to radon from the ground or, in some cases, from building components including unprocessed natural materials.

Indication of the potential significance of radon in the general building stock came with the realization in the 1970s of the health implications of very high concentrations in Swedish homes built using lightweight concretes incorporating alum shale as aggregate. This shale had extremely high radium content, causing high radon emanation rates from the finished concrete, which—together with low ventilation rates prompted by the interest in reducing energy use—resulted in high airborne concentrations in this segment of the housing stock. Ironically, it has subsequently been found in Sweden that the bulk of radon in the housing stock comes from the ground. Furthermore, monitoring in various countries has indicated that even average indoor concentrations are significant from the point of view of environmental risk. And, indeed, although changes in the ventilation rate can affect the indoor concentration significantly, the primary determinant of whether or not a particular indoor environment has high levels is, for many classes of buildings, the rate of radon entry.

Because of the apparent health implications, the early work on indoor concentrations has given rise to a broad range of research characterizing ^{222}Rn and its decay products indoors. This work has included significant monitoring programs in homes, investigation of the sources of indoor radon, study of the behavior of the decay products, and development of techniques for controlling indoor concentrations. In addition, radiobiologists and epidemiologists have begun to apply dosimetric and dose-response data explicitly to the problem of environmental exposures. These international efforts have resulted in an extensive literature, major collections of which are indicated in Table 1.1, but with a comparable number of

TABLE 1.1   Major Collections Containing Indoor Radon Articles[a,b]

Natural Radiation Environment III, proceedings of Symposium, Houston, Texas, April 1978. (Edited by T. Gesell and W. M. Lowder)—Technical Information Center (CONF-780422), Springfield, Virginia, 1980.

Radon and Radon Daughters in Urban Communities Associated with Uranium Mining and Processing, proceedings of three AECB Workshops in Ontario, Canada, 1978–1980— Atomic Energy Control Board, Ottawa, Canada, 1978–1980.

Assessment of Radon and Daughter Exposure and Related Biological Effects, proceedings of Specialist Meeting, Rome, Italy, March 1980. (Edited by G. F. Clemente, A. V. Nero, F. Steinhäusler, and M. E. Wrenn)—RD Press, Salt Lake City, Utah, 1982.

Natural Radiation Environment, proceedings of Second Special Symposium on Natural Radiation Environment, Bombay, India, January 1981. (Edited by K. G. Vohra, U. C. Mishra, K. C. Pillai, and S. Sadasivan)—Wiley Eastern Limited, New Delhi, 1982.

Indoor Air Pollution, proceedings of the International Symposium on Indoor Air Pollution, Health and Energy Conservation, Amherst, Massachusetts, October 1981. (Edited by J. Spengler, C. Hollowell, D. Moschandreas, and O. Fanger)—Special Issue of *Environment International,* **8** (No. 1–6), 1982.

Indoor Radon. (Edited by A. V. Nero and W. M. Lowder)—Special Issue of *Health Physics,* **45** (No. 2), August 1983.

Radon—Radon Progeny Measurements, proceedings of International Meeting, Montgomery, Alabama, August 1981—U.S. Environmental Protection Agency (EPA 520/5-83/021), Washington, DC, 1983.

Indoor Exposure to Natural Radiation and Associated Risk Assessment, proceedings of International Seminar, Anacapri, Italy, October 1983. (Edited by G. F. Clemente, H. Eriskat, M. C. O'Riordan, and J. Sinnaeve)—*Radiation Protection Dosimetry,* **7** (No. 1–4), 1984.

Exposure to Enhanced Natural Radiation and Its Regulatory Implications, proceedings of Seminar, Maastricht, Netherlands, March 1985. (Edited by B. Bosnjakovic, P. H. van Dijkum, M. C. O'Riordan, and J. Sinnaeve)—Special Issue of *Science of the Total Environment,* **45,** October 1985.

papers scattered among a wide variety of journals and conference proceedings. This book is intended to be a substantive review of our growing understanding of radon and its decay products in indoor air.

Another result of the apparently large health implications of indoor radon has been substantial attention to the development of policies and strategies for preventing or eliminating excessive concentrations. Underlying this question is some specification, regulatory or advisory, of what constitutes "acceptable" versus "unacceptable" concentrations. Many who are newly initiated to the radon question are wont to refer to some particular agency's (or country's) "standard" for indoor radon; most often the standard indicated is not a standard at all, but rather a guideline developed for some specific circumstance. (In rare cases, it actually is a regulatory standard, but narrowly drawn and not generally applicable to "indoor radon.") Similarly, a naive strategy for identifying and controlling excessive concentrations tends to rely on costly or inefficient survey or remedial techniques, as well as having no well-defined allocation of responsibility. Questions of standards and strategies are treated in the last chapter of this book. Although such issues are not the primary focus of this volume, we hope that the detailed treatment of radon

TABLE 1.1 (*Continued*)

Indoor Radon, proceedings of APCA International Specialty Conference, Philadelphia,
   Pennsylvania, February 1986—Air Pollution Control Association, Pittsburgh (SP-54),
   1986.
Indoor Air Quality, based on the Third International Conference on Indoor Air Quality and
   Climate, Stockholm, August 1984. (Edited by B. Berglund, U. Bergland, T. Lindvall, J.
   Spengler, and J. Sundell)—Special Issue of *Environment International,* **12,** (Nos. 1–4),
   1986; more of the radon papers are in *Radon, Passive Smoking, Particulates and Housing
   Epidemiology,* Vol. 2 of *Indoor Air* (Edited by B. Berglund, T. Lindvall, and J. Sundell),
   Swedish Council for Building Research, Stockholm, 1984.
Radon and Its Decay Products: Occurrence, Properties and Health Effects, proceedings of
   ACS Symposium, New York City, New York, April 1986. (Edited by P.K. Hopke)—
   Symposium Series 331, American Chemical Society, Washington, DC, 1987.

Major Reviews

The Effects on Populations of Exposure to Low Levels of Ionizing Radiation (Committee on
   the Biological Effects of Ionizing Radiation[c])—National Academy of Sciences,
   Washington, DC, 1980.
Indoor Pollutants (Committee on Indoor Pollutants)—National Academy Press, Washington,
   DC, 1981.
Ionizing Radiation: Sources and Biological Effects (United Nations Scientific Committee on
   the Effects of Atomic Radiation)—United Nations, New York, 1982.
*Evaluation of Occupational and Environmental Exposures to Radon and Radon Daughters in
   the United States*—Report No. 78, National Council on Radiation Protection and
   Measurements, Bethesda, Maryland, 1984.

[a] For references on suggested radon standards, see Chapter 12.
[b] Two major international meetings during 1987 will result in significant collections of indoor radon articles:
The Fourth International Conference on Indoor Air Quality and Climate (Berlin, August 17–21, 1987) and
the Natural Radiation Environment IV (Lisbon, December 7–11, 1987). Both these international conferences can be expected to continue on a periodic basis.
[c] The Committee has recently developed a report on alpha radiation: *Health Risks of Radon and other
Internally Deposited Alpha Emitters,* in press.

and its decay products that forms the core of this book will provide a fertile ground
on which to develop policy alternatives and realistic strategies for controlling indoor radon.

2 FUNDAMENTALS

2.1 Characteristics of Radon and Its Decay Products

A principal characteristic of radon that gives it more radiological significance than
earlier members of the uranium (and thorium) decay chains is the fact that it is a
noble gas. As such, once it is formed in radium-bearing material, a radon atom is
relatively free to move, provided it first reaches the material's pore space (typically
by recoil from the parent radium atom's emission of an alpha particle). Once in
the pore space, macroscopic transport of radon is possible, either by molecular
diffusion or by flow of the fluid in the pore space. Radon can therefore reach air

or water to which humans have access, provided that transport is sufficiently rapid to be completed before the radon decays.

Formed in the ^{238}U decay chain (Fig. 1.2) from decay of ^{226}Ra, ^{222}Rn is the most important radon isotope because it has the longest half-life, 3.8 days. This is long enough that much of the ^{222}Rn formed either in building materials or in the ground within approximately a meter of building understructures can reach the indoor environment. Similarly, much of the ^{222}Rn formed within about a meter of the earth's surface reaches the outdoor atmosphere, although this has less radiological significance than that reaching indoor environments, which have relatively small volumes compared with the contributing source material. In some cases, whether for the indoor or outdoor environment, radon from much larger distances than a meter can be important if high-permeability transport routes (such as gravelly soil or fissures in the ground) are available.

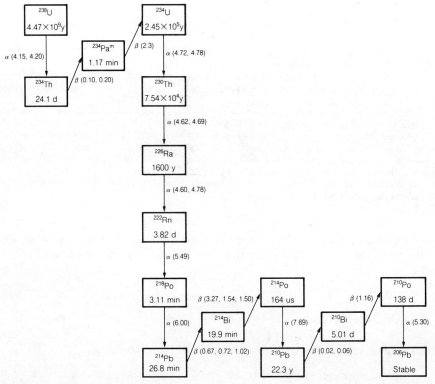

Figure 1.2. ^{238}U decay chain, including ^{222}Rn and its decay products. ^{222}Rn, its parent ^{226}Ra, and its decay products are members of the ^{238}U decay series. Airborne concentrations of ^{218}Po, ^{214}Pb, and ^{214}Bi are of prime radiological interest owing to their potential for retention in the lung, leading to subsequent irradiation by the alpha decays of ^{218}Po and ^{214}Po. Half-lives (in boxes) and alpha energies (in MeV) from Ref. 57. Beta end-point energies (in MeV) from Ref. 83 (except for ^{234}Th and ^{234}Pa^m, from Ref. 84. See Section 8.4 for comparable ^{232}Th decay chain (given in Fig. 1.9). Figure courtesy of Lawrence Berkeley Laboratory.

In contrast, although about as much ^{220}Rn (sometimes called thoron) activity is formed (in this case from decay of ^{224}Ra, a member of the ^{232}Th decay chain—see Section 8.4 on ^{220}Rn), substantially less reaches air because its short half-life (56 s) limits the distance it can travel before decay.* Finally, very little of another radon isotope, ^{219}Rn, is present in air because the ^{235}U decay chain, of which it is a member, has a natural abundance that is a factor of 100 lower and because of ^{219}Rn's short half-life (4 s).

The second important characteristic of radon is that it decays to radionuclides that are chemically active and relatively short-lived. As indicated in Fig. 1.2, the four radionuclides following decay of ^{222}Rn have half-lives of less than 30 min, so that—if collected in the lung on being inhaled—they are likely to decay to ^{210}Pb before removal by lung clearance mechanisms. (Similarly, ^{220}Rn begins a series of relatively short-lived isotopes; the most significant dose arises from the inhalation of ^{212}Pb, which has a half-life of 10.6 h.)

The radiation released on decay of the short-lived decay products imparts the lung dose to which increased risk of lung cancer is attributed. The alpha radiation from the polonium isotopes contributes the radiologically significant dose, primarily because alpha particles deposit their energy within such a small thickness of tissue. As a result, the alpha energy is deposited in the relatively sensitive lung lining and also has a dense deposition pattern, which has much greater biological impact.

The concentration of (short-lived) decay products in air is ordinarily not given in terms of individual decay-product concentrations, but rather by a collective concentration that is normalized to the amount of alpha decay energy that will ultimately result from the mixture of decay products that is present. This quantity is the "equilibrium-equivalent" decay-product concentration (EEDC),† the amount of each decay product necessary to collectively have the same potential alpha-energy concentration (PAEC) that is actually present. (The decay-product concentration can also be given in terms of the PAEC itself. See Section 8.1 of this chapter on quantities and units.) The ratio of EEDC to radon concentration is the equilibrium factor, equal to 1 if radon and all its decay products are in radioactive equilibrium (and therefore have the same radioactivity concentration), but in the range of 0.2–0.6 for most indoor atmospheres and somewhat higher outdoors.

For a given indoor radon concentration, the concentrations of the decay prod-

---

*Although indoor concentrations of the ^{220}Rn gas itself are ordinarily much less than those of ^{222}Rn, scattered data (cf. Section 8.4 on ^{220}Rn) suggest that, at least in buildings with average or below-average ^{222}Rn concentrations, the potential alpha-energy concentration (PAEC) of ^{220}Rn decay products—while ordinarily less than that from ^{222}Rn decay products—can be a significant fraction of the total PAEC. Unfortunately, too little information is available to assess reliably the overall prevalence or importance of ^{220}Rn and its decay products, except to say that the PAEC has rarely, if ever, been found to approach the higher levels found for ^{222}Rn. As discussed later, results from measurements of indoor concentrations are consistent with a picture where ^{222}Rn transport is dominated by pressure-driven flow, and ^{220}Rn transport by diffusion.

†This quantity is often called the equilibrium-equivalent radon concentration, a practice that is avoided here because it is actually a measure of the decay-product concentration.

ucts can vary over a substantial range, since they are removed from the air, not only by radioactive decay, but also by ventilation and by reactions with the structure and its furnishings. An additional and important manifestation of their chemical activity is that the decay products can form small airborne agglomerates and can attach to previously existing particles. Such characteristics of the airborne decay products affect the rate at which they deposit on walls and furnishings, the pattern and degree of deposition in the lung, and, ultimately, the magnitude and distribution of the associated radiation dose.

2.2   Factors Affecting Indoor Concentrations

The indoor concentration of radon and its decay products, or of any other airborne pollutant, depends on three factors: the entry or production rate from various sources, the ventilation rate, and the rates of chemical or physical transformation or removal. Because of its relatively long half-life and lack of chemical activity, ^{222}Rn itself acts much like a stable pollutant whose indoor concentration is determined by only two factors, the entry rate and the ventilation rate. In contrast, the behavior of the decay products is much more complex, depending on the radon that is present, the ventilation rate, and the interplay among radioactive decay, chemical reactivity, particle concentrations, and the nature of the boundary layer between the indoor atmosphere and the surfaces that enclose it. Nonetheless, as a practical matter, the decay-product concentration is indicated approximately by the radon concentration, which is determined by source and ventilation characteristics. The influence of these factors on indoor concentrations is discussed here briefly. In addition, Section 8.2 treats the question of ventilation rates per se.

Both excessive entry rates and decreased ventilation rates appear to be important causes of the high concentrations found in Swedish homes, which constituted a signal that scientists in other countries should investigate radon concentrations in their own building stocks. It is important to realize that extensive research on other aspects of indoor air quality was also beginning about the same time (see citations in Table 1.1), because of the discovery that several classes of pollution could occur indoors at higher levels than outdoors. For example, the by-products of combustion—such as carbon monoxide, nitrogen oxides, and particulates—are primary pollutants from the point of view of outdoor air quality. But concentrations are often much higher indoors, owing to the presence of gas stoves, kerosene space heaters, and other appliances that are not vented effectively to the outdoors (1, 2). Similarly, although organic chemicals of various kinds are regulated in outdoor air and around toxic waste dumps, concentrations can be much higher indoors, again because of the presence of indoor sources (3, 4). In the United States, much of the research on indoor air quality began because of the fear that energy-conservation measures might raise levels of such pollutants.

The basis of this concern may be seen by considering the steady-state concentration of a nonreactive gas entering an interior space from effectively internal sources (including the ground) at a fixed rate per unit volume, S_V. The concentration in this case is easily shown to be

$$I = (S_V + I_o\lambda_v)/(\lambda_v + d) \tag{1}$$

where λ_v is the ventilation rate, I_o is the concentration in outdoor air, and d is the decay rate of the gas (if applicable). For typical ventilation rates, greater than 0.1 h^{-1}, the decay rate of ^{222}Rn (0.0076 h^{-1}) can be ignored in this equation, so that $I - I_o = S_V/\lambda_v$. This simplifies even further, to $I = S_V/\lambda_v$, when—as is often the case—the outdoor concentration is much smaller than the indoor.

This expression does not encompass recently understood and important aspects of radon behavior, including time-dependent and interactive phenomena, as discussed in later sections. Moreover, as is obvious, it cannot be used to describe the behavior of radon decay products, whose concentrations are determined by a number of interdependent reaction rates, as described qualitatively below and in more detail in succeeding chapters. Nonetheless, it is useful for specific analytical purposes, an obvious example being that, for a fixed source strength, a decrease in the ventilation rate—e.g., to save energy—will result in a corresponding increase in the indoor concentration.

However, the relative importance of source strengths in determining indoor radon concentrations became clear in initial studies of concentrations and ventilation rates in U.S. homes. Earlier work had already indicated significant concentrations of ^{222}Rn and its decay products in U.S. homes (5), and subsequent work had confirmed that, with supply of differing amounts of mechanical ventilation in a given house, the radon concentration varied as the inverse of the ventilation rate (6). But results from simultaneous ^{222}Rn and ventilation-rate measurements in several groups of homes showed no apparent correlation between these two parameters (7). As shown in Figure 1.3, the radon concentrations and ventilation rates for each sample group showed an approximately order-of-magnitude range; for the combined sample of about 100 homes, the concentration showed a significantly larger variability than the ventilation rate. If the ventilation rate λ_v and source strength S_V were independent in this sample of houses, and if the range of concentrations observed were caused primarily by differences in ventilation rate, then—because $I = S_V/\lambda_v$ takes a linear form $\ln I = \ln S_V - \ln \lambda_v$, on a logarithmic plot—the data points of Figure 1.3 would cluster around a straight line with slope -1. No such correlation is apparent. The relative range and independence of these two quantities suggested that the source strength was the dominant determinant of the wide range of concentrations observed in U.S. housing.

Such indications have prompted substantial work in understanding the size and variability of radon entry rates, as discussed below. However, it is important to emphasize that other factors still play an important role: ventilation rates vary substantially within the housing stock, which is, of course, one of the major incentives for past and current efforts to increase the efficiency of energy use in buildings. (In the United States, an added incentive is that even the average ventilation rate—see Section 8.2—is relatively high compared with rates in many countries.) And, even for a given radon concentration, the concentrations and physical state of the decay products—which account for the health effects of principal concern—can vary significantly. We turn now to a brief review of indoor

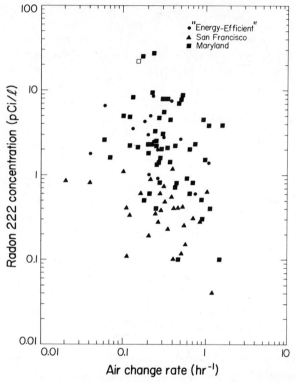

Figure 1.3. ^{222}Rn concentrations and air exchange rates measured in 98 U.S. residences. The results shown are from three survey groups: "energy-efficient" houses in the United States and (one) in Canada; conventional houses in the San Francisco area; and conventional houses in a community in rural Maryland. Data from Ref. 7.

^{222}Rn concentrations, after which we shall examine more closely the factors affecting indoor levels. Concentrations of ^{220}Rn and its decay products are treated in Section 8.4.

3   INDOOR CONCENTRATIONS

Since identification of ^{222}Rn and its decay products as potentially important indoor pollutants, a large number of efforts have been undertaken actually measuring concentrations in homes. In a few countries, mostly European, these efforts have even included surveys in statistically designed samples of the housing stock. Taken together, monitoring efforts to date provide a useful appreciation of residential radon concentrations in—not only Europe—but even the United States, where a wide variety of small or local survey efforts have been completed. Data are less complete for commercial and public buildings, although a variety of information can be brought to bear to suggest the approximate scale of radon concentrations in such environments.

This section briefly reviews the results of indoor radon surveys, primarily those performed in residences. No attempt is made to mention the many specific studies that have been performed. In particular, for residences—the focus of large numbers of efforts—only the few surveys or analyses that are representative of a large segment of the housing stock are discussed explicitly. Results from a significant number of individual surveys may be found in the major references given in Table 1.1 and in numerous individual journal articles and reports. Most of the results discussed here are summarized in Table 1.2.

It is also worth noting the tendency of the research community to measure radon concentrations in survey efforts, rather than decay-product concentrations. This tendency arises largely from the availability of reasonably reliable and very simple integrating etched-track radon monitors (see, for example, Ref. 8), a significant contrast to the state of decay-product monitoring. (An alternative technique being used in many shorter-term studies is based on collection of radon for a few days in charcoal cannisters; see, for example, Ref. 9.) Fortunately, given a reasonable understanding of the relationship between radon and its decay products and an awareness of the fact that the decay-product-to-radon ratio (typically in the range of 0.2–0.8) does not vary as widely as radon concentrations, measurement of radon is a reasonable indicator of decay-product concentrations and is a very effective tool in survey efforts. This is analogous to the situation for many other pollutants: for example, although health effects associated with NO_2 exposures may have a substantial dependence on peak (rather than average) concentrations, an integrating sampler can be a very effective survey instrument, provided that associated studies examine relationships between average and peak concentrations under well-characterized conditions. As seen below, another incentive for emphasizing the radon concentrations per se is that this parameter appears to be a relatively direct indicator for use in strategies for identifying and controlling excessive concentrations, and, as discussed in Chapter 7, it may actually be a more consistent indicator of dose than the decay-product concentration.

3.1 Concentrations in North American Housing

Despite a broad range of U.S. efforts to characterize indoor radon, including a substantial number of studies that have included measurements in existing U.S. homes, there has been no direct broad-scale determination of the concentrations to which the U.S. population is exposed. The numerous U.S. studies have varied significantly in incentives, scientific objectives, selection of homes, and measurement procedures. The results from these studies therefore vary significantly, as do the conclusions that may be drawn from them. An obvious solution to this difficulty would be to carry out measurements in a valid statistical sampling of U.S. homes. From even an approximate evaluation of the data already in hand, it is clear that measurements in on the order of 1000 homes would determine the mean concen-

TABLE 1.2 Distribution of ^{222}Rn Concentrations in Various Countries

Country	No. of homes monitored	Type	Concentration (Bq/m³) GM	Concentration (Bq/m³) AM	GSD or % of tail	Notes	Ref.
U.S.	817	Single-family	33	55	2.8	Aggregated 22 data sets, adjusting to annual-avg.	10
Canada	453		38	54	2.36	Physics professors	11
	9999		13		2.7	Median values from 14 city surveys; mostly basement values; PAEC converted assuming equil. factor = 0.5.	14
Sweden	500	Detached	69	122	2% > 800 Bq/m³	Built before 1975	15
		Apartments	53	85	0.5% > 800 Bq/m³		
Denmark	22	Single-family Flats		70		Preliminary surveys; average of winter and summer means	18
Finland	2000	Small houses	64	82	2% > 800 Bq/m³		17
F.R.G.	6000		40	49	1.8		20
Netherlands	1000		24		1.6	High levels show excess above lognormal	22
Belgium	79		41		1.7	Preliminary national survey	79
France	765		44	76		Incomplete natl. survey	80
U.K.	2000		15	25	2% > 200 Bq/m³	Living areas; bedrooms had GM of 11 Bq/m³	21
					2.6		
Ireland	250		43		10% > 100 Bq/m³	Preliminary survey	81
Japan	251		19		2% > 100 Bq/m³	Composite of 4 city surveys	82

GM = geometric mean
GSD = geometric standard deviation
AM = arithmetic mean

tration very accurately and ascertain the fraction of homes at high concentrations (say, 10 times the mean) to a reasonable accuracy.

However, regardless of such an effort, the data already available are quite substantial, including tens of data sets from a wide variety of studies, with the precise number depending on the criteria for inclusion. It has been clear for some time that a systematic analysis of available data would have considerable value, and such an analysis has been performed on data available as of 1984–1985 (10). This analysis explicitly considered important differences between the studies and aggregated the various data sets, using both nonparametric and lognormal representations to yield a nominal radon distribution for single-family houses (the dominant type of residence) in the United States. Figure 1.1 shows the probability distribution obtained from direct aggregation of 19 of the data sets for which individual data were available. This particular aggregation, although not suitable for drawing conclusions about annual-average concentrations, indicates the substantial conformance of indoor radon concentrations to a lognormal representation, a result that has been observed in many individual studies.

The analysis examined a total of 38 data sets, corresponding to different areas (usually a state or urban area) of the United States. A significant number of these sets arose from monitoring effects that were prompted by some prior knowledge of a potential for elevated concentrations. However, the main conclusions of the analysis were based on 22 data sets apparently lacking such prior indication. In either case (i.e., the 38 sets or the 22-set grouping), the geometric mean (GM) concentrations from the sets ranged from 11 to 210 Bq/m^3 (actually, 0.3–5.7 pCi/L, since *all* of these studies used the traditional units). Geometric standard deviations (GSDs) ranged from 1.3 to 4 among all 38 sets.

The results of aggregating these sets in different manners are quite robust, with the main distinction being simply that aggregations utilizing the full 38 sets yielded a somewhat higher aggregate mean than those including only the 22 "unbiased" sets. The overall result, relying on the 22-set aggregations (and including a normalization of data taken only during heating seasons to obtain an estimate of yearlong averages) is a distribution of annual-average ^{222}Rn concentrations that averages 55 Bq/m^3 (1.5 pCi/L) and that has a long tail with 1–3% of homes exceeding 300 Bq/m^3 (8 pCi/L). The analysis indicates that 7% (or about 4 million) of the U.S. single-family housing stock have concentrations greater than 150 Bq/m^3 (4 pCi/L). Alternatively, the distribution can be expressed as a lognormal function with a GM of 33 Bq/m^3 (0.9 pCi/L) and a GSD of 2.8. This result can only be associated with the portion of the housing stock consisting of single-family houses, since 99% of the data are drawn from such homes. However, this is the dominant element of the U.S. housing stock, and the results indicate that on the order of a million homes in the United States have annual-average ^{222}Rn concentrations of 300 Bq/m^3 or more. (Another interesting observation from this analysis is that the geometric means of the "unbiased" 22 sets are themselves lognormally distributed, with a GSD of 2.0. This index demonstrates the substantial variability of mean indoor radon concentrations from one area to another.)

Currently, results from studies involving larger numbers of homes, often selected on a statistical basis or covering a larger portion of the United States, are beginning to become available. A notable example is a study that performed integrated year-long measurements in the homes of approximately 450 physics faculty at about 100 colleges and universities across the United States (11). The ^{222}Rn concentrations so obtained average 54 Bq/m^3 (1.47 pCi/L) and fit a lognormal distribution admirably well, with a GM and GSD of 38 Bq/m^3 and 2.36, respectively. This implies that 0.8% of homes have concentrations greater than 300 Bq/m^3, at the low end of the range estimated from the analysis discussed above. On the other hand, the fraction above 150 Bq/m^3, 6%, is very close to the earlier result. Although a study of homes of physics faculty cannot be construed to be a representative sampling of U.S. homes (a problem suffered also by the aggregate analysis just discussed), this study has the advantage that the homes are widely distributed across the United States and that the measurement protocol determined directly a year-long average concentration. The averages from the 100 or so institutions are themselves lognormally distributed, with a GM of 46 Bq/m^3 and a GSD of 1.75. Interestingly, the highest average from both this study and the aggregate analysis above occurred in the state of North Dakota.

This suggests the need to recognize that the broad distributions discussed here do not of themselves reveal the much higher distributions that may occur in specific areas. For example, both studies just referred to indicate that areas of North Dakota have average concentrations much higher than the U.S. mean, and a correspondingly higher portion of houses exceeding any particular concentration. More recently, two other such areas have been identified, one in the Spokane River Valley of Washington and Idaho, where the average winter concentration in 46 homes was found to be 500 Bq/m^3 (13.3 pCi/L), with 20 of the houses exceeding 300 Bq/m^3 (12). At about the same time, astounding concentrations were found in eastern Pennsylvania (a state that was already known to have very high levels in some locales) (13). Although no dependable frequency distribution can be extracted from the results of monitoring about 4000 homes in this area, the average appears to be similar to the Spokane results, but with a much larger number of houses involved and with indoor radon concentrations as high as 100,000 Bq/m^3. An exceptional concentration of high levels has also been found in the town of Clinton, New Jersey, where about half of approximately 100 houses monitored in one neighborhood had winter concentrations exceeding 7500 Bq/m^3.

A significant number of the earlier studies analyzed in Ref. 10 measured the concentration of decay products instead of radon. One of these in particular (5) measured both concentrations averaged over week-long periods, thereby determining directly an effective equilibrium ratio, which was found to range from 0.31 to 0.82 among the houses examined. As is evident from the measurements from other countries, discussed below, there is significant evidence that equilibrium ratios tend to average about 0.4 among samples of housing, with significant variability from one time to another, from one house to another, and perhaps some differences from one region or country to another.

One of the earliest large studies was conducted in Canada, where an approximate idea of indoor concentrations has been obtained by performing grab-sample measurements in a large number of homes (9999) across that country (14). Rather than being a representative sampling, homes were selected from 14 of Canada's largest cities, therefore directly representing a major portion of the housing stock. The geometric mean EEDC varied from 3 to 13 Bq/m^3 among these cities, the median being 7 Bq/m^3. The median GSD was about 2.7. These results cannot, however, be thought of as representing the living-space average of these homes, since the preferred sampling site was chosen to be the basement. (The ^{222}Rn concentrations were also measured, but are suspect in view of the very large GSD obtained, a median of 4.0 among the 14 cities, and the fact that measurements were performed in basements.)

3.2 Residential Concentrations in Europe

Significant efforts to determine indoor radon concentrations have been conducted in numerous European countries. However, in only a few have these efforts been designed to provide representative information on concentrations in the housing stock as a whole. The results from studies designed, more or less, to meet this objective, differ to a significant, but understandable, degree from one country to another.

Sweden, a principal in inciting the wide interest in radon, has more recently completed a country-wide survey, utilizing 2-week passive ^{222}Rn measurements in about 500 homes built before 1975 (15). The results averaged 122 Bq/m^3 (GM 69 Bq/m^3) for 315 detached houses and 85 Bq/m^3 (GM 53 Bq/m^3) for 191 apartments. The distributions are approximately lognormal, with 10% of the results over 266 Bq/m^3 (detached) or 187 Bq/m^3 (apartments). Overall, concentrations are higher than for countries outside Scandinavia, with about 2% of detached homes and 0.5% of apartments estimated to have ^{222}Rn concentrations exceeding 800 Bq/m^3—comparable to their remedial action level of 400 Bq/m^3 EEDC, assuming a typical equilibrium factor of 0.5. A supplementary study of detached houses built since 1975 yielded a GM similar to that for the larger study, but with a smaller fraction at high concentrations (16).

Preliminary results from measurements in more than 2000 houses in Finland yield a GM of 64 Bq/m^3 and about 2% greater than 800 Bq/m^3, similar to the Swedish single-family results (17); a strong geographical dependence was observed. Results from a small sampling in Denmark show somewhat lower concentrations in that country, e.g., average (not GM) concentrations in single-family dwellings of 88 Bq/m^3 in winter and 24 Bq/m^3 in summer (18). However, some of the apparent difference may arise from differences in measurement period.

Results from a survey of about 6000 homes in the Federal Republic of Germany using etched-track ^{222}Rn detectors have recently become available, yielding a GM of 40 Bq/m^3 and GSD of 1.8 (19). In spite of the fact that a larger number appeared at high concentrations than indicated by these lognormal parameters, only

10 (0.2%) of the homes sampled had concentrations exceeding 500 Bq/m^3. Other results from the FRG indicate an equilibrium factor of 0.3 indoors and 0.4 outdoors (20).

A survey mounted in the United Kingdom has measured ^{222}Rn concentrations in about 2000 homes, yielding a GM of 15 Bq/m^3 and GSD of 2.6 for living areas (11 Bq/m^3 and 2.5 for bedrooms). The ratio of summer to winter concentrations was found to be 0.51 in living areas and 0.53 in bedrooms. Concentrations substantially higher than these overall values have been found in specific areas, such as Cornwall (21).

Measurement of ^{222}Rn concentrations in about 1000 dwellings in the Netherlands gave a distribution well represented (except for an excess of high concentrations) by a lognormal function with GM 24 Bq/m^3 and GSD 1.6 (22).

In Europe, it is also important to realize that many of the countries mentioned have identified areas or portions of the housing stock with exceptionally high concentrations. As noted earlier, it was housing with concretes using alum-shale as aggregate that drew initial attention to indoor radon as a problem, but more recently radon from the ground has been identified as the primary source in Swedish housing, and this varies substantially from one area to another. In Finland, a study on the south coast found averages in the 31 locales surveyed to range from 95 to 1200 Bq/m^3, with the total sample averaging 370 Bq/m^3 and 12% of houses exceeding 800 Bq/m^3 (23). As a final example, the average from Cornwall was 390 Bq/m^3, 15 times the national average for the United Kingdom (21).

More limited information is available from a number of other countries. Except for special local areas, none of the results exceed the distribution found for the Scandinavian countries. And some approach the considerably lower levels characteristic of the outdoors, with average concentrations in the vicinity of 10 Bq/m^3.

3.3 Other Buildings

Very few data are available on radon concentrations in buildings other than residences. However, the same range of radon sources contributing to residential radon also contribute—to a greater or lesser degree—to levels in other buildings. Hence, it is to be expected that the minimum concentration observed in such buildings is the outdoor level—averaging about 10 Bq/m^3 of ^{222}Rn, as indicated in Section 8.3—but that higher levels, even in the range of those in residences, should be the norm. To the extent that structures such as hospitals or office buildings have a larger number of stories and higher ventilation rates than residences, we would expect lower concentrations.

Only a small number of measurements in other buildings—whether offices, stores, hospitals, or schools—have actually been performed, and virtually no statistically meaningful data have been developed. It is, nonetheless, worth mentioning two substantial studies from the United States as examples. One of these was conducted in the Pittsburgh, Pennsylvania, area, using grab-sample measurements taken during occupancy (an important issue if ventilation systems are turned off during unoccupied hours) in schools, stores, and other public and commercial buildings (24). Average concentrations for various groups of buildings, many including on the order of 100 measurements, were in the vicinity of 15–20 Bq/m³, slightly higher than the outdoor concentrations measured (about 10 Bq/m³), and much less than the annual-average concentrations found in a local survey of residential levels, about 96 Bq/m³. A survey of 38 office buildings in the Pacific Northwestern United States found concentrations to average 11, 26, and 44 Bq/m³

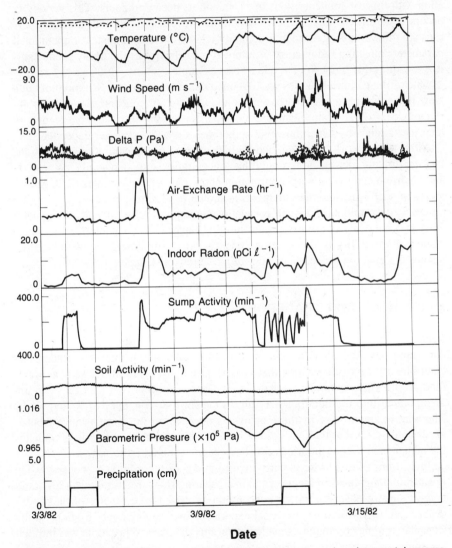

Figure 1.4. Variability of ²²²Rn concentration, ventilation rate, and environmental parameters in a house with a basement. These data were accumulated over a 2-week period during a several-month experiment examining the dependence of radon entry on environmental factors. From Ref. 27.

for the three cities included (25). These results, obtained with integrating samplers, are somewhat lower than comparable residential concentrations in the respective areas.

3.4   Time Dependence of Indoor Concentrations

Numerous measurements of radon in dwellings have indicated the substantial variation with time of concentrations of ^{222}Rn and its decay products. This variability occurs with time of day, weather conditions, or season. Without ascribing any cause to this variability—which is certainly related to environmental or operational parameters affecting radon entry or removal (or behavior of the decay products)—it is useful at this point to give one or two examples.

One of the earlier examples was obtained using continuous ^{222}Rn monitors in a New Jersey house, measuring basement and upper-floor concentrations over a period of weeks (26). A significant diurnal dependence was observed, consistent with later measurements, which however sometimes showed a stronger dependence.

More recent work has examined the dependence of concentrations on various factors, directly measuring not only the concentration, but also source parameters and environmental factors affecting radon entry and ventilation rates (27). An example of such real-time measurements is shown in Figure 1.4.

Detailed examination of such correlations is important for understanding radon entry and removal, as discussed later in this chapter and in Chapter 2. An appreciation of variability is also a key element in proper interpretation of monitoring results and effective selection of control measures (cf. Chapter 12).

4   SOURCES AND TRANSPORT

Radon arises from trace concentrations of radium in the earth's crust, and indoor concentrations depend on access of this radon to building interiors. Radon can enter directly from soil or rock that is still in the crust, via utilities such as water (and, in principle, natural gas) that carry radon, or from crustal materials that are incorporated into the building structure in the form of concrete, rock, and brick. The relative importance of these pathways depends on the circumstances, but it has become clear that the first—direct ingress from the soil—ordinarily dominates the higher indoor concentrations that have been observed in homes.

Indications of this arose in early investigations of radon in U.S. houses, when it was found that measurements of radon emanating from structural materials could not account for observed indoor concentrations, based on estimates of the air exchange rate (5). Moreover, practical experience in reducing concentrations in the Canadian mining communities made it clear that the major entry route was through the house understructure, at least in these houses.

A clearer picture emerged from the distribution of entry rates inferred from direct measurements of radon concentration and ventilation rate (such as the data shown in Fig. 1.3). Figure 1.5 shows such entry-rate distributions from various

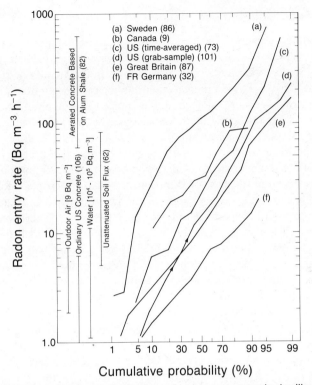

Figure 1.5. Cumulative frequency distributions of radon entry rates in dwellings. The entry rate is determined from the product of simultaneously measured radon concentration and ventilation rate. The number of residences in each sample is indicated in parentheses. The references from which these results are taken are: (a) 28, (b) 71, (c) 6, 27, 35, 72–74, (d) 7, (e) 75, and (f) 76. The bars at the left indicate the range of contributions expected from a variety of sources, with assumptions indicated in brackets. For each source, we have assumed a single-story house of wood-frame construction with a 0.2-m thick concrete-slab floor. The floor area and ceiling height are assumed to be 100 m^2 and 2.4 m, respectively; water usage is assumed to be 1.2 m^3/day, with a use-weighted transfer efficiency for radon to air of 0.55; and the ventilation rate is assumed to be in the range 0.2–0.8 h^{-1}. References for estimates of source contributions are: outdoor air (62), U.S. concrete (29), alum-shale concrete (66); water (31); and soil flux (30). Figure taken from Ref. 77.

countries, as well as indicating the potential contribution of various sources. Although building materials were first suspected as the major source in the United States, based on the experience in Europe (e.g., Ref. 28), the initial U.S. results strongly suggested that the soil must be the major source (7). Understanding how the rate of radon entry could be approximately equal to the unimpeded flux from the ground (i.e., in the absence of the house) has been a major focus of research on radon entry, in both North America and Europe.

This section discusses briefly the current state of knowledge of radon sources and transport. Far more comprehensive treatments are given in Chapters 2, 3, and 4.

4.1 Soil and Building Materials

Understanding the radon mass balance for a building requires specific consideration of the various sources. As indicated in Figure 1.5, a median (or GM) entry rate for U.S. single-family houses appears to be in the vicinity of 20 Bq m^{-3} h^{-1} (0.5 pCi L^{-1} h^{-1}). Based on emanation rate measurements from U.S. concretes (29), one might expect emissions from this source to account for a median of about 2-3 Bq m^{-3} h^{-1}, far below the rate observed. On the other hand, the potential contribution from unattenuated soil flux, a median of about 25 Bq m^{-3} h^{-1} (based on Ref. 30), corresponds much more closely with the indoor observations. However, houses have understructures that might be expected to impede substantially the ingress of radon, at least by diffusion, the main mechanism for causing the observed fluxes from uncovered soil. As discussed in detail in Chapter 2 (and in Ref. 31), although transport via diffusion accounts well for observed fluxes from building materials and exposed soil and could account for small fluxes from the soil through some understructure materials (such as concrete), diffusion cannot account for the total entry rates observed in single-family houses. Another mechanism must account for the efficiency with which radon from soil enters such homes. It appears that this mechanism is bulk flow of soil gas driven by small pressure differences between the lower part of the house interior and the outdoors.

As discussed in Section 8.2 on ventilation rates, pressure differences of only a few Pascals—i.e., of the order of a ten-thousandth of an atmosphere—arise from winds and indoor–outdoor temperature differences and are precisely the cause of ventilation in homes during seasons when the windows are closed. These same pressure differences can, in principle, drive the small flows of soil gas needed to account for the observed rate of radon entry into homes: soil gas contains enough radon that, on the average, only 0.1% of infiltrating air would have to be drawn from the soil to account for observed indoor concentrations (31).

As discussed more fully in Chapter 2, recent work has begun to characterize directly and systematically the potential for pressure differences to cause entry of radon via soil gas, probably through imperfections and penetrations in the house understructure that permit passage of the relatively small amount of soil gas required. A study of radon entry in a single family house with a basement (see Fig. 1.4) analyzed the entry rate versus the ventilation rate, measured over a period of months, and concluded that entry could usefully be represented by a sum of two components: one—the smaller—independent of ventilation rate, much as diffusion would be, and a larger term proportional to ventilation rate, as pressure-driven flow might be (27). Moreover, the observed pressure and soil parameters appeared consistent with the soil-gas flow rate that was implied by the measured concentrations and ventilation rates. In addition, theoretical simulations of transport (e.g., Ref. 32) are helping to form a fundamental picture. Finally, recent experiments have directly observed, in houses with basements, the underground depressurization implied by this picture and have monitored underground soil-gas movement by injecting and monitoring tracers (33). A different kind of experiment—practical experience with remedial measures in such areas as Eastern Pennsylvania (34) and the Spokane River Valley (12), using techniques such as those discussed in Chapter 10—is confirming and providing new information on the flow of radon-bearing air through house understructures. It is interesting to note that these results may also have significant implications for entry of other pollutants from the soil.

The studies of houses with basements have given results that may also apply in large part to slab-on-grade structures, where the pressure difference generated can still draw soil gas through any penetrations in or around the slab. However, few direct measurements in such structures have been performed. The other understructure type of substantial importance is the crawl space, which to some extent isolates the interior from the soil—at least with respect to pressure-driven flow between the two. Limited measurements of the transport efficiency of radon through crawl spaces yield the result that a substantial portion of the radon leaving uncovered soil manages to enter the interior, even if vents are open to permit natural ventilation of the space (35).

In retrospect, this is not entirely surprising, since the stack effect will tend to draw infiltrating air into the home from the crawl space, which can retain radon from the soil in conditions where winds are not sufficient to flush it to the outdoors via the vents. Furthermore, for structures where the vents are sealed shut, e.g., to save energy, it is conceivable that the crawl space still provides sufficient connection between the house interior and the soil that pressure-driven flow can enhance the flux from the soil above levels associated merely with diffusion; the work reported in Ref. 35 may have observed this effect. Another observation from this study is that energy conservation efforts that focus on tightening the floor above a crawl space can significantly reduce infiltration rates, while reducing radon entry a corresponding amount, as a result of which indoor concentrations are little affected.

Thus, sufficient mechanisms exist to account for the substantial amount of radon that appears to enter single-family homes from the soil, apparently without great regard to substructure type. However, this does not imply that other sources of radon are unimportant. As discussed in Chapter 3, it is clear that materials utilized in a building structure *can* contribute substantial indoor concentrations, although this is not usually the case (even for natural stone that has higher-than-average radium content). Moreover, in buildings that are relatively isolated from the ground, such as multistory apartment buildings, indoor concentrations are expected to be lower than average—as is often the case in central European dwellings—and to arise primarily from the building materials and from radon in outdoor air.

4.2 Water

Probably more important than building materials as a source of radon in certain parts of the housing stock is domestic water drawn from underground sources. Surface waters have radon concentrations too small to affect indoor levels when used domestically, but ground water is in a good position to accumulate radon generated within the earth's crust. As a result, very high radon concentrations can sometimes be found in associated water supplies. For example, a survey of ^{222}Rn concentrations in well-water in Maine found a range of 7×10^2 to 7×10^6 Bq/m^3 (20–180,000 pCi/L), whereas wells in granitic areas were found to average 8×10^5 Bq/m^3 (36). With normal water use, the radon entering indoor air from water with such high concentrations can be expected to be significant.

Examinations of the overall potential contribution of water-borne radon to indoor concentrations have tended to be no more sophisticated than to consider typical water use rates, house volumes, and ventilation rates, yielding a ratio of radon in air to radon in the water supply of about 10^{-4}. However, it is possible to make a more realistic estimate of the distribution of the air-to-water ratio, using more detailed distributional information (rather than just averages) on water use rates, efficiency of radon release from domestic water used in various ways, house volumes, and ventilation rates. Such an analysis of U.S. data for single-family houses yields a ratio with a lognormal distribution having a GM of 0.65×10^{-4} and a GSD of 2.88, as discussed in Chapter 4. Taken together with recently developed data on ^{222}Rn in public water supplies (37), such a distribution permits quantitative assessment of the contribution of public water supplies to indoor radon concentrations. The result of such an assessment is that such supplies contribute an average of approximately 1 Bq/m^3 (0.03 pCi/L) in the 30% of U.S. homes served by ground water, only about 2% of the average indoor concentration in U.S. single-family homes.

However, the very high water-borne concentrations that are sometimes found— particularly from private wells—must be expected to contribute much larger airborne concentrations in the homes affected. Using the few data that are available for the approximately 18% of the U.S. population using private wells, the indoor contribution from water for this segment of the housing stock can be estimated to average about 20 Bq/m^3. About 10% of the houses served by these wells (totaling about 2% of the U.S. housing stock) are estimated to have indoor concentrations from water of 40 Bq/m^3 or more. Although these estimates for radon from private wells cannot be regarded as reliable, they suggest that the portion of the population using private wells may be experiencing significantly higher radon exposures than average, particularly in areas with high radon activity in water.

4.3   Summary of Source Contributions

We can thus point to the major sources of radon present in indoor environments. For single-family houses and other structures of one or two stories, the ground constitutes the principal source, but with a noticeable portion entering with outdoor air, i.e., on the order of 10 Bq/m^3. However, there are circumstances in which the building materials or domestic water supplies are important. In contrast, in high-rise buildings, including apartments, the ground is of lesser importance, and the amount of radium-bearing building materials per unit volume is larger, so that outdoor air and the building materials are typically the dominant contributors, al-

TABLE 1.3   Approximate Contributions of Various Sources to Observed Average Radon Concentrations[a]

Source	Single-family houses, Bq/m^3 (pCi/L)	High-rise apartments, Bq/m^3 (pCi/L)
Soil potential (based on flux measurements)	55 (1.5)	>0 (>0)
Water (public supplies)[b]	0.4 (0.01)	0.4 (0.01)
Building materials[c]	2 (0.05)	4 (0.1)
Outdoor air	10 (0.25)	10 (0.25)
Observed indoor concentrations	55 (1.5)	12? (0.3?)

[a]In each case, the arithmetic mean is shown, based on entry rates (or, in the case of outdoor air, concentrations) discussed in the text and on an air exchange rate of 0.5 h^{-1}.
[b]Indicated water contribution applies to 80% of U.S. population served by public supplies. Contribution may average 20 Bq/m^3 in homes using private wells, with even higher contributions in high-activity areas.
[c]The contribution of building material in single-family houses corresponds to a slightly smaller geometric mean entry rate than that estimated in the text because not all houses are slab-on-grade or one-story. A higher contribution to apartment air is suggested on the presumption that, on the average, high-rise apartments have a larger amount of radium-bearing material per unit volume than do single-family homes.

though the ground and water supplies can be important in some cases. Other potential sources, such as natural gas, ordinarily contribute negligible amounts by comparison (38, 39).

For a specific set of assumptions, characteristic of U.S. buildings, Table 1.3 indicates the approximate average contribution of various sources to the indoor concentration for single-family buildings and (to the extent data are available) for apartments. For comparison, the observed concentrations are also given. Note that, considering the uncertainties involved, the presumed contributions are consistent with the observed levels, i.e., an average of 55 Bq/m^3 in single-family houses and a substantially smaller concentration in high-rise apartments.

5   BEHAVIOR OF THE DECAY PRODUCTS

Even for a given amount of ^{222}Rn, the concentrations of its decay products and their physical state can vary considerably. What particularly distinguishes the decay products from ^{222}Rn itself is their chemical activity: the decay products can attach to airborne particles, to indoor (macroscopic) surfaces, and to the human respiratory tract, where they can deposit either directly or after attachment to airborne particles. In addition, the detailed behavior and health significance of the decay products is greatly influenced by their half-lives and decay modes, indicated in Figure 1.2. The alpha decays imparting the radiation dose of greatest significance are those of ^{218}Po and ^{214}Po, for the ^{222}Rn series. (The comparable isotopes for the ^{220}Rn series are ^{212}Bi and ^{212}Po, as indicated in Section 8.4.) The overall concentration of decay products, given by the potential alpha-energy concentration (PAEC) or the equilibrium-equivalent decay-product concentration (EEDC), depends on the concentrations of the first three decay products (^{218}Po, ^{214}Pb, and ^{214}Bi) for the 222 series (and on ^{212}Pb and—to a minor extent ^{212}Bi—for the 220 series) and on the amount of polonium alpha energy that each will yield (see Section 8.1 on quantities and units).

Understanding the behavior of the decay products is needed, not just to satisfy a general scientific interest in the relationship between indoor radon concentrations and decay-product concentrations, but specifically to provide a quantitative basis for characterizing the radiological implications of decay-product exposures and for indicating the potential utility of control measures aimed at modifying concentrations of the decay products. Although the discussion of this section focuses primarily on behavior of ^{222}Rn decay products, the same considerations apply in the main to the ^{220}Rn series. At a few points in the discussion, critical differences are indicated.

5.1 General Considerations

In an atmosphere where the concentration of radon is stable and where each decay product, once formed, is removed only by radioactive decay, radon and its decay products would be in a state of equilibrium, all having the same (radioactivity) concentration. In an indoor atmosphere where air is exchanged at some fixed ventilation rate, not only is the radon concentration less than it would otherwise be, but the concentrations of the decay products are reduced relative to that of radon because of removal by ventilation.

However, the behavior of the decay products, as suggested above, is further complicated by their chemical activity: the fact that the decay products can attach to particles or surfaces, and that these attachment rates can vary with conditions, makes general characterization of the state of the decay products—and of its dependence on ventilation rate, particle concentrations, and other factors—exceedingly complex. However, since we are dealing with only a few species, whose rate of production from early members of the decay chain is determined solely by known half-lives, it is still possible to specify a relatively straightforward framework for considering the behavior of the decay products.

Figure 1.6 illustrates, for an unspecified decay product (or "progeny"), various mechanisms for changing the state or presence of the decay product, other than radioactive decay itself. Because the deposition rates for the decay products depend strongly on whether or not they are attached to particles—and even on the particle characteristics—airborne particles play a crucial role in determining the concentrations that are present in air, and potentially on the radiation dose that results from a given concentration. Given the parameters that are indicated in Figure 1.6, one can write down a system of conservation-of-mass equations, following Ref. 40, that determine the concentrations based on given rate constants or—conversely—that can determine the rate constants from experiments that measure individual decay-product concentrations. Practical application of such a theoretical framework usually requires assumptions that simplify the picture. One of the usual sim-

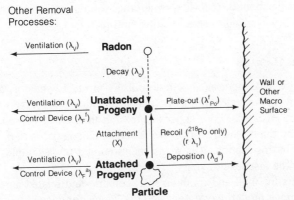

Figure 1.6. Decay-product removal mechanisms (other than radioactive decay) and associated rate constants. Once created by decay of its parent, a decay product (or "progeny") may attach to an airborne particle, a process that is usually considered to be reversible for ^{218}Po because of the substantial recoil energy associated with alpha decay. Whether attached or not, a decay product can be removed from the indoor air by plateout/deposition on indoor surfaces, by ventilation, by an air-cleaning device, or by radioactive decay.

plifications is consideration only of a single well-mixed space. Another is lack of differentiation of rate constants on the basis of aerosol size or chemical composition.

These simplifications aside, key issues of interest are the rates of attachment of the decay products to particles, as well as the rate at which free and attached decay products deposit on walls. (In many cases, deposition is parameterized in terms of the "deposition velocity," which is defined as the ratio of the flux toward the surface to the concentration in the volume, which—in turn—equals the deposition rate times the volume-to-surface ratio for the space under consideration.)

By way of perspective, whereas typical ventilation rates are on the order of 0.5 h^{-1} and decay-product radioactive decay constants range from 1.6 h^{-1} for ^{214}Bi to 14 h^{-1} for ^{218}Po, rates of attachment to particles, for typical particle concentrations, appear to be on the order of 50 h^{-1}, with slightly lower rates—perhaps 15 h^{-1}—for plateout of unattached decay products onto interior surfaces. In contrast, rates for deposition onto walls of airborne particles and therefore of attached decay products are very low, on the order of 0.1 h^{-1}. Lowering the particle concentration tends to result in a higher overall rate of deposition onto the walls (because a higher proportion of the decay products are unattached) and a lower equilibrium factor. This condition can, of course, be attained by use of particle-cleaning devices, which also directly remove decay products from the air. However, the advantage indicated by the lower equilibrium factors and lower EEDC may be balanced by the fact that a higher fraction of the EEDC is associated with unattached decay products, which appear to cause a more significant dose to the lung epithelium than the same amount of attached decay products.

(By way of comparison, the decay rate for ^{212}Pb, the most important ^{220}Rn decay product, is about 0.07 h^{-1}, so small that ventilation and other removal processes almost always lead to small equilibrium factors.)

5.2 Recent Results

The complexity and importance of radon decay-product behavior, as well as the potential interest in air cleaning as a control technique, has given rise to a substantial amount of work—both experimental and theoretical—on characterization of the decay products. Such work is reviewed in Chapters 5 and 6, as well as in Refs. 41–43. In this section, it is worth mentioning a few examples of important progress over the last several years.

Experiments in small and room-sized chambers, and related analysis in terms of a room-average model, have suggested the values for deposition rates indicated above (44, 45). This and earlier work—in particular, diffusion tube measurements (46)—has demonstrated that the rate at which "unattached" decay products plate out, although very high compared with particle deposition rates, is smaller than would occur if the decay products were present in the form of single unattached atoms (which would have a very high diffusion constant). The resulting conclusion, that an unattached decay product is actually a cluster of atoms including a decay-product atom, appears to be confirmed in experiments that measure the size distribution of decay products: they appear to divide into two regimes, one mode having a median diameter of about 100 nm, as might be expected based on the size distribution of particles typically present in a room, and a smaller fraction with median diameter in the vicinity of 10 nm, perhaps an order of magnitude greater than the size of a single ^{218}Po atom (47).

Considering what is known about the behavior of radon decay products, estimates have also been made of the effect of air-cleaning devices on the radiation dose to the lung. Such estimates suggest that the radical reduction in decay-product concentration (given as EEDC or PAEC) that is possible by air cleaning may not cause a corresponding decrease in effective dose and in health effects; it is even possible that there is no decrease at all (48). On the other hand, a detailed review of dosimetric models yields the result that, although the EEDC (or, equivalently, the PAEC) is an imperfect measure of dose and—ultimately—of potential health effects, it is still a reasonably good indicator, assuming that parameters are in the normal range (49). These results seem to suggest that—to the extent that air-cleaning devices result in particle concentrations outside the normal range—there is the potential that the EEDC (or PAEC) is no longer a good indicator of dose. Furthermore, more recent dosimetric studies suggest that, even for variability in decay product state caused by normal differences in particle concentration, the ^{222}Rn concentration may be a better indicator of effective dose equivalent than the EEDC (see Chapter 7).

Finally, Figure 1.6 does not explicitly indicate one of the potentially substantial influences on decay-product behavior, i.e., the fact that air within a room moves and that the pattern and rate of air movement can strongly affect deposition rates. Recent advances in modeling of air movement have made it possible to begin removing the simplifying assumption ordinarily used for simulation of decay-product behavior, that of a well-mixed room. The more detailed formulation permits treatment of the boundary layer more realistically, thereby providing a basis for determining the manner in which plateout rate (or deposition velocity) depends on conditions in the room, especially near the wall (50).

The importance, not only of ventilation rate, but also of other aspects of air movement, indicates the need to consider in detail the manner in which buildings operate as a basis for understanding the behavior of radon decay products. A comparable conclusion arises in trying to understand how radon enters buildings; i.e., it has become clear that the building is not a passive object into which radon diffuses, but actively contributes to the entry of radon. And, indeed, both these issues—radon entry and decay-product behavior—are linked to the question of ventilation and air movement in a more subtle way than was initially envisioned: whereas the ventilation rate might be thought to influence indoor concentrations primarily by removing radon from the building interior and, to a lesser extent, by some reduction in the equilibrium factor, we have found that the same factors that account for infiltration affect radon entry decisively and that comparable factors driving indoor air movement substantially affect decay-product behavior. Considering also the chemistry of the decay products, we see that properly understanding the behavior of radon and its decay products (as well as other pollutants) in buildings requires treatment of the problem as one of indoor atmospheric science, where airborne concentrations have a temporal and spatial dependence determined by sources and sinks, specific chemical and physical reactions, and complex indoor and outdoor wind fields.

6 HEALTH EFFECTS

The ultimate reason for all the work reviewed in this volume is the potential for exposures to radon decay products to cause ill effects among humans. A primary basis for this concern has been the increased incidence of lung cancer among mine workers exposed to higher-than-average levels of ^{222}Rn decay products, but several kinds of studies provide information on the effects of decay-product exposures. Together, these lead to some estimation (quantitative or otherwise) of the risk of lung cancer from indoor exposures and of the importance of this risk relative to other environmental insults.

6.1 Types and Results of Health Studies

Studies of the effects of radiation generally fall into two categories. The first consists of epidemiological studies of humans exposed to radiation in the workplace, in the course of medical procedures, or in the environment, either natural or modified, the last including the extreme case of the Japanese nuclear bomb victims. The second class consists of a variety of laboratory studies, including animal tests and cellular or physiological human studies. The principal classes of studies of the effects of radon decay products are epidemiological studies of miners and laboratory studies of animals, both subjected to relatively high exposures of ^{222}Rn decay products. In addition, a much broader range of studies, involving other types of radiation exposures and other types of biomedical investigations, contribute to a broader base of knowledge in the context of which the information specific to decay-product exposures is interpreted. A principal example is the recent effort to understand in detail the nature and site of the radiation doses resulting from inhalation of airborne decay products. The dosimetry of ^{222}Rn decay products, the evidence from human epidemiology, and the results from animal studies are discussed in detail in Chapters 7, 8, and 9 of this volume. It is useful to note here the relationship among these research areas.

The miner studies offer a direct, although flawed, indication of the relationship between exposures and increased incidence of lung cancer. The principal study groups have been underground uranium miners in the United States, Czechoslovakia, and Canada, and iron, zinc, and lead miners in Sweden. The results of these studies, given in terms of increased risk per unit exposure or its equivalent, differ significantly among themselves, as indicated in Figure 1.7, where the incidence (following exposure) per unit exposure from various studies is plotted against the estimated cumulative exposure of the groups of workers examined in each study. The factors potentially contributing to differing values for dose-response factors are numerous, including differences in methods of analysis, inconsistency or error in the estimation of exposures, and differences in the presence of cofactors (such

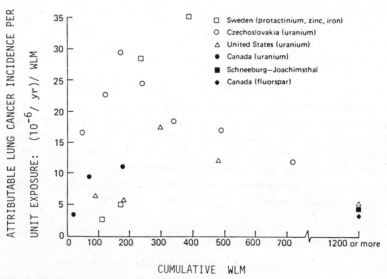

Figure 1.7. Attributable lung cancer incidence per unit exposure versus cumulative exposure as determined from miner studies. For most human data available, the figure shows the excess chance of cancer (in each year of follow-up) per unit exposure (in WLM) versus the cumulative exposure (in WLM) for each miner group. Adapted from Ref. 78.

as diesel exhaust and ore dust), as well as the potential for a genuine dependence of the dose-response factor on cumulative exposure or on exposure rate.

Given the number of such factors, the apparent range in values is not surprising. Note that paying most attention to the data between about 100 WLM and 500 WLM (thereby neglecting the low-exposure data, which become less significant statistically as the exposure decreases, and the high-exposure end, where the risk per unit exposure appears to decrease), we are left with a range of roughly 5–35 lung cancers per year per WLM per million people. Taking an approximate median of 12, this means that for each WLM of total exposure an individual would suffer an attributable risk of 12×10^{-6} per year thereafter (or perhaps only after the latency period for appearance of lung cancer, this being one of the ambiguities of the studies). Given in terms of SI units, not often used in this context, the $12 \times 10^{-6} \, y^{-1} \, WLM^{-1}$ individual annual risk per unit exposure becomes (see Section 8.1 on quantities and units) $0.9 \times 10^{-6} \, y^{-1} (J \, m^{-3} \, s)^{-1}$. (For convenience, the combination $J \, m^{-3} \, s$ is maintained as a unit of exposure.) Assuming, as is typically done (51), that this attributable risk applies to a 30-year period of expression, this implies an individual lifetime risk per unit exposure of about $2.8 \times 10^{-5} (J \, m^{-3} \, s)^{-1}$ (or $3.6 \times 10^{-4} \, WLM^{-1}$). Various groups have considered the results from these studies, and—given the fact that they all utilize basically the same results—it is not surprising that they should arrive at similar values for the risk per unit exposure. The reader is referred not only to Chapter 8 in this volume, but also to a series of papers presented at the 1983 international conference at Anacapri (49, 52, 53). Nonetheless, the "modest" differences in risk estimates—say a factor of 2 to 4—can have substantial implications when considering the importance of radon exposures and strategies for controlling them (cf. Chapter 12).

Aside from the statistical uncertainties associated with the risk factor cited above, there are lingering underlying problems that have not been fully resolved. A major example is whether there is a synergism between decay-product exposures and smoking, or—put another way—whether the decay-product risk factor depends on smoking or smoking history. A related issue is whether a risk factor cited in "absolute" terms as above is better or worse than a "relative" risk factor, giving the attributable risk as a fraction of the "background" risk of lung cancer. In such terms, the rate of appearance of lung cancer appears to increase by about 1% per WLM exposure, or 0.08% per $J \, m^{-3} \, s$ (53).

A major tool for examining such issues, and in general for permitting controlled experiments on factors affecting risk, is the use of animal studies wherein disease incidence or physiological change in groups of animals inhaling radon decay products is compared with rates in control groups. Chapter 9 treats these studies in detail, including major efforts using (Beagle) dogs, rats, and hamsters as subjects. Reference 51 contains an earlier and useful summary of the animal studies.

The animal studies not only provide information on disease incidence as a function of exposure, but also provide a convenient means for investigating the detailed dosimetry of decay-product exposure, i.e., the manner in which the decay products deposit in the airways and the nature of the resulting radiation dose. Investigations of these matters are also carried out in humans. In fact, in recent years sufficient information has been accumulated about the structure and behavior of the human lung, as well as about the characteristics of airborne ^{222}Rn decay products, that it has become feasible to calculate the detailed pattern of deposition and exposure as a function of pulmonary characteristics and decay-product/particle mixture. Several of the references cited above treat this question in detail, as does Chapter 7 of this volume.

A principal result of these detailed dosimetric studies is the ability to construct a rational framework within which to consider differing types of studies and to extend the results to conditions other than those actually present in the studies. For the present purpose, this offers two advantages: (i) it permits intercomparison of the results of studies of different types or undertaken under different conditions; and (ii) it permits application of these results to exposures in the site of present interest, the indoor environment.

6.2   Risk from Indoor Exposures

Numerous investigators have recently examined the applicability of dose-response data from the miner studies to environmental and, in particular, indoor exposures. This requires consideration of a number of factors, including a population that is much broader in its constitution than the miner population, which tends to be healthy males in the prime of life. In addition, the miners were engaged in a higher level of physical activity during exposure, therefore with higher breathing rates, than the average level of the general population. Finally, the mine atmosphere contains a different mix of substances than an ordinary indoor environment, with the amount and size distribution of airborne particulates being of special interest.

A number of papers have examined such issues, as does Chapter 7. The typical result is the conclusion that the dose-response factor derived from the miner studies can be applied relatively directly to environmental exposures. A relatively straight-forward calculation indicates the size of those exposures: an average indoor ^{222}Rn concentration of, say, 50 Bq/m^3 implies, for an equilibrium factor of 0.4, an average decay-product concentration of 20 Bq/m^3. If two-thirds of a 70-year life-time is spent in this concentration, the lifetime exposure is 933 Bq m^{-3} y or (see Section 8.1 on quantities and units) 164 J m^{-3} s (12.6 WLM). (If the other third of a life is spent at about 5 Bq/m^3 EEDC, a quarter of the indoor value, the total exposure is in the vicinity of 1000 Bq m^{-3} y, 180 J m^{-3} s, or 14 WLM.) Using the nominal lifetime risk per unit exposure given above, 2.8×10^{-5} (J m^{-3} s)$^{-1}$, this exposure implies an associated lifetime risk of 0.5% (neglecting detailed consideration of the population's age distribution, smoking habits, and other characteristics). In point of fact, this risk (and risk factor) are slightly higher than that suggested by reviews under the auspices of national and international radiation protection organizations (49, 51), but somewhat lower than that used by the U.S. Environmental Protection Agency (54). This risk, if applied uncritically to the U.S. population of 230 million, implies that 1 million of them might contract lung cancer as a result of ^{222}Rn decay-product exposures, or that about 10–15% of the current annual incidence of 120,000 is due to this exposure (as compared with 14% implied by the relative risk factor cited above).

These estimates are quite uncertain, because of uncertainty in both the primary studies of the miners and the applicability of those results to environmental exposures of the general population. One aspect of this applicability issue is that the average exposure just cited, 1000 Bq m^{-3} y, or 14 WLM, is well below the range where the epidemiological data have much statistical significance. On the other hand, this is not true of the higher levels found indoors. Lifetime exposure to an EEDC of 120 Bq/m^3 (associated with 300 Bq/m^3 ^{222}Rn) implies a total exposure of 5600 Bq m^{-3} y or 9.8×10^2 J m^{-3} s (76 WLM). This exceeds exposures typical of present-day underground uranium miners and is in an exposure range where the associated lifetime risk, estimated to be 2–3%, assumes much more significance because there is no longer a need to extrapolate to low doses.

Regardless of the precise estimates, it is useful to put such risks in perspective relative to those from other environmental exposures. First, these exposures exceed those from other types of environmental radiation. Considering the population at high risk (e.g., in the million U.S. homes with ^{222}Rn concentrations of 300 Bq/m^3 or more), these exposures far exceed in significance even those accumulated in occupational settings, e.g., uranium mines, nuclear power plants, or medical facilities. Second, the average risk, whether 0.2 or 0.5%, far exceeds the levels at which other types of environmental exposures—such as those from outdoor airborne pollutants or toxic wastes—are considered to be significant. Regulatory investigation and even action often begins at lifetime risk levels in the range of 10^{-5}–10^{-6}, a factor of a thousand below the estimated average risk from ^{222}Rn decay products, and even further below the 1+% risk of the heavily exposed portion of the population. This is especially ironic considering that, however uncertain the estimates of risk from decay-product exposures might be, they are much less uncertain than the estimates for other exposures, e.g., to potentially carcinogenic chemicals. The estimates for such chemicals are typically based on animal tests at exposures thousands of times higher than human exposures, with assumptions that are purposely selected to overestimate the risk in order to be conservative in protecting the public. A further irony is that concentrations of such chemicals may be much higher in the indoor environment than outdoors, where the main regulatory attention is focussed.

7 IDENTIFYING AND CONTROLLING INDOOR CONCENTRATIONS

Given the apparent importance of indoor exposures to ^{222}Rn decay products, an immediate question is how to assure that the levels to which the population is exposed are acceptable. The answer to this question entails several related issues, including the narrow ones of measurement and control techniques and the broader problem of formulating a control strategy.

7.1   Measurement Techniques

Measurement of the airborne concentration of radon or its decay products is based on detection of the radiation associated with radioactive decay. This radiation includes, not only the alpha and beta radiation indicated in Figure 1.1, but X or gamma radiation from transition of the decay product from the ''excited'' state in which it is left to its ''ground'' or unexcited state. Any of these forms of radiation is capable of creating ions in materials through which it passes, and measurement methods are based on detection of this ionization or its aftermath.

In spite of this uniformity in the basic principle of detection, practical measurement techniques take widely different forms, substantially affecting their range of application. Specific techniques are designed for measuring the concentration of radon, the EEDC, or, indeed, the concentration of individual decay products. Some techniques are suitable for short-term measurements, where a ''grab'' sample of air is taken, or for continuous real-time measurements, where repeated samples are taken. Other techniques are designed for intermediate to long-term sampling, where only the average concentration is sought. Some techniques may be self-contained, requiring the presence of a moderate to large piece of equipment at the site of measurement, whereas other techniques deploy a small sampler or detector, which must be returned to a central laboratory for analysis. Finally, some techniques are inexpensive or easy to use, whereas others are suitable for use only in the context of experiments carried out by experienced scientists.

Measurement techniques are treated briefly in the appendix to this book, and also in a number of specific instrumentation reviews (55, 56). As an illustration, however, it is worth mentioning three widely used techniques that are suitable for use in monitoring large numbers of houses:

1. Grab-sample monitoring for either ^{222}Rn or its decay products can be performed using highly-portable self-contained instruments that use a scintillation material to measure alpha particles emitted in a small collection cell (for ^{222}Rn) or from a filter (for the decay products). The entire measurement is completed within some tens of minutes, therefore only giving the concentration at a specific time. Considering the potential variability of concentration with time, this does not give a direct measure of the average exposure rate in a home.

2. A charcoal sampler with dimensions on the order of 10 cm can be used to collect ^{222}Rn over a period of a day to a week, then sealed and returned to a laboratory, where the gamma radiation from decay products contained in the sampler can be measured (9). This technique is not suitable for more than 1 week: late in this period much of the ^{222}Rn collected at the beginning will be gone because of its 3.8-day half-life.

3. An etched-track detector with dimensions of only about 3–4 cm can be placed in a home for periods from weeks to a year, then returned to a laboratory where the plastic detector material is etched to show tracks left by the passage of alpha particles from the decay of ^{222}Rn and its decay products (8). As ordinarily deployed, such detectors have a filter permitting entry of ^{222}Rn, but not its decay

products (for which it is difficult to calibrate the device). This technique has the advantage of giving a long-term average concentration, which, however, might be considered a disadvantage if a quick result is desired.

In the context of a program for identifying and reducing excessive concentrations, the suitability of each of these techniques would depend on the objective of any particular measurement, as discussed in Chapter 12.

7.2 Control Techniques

The techniques available for controlling indoor concentrations of ^{222}Rn and its decay products correspond quite closely to the basic factors found to affect concentrations. For several of the major classes of indoor pollution—whether radon, combustion products, or airborne chemicals—these factors include the source strengths (or entry rates) for the pollutants of interest, the ventilation rate (and pattern), and reactions of the pollutants with each other and with the building or its contents. For each pollutant class, concentrations appear to be distributed approximately lognormally, and the largest contributor to the width of the distribution is typically the source strength, but, in each case, variability in ventilation rates and in reaction rates contributes significantly. For the case of radon, as for the other pollutants, it appears that control techniques altering the entry rate offer greater potential reduction than other techniques.

The strong variability found in radon entry rates suggests the efficacy of a control program aimed at minimizing entry rates, particularly where they are large. Considering the importance of pressure-driven flow of soil gas into houses through their understructures, substantial attention has been given in recent years to the potential for reducing this flow. It is clear that the use of better barriers, sealants, and construction techniques can have a significant effect on the radon entry rate, but this potential appears limited in most cases, one reason being that a substantial pressure-driven entry rate can persist if only a few passages for soil gas remain or if new imperfections appear as a result of slight movement of the house understructure.

An alternative approach that has the potential for reduction of entry rates by large factors is to apply a technique that reduces (or increases) the air pressure immediately under the house, thereby disrupting the flow of air that carries radon from underlying soil into the house. This might be thought of as offering an alternative route for the radon flux from the ground (or creating a pressure barrier). And, indeed, in certain cases where the main entry route is highly localized, as through a drain tile and sump system, what one does is provide local venting to the outdoors. In the more general case of a basement (or slab-on-grade), one or a few pipes with a small fan to depressurize (or, sometimes, pressurize) the material (preferably gravel) immediately below the concrete floor can greatly reduce the radon entry rate. In the case of crawl spaces, active ventilation of the space below the house can easily be accomplished, although—as noted above—careful sealing of the floor may be quite practical in this case.

For situations where large entry rates are responsible for excessive indoor concentrations, such entry reduction techniques appear ordinarily to have the greatest potential effect. However, there are also circumstances where increases in ventilation rate are appropriate, whether because the ventilation rate in question is unusually low, because source reduction techniques do not appear effective for the case at hand (e.g., if the source is unusual building materials incorporated into the structure), or because—in rare cases of extremely high concentrations—an immediate, if only temporary, solution is required. The primary limitation of increased ventilation rates, especially in homes with very high concentrations, is that reduction of indoor concentrations by large factors will require increases in the ventilation by large factors, which is often impractical, uncomfortable, or too expensive, at least for the long term. For homes where only modest reductions are sought, ventilation rate increases are quite practical, including use of mechanical systems that recover energy that would otherwise be lost—either by incorporation of an air-to-air heat exchanger between incoming and outgoing air streams or by simple recovery of heat from exhaust air. (However, an exhaust ventilation system has to be used with some care, since it may result in increased depressurization of the house and larger radon entry rates.)

An alternative means of control is, of course, use of air-cleaning systems to remove the decay products. The most common of these employ particle removal techniques such as filtration and electrostatic precipitation. However, although the better devices using such techniques can substantially reduce the decay-product concentrations as measured by EEDC or PAEC, their effect on the dose to the lung is far from clear. As a result, it is generally thought that source-strength reduction is the best control technique, with the next best option being increased ventilation rates.

7.3 Strategies

Knowledge of measurement techniques and methods for control does not constitute a strategy for identifying and controlling excessive concentrations. Identification and control can be achieved only in a more general framework that embodies the objectives to be met and the overall strategy for achieving them. In this context, specific measurement and control techniques are merely the tactics or tools for a campaign against the radon problem. The fundamental elements of a control strategy are discussed in more detail in Chapter 12, but it is worth emphasizing here that two of the elements are mainly technical and two are mainly questions of valuation and responsibility. The technical elements are (i) developing the actual scheme for identifying areas and individual houses with high concentrations, and (ii) formulation of a logical structure for choosing what control technique(s) should be attempted in each type of situation. Just as important are (iii) that some agreement be reached on the objectives of the strategy, usually embodied in a structure of concentration limits (or guidelines) or comparable devices, and (iv) that responsibility (both scientific and fiscal) be allocated for locating houses with excessive levels and for implementing the appropriate control measures. Improvements in scientific understanding and technical capabilities are prerequisites for coping with the problem of indoor radon. But little can be done effectively without carefully framing various objectives and creating an overall strategy suited to achieving them.

7.4 Future Developments

As is clear from the discussion in this chapter and from the material in the body of this book, a great deal is known about the causes, concentrations, consequences, and control of indoor radon. We have a functional, albeit preliminary, appreciation of indoor levels and their distribution. We understand in principle how various sources contribute to these levels. The evidence from health studies is sufficient to permit a tentative assessment of the risk. Although the assessment is tentative, it is sounder than estimates made for most other environmental exposures, and indicates that the risk involved is larger than for most other enviromental exposures. Substantial progress has been made in developing techniques to reduce indoor radon concentrations where they might otherwise be excessive.

Our current understanding is an incentive and a basis for formulating an attack on the ''radon problem.'' A preliminary element of that attack is, of course a more intensive research effort, prompted by recognition of the potential importance of indoor radon exposures and by the need for a more comprehensive understanding of radon behavior and associated health effects. During the 1980s, a substantial upgrading of the research effort occurred, as evidenced for example by the institution of broad programs sponsored by the Commission of the European Communities—as well as efforts occurring both cooperatively and independently in various countries—and by the substantial increase in U.S. efforts sponsored by the Department of Energy, the Environmental Protection Agency, and by many states in the wake of the discoveries on or near the Reading Prong. The recent surge of activity has added significantly to our knowledge of the concentrations and behavior of radon and its decay products, although not to a degree that the overall picture has changed in a qualitative way. Similarly, there is now an increased commitment to investigation of the mechanisms and risks of lung cancer induction from decay product exposures; however, it is not expected that these efforts will radically alter our appreciation of the risks in the near future, although they might ultimately contribute substantially to understanding the basic mechanisms of carcinogenesis. A brief look at current work on radon gives some indication of the directions that might be expected for the future.

With respect to concentrations, we have recently seen a vast increase in the number of homes in which monitoring has been performed, particularly in the United States. The resulting increase in the amount of data available has not improved our knowledge of the concentration distribution, however; it has even misled the public and many scientists. For example, a recently reported data base of 60,000 results from etched-track measurements in the United States (85) gives a much higher average radon concentration than the results discussed in this chapter, as well as a much larger fraction exceeding $150 \ \mathrm{Bq/m^3}$ (4 pCi/L). Even analyzing only a restricted data set to avoid the effect of oversampling in states with large monitoring efforts (such as Pennsylvania and New Jersey), the average concentration is found to be 152 Bq/m³ (4.1 pCi/L), far larger than the 55 Bq/m³ (1.5 pCi/L) discussed in Section 3.1. In addition, about 20% of the restricted sample is found to exceed 150 Bq/m³ (4 pCi/L). However, the data include many results from sampling in basements and are not corrected to annual-average concentrations, for which reasons they are comparable neither to the results from Refs. 10 and 11 nor to the 4-pCi/L limit recommended by the U.S. Environmental Protection Agency (cf. Chapter 12), which applies to the average indoor concentration experienced by the occupants. Furthermore, the data provide no identification of multiple detectors placed in the same house. In the absence of sufficient information to make proper corrections associated with these factors, one can only make crude estimates, based on other information, on the potential size of these corrections. Such estimates indicate that the average indicated above, about 152 Bq/m³, is *approximately* a factor of 2 too high. Considering the large uncertainties in the resulting average, about 75 Bq/m³, this is consistent with the average previously found (which has smaller uncertainties), 55 Bq/m³. Similarly, the (corrected) fraction of homes with annual–average living-space concentrations exceeding 150 Bq/m³ would be far smaller than 20%, thus effectively eliminating the contrast with the previous result of about 6%. Results from current carefully designed surveys appear to be consistent with the results of Refs. 10 and 11, to the extent there is overlap. For example, preliminary results from a 2400-home survey in New York State (86) indicate an average concentration of 1.4 pCi/L (52 Bq/m³) and only 5% exceed 4 pCi/L (150 Bq/m³), even though the initial data are from wintertime measurements. Results from many other state surveys are beginning to become available, but unfortunately without the corrections to annual-average living-space concentration that are necessary to yield a useful concentration distribution or a comparison to recommended limits. As discussed in Chapter 12, monitoring results, to be useful, often need to be adjusted significantly to yield the average concentration to which occupants are exposed.

It should also be noted that substantial numbers of homes having extremely high concentrations, in the range of 2000 to 50,000 Bq/m³ (54–1350 pCi/L), have been found in the Reading Prong area of Pennsylvania and in adjoining areas of New Jersey, raising the possibility that the lognormal distribution from Ref. 10 may significantly underestimate the number of homes at very high levels. One way of viewing this possibility is that, when considering the extreme tail of the distribution, a relatively small number of homes—potentially arising from one or a few areas—can cause a radical divergence from lognormality. Alternatively, it must be remembered that many of the high-concentration results arise from wintertime measurements, often obtained in basements, and that—in the extreme tail—application of correction factors of 2 or so to the concentrations measured can change the fraction in the tail by more than an order of magnitude. Nonetheless, the incidence at high concentrations is both extremely interesting scientifically and very distressing for the occupants. To cite an extreme case, data from 103 homes monitored in Clinton, New Jersey, if plotted to yield lognormal parameters, are found to be characterized well by a geometric mean of 100 pCi/L (3700 Bq/m^3) and a geometric standard deviation of 5.0, both startlingly large numbers (87). Given the scope of the efforts in the United States, an unusually complete picture of the concentration distribution, particularly in the extreme tail, can be expected to develop.

It is interesting to note, too, that many of the homes in Clinton were slab-on-grade, confirming the suspicion voiced in Chapter 2 that the physical factors affecting indoor concentrations in such homes are essentially similar to those for houses with basements. Other current work is confirming and developing our basic picture of radon entry. In addition to efforts devoted directly to reducing levels in homes where they are found to be excessive, experiments have been initiated to investigate in detail the generation and transport of radon, including the influence of environmental factors and the effectiveness of control techniques. The prototype of such intensive studies has focused on a small number of homes in New Jersey, each heavily instrumented to monitor key concentrations and related parameters over a period of a year as a basis for extracting more detailed information on the process of radon entry (88). Related experiments elsewhere can be expected to examine various aspects of radon entry in both existing and new homes.

Corresponding theoretical efforts are also significant, as noted in Chapter 2. A simple model for the pressures driving radon entry, as well as ventilation rates, has recently been used for examining the effect on concentrations of ventilation characteristics (including exhaust ventilation), understructure type, and soil characteristics (89). In addition, a more complete finite-difference model has been used to simulate radon entry, including the effects of a soil type in the immediate vicinity of the basement that differs from that further away (90). The next step is to extend modeling to consider more heterogeneous configurations in respect to substructure and soil, even including two-phase effects involving the interaction of water and soil gas.

Related to this physical understanding and to the needs of control programs are efforts to understand how various kinds of physical data are correlated with indoor concentrations and how they may be used as a geographic predictor thereof. These include field studies attempting to examine such correlations (e.g., Ref. 91), which often find them to be weak. In parallel with these efforts, examination of preexisting data, such as aerial radiation surveys, aims at developing elements of a predictive capability needed for locating areas likely to have higher-than-average radon concentrations (e.g., Ref. 92).

In the area of health effects, progress has been made recently in lung dosimetry and in animal studies; these results are reported in Chapters 7 and 9, respectively. The situation is somewhat different for epidemiological studies, where few new studies have been reported in recent years, and where the most significant developments have been retrospective analyses of the nature and significance of the results, such as is done in Chapter 9. As indicated there in an editors' note, recent assessments have not provided the convergence one might wish in dose-response factors applying to public exposures to radon's decay products. Moreover, epidemiological studies conducted among the general public will have difficulty providing new, quantitative estimates of the dose-response provided by utilization of the miner data, unless the dose-response factor is larger than estimated by most scientists.

Finally, greater experience with application of control techniques (largely those described in Chapter 10 for reducing radon entry rates, but also those for removal from indoor air discussed in Chapter 11) can be expected to improve the effectiveness of techniques, as well as reducing their cost and sharpening the process by which appropriate techniques are chosen for each circumstance. In addition, an improved understanding of the behavior of radon, as well as of the health effects of exposures, can provide a more complete basis for selecting control objectives and for identifying areas or homes that have excessive concentrations.

8   APPENDIX

8.1   Radioactive Quantities and Units of Measure

Amounts of radioactive material can be specified in principle by either mass or activity, the latter being more conventional. The activity is the actual rate at which atoms decay radioactively, and the standard international (SI) unit for activity is the Becquerel (Bq), equal to a decay rate of one per second (s^{-1}). This unit (or its traditional equivalent, the Curie) is adequate for expressing activity and (activity) concentration, not only for radon, but also for its decay products and any combination of them. The present work utilizes SI units primarily, but traditional units are defined below in terms of the modern units. In the text, the older units are sometimes given parenthetically or when citing work that is difficult to translate without modifying sense or quantitative results.

For decay products, the collective quantity of most use is the equilibrium-equivalent decay-product concentration (EEDC). Based on the alpha decay energies and half-lives of the ^{222}Rn decay series given in Ref. 57 (see Fig. 1.2), the EEDC is given in terms of the individual decay-product concentrations as

$$\text{EEDC}_{222} = 0.106 \times I(^{218}\text{Po}) + 0.513 \times I(^{214}\text{Pb}) + 0.381 \times I(^{214}\text{Bi}) \quad (2)$$

with concentrations of each decay product (and of the EEDC) given in Bq/m^3 or pCi/L. (The ^{214}Po concentration does not contribute significantly to this expression because of its very short half-life, causing very few ^{214}Po atoms to be present in air as compared with the other short-lived decay products. However, the ^{214}Po alpha energy is the largest contributor to the coefficients in this expression, since the presence of each of the previous three decay products implies a ^{214}Po decay.) The analogous expression for the ^{220}Rn series, based on data from Ref. 57 (cf. Section 8.4), is

$$\text{EEDC}_{220} = 0.913 \times I(^{212}\text{Pb}) + 0.087 \times I(^{212}\text{Bi}) \quad (3)$$

(^{216}Po and ^{212}Po do not contribute directly to this expression—again, because of their very short half-lives—even though ^{212}Po contributes the dominant alpha energy.)

Historically, the potential alpha-energy concentration (PAEC) itself was used as the measure of decay-product concentration, with the standard unit being working level (WL). The corresponding SI unit is that of energy per unit volume, J/m^3, and PAEC = EEDC $\times$ 5.57×10^{-9} J/Bq (or 1287 MeV/pCi) for the ^{222}Rn series. (The corresponding factor for the ^{220}Rn series is 7.56×10^{-8} J/Bq, or 1.75×10^4 MeV/pCi.) In any case, the PAEC is effectively supplanted by the EEDC (i.e., the decay-product concentration itself), except possibly in specifying exposures. (Note that in one respect the PAEC is a more effective measure of concentration than the EEDC; i.e., in comparing ^{222}Rn and ^{220}Rn: per unit radioactivity, the ^{220}Rn decay products carry 13.6 times as much PAEC as the ^{222}Rn decay products.)

The basic measure of exposure is essentially the product of concentration (or its equivalent) and time. EEDC $\times$ time has units of Bq m^{-3} s, although hour, month, or year might also be used as the unit of time. PAEC $\times$ time has SI units of J m^{-3} s, but the traditional units are working-level hour (WLH) or—more frequently—working-level month (WLM), equal to 173 WLH. Exposure rate, in the SI units, simply reduces to average EEDC (or alternatively PAEC), but in the old units is usually WLM/y.

Table 1.4 lists conversion factors between SI and traditional units.

8.2 Ventilation Rates: Distribution and Dependence

A key factor affecting indoor pollutant concentrations is the ventilation rate. Characterizing ventilation rates in buildings can be difficult, since many buildings are complex structures, and paths and rates of air movement can depend substantially on location and time. Even considering only homes, the question is complicated, both because of the wide variety of housing structures and because—even for a given (and even simple) structure type—the pattern of air movement is complex.

TABLE 1.4 SI Units and Equivalents for Traditional Units[a]

Parameter, SI unit	Conversion for traditional unit
Activity, Bq	1 Ci = 3.7×10^{10} Bq (1 pCi = 0.037 Bq)
Concentration, Bq m^{-3}	1 pCi/L = 37 Bq m^{-3}
PAEC, J m^{-3}	1 WL = 1.3×10^5 MeV/L = 2.08×10^{-5} J m^{-3}
EEDC$_{222}$, Bq m^{-3}	1 WL (PAEC) = 3740 Bq m^{-3}
EEDC$_{220}$, Bq m^{-3}	1 WL (PAEC) = 276 Bq m^{-3}
Exposure, J m^{-3} s	1 WLM = 12.97 J m^{-3} s
Exposure, Bq m^{-3} y	1 WLM = 73.9 Bq m^{-3} y
Exposure rate, J m^{-3}	1 WLM/y = 4.11×10^{-7} J m^{-3}
Exposure rate, Bq m^{-3}	1 WLM/y = 73.9 Bq m^{-3}

[a]The data on which these conversions are based are taken from Ref. 57.

These complexities have substantial implications for the behavior of any reactive species, including radon decay products, and for the manner and degree of radon entry, as described elsewhere in this chapter.

Nevertheless, restricting attention to homes—consisting of relatively self-contained living units—simplifies the picture sufficiently that the ventilation rate has a less ambiguous meaning (although even this can be complicated in the case of multiapartment buildings in which air is recirculated among different units). Moreover, the rate can actually be measured relatively directly. For example, the ventilation rate measurements contributing to Figure 1.3 were performed by injecting a tracer gas, sulfur hexafluoride (SF_6), into each house, then—after a mixing time—measuring the concentration as a function of time using an infrared analyzer: the ventilation rate equals the rate of decay of the tracer concentration. And in a current passive measurement technique, a tracer is released from a small source at a constant rate and a collecting monitor, consisting of a diffusion tube and an absorber (characteristic of a number of techniques for passive sampling of gaseous pollutants indoors), measures the average concentration during the time this system is deployed (58): this measured value is then proportional, in first order, to the average of the inverse of the ventilation rate, $I_{tracer} = S_V(1/\lambda_v)_{average}$.

The results of such measurements confirm the expectation that ventilation rates vary substantially from one country to another, from one class of buildings to another, and even within the same general structural class, e.g., single-family houses or multiunit apartment buildings. Still, for most homes in the United States (and many industrialized nations), the average ventilation rate during seasons when the windows are kept mostly closed lies in the range 0.1–1 h^{-1}. This total ventilation rate is made up of three components: infiltration of air through small openings or imperfections in the building shell, exchange of air through windows or doors that are partially or temporarily open, and ventilation supplied mechanically by exhaust fans or other systems. Each of these components varies with time, not only from one season to another, but also from one day to the next, and even over shorter periods. As a result, the total ventilation rate has a significant time dependence, even within a single building. Even during the heating season, when—for many homes—infiltration supplies most of the ventilation, substantial variability occurs, as noted below.

It is important, in considering the results of ventilation rate measurements, to pay attention to what component of the ventilation the monitoring protocol was designed to measure. For example, the basic tracer injection technique mentioned above is often employed with windows closed, therefore measuring only the infiltration rate, often the dominant winter component. In contrast, the integrating passive technique measures the average inverse *total* ventilation rate.

Like the radon concentrations discussed in this chapter, measurements of infiltration rate in any sample of buildings are often found to be distributed lognormally; i.e., the distribution of the log of the ventilation rate is approximately "normal" or Gaussian. An example of this is a set of measurements taken in 200 single-family houses in several cities of the United States, where weatherization programs were taking place (59). The average infiltration rate was found to be 1.1 h^{-1}, and a more recent determination of the geometric mean and standard deviation yields 0.90 and 2.13, respectively, as discussed in Chapter 4. Considering the age and condition of these houses, their infiltration rates are higher than the average U.S. value, which in turn is significantly higher than in northern European countries, where substantial energy-saving efforts appear to have effected significant reduction in infiltration rates.

In recent years, the processes driving infiltration rates in homes have come to be better understood, and even embodied in relatively simple quantitative models. Basically, we now know that infiltration occurs because of air convection into and out of the house, driven by small pressures across the building shell arising from two factors: winds, which obviously exert small—although complex—forces on the building and its surroundings (specifically, the ground), and temperature differences between indoors and outdoors. During the heating season, this temperature difference causes a "stack" effect (much as in a fireplace and chimney), such that air is drawn in near the bottom of the structure and forced out toward the top. The pressure differences caused by winds and temperature differences are roughly comparable in size, averaging on the order of a few Pascals (with higher values in relatively severe climates). Because the size and pattern of the associated pressures vary markedly from one time to another, it is not surprising that infiltration rates also vary substantially.

A number of groups have formulated models giving the infiltration rates in terms of the pertinent environmental parameters, and their success is reviewed in a recent publication of the Air Infiltration Centre (60). As successful as any model— even complex ones—is a simple parameterization of the infiltration rate in terms of the wind speed V, the temperature difference dT, and an effective "leakage area" A_o. In these terms, the infiltration component of the ventilation rate may be expressed as

$$v_i = A_o \left[\left(f_w V \right)^2 + \left(f_s dT^{1/2} \right)^2 \right]^{1/2} \tag{4}$$

where f_w is a parameter accounting for local and terrain shielding effects, the distribution of leakage area around the building envelope, and the height of the building relative to the height at which the wind speed is measured; f_s is a stack parameter accounting for the building height and the distribution of leakage area (61). Using this model together with applicable meteorological information, heating-season infiltration rates have been estimated from measurements performed in 200 houses distributed throughout the United States and Canada. The average was found to be 0.67 h^{-1} (with a significantly lower value, 0.48 h^{-1}, found for houses less than 2 years old at the time of measurement).

8.3 Outdoor Concentrations of Radon and Its Decay Products

During the last two or three decades, a significant effort has been devoted to monitoring of outdoor radon concentrations, either as part of the overall characterization of environmental radiation exposures or to determine environmental radon levels as a contrast to those in occupational or indoor settings. A recent paper by Gesell reviews and analyzes the results from such efforts, examining the variability of outdoor ^{222}Rn concentrations with time of day, season, altitude, and location (62).

The magnitude and behavior of outdoor concentrations is indicated by Figure 1.8, where continuous measurements taken at three locations are seen to yield concentrations (averaged over approximately 1 month) in the range of 4–15 Bq/m^3 (0.1–0.4 pCi/L), with a significant seasonal variation whose behavior differed among the locations. Examining the same data versus time of day yields average concentrations having a substantial diurnal variability (roughly a factor-of-two range in each case), with the lowest values occurring at noon or soon thereafter and the highest in the middle of the night or early morning. The observed variation with time can be attributed to differences in environmental conditions, affecting not only the movement of radon out of the ground, but also—and probably more importantly—the rapidity of mixing in the atmosphere. This mixing determines the height dependence of concentration, which varies only modestly over distances comparable to the height of buildings (e.g., about a factor of 2 from 1 to 100 m or from 0.01 to 1 m height above the ground).

Significantly higher and lower values than found in Figure 1.8 have been found at other locations, e.g., averages of 28 Bq/m^3 in Grand Junction and 0.5–1 Bq/m^3

SEASONAL VARIATION

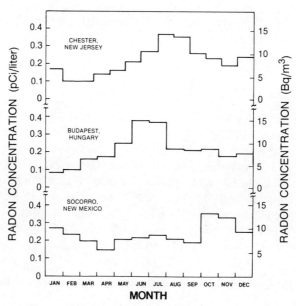

Figure 1.8. Year-long variability of atmospheric ^{222}Rn concentration. Measurements were performed 1 m above the ground in three different locations. Adapted from Ref. 62, Figure 1, by permission.

in Alaska; low values also occur in areas substantially influenced by marine air. Moreover, instantaneous values can also vary markedly from the averages. Gesell suggests that the mean value for the contiguous United States lies between 0.1 and 0.4 pCi/L (4–15 Bq/m^3), probably in the vicinity of 0.25 pCi/L (10 Bq/m^3). Data from other countries are similar.

Some information is also available on the decay products in outdoor air, where— because of the relative absence of surfaces (compared with indoors)—one might expect higher equilibrium ratios. For example, measurements in New York yielded ratios around 0.45 (with the uncombined fraction of ^{218}Po at 9%) at a rural location and 0.40 (uncombined fraction at 5%) on a city sidewalk (63). Subsequent measurements outside eight houses in New York and New Jersey gave mean equilibrium ratios averaging 0.79, considerably higher than the indoor ratios measured (5). More recent data (cf. Table 1.5) yield an equilibrium factor of 0.56 (64).

A ^{222}Rn concentration of 10 Bq/m^3, although completely negligible compared with the higher indoor values observed, is still significant compared with typical indoor concentrations. Therefore, the outdoor contribution has to be considered in making precise estimates of human exposures to ^{222}Rn decay products. It also has to be considered in examining the sources of radon found indoors: the approximately 10 Bq/m^3 coming in with outdoor air is approximately 20% of the average ^{222}Rn concentration observed in U.S. single-family homes and an even larger percentage of concentrations in other types of buildings.

8.4 Radon-220 and Its Decay Products

Our present understanding of the occurrence and behavior of ^{220}Rn and its decay products is very limited compared with our knowledge of the ^{222}Rn series. Not nearly as much effort has been devoted to ^{220}Rn characterization, because preliminary and modest evidence—both theoretical and experimental—suggests that airborne concentrations of ^{220}Rn and its decay products are not as important from a radiological point of view as their more common relatives. This occurs in spite of the fact that the ^{232}Th decay series, shown in Figure 1.9, has approximately the same (activity) concentration in the earth's crust as the ^{238}U series, about 25 Bq/kg (65, 66). (See also Chapter 2, Section 3.1.)

The differences have to do partly with the short half-life of ^{220}Rn, 1 min as compared with 4 d for ^{222}Rn, and partly with the details of radon and decay product behavior in the indoor or outdoor environment and inside the lung. The first factor sharply limits the time available for transport from the source material, so that only a small thickness of building material or soil serves as an effective source for ^{220}Rn entering the atmospheric environment, indoors or outdoors. The second affects the concentrations present in the air and the dose delivered by the decay products that deposit in the lung. The net result of all these factors is that—at least for indoor ^{222}Rn concentrations in the normal range—the ^{220}Rn decay products (in particular, ^{212}Pb) appear—on the basis of limited evidence—to have a potential alpha-energy concentration (PAEC) that is less than, but still significant, compared with that from the ^{222}Rn series. However, the PAEC itself does not reflect the

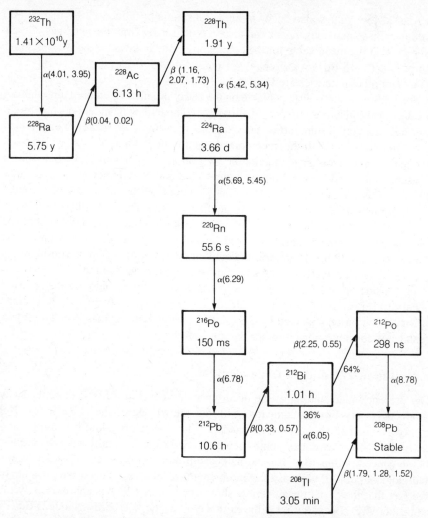

Figure 1.9. ^{232}Th decay chain, including ^{220}Rn and its decay products. Airborne concentrations of ^{212}Pb and ^{212}Bi are of prime radiological interest because of their potential for retention in the lung, leading to subsequent irradiation by the alpha decay of ^{212}Bi or ^{212}Po. Cf. Figure 1.2 for ^{238}U decay chain. Half-lives and alpha energies (in MeV) from Ref. 57; beta end-point energies (in MeV) from Ref. 83.

present understanding that a given amount of alpha energy from the ^{222}Rn series has substantially more biological impact than alpha energy from the ^{220}Rn series (cf. Chapter 7).

We consider first the concentrations expected if transport from the source to the air were dominated by diffusion for both these radon isotopes, as is likely to be the case outdoors. The depth of soil serving as a source is then indicated by the diffusion length, which is proportional to the square root of the half-life. The ratio of the ^{220}Rn to ^{222}Rn half-lives is $1/5940$ (i.e., 55.6 s$/3.82$ d), yielding $1/77$ as the diffusion length ratio. This indicates the relative depth cleared per characteristic time, which is given by the half-life itself. Since the activity concentration in the soil is similar for the ^{232}Th and ^{238}U series, the relative rate at which ^{220}Rn and ^{222}Rn activity escapes from the surface of the source material is the relative thickness cleared $(1/77)$ divided by the relative time scale $(1/5940)$, yielding a factor of 77. Thus, much more ^{220}Rn activity is expected to escape than ^{222}Rn activity! (However, because of the difference in half-lives, this greater activity is supported by only $1/77$th as many atoms.) In contrast, it is easy to show that—if the transport mechanism is pressure-driven flow of air through the source material and into the open air—the rate at which activity leaves the surface is the *same* for the two isotopes. (In this case, only $1/5940$th as many ^{220}Rn atoms escape.)

For a typical ventilation rate of 1 h^{-1}, the assumption of pure diffusion (with no barriers between the source and the air) can therefore be shown, using Equation 1, to imply about twice as much ^{220}Rn activity in indoor air as ^{222}Rn. As we shall see, the observed ratio is not usually this large. However, for outdoor air, the correspondence is reasonably good. For example, a review by Schery (64) of ^{220}Rn and its decay products indoors cites typical fluxes from open soil of 2 Bq m^{-2} s^{-1} for ^{220}Rn and 0.016 Bq m^{-2} s^{-1} for ^{222}Rn, a ratio that is only slightly larger than the factor of 77 suggested above. Based on a simple eddy diffusion model to represent the transport of radon upward into the atmosphere, he concludes that the concentrations of ^{220}Rn and ^{222}Rn 1 m above the ground ought to be 9 and 6 Bq/m^3, respectively, compared with his (limited) measurement results of 16 and 6 Bq/m^3, respectively. He notes that his tentative result of 4.6 nJ/m^3 for PAEC$_{212}$ (the PAEC from ^{212}Pb, the primary ^{220}Rn decay product: see Section 8.1 on quantities and units), versus 20 nJ/m^3 for PAEC$_{222}$ (the PAEC from the ^{222}Rn decay products), compare reasonably with more extensive measurements made in the Federal Republic of Germany (67). (These results imply an equilibrium factor for ^{220}Rn decay products that is extremely small—not surprising considering the relative half-lives of ^{220}Rn and ^{212}Pb—and an equilibrium factor for ^{222}Rn decay products greater than 0.5.)

The data on indoor concentrations are limited and more difficult to interpret. A number of workers cite results for the ratio of PAEC$_{220}$ to PAEC$_{222}$ centering around 0.5. See, for example, European data ranging from 0.3 to 0.8, summarized in Ref. 68 and North American results from Elliott Lake, Canada, of 0.3 (69) and for the United States of 0.6 (70). These results indicate the potential significance of the ^{220}Rn series indoors. However, our understanding of the factors affecting the ^{220}Rn concentrations, both absolutely and relative to ^{222}Rn, is tentative at best.

For example, if entry of both radon isotopes is diffusion-dominated, as has been supposed in some classes of European housing (particularly apartment structures), and concentrations in the source materials are similar, then indoor radon concentrations ought to be similar for the two isotopes (as noted earlier), the activity concentration of the decay products ought to be a factor of 5 or so less for ^{220}Rn than for ^{222}Rn (because the long half-life of ^{212}Pb causes most of it to be removed by ventilation or deposition rather than by decay), and the PAEC$_{220}$ ought to be greater than the $PAEC_{222}$ by a modest factor, e.g., 2 or 3. Even in European housing the ratio is closer to 0.5, suggesting significant differences in the source concentrations or generation parameters for the two isotopes, barriers to the presumed diffusion process, other mechanisms for radon entry, or unaccounted-for differences in the decay-product behavior.

One difficulty is obvious; i.e., at the concentrations typical of European apartment structures, the ^{222}Rn entering the indoor air from structural materials can almost be equaled by that entering from the outdoor air. In contrast, the ^{220}Rn half-life is so short compared with ventilation time constants that no comparable contribution arises for this isotope.

Another factor to be considered is the more interesting one that pressure-driven flow has been shown to be the dominant contributor to indoor ^{222}Rn for many types of structures and may also be significant for ^{220}Rn. For homes such as those that dominate the U.S. housing stock, little diffusion from the floor and wall material is expected in any case (because of the use of wood and the painting of other types of materials), so that some other entry route is likely to dominate observed concentrations of the ^{220}Rn series. As indicated above, comparable concentrations in the source materials would imply similar activity entry rates for a pure flow process. Because of the relative size of decay rates and typical ventilation rates, this would imply ^{220}Rn concentrations only about 2% of ^{222}Rn concentrations (and, using the same argument as above) a similar ratio of PAECs. Thus, the concentration ratios expected differ by about two orders of magnitude, depending on whether diffusion or flow is the presumed mechanism, and the actual observation—in both European and American housing—lies approximately at the geometric mean. This suggests the dominance of different entry mechanisms for the two isotopes or a combination of diffusion and flow applying to both, a possibility that was indicated in the early work on pressure-driven flow (27).

However, the measurements of Schery in U.S. buildings (70) also afford the possibility for an interesting comparison, indicated in Table 1.5. There are indicated the results of outdoor measurements cited above, as well as the average indoor $PAEC_{212}$ and $PAEC_{222}$ from Schery's 68 measurements in buildings in 21 states. The detailed data show a significant correlation between these two parameters (in contrast to the work of Ref. 69), suggesting the possibility of common

TABLE 1.5   Comparative Concentrations of ^{220}Rn and ^{222}Rn and Their Decay Products[a]

	Outdoor (1 m height)		Indoor	
	Rn (Bq/m³)	PAEC (nJ/m³)	Rn (Bq/m³)	PAEC (nJ/m³)
^{220}Rn Series	16	5[b]	3–4[c]	21[b]
^{222}Rn Series	6	20	15–20[d]	44

[a] Based on Refs. 64, 70.
[b] These are only the PAECs for ^{212}Pb, the dominant contributor of the ^{220}Rn decay products.
[c] Estimated from Fig. 3 in Ref. 70.
[d] Estimated from PAEC (44 nJ/m³) assuming an equilibrium factor of 0.4–0.5.

entry mechanisms (or, of course, common removal mechanisms). Also shown are estimates of the indoor radon concentrations, based on the $PAEC_{222}$ for ^{222}Rn and on one of Schery's illustrations for the ^{220}Rn. These concentrations are in good agreement with his average $^{220}Rn/^{222}Rn$ ratio of 0.23, which is—consistent with the comments above—at the (geometric) midpoint between the expectations for purely diffusion and purely flow entry mechanisms.

However, the ^{222}Rn concentration estimate is considerably less than the average concentration in U.S. single-family homes suggested on the basis of the studies discussed in the body of this chapter, i.e., 55 Bq/m^3. This estimate may be so low because the equilibrium factor during Schery's measurements was considerably lower than the 0.4–0.5 assumed in converting his mean $PAEC_{222}$ to a ^{222}Rn concentration (cf. Table 1.4). A mean equilibrium factor of 0.15 (S. D. Schery, personal communication) for these measurements yields, instead of 15–20 Bq/m^3, an estimated mean ^{222}Rn concentration near 50 Bq/m^3, consistent with other results from the United States. We are then left with the puzzle as to why the equilibrium factor for the ^{222}Rn decay products was so low compared with means found in other studies.

Furthermore, it is interesting to note the relative sizes of the PAECs cited in the table. The indoor $PAEC_{222}$ is clearly the largest, and the indoor $PAEC_{212}$ is comparable to the *outdoor* $PAEC_{222}$. Since—as noted in Ref. 64 and discussed more thoroughly in Chapter 7—a given PAEC from the ^{220}Rn series is thought to have much less significance than a comparable PAEC from the ^{222}Rn decay products, it appears that indoor concentrations of the 220 series are less significant even than outdoor radon concentrations. Nonetheless, the possible health significance is not to be ignored, and, indeed, understanding better the behavior of the ^{220}Rn series presents not only an interesting scientific problem, but even a tool by which to explore more fully the mechanisms for transport of the radon isotopes into the indoor environment.

REFERENCES

1. Girman, J. R., Apte, M. G., Traynor, G. W., Allen, J. R., and Hollowell, C. D. (1982). Pollutant emission rates from indoor combustion appliances and sidestream cigarette smoke, *Environ. Int.*, **8**, 213.

2. Spengler, J. D., and Sexton, K. (1983). Indoor air pollution: A public health perspective, *Science*, **221**, 9.

3. Miksch, R. R., Hollowell, C. D., and Schmidt, H. E. (1982). Trace organic chemical contaminants in office spaces, *Environ. Int.*, **8**, 129.

4. McCann, J., Horn, L., Girman, J. R., and Nero, A. V. Potential risks from exposure to organic carcinogens in indoor air. In Sanbhu, S. S., de Marini, D. M., Mass, M. J., Moore, M. M., and Mumford, J. S. (eds.), *Short-Term Bioassays in the Analysis of Complex Environmental Mixtures*, Plenum, New York, in press.

5. George, A. C., and Breslin, A. J. (1980). The distribution of ambient radon and radon

daughters in residential buildings in the New Jersey–New York area. In Gesell, T. F., and Lowder, W. M. (eds.), *Natural Radiation Environment III*, Tech. Info. Ctr/DOE CONF-780422, Springfield, VA, p. 1272.

6. Nazaroff, W. W., Boegel, M. L., Hollowell, C. D., and Roseme, G. D. (1981). The use of mechanical ventilation with heat recovery for controlling radon and radon-daughter concentrations in houses, *Atmos. Environ.*, **15**, 263.

7. Nero, A. V., Berk, J. V., Boegel, M. L., Hollowell, C. D., Ingersoll, J. G., and Nazaroff, W. W. (1983). Radon concentrations and infiltration rates measured in conventional and energy-efficient houses, *Health Phys.*, **45**, 401.

8. Alter, H. W., and Fleischer, R. L. (1981). Passive integrating radon monitor for environmental monitoring, *Health Phys.*, **40**, 693.

9. Cohen, B. L., and Cohen, E. S. (1983). Theory and practice of radon monitoring with charcoal adsorption, *Health Phys.*, **45**, 501.

10. Nero, A. V., Schwehr, M. B., Nazaroff, W. W., and Revzan, K. L. (1986). Distribution of airborne radon-222 concentrations in U.S. homes, *Science*, **234**, 992.

11. Cohen, B. L. (1986). A national survey of ^{222}Rn in U.S. homes and correlating factors, *Health Phys.*, **51**, 175.

12. Turk, B. H., Prill, R. J., Fisk, W. J., Grimsrud, D. T., Moed, B. A., and Sextro, R. G. (1986). Radon and remedial action in Spokane River Valley residences: An interim report, report LBL-21399, Lawrence Berkeley Laboratory, Berkeley, CA.

13. Sachs, H. M., Hernandez, T. L., and Ring, J. W. (1982). Regional geology and radon variability in buildings, *Environ. Int.*, **8**, 97.

14. McGregor, R. G., Vasudev, P., Létourneau, E. G., McCullough, R. S., Prantl, F. A., and Taniguchi, H. (1980). Background concentrations of radon and radon daughters in Canadian homes, *Health Phys.*, **39**, 285.

15. Swedjemark, G. A., and Mjönes, L. (1984). Radon and radon daughter concentrations in Swedish homes, *Radiat. Prot. Dosim.*, **7**, 341.

16. Swedjemark, G. A., and Mjönes, L. (1984). Exposure of the Swedish population to radon daughters. In Berglund, B., Lindvall, T., and Sundell, J. (eds.), *Indoor Air: Radon, Passive Smoking, Particulates and Housing Epidemiology*, Vol. 2, Swedish Council for Building Research, Stockholm, p. 37.

17. Castrén, O., Winqvist, K., Mäkeläinen, I., and Voutilainen, A. (1984). Radon measurements in Finnish houses, *Radiat. Prot. Dosim.*, **7**, 333.

18. Sørensen, A., Bøtter-Jensen, L., Majborn, B., and Nielsen, S. P. (1985). A pilot study of natural radiation in Danish homes, *Sci. Total Environ.*, **45**, 351.

19. Schmeir, H., and Wicke, A. (1985). Results from a survey of indoor radon exposures in the Federal Republic of Germany, *Sci. Total Environ.*, **45**, 307.

20. Keller, G., and Folkerts, K. H. (1984). A study on indoor radon. In Berglund, B., Lindvall, T., and Sundell, J. (eds.), *Indoor Air: Radon, Passive Smoking, Particulates and Housing Epidemiology*, Vol. 2, Swedish Council for Building Research, Stockholm, p. 149.

21. Green, B. M. R., Brown, L., Cliff, K. D., Driscoll, C. M. H., Miles, J. C., and Wrixon, A. D. (1985). Surveys of natural radiation exposure in UK dwellings with passive and active measurement techniques, *Sci. Total Environ.*, **45**, 459.

22. Put, L. W., and de Meijer, R. J. (1984). Survey of radon concentrations in Dutch dwellings. In Berglund, B., Lindvall, T., and Sundell, J. (eds.), *Indoor Air: Radon,*

Passive Smoking, Particulates and Housing Epidemiology, Vol. 2, Swedish Council for Building Research, Stockholm, p. 49.

23. Castrén, O., Voutilainen, A., Winqvist, K., and Mäkeläinen, I. (1985). Studies of high indoor radon areas in Finland, *Sci. Total Environ.*, **45**, 311.

24. Cohen, B. L., Kulwicki, D. R., Warner, K. R., Jr., and Grassi, C. L. (1984). Radon concentrations inside public and commercial buildings in the Pittsburgh area, *Health Phys.*, **47**, 399.

25. Turk, B. H., Brown, J. T., Geisling-Sobotka, K., Grimsrud, D. T., Harrison, J., Koonce, J. F., and Revzan, K. L. (1986). Indoor air quality and ventilation measurements in 38 Pacific Northwest commercial buildings, report LBL-21453, Lawrence Berkeley Laboratory, Berkeley, CA.

26. Spitz, H. B., Wrenn, M. E., and Cohen, N. (1980). Diurnal variation of radon measured indoors and outdoors in Grand Junction, Colorado and Teaneck, New Jersey and the influence that ventilation has upon the buildup of radon daughters. In Gesell, T. F., and Lowder, W. M. (eds.), *Natural Radiation Environment III*, US Dept. of Energy, CONF-780422, Springfield, VA, p. 1308.

27. Nazaroff, W. W., Feustel, H., Nero, A. V., Revzan, K. L., Grimsrud, D. T., Essling, M. A., and Toohey, R. E. (1985). Radon transport into a detached one-story house with a basement, *Atmos. Environ.*, **19**, 31.

28. Hildingson, O. (1982). Radon measurements in 12,000 Swedish homes, *Environ. Int.*, **8**, 67.

29. Ingersoll, J. G. (1983). A survey of radionuclide contents and radon emanation rates in building materials used in the U.S., *Health Phys.*, **45**, 363.

30. Wilkening, M. H., Clements, W. E., and Stanley, D. (1972). Radon-222 flux measurements in widely separated regions. In Adams, J. A. S., Lowder, W. M., and Gesell, T. F. (eds.), *Natural Radiation Environment II*, Conf-720805, National Technical Information Service, Springfield, VA, p. 717.

31. Nero, A. V., and Nazaroff, W. W. (1984). Characterising the source of radon indoors, *Radiat. Prot. Dosim.*, **7**, 23.

32. DSMA Atcon Ltd. (1983). Review of existing instrumentation and evaluation of possibilities for research and development of instrumentation to determine future levels of radon at a proposed building site, report INFO-0096, Atomic Energy Control Board, Ottawa, Canada.

33. Nazaroff, W. W., Lewis, S. R., Doyle, S. M., Moed, B. A., and Nero, A. V. (1987). Experiments on pollutant transport from soil into residential basements by pressure-driven air flow, *Environ. Sci. Technol.*, **21**, 459.

34. Henschel, D. B., and Scott, A. G. (1986). The EPA program to demonstrate mitigation measures for indoor radon: Initial results. In *Indoor Radon*, Proc. APCA Int. Specialty Conf., Philadelphia, Air Pollution Control Association, Pittsburgh, PA.

35. Nazaroff, W. W., and Doyle, S. M. (1985). Radon entry into houses having a crawl space, *Health Phys.*, **48**, 265.

36. Hess, C. T., Weiffenbach, C. V., and Norton, S. A. (1983). Environmental radon and cancer correlations in Maine, *Health Phys.*, **45**, 339.

37. Horton, T. R. (1985). Nationwide occurrence of radon and other natural radioactivity in public water supplies, report EPA 520/5-85-008, U.S. Environmental Protection Agency, Eastern Environmental Radiation Facility, Montgomery, AL.

38. Gesell, T. F. (1973). Some radiological aspects of radon-222 in liquified petroleum gas. In Stanley, R. E., and Moghissi, A. A. (eds.), *Noble Gases*, U.S. Energy Research & Dev. Admin., CONF-730915, Las Vegas, NV, p. 612.

39. Johnson, R. H., Bernhardt, D. E., Nelson, N. S., and Galley, H. W. (1973). Radiological health significance of radon in natural gas. In Stanley, R. E., and Moghissi, A. A. (eds.), *Noble Gases*, U.S. Energy Research & Dev. Admin., CONF-730915, Las Vegas, NV, p. 532.

40. Jacobi, W. (1972). Activity and potential alpha energy of radon 222 and radon 220 daughters in different air atmospheres, *Health Phys.*, **22**, 441.

41. Bruno, R. C. (1983). Verifying a model of radon decay product behavior indoors, *Health Phys.*, **45**, 471.

42. Porstendörfer, J. (1984). Behaviour of radon daughter products in indoor air, *Radiat. Prot. Dosim.*, **7**, 107.

43. Offermann, F. J., Sextro, R. G., Fisk, W. J., Nazaroff, W. W., Nero, A. V., Revzan, K. L., and Yater, J. (1984). Control of respirable particles and radon progeny with portable air cleaners, report LBL-16659, Lawrence Berkeley Laboratory, Berkeley, CA.

44. George, A. C., Knutson, E. O., and Tu, K. W. (1983). Radon daughter plateout—I. Measurements, *Health Phys*, **45**, 439.

45. Knutson, E. O., George, A. C., Frey, J. J., and Koh, B. R. (1983). Radon daughter plateout—II. Prediction model, *Health Phys.*, **45**, 445.

46. Busigin, A., van der Vooren, A. W., Babcock, J. C., and Phillips, C. R. (1981). The nature of unattached RaA (^{218}Po) particles, *Health Phys.*, **40**, 333.

47. Knutson, E. O., George, A. C., Knuth, R. H., and Koh, B. R. (1984). Measurements of radon daughter particle size, *Ratiat. Prot. Dosim.*, **7**, 121.

48. Jonassen, N. (1984). Removal of radon daughters by filtration and electric fields, *Radiat. Prot. Dosim.*, **7**, 407.

49. James, A. C. (1984). Dosimetric approaches to risk assessment for indoor exposure to radon daughters, *Radiat. Prot. Dosim.*, **7**, 353.

50. Schiller, G. A., Nero, A. V., Revzan, K. L., and Tien, C. L. (1984). Radon decay-product behavior indoors: Numerical modeling of convection effects, Report LBL-17609, Lawrence Berkeley Laboratory, Berkeley, CA.

51. Evaluation of occupational and environmental exposures to radon and radon daughters in the United States (1984). Report No. 78, National Council on Radiation Protection and Measurements, Bethesda, MD.

52. Harley, N. H. (1984). Comparing radon daughter dose: Environmental versus underground exposure, *Radiat. Prot. Dosim.*, **7**, 371.

53. Jacobi, W. (1984). Possible lung cancer risk from indoor exposure to radon daughters, *Radiat. Prot. Dosim.*, **7**, 395.

54. Ellett, W. H. (1985). Epidemiology and risk assessment: Testing models for radon-induced lung cancer. In Gammage, R. B., and Kay, S. V. (eds.), *Indoor Air and Human Health*, Lewis Publishers, Chelsea, MI, p. 102.

55. Budnitz, R. J. (1974). Radon-222 and its daughters—A review of instrumentation for occupational and environmental monitoring, *Health Phys.*, **26**, 145.

56. George, A. C. (1980). Radon and radon daughter field measurements. In Proc. Seminar

on Traceability for Ionizing Radiation Measurements, National Bureau of Standards, Washington, DC.

57. Browne, E., and Firestone, R. B. (1986). *Table of Radioactive Isotopes* (V. S. Shirley, ed.), Wiley-Interscience, New York.

58. Dietz, R. N., and Cote, E. A. (1982). Air infiltration measurements in a home using a convenient perfluorocarbon tracer technique, *Environ. Int.*, **8**, 419.

59. Grot, R. A., and Clark, R. E. (1981). Air leakage characteristics and weatherization techniques for low-income housing. In Thermal performance of the exterior envelopes of buildings, report ASHRAE SP28, American Society of Heating, Refrigerating and Air Conditioning Engineers, New York.

60. Liddament, M., and Allen, C. (1983). The validation and comparison of mathematical models of air infiltration, technical note AIC 11, Air Infiltration Centre, Bracknell, Great Britain.

61. Grimsrud, D. T., Modera, M. P., and Sherman, M. H. (1982). A predictive air infiltration model—long-term field test validation, *ASHRAE Trans.*, **88**, 1351.

62. Gesell, T. F. (1983). Background atmospheric ^{222}Rn concentrations outdoors and indoors: A review, *Health Phys.*, **45**, 289.

63. George, A. C. (1972). Indoor and outdoor measurements of natural radon and radon decay products in New York City air. In Adams, J. A. S., Lowder, W. M., and Gesell, T. F. (eds.), *Natural Radiation Environment II*, CONF-720805, National Technical Information Service, Springfield, VA, p. 741.

64. Schery, S. D. (1986). Studies of thoron and thoron progeny: indications for transport of radioactivity from soil to indoor air. In *Indoor Radon*, Proc. APCA Int. Specialty Conf., Philadelphia, Air Pollution Control Association, Pittsburgh, PA.

65. Nero, A. V. (1983). Airborne radionuclides and radiation in buildings: A review, *Health Phys.*, **45**, 303.

66. United Nations Scientific Committee on the Effects of Atomic Radiation (1982). Ionizing radiation: Sources and biological effects, United Nations, New York.

67. Keller, G., Folkerts, K. H., and Muth, H. (1982). Activity concentrations of 222-Rn, 220-Rn, and their decay products in German dwellings, dose calculations and estimate of risk, *Radiat. Environ. Biophys.*, **7**, 263, cited in Ref. 64.

68. Tóth, Á. (1984). A simple field method for determination of ^{220}Rn and ^{222}Rn daughter energy concentrations in room air, *Radiat. Prot. Dosim.*, **7**, 247.

69. Gunning, C., and Scott, A. G. (1982). Radon and thoron daughters in housing, *Health Phys.*, **42**, 527.

70. Schery, S. D. (1985). Measurements of airborne ^{212}Pb and ^{220}Rn concentrations at varied indoor locations within the United States, *Health Phys.*, **49**, 1061.

71. Smith, D. (1979). Ventilation rates and their influence on equilibrium factor, in Second Workshop on Radon and Radon Daughters in Urban Communities Associated with Uranium Mining and Processing, Atomic Energy Control Board, Ottawa.

72. Doyle, S. M., Nazaroff, W. W., and Nero, A. V. (1984). Time-averaged indoor radon concentrations and infiltration rates sampled in four U.S. cities, *Health Phys.*, **47**, 579.

73. Nazaroff, W. W., Boegel, M. L., and Nero, A. V. (1983). Measuring radon source magnitude in residential buildings. In Proc. International Meeting on Radon-Radon Progeny Measurements, report EPA 520/5-83/021, U.S. Environmental Protection Agency, Washington, DC, p. 101.

74. Nazaroff, W. W., Offermann, F. J., and Robb, A. W. (1983). Automated system for measuring air-exchange rate and radon concentration in houses, *Health Phys.*, **45**, 525.

75. Cliff, K. D. (1978). Assessment of airborne radon daughter concentrations in dwellings in Great Britain, *Phys. Med. Biol.*, **23**, 696.

76. Wicke, A. (1979). Untersuchungen zur Frage der Naturlichen Radioktivitat der Luft in Wohn- und Aufenthaltstraumen, Ph.D. thesis, Justus Liebig Universitat, Giessen.

77. Nazaroff, W. W., and Nero, A.V. (1984). Transport of radon from soil into residences. In Berglund, B., Lindvall, T., and Sundell, J. (eds.), *Indoor Air: Radon, Passive Smoking, Particulates and Housing Epidemiology*, Vol. 2, Swedish Council for Building Research, Stockholm, p. 15.

78. *Indoor Pollutants* (1981). National Academy of Sciences, Washington, DC.

79. Poffijn, A., Marijns, R., Vanmarcke, H., and Uyttenhuve, J. (1985). Results of a preliminary survey on radon in Belgium, *Sci. Total Environ.*, **45**, 335.

80. Rannou, A., Madelmont, C., and Renouard, H. (1985). Survey of natural radiation in France, *Sci. Total Environ.*, **45**, 467.

81. McAulay, I. R., and McLaughlin, J. P. (1985). Indoor radiation levels in Ireland, *Sci. Total Environ.*, **45**, 319.

82. Aoyama, T., Yonehara, H., Sakanoue, M., Kobayashi, S., Iwasaki, T., Mifune, M., Radford, E. P., and Kato, H. (1987). Long-term measurements of radon concentrations in the living environments in Japan: A preliminary report. In P. K. Hopke (ed.), *Radon and Its Decay Products: Occurrence, Properties, and Health Effects*, ACS Symposium Series 331, American Chemical Society, Washington, DC, p. 124.

83. National Council on Radiation Protection and Measurements (1985). *A Handbook of Radioactivity Measurement Procedures*, 2nd ed. Report No. 58, National Council on Radiation Protection and Measurements, Bethesda, MD.

84. Lederer, C. M., and Shirley, V. S. (1978). *Table of Isotopes*, 7th ed., Wiley-Interscience, New York.

85. Alter, H. W., and Oswald, R. A. (1987). Nationwide distribution of indoor radon concentrations: A preliminary data base, *J. Air Pollution Control Ass.* **37**, 227.

86. New York State Energy Research and Development Authority (1986). News release of December 4, NYSERDA, Albany, NY.

87. Nero, A. V., Revzan, K. L., and Sextro, R. G. (1987). Appraisal of the U.S. data on indoor radon concentrations. In Proc. of Fourth International Symposium on the Natural Radiation Environment, Lisbon, Dec. 7–11, 1987 (and to be published *Radiation Protection Dosimetry*).

88. Sextro, R. G., Harrison, J., Moed, B.A., Revzan, K. L., Turk, B. H., et al. (1987). An intensive study of radon and remedial measures in New Jersey homes: preliminary results. In Fourth Int. Conference on Indoor Air Quality and Climate, Berlin, Aug. 17–21, 1987.

89. Mowris, R. J., and Fisk, W. J. (1987). Modeling the effects of exhaust ventilation on radon entry rates and indoor radon concentrations, Lawrence Berkeley Laboratory report LBL-22939, Berkely, CA (submitted to *Health Physics*).

90. Loureiro, C. de O. (1987). *Simulation of the Steady-State Transport of Radon from Soil into Houses with Basements Under Constant Negative Pressure*. Ph.D. Dissertation, Environmental Health Sciences, Univ. of Michigan, Ann Arbor, MI.

91. Steck, D. J. (1987). Geological variation of radon sources and indoor radon along the southwestern edge of the Canadian shield. In Fourth Int. Conference on Indoor Air Quality and Climate, Berlin, Aug. 17–21, 1987.

92. Revzan, K. L. and Nero, A. V. (1987). Mapping surficial radium content of U. S. soil as a partial indicator of indoor radon concentrations. In Fourth Int. Symposium on Natural Radiation Environment, Lisbon, Dec. 7–11, 1987.

PART ONE

SOURCES AND TRANSPORT PROCESSES

▬ 2

Soil as a Source of Indoor Radon: Generation, Migration, and Entry

WILLIAM W. NAZAROFF

Environmental Engineering Science, California Institute of Technology, Pasadena, California

Indoor Environment Program, Lawrence Berkeley Laboratory, University of California, Berkeley, California

BARBARA A. MOED and RICHARD G. SEXTRO

Indoor Environment Program, Lawrence Berkeley Laboratory, University of California, Berkeley, California

1 INTRODUCTION

Soil and rock are the source of most radon to which people are exposed. In fact, the only other sources of significance are building materials, and even these generate radon because of radium that originated in the earth (or to a small degree from predecessor radioisotopes that originated in the earth themselves). In discussing radon sources, then, it is common and convenient to distinguish not only among the materials that contain the radium that leads to indoor radon, but also among the agents and pathways by which radon enters. When we speak of soil as the source of indoor radon, we implicitly mean that portion of the total indoor radon concentration which originates in the earthen material underlying the structure and moves directly through the building substructure and into the indoor air. That movement is generally restricted to distances of several meters or less and must occur within several half-lives of radon, i.e., within a few weeks.

The other agents by which radon generated in the soil may enter indoor air are potable water (discussed in Chapter 4) and outdoor air and natural gas (discussed in Chapter 1). For countries in which high indoor radon levels are common, including Canada, the United States, and Sweden, there is growing evidence that the source of most radon at levels of concern in indoor air is the underlying soil from which radon directly enters the building substructure by a combination of convective and diffusive transport. Such evidence may be grouped into three categories: (i) efforts to account for indoor radon concentrations by balancing rates of entry and removal (1, 2), (ii) remedial measures taken to lower high indoor radon concentrations (3–5), and (iii) theoretical studies of radon migration from soil into buildings (6, 7).

An understanding of the sources and transport processes accounting for radon in indoor air is of considerable importance. Radon levels may be unacceptably high in a substantial proportion of the housing stock in developed countries. In the United States, for example, it has been estimated that one to four million homes have radon concentrations exceeding recently recommended guidelines (8). Furthermore, of the two major factors that determine indoor concentrations—the radon entry rate and the ventilation rate—the entry rate appears to be more variable and hence the more important factor in determining which houses have high levels. Thus, identifying houses with high levels, designing optimal control measures, and predicting the impact of changes in building construction practice on indoor radon concentrations—all depend on knowledge of radon sources.

This chapter is concerned extensively with the transport mechanisms by which radon migrates in soil air and through building substructures. The discussion necessitates a summary of some important characteristics of soil: grain size, permeability, porosity, and moisture content. The mechanisms of radon generation in soil and entry into soil pore space are described. Then some relevant features of building construction and operation that relate to radon entry are discussed. Of particular importance are substructure design, the location and size of substructure penetrations, and operations, such as the use of a fireplace, that may lead to a lowering of the pressure in the structure relative to the outdoors. The physics of radon migration in soil is discussed, including the mechanisms that generate pressure gradients in the soil and lead to convective transport of radon. The relationship between indoor radon concentration and air-exchange rate is explored. Understanding this relationship is necessary to properly interpret the results of field measurements and to accurately predict the effect of changes in building operation on the indoor concentration. The final section illustrates one application of a detailed understanding of soil as a source of indoor radon: identification of areas for which high indoor radon concentrations are likely on the basis of geological and geographical data collected for other purposes.

The focus of the present discussion is on the most abundant radon isotope, ^{222}Rn, and on the building practices used for single-family dwellings in the United States. Thoron (^{220}Rn), the other radon isotope of some importance, is discussed to a lesser degree. Although on average it is generated at the same rate in soil as ^{222}Rn, its much shorter half-life leads to a much shorter transport range and generally lower concentrations indoors. The discussion is, for the most part, sufficiently general that the extension to other building types follows once the key building characteristics are identified. Control techniques for preventing the direct entry of radon from soil are discussed extensively in Chapter 10 and consequently are not treated here.

A schematic representation of the key elements of soil as a source of indoor radon is presented in Figure 2.1. It is useful to distinguish two main concepts.

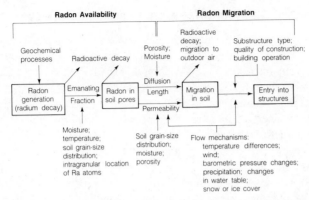

Figure 2.1. Schematic representation of radon production and migration in soil and its entry into buildings.

"Radon availability" identifies the factors that influence the concentration of radon in soil air in the absence of structures. These parameters determine the source potential of the soil. "Radon migration" groups the factors that determine the movement of radon from the soil air into buildings. This element depends on both soil and building-related factors. Both concepts contribute to the process by which soil serves as a source of indoor radon. They combine in a manner that is roughly multiplicative: soil is a small source of indoor radon if either the rate of generation of radon in the soil pores or the rate of transport of radon from the soil into the building is small.

In Figure 2.1, the boxes represent the major states of radon from its generation in soil to its entry into a building; labels on horizontal arrows indicate a characteristic of the soil that is a measure of how readily radon moves from one state to the next; labels on vertical arrows indicate parameters and processes that significantly influence the rate or transition from one state to another. Labels on diagonal arrows indicate paths by which radon generated in soil may fail to enter a building. Among many features of this representation, one may note that moisture plays a role at several steps in the process.

2 PHYSICAL CHARACTERISTICS OF SOIL

As might be expected, the physical characteristics of a soil play key roles in determining the radon concentration in nearby buildings. Many of these characteristics have been widely investigated for other purposes by civil engineers (9, 10), agronomists (11), petroleum engineers (12–14), and groundwater hydrodynamicists. Consequently, it is instructive to briefly review the information from these fields that is relevant to indoor radon. Important factors relating to radon production in soil are outside the scope of these fields and are discussed in Section 3.

2.1   Grain-Size Distribution, Porosity, and Moisture Content

Soils have two major volume fractions. The solid fraction consists mainly of mineral grains of a wide range of sizes, and also includes a small amount of organic matter. The void fraction consists of liquid, usually water, and gas. The gas is generally similar in composition to air. The void fraction is also known as the soil porosity, and the volume fraction of water is often called the moisture content. A soil is saturated when the moisture content equals the porosity.

Soils are classified according to the size distribution of the solid grains, with the major divisions being clay, silt, and sand. Characteristic particle sizes for each class are given in Table 2.1. Grains larger than sand and up to 15 cm in diameter are classified as gravel. In contrast to the larger particles, which are formed by mechanical weathering, clays are formed by chemical processes. Because of their small size and active surfaces, they may interact in a complex manner with other grains and with water. Consequently, they exhibit macroscopic properties, particularly sorption of radioisotopes and interaction with water, that are quite different than those of silts and sands.

Apart from this distinction in the formation process between clays and other soil types, the physical characteristics of soil pertaining to fluid flow vary widely with grain size distribution. However, attempts to predict these characteristics for a particular soil on the basis of grain size distribution have not been very successful. Discussions of such efforts may be found in the literature (12–15). Here, we present some representative data and simple analytical results as a basis for making numerical estimates of radon migration rates through soil.

Soil porosities are commonly in the vicinity of 0.5. By comparison, uniformly sized spheres have a porosity between 0.26 (close packing) and 0.48 (open packing). Because of the greater tendency for small particles to "bridge," clays tend to have higher porosities than sands. Poorly sorted soils, that is, having a wide range of grain sizes, may have porosities of 0.3 or less.

The pore space within soils may be thought of, paradoxically, as both continuous and discrete: large pores are connected by narrower channels. The pore space has two major components: the "textural" pore space, always present, which results from the random packing of the soil particles; and "structural" pore space, present only in well-aggregated soils, which exists between the soil aggregates. Transient aggregates may form owing to cracking upon drying in soils containing a high percentage of clay-sized particles. Long-lived aggregates, which withstand

TABLE 2.1   Representative Values of Physical Characteristics of Soil

Type	Grain size (μm)	Porosity	Field capacity, saturation (%)[a]	Wilting point, saturation (%)[a]
Sand	60–2000	0.4	15	5
Silt	2–60	0.5	58	10
Clay	<2	0.6	68	48

[a]A saturation of 100% means that the entire pore volume is filled with water.
Source: Ref. 17.

wetting cycles, tend to form in soils containing much colloidal and organic material (16).

The moisture content of a soil not only depends on the grain-size distribution, but may be highly variable over time. A variety of physical effects control the migration of liquid water in the soil pores. These forces form the basis for distinguishing among the components of the liquid phase (11). For our purposes, a classification system with three categories is most useful. The "hygroscopic" component of soil water is adsorbed on the grain surfaces by local electrostatic forces. This component is the most tightly bound and may be retained for relatively long time periods even when the soil is otherwise dry. It is particularly important in clays owing to the small grain size, the polar nature of water molecules, and the crystalline structure of the clay particles. The "capillary" component of soil water is held in small pores and in a film around the particles by surface tension. The most variable component is termed "gravitational" water—that contained in the large pores—which is free to move under the influence of gravity.

Some understanding of the magnitude of these components for different soil types may be gained from the parameters "field capacity" and "wilting point" (17). The field capacity refers to the volume fraction of water in soil after it has been thoroughly wetted, then drained for about 2 days. The wilting point refers to the moisture content at which test plants growing on the soil wilt and do not recover if their leaves are kept in a humid atmosphere overnight. These can be expressed in terms of the saturation percent or volume percent, determined with respect to the pore volume or total volume, respectively. As with porosity, both parameters increase with decreasing particle size. Typical values for the field capacity and for the wilting point are presented in Table 2.1.

Moisture content is a very important factor for radon emanation and migration in soil. For a well-drained soil, the void volume contains water in the smaller pores and air in the larger pores. As discussed in Section 3.2, the capillary water increases the radon emanation fraction by absorbing the recoil energy of the newly formed atom. However, this water does not increase the resistance of the soil to airflow to a great degree since it is the larger pores that make the dominant contribution.

2.2 Permeability

One of the most important physical characteristics of soil pertinent to indoor radon is its permeability, i.e., how readily a fluid—in this case air—may flow through it. Permeability relates the apparent velocity of fluid flow through the soil pores to the pressure gradient. This relationship, described by Darcy's law, is discussed in detail in Section 5.2. Here, our attention is focused on the range of values of soil permeability and the factors that may affect it.

The importance of soil permeability in the study of indoor radon arises from the very broad range of values it assumes: as shown in Figure 2.2, the permeability of common soils in the absence of structural pores may span more than 10 orders of magnitude. We shall see that at the lower end of this range, molecular diffusion

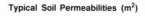

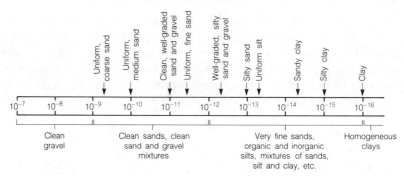

Figure 2.2. Permeability (m²) of representative soil types. Data from Terzaghi, K., and Peck, R. B. (1967). *Soil Mechanics in Engineering Practice,* 2nd ed., Wiley, New York; Tuma, J. J., and Abdel-Hady, M. (1973). *Engineering Soil Mechanics,* Prentice-Hall, Englewood Cliffs, NJ, p. 102.

becomes the dominant process by which radon migrates through soil near build-ings. At the upper end of this range, convective flow is the dominant radon trans-port mechanism. Since the convective flow rate increases with increasing perme-ability, and since the radon entry rate increases with convective flow of soil air into the substructure, the potential for radon entry is expected to increase mono-tonically with permeability for large grained soils. The actual entry rates are influ-enced by the characteristics of the building shell and the building operation.

Conceptually, permeability is based on the macroscopic properties of soil, i.e., the bulk volume flux of a fluid for a given pressure differential. This bulk property clearly depends on the microscopic characteristics of the soil: the size, shape, number, and orientation of pores, in particular, and the moisture content. Larger-grained soils generally have higher permeabilities: their pores are larger, and con-sequently the frictional resistance to fluid flow at the surface of the grains is of lesser importance than it is in fine-grained soils. Beyond this qualitative under-standing, there has been considerable research toward establishing relationships between physical parameters of a porous medium and its permeability. The ap-proaches have included empirical correlations, simplified physical modeling, and statistical theories. As discussed by Scheidegger (12), probably the most widely accepted approach to linking geometrical properties of a porous medium with its permeability was first developed by Kozeny. His approach was to solve the Navier-Stokes equation, which describes the momentum balance in a fluid, for an assem-blage of channels of various cross-sections, but of constant length. When the re-sulting flow is compared with Darcy's law, the following expression for permea-bility is obtained:

$$k = \frac{c\epsilon^3}{TS^2} \qquad (1)$$

where c is a constant that depends on the pore shape and, theoretically, varies between 0.5 and 0.67; ϵ is the porosity; T is the tortuosity, an empirical factor greater than or equal to 1.0 that accounts for the fact that the flow channels are not straight; and S is the specific surface area. For uniform, spherical particles

$$S = \frac{6(1 - \epsilon)}{d} \tag{2}$$

where d is the particle diameter.

For uniformly sized particles, we see that the permeability varies approximately as the square of the particle diameter. In Table 2.2 we present representative permeabilities for the three main soil types based on this equation. In comparing these results with Figure 2.2, we see that the representative permeabilities show the same general dependence on particle size as indicated by the characteristic data.

The Kozeny theory applies only to a soil completely saturated with the fluid of interest. For the case at hand, this means a soil with a small moisture content. In general, the permeability of soil is dependent on the degree of saturation of the fluid, especially within the large pores. Recognition of this dependence has led to the use of the term "relative permeability," which is defined as the ratio of the effective permeability at a given saturation to the permeability when the saturation is 100% for the fluid of interest (18). Studying variations in relative permeability with percent saturation improves our understanding of the influence of moisture content on the air permeability of soils.

Figure 2.3 shows the relative permeability for air (k_{ra}) and water (k_{rw}) as functions of water saturation for a loamy sand. An important point is illustrated here: for this soil, the value of the air permeability remains roughly constant and equal to that for the soil when dry, until water fills a large fraction, about 42%, of the pore space. For the surface and subsurface samples studied, the percent saturation at field capacity was 43% and 47%, respectively, suggesting that the air permeability, for sandy soils, is not strongly affected by changes in moisture content below the field capacity. As moisture content increases above field capacity, the large pores begin to fill with water, and the reduction in air permeability is large. Other studies have shown that the air permeability at field capacity ranges from 0.6 to 0.8 of that of the dry medium (19, 20).

The influence of moisture content below field capacity on the air permeability is greater for clayey soils than for sandy soils for two reasons: the mean pore size

TABLE 2.2 Representative Permeabilities (k) Based on Kozeny Theory[a]

Soil type	d (μm)	ϵ	S (m^{-1})	k (m^2)
Clay	1	0.6	2×10^6	1×10^{-14}
Silt	20	0.5	2×10^5	1×10^{-12}
Sand	200	0.4	2×10^4	4×10^{-11}

[a]$c = 0.5$; $T = 1/\epsilon$ (117); d = particle diameter; ϵ = porosity; S = specific surface area.

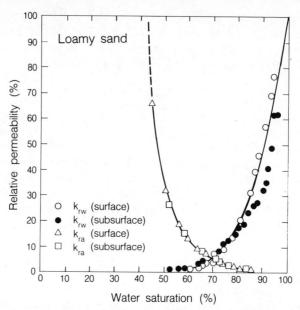

Figure 2.3. Relative permeability of loamy sand for air (k_{ra}) and water (k_{rw}) as a function of water saturation.

is smaller than in sands, so that at field capacity there is a greater tendency for pore blockage in clayey soils; and clayey, or cohesive, soils develop aggregates between which most of the fluid flow occurs (21–23). The formation of aggregates is, as mentioned above, strongly influenced by moisture content.

A further important consideration is the possibility of chemical interactions between soil grains and water. Such interactions tend to retard the flow of water through the soil. Consequently, the apparent intrinsic permeability for water flow through soil may be lower than that for airflow through soil. Since most measurements of the permeability of soil have used water as the fluid, there may be a systematic underestimation in applying these data to the analysis of radon migration in soil.

In addition to the complicating effect of soil moisture, theoretical analyses, such as that due to Kozeny, invariably reflect analyses on a porous medium that is an idealization from even the most regular soil. Undisturbed soils exhibit many complicating features. All soils consist of a distribution of particle sizes, and both the breadth of the distribution and its shape may affect permeability in a way that is not adequately described by the specific surface area. Another factor that may be of particular importance in considering soil as a source of indoor radon is anisotropy in soil permeability. For example, because sedimentary beds are deposited in layers with particles settling under the combined forces of gravity and fluid drag, one might generally expect the permeability of an undisturbed sedimentary soil to be greater in the horizontal than in the vertical direction. One might further expect this effect to be enhanced for platelike clay minerals, as compared to more rounded sand grains. Directional permeability measurements have been made on samples of water-bearing consolidated soils consisting of sand, silt, and clay. The results showed higher horizontal permeabilities by factors of 1.4–7, depending on the site (24). Similar measurements were made on settled sand and limestone samples. Again, where there were differences, the horizontal permeability was higher, but typically by only 20% for these cases. Differences between horizontal and vertical permeabilities of less than an order of magnitude may not be significant, given the range of permeability values. However, differences of a factor of 1000 have been measured (25). The significance for radon entry is this: a higher permeability in the horizontal than in the vertical direction may lead to a larger volume of soil providing radon for the structure.

Structural pore space, when present, strongly influences the permeability of soil and may impart to soils that are texturally clays and clay loams permeabilities similar to those of coarse sands (26). The presence of biopores—penetrations in the soil due to animal or plant activity—may also increase the permeability of fine- and medium-textured soils to values similar to those associated with coarse-textured soils (27).

Whatever complications exist in assessing the behavior of undisturbed soils from theoretical analyses are amplified in investigating radon entry into buildings. Here the nearby soils have often been disturbed and redistributed during construction, and the roots of landscaping vegetation may increase the local permeability. Nevertheless, these effects may be of secondary importance relative to the very large effect of particle size on permeability. Consequently, simple on-site measurements or relevant data from published sources on soil grain-size distribution or permeability may be of considerable use in strategies and techniques for identifying buildings with high concentrations.

2.3 Diffusivity

Owing to random molecular motions, there is a tendency for a substance to migrate down its concentration gradient in a material. As is discussed in Section 5.1, this tendency is described by Fick's law, which relates a concentration gradient to a flux. The coefficient relating these parameters is termed the molecular diffusivity, or diffusion coefficient. In a porous medium, it is a property of the fluid in the pores, the pore structure, and the diffusing species.

For a porous material there are as many as four ways in which Fick's law may be written, depending on whether one uses bulk or pore volume to determine concentration and bulk or pore area to determine flux density; different diffusion coefficients result, and the symbols and terminology have not become standardized in the literature. The "bulk" diffusion coefficient, herein denoted D, relates the gradient of the interstitial concentration of the diffusing species to the flux density across a *geometric* or *superficial* area. The "effective" or "interstitial" diffusion coefficient, denoted D_e, relates the gradient of the interstitial concentration to the flux density across the *pore* area. (Note that this is equivalent to the coefficient that relates the gradient of the bulk concentration to the flux density across the geometric area. The fourth possible formulation has, fortunately, not been used.) These coefficients are related by the porosity, ϵ:

$$D = D_e \epsilon \tag{3}$$

The diffusion of radon in soil has been investigated for several purposes. Globally, the movement of radon from soil into the atmosphere appears to be primarily due to molecular diffusion (28). Since little radon is emitted from oceans, it has been used as an atmospheric tracer for continental air masses (29). Another interest in which radon diffusivity in soil arises is uranium exploration: by mapping soil gas concentrations of radon near the surface, one may be able to identify subsurface deposits of soils enriched in uranium (30). Diffusion of radon through soil has recently been investigated in connection with the use of earthen covers to retard the release of radon into the atmosphere from uranium mill-tailings piles (31, 32). Radon diffusion in soil has also been studied in connection with earthquake prediction (33).

The results of several measurements of the radon diffusion coefficient in soil are summarized in Table 2.3. The upper bound is given by the diffusion coefficient of radon in open air (denoted D_o), 1.2×10^{-5} m^2 s^{-1} (34). Typically, the effective diffusion coefficient of radon in soil of low moisture content is 10^{-6} m^2 s^{-1}.

As in the case of permeability, there have been numerous attempts to relate the diffusivity ratio D/D_o to the physical parameters, particularly ϵ, of the porous medium. From work on CO_2 migration in soils, Buckingham (35) proposed the correlation

$$\frac{D}{D_o} = \epsilon^2 \tag{4}$$

Later Penman (36), studying a wide range of porous materials, obtained the correlation

$$\frac{D}{D_o} = 0.66\epsilon \qquad 0.0 < \epsilon < 0.6 \tag{5}$$

Currie (37) discussed other correlations and reported on experiments showing that such correlations must account for the shape of the grains. He concluded that a correlation of the form

$$\frac{D}{D_o} = \gamma \epsilon^\mu, \tag{6}$$

where γ and μ are properties of the material, fit data from a wide range of media.

Water plays an important role in influencing the radon diffusion coefficient in soil. In a saturated soil, the radon diffusion coefficient may be reduced to $2 \times$

TABLE 2.3 Effective Diffusion Coefficients for Radon in Soil

Soil description	Ref.	D_e (m^2 s^{-1})	Comments
Mill tailings (2 samples)	32	$(5.4-7.2) \times 10^{-6}$	Moisture content 0.7–1.5% dry weight
Eluvial-detrital granodiorite	38	4.5×10^{-6}	Dry
Silty sandy clay	32	2.7×10^{-6}	Moisture content 1.5% dry weight
		2.5×10^{-7}	Moisture content 10.5% dry weight
		6.0×10^{-8}	Moisture content 17.3% dry weight
Compacted silty sands (12 samples)	31	$(3.0 \pm 1.3) \times 10^{-6}$	Porosity = 0.29–0.36; Saturation = 0.05–0.34
Compacted clayey sands (12 samples)	31	$(3.2 \pm 1.5) \times 10^{-6}$	Porosity = 0.32–0.39; Saturation = 0.09–0.55
Compacted inorganic clays (5 samples)	31	$(2.5 \pm 1.0) \times 10^{-6}$	Porosity = 0.32–0.43; Saturation = 0.06–0.34
Diluvium of metamorphic rocks	38	1.8×10^{-6}	Dry
Eluvial-detrital deposits of granite	38	1.5×10^{-6}	Dry
Loams	38	8×10^{-7}	Dry
Varved clays	38	7×10^{-7}	Dry
Mud	38	5.7×10^{-10}	37% Moisture
Mud	38	2.2×10^{-10}	85% Moisture

10^{-10} m^2 s^{-1} (38). This value is so much lower than that in air that, for practical purposes, we can view the effect of water on the radon diffusion coefficient in soil as blocking a fraction of the available pore space. The results of one study of the radon diffusion coefficient as a function of the fraction of pore space filled with water are presented in Figure 2.4. For low moisture contents, water is predominantly on grain surfaces and in small pores. Since transport through the larger pores dominates, the diffusion coefficient is a weak function of moisture content. As the soil nears saturation, the larger pores become occluded and the rate of reduction in diffusion coefficient with increasing moisture content grows.

Currie (39) investigated the relationship between moisture content of porous materials and the bulk diffusivity of hydrogen. He classified materials according to whether or not the grains had an internal pore structure: sand, for example, constituted a solid particle system, whereas a soil containing much clay was considered a ''crumbly'' particle system. He found that the behavior of these two types differed, particularly when nearly dry. In this case, the diffusivity depended very slightly on moisture in the crumbly particle system, but strongly on moisture in the solid particle system. He interpreted these data as indicating that the moisture in the crumbly particle system was taken up in the internal pores of the particles and, hence, had little influence on diffusive transport through the sample, which was dominantly through the larger pores. Once the internal pores were saturated, the solid and crumbly particle systems behaved similarly, with the dependence of diffusivity on moisture well represented by

$$\frac{D_w}{D} = \left[\frac{\epsilon_a}{\epsilon}\right]^{\sigma} \tag{7}$$

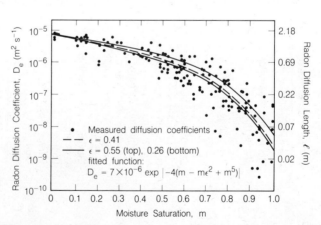

Figure 2.4. Effect of soil moisture content on radon diffusivity. Moisture saturation (m) is the fraction of pore volume filled with water. The porosity is indicated by ϵ. Reproduced from Rogers, V. C., Nielson, K. K., and Kalkwarf, D. R. (1984). Radon attenuation handbook for uranium mill tailings cover design, report NUREG/CR-3533, US Nuclear Regulatory Commission, used by permission.

with σ approximately equal to 4. In this equation D_w is the bulk diffusion coefficient of the wet soil, and ϵ_a is the air-filled porosity (air volume divided by total volume).

The diffusion coefficient for the other isotopes of radon has been observed to be comparable to that for ^{222}Rn.

3   RADON PRODUCTION IN SOIL

This section focuses on the characteristics of soil that influence the rate of radon emanation into the pore air of the soil. We consider two parameters: the radium content and the emanation coefficient.

3.1   Radium Content

The radium content of the soil is typically given as an activity concentration per unit mass. The radium content in these terms is equivalent to the total production rate of radon in the soil, with 1 Bq kg^{-1} of radium yielding radon at a rate of 1 atom kg^{-1} s^{-1}.

Table 2.4 and Figure 2.5 present data on ^{226}Ra and ^{232}Th concentrations in surface soils. The data in Figure 2.5 are based on aerial measurements of ^{214}Bi gamma emissions (40). These data reflect the strength of such emissions from a depth of up to 0.5 m of soil. Two factors may systematically bias these results. First, a fraction of the radon produced in the soil migrates into the atmosphere: hence, the bismuth activity near the surface of a uniform soil is lower than its radium activity. Second, soil bulk density varies (but not proportionately) with moisture content, and gamma attenuation is directly related to density. Consequently, aerial gamma measurements of a given soil are inversely related to its moisture content. The exposure rate above a soil containing 50% water by weight is 36% lower than that above the same soil when dry (41). Since the calibration pads for the aerial detectors contained 20–30% water, the measurements can be in error by up to 20% owing to this effect.

The data in Table 2.4 result from measurements of gamma activity of soil samples collected primarily along U.S. interstate highways (42). The ^{226}Ra content was determined primarily from ^{214}Bi emissions from samples that had been sealed and stored long enough for ^{214}Bi to come to equilibrium with its radium precursor. Data on ^{232}Th, the primordial precursor of ^{220}Rn, reflect gamma emissions from a combination of its decay products. The longest-lived species in the chain from ^{232}Th to ^{220}Rn is ^{228}Ra, with a half-life of 5.7 years, very short in terms of geological time scales. Hence, the ^{232}Th content of a soil is a good indicator of its rate of production of ^{220}Rn.

The radium content of soils tends to reflect the radium content of the rocks from which the soil formed. Table 2.5 summarizes the ^{226}Ra and ^{224}Ra content of rocks. These data are a compilation of over 2500 laboratory-based γ-spectrometric anal-

TABLE 2.4 ^{226}Ra and ^{232}Th Concentrations in Surface Soils

State	No. samples[a]	^{226}Ra (Bq kg^{-1})[b]	^{232}Th (Bq kg^{-1})[b]
Alabama	8	30 (17–52)	28 (13–56)
Alaska	6 (7)	24 (16–34)	32 (7–85)
Arizona	6	35 (9–74)	23 (7–48)
Arkansas	0 (1)		59
California	3	28 (9–48)	20 (11–28)
Colorado	32 (20)	52 (18–126)	48 (4–115)
Delaware	2	43 (41–44)	44
Florida	11 (10)	31 (9–85)	9 (4–14)
Georgia	9	33 (17–59)	41 (10–126)
Idaho	12 (13)	41 (24–59)	44 (16–70)
Illinois	7 (8)	36 (24–44)	36 (18–44)
Indiana	2	39 (37–41)	43 (41–44)
Kansas	6 (4)	36 (13–52)	48 (12–59)
Kentucky	13 (12)	56 (30–155)	44 (33–56)
Louisiana	2	26 (21–31)	24 (22–26)
Maryland	6	27(18–44)	26 (18–32)
Michigan	10	41 (17–74)	21 (9–30)
Mississippi	3	44 (28–59)	41 (30–63)
Missouri	10	41 (11–52)	37 (12–48)
Nevada	6	56 (33–74)	56 (23–111)
New Jersey	24 (23)	32 (9–52)	33 (11–56)
New Mexico	13	56 (27–100)	35 (18–67)
New York	6	31 (18–44)	26 (15–41)
North Carolina	8	29 (18–44)	34 (16–56)
Ohio	12	56 (30–93)	37 (26–56)
Oregon	8 (9)	30 (9–78)	27 (16–56)
Pennsylvania	33	44 (17–89)	41 (14–63)
Tennessee	10 (11)	41 (24–52)	35 (24–56)
Texas	10	33 (20–52)	27 (15–41)
Utah	32 (28)	48 (20–70)	41 (7–85)
Virginia	13	31 (22–41)	32 (16–52)
West Virginia	11	48 (29–59)	52 (41–59)
Wyoming	13 (12)	37 (24–63)	41 (22–67)
All samples	327 (331)	41 (9–155)	36 (4–126)

[a]Where two numbers are given, the one in parentheses applies to ^{232}Th.
[b]Arithmetic mean (range of values in parens).
Source: Ref. 42.

yses reported in English-language publications (43). The radium concentrations within each rock class except the intermediate extrusives were found to be distributed lognormally. Radium contents tended to decrease with silica contents in extrusive and intrusive igneous rocks, with the exception of alkali feldspathoidal rocks, which are rare. The extremely high ^{226}Ra contents listed in the ranges within the chemical sedimentary and shale classes are undoubtedly due to phosphates and black shales, respectively. The mean values for rocks excluding alkali rocks in

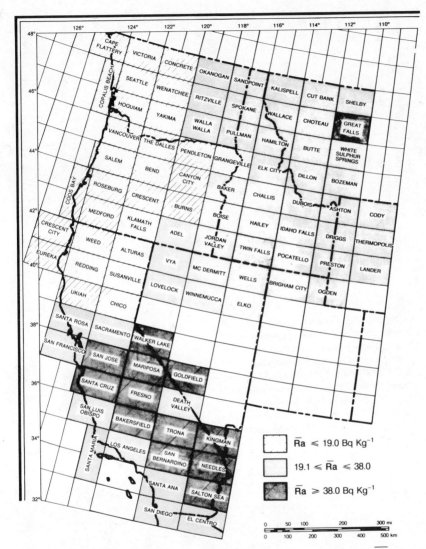

Figure 2.5. Geographical distribution of mean ^{226}Ra content by quadrangle, $\overline{\text{Ra}}$, of surface soils for the Western United States. These results are based on an analysis of aerial radiometric data. Reproduced from Ref. 40.

Table 2.5 tend to support the data for soils given in Table 2.4; the ranges suggest that the range of Ra concentrations, even in soils distant from U mining and milling sites, is probably larger than indicated in Table 2.4.

In combination, these studies suggest that surface soils in the United States typically contain 10–100 Bq/kg of both ^{226}Ra and ^{224}Ra.

Values much higher than the range given by these studies have been found in soils near uranium mining areas and mill-tailings piles. For example, Powers et

TABLE 2.5 Radium Concentrations in Rocks

Rock class[b]	Example	^{226}Ra (Bq kg^{-1}) No. samples	Mean[c]	Range	^{228}Ra (Bq kg^{-1})[a] No. samples	Mean[c]	Range
Acid extrusives	Rhyolite	131	71	10–285	131	91	4–470
Acid intrusives	Granite	569	78	1–372	573	111	0.4–1025
Intermediate extrusives	Andesite	71	26	2–64	71	27	2–113
Intermediate intrusives	Diorite	271	40	1–285	273	49	2–429
Basic extrusives	Basalt	77	11	0.4–41	77	10	0.2–36
Basic intrusives	Gabbro	119	10	0.1–71	110	9	0.1–61
Ultrabasic rocks	Dunite	31	4	0–20	30	6	0–30
Alkali feldspathoidal intermediate extrusives	Phonolite	138	368	24–769	139	543	38–1073
Alkali feldspathoidal intermediate intrusives	Syenite	75	692	4–8930	75	5	2–3560
Alkali basic extrusives	Nephelinite	27	29	6–149	27	36	8–2670
Alkali basic intrusives	Foidite	8	29	5–67	34	8	11–81
Chemical sedimentary rocks[d]	Evaporites	243	45	0.4–335	239	60	0.1–535
Carbonates	Limestone	141	25	0.4–223	131	7	0–45
Detrital sedimentary rocks[e]		412	60	1–992	411	50	0.8–1466
Clay		40	50	14–198	40	35	8–223
Shale		174	73	11–992	174	66	21–158
Sandstone and conglomerate		198	51	1–770	198	39	3–919
Metamorphosed igneous rocks	Gneiss	138	50	1–1835	138	60	0.4–421
Metamorphosed sedimentary rocks	Schist	207	37	1–657	208	49	0.4–368

[a]Because of the short half-lives of ^{228}Ac (6.1 h), ^{228}Th (1.9 y), and ^{224}Ra (3.7 d), one expects ^{224}Ra to be in equilibrium with ^{228}Ra.
[b]Rocks are classified on the bases of whole-rock silica content (acid > intermediate > basic > ultrabasic) and alkali and calcic feldspar mineralogy.
[c]Arithmetic mean.
[d]Includes carbonates.
[e]Includes clay, shale, sandstone, and conglomerates.
Source: Ref. 43.

72

al. (44) found a range of 15–1700 Bq/kg of ^{226}Ra for 28 samples collected near uranium mining and milling areas in Wyoming, New Mexico, and South Dakota. In Jaduguda, Bihar, India, an area with known deposits of uraniferous materials, ^{226}Ra concentrations of 40–200 Bq/kg were reported (45). Sixty-three samples from Canada collected near the surface of two mill-tailings piles contained a mean ^{226}Ra concentration of 1760 Bq/kg (46).

3.2 Emanation Coefficient

Only a fraction of the radon generated in soil ever leaves the solid grains and enters the pore volume of the soil. This fraction is known as the ''emanation coefficient'' or, alternatively, ''emanating fraction'' or ''emanating power.''

Experimental measurements of the emanation coefficient of rocks and soils have been made by many investigators. These data, summarized in Table 2.6, indicate an approximate range of 0.05–0.7 for soil. We have some understanding of the basic physical processes leading to radon emanation from soil (see Fig. 2.6); however, measured emanation coefficients are considerably higher than predicted by simple physical models.

Conservation of linear momentum dictates that, upon being created by the alpha decay of radium, ^{222}Rn and ^{220}Rn atoms possess kinetic energies of 86 and 103 keV, respectively (47). The newly formed atom travels from its site of generation until its energy is transferred to the host material. The distance traveled depends on the density and composition of the material. The range of ^{222}Rn is 0.02–0.07 μm for common minerals, 0.1 μm for water, and 63 μm in air; the range of ^{220}Rn in air is 83 μm (48).

The emanation coefficient is considered to have three components: direct recoil, indirect recoil, and diffusion. These components arise from the locations of the end points of the path of the recoiling radon atoms. The direct recoil fraction refers to radon atoms that terminate their recoil in the fluid-filled pore space. Atoms that leave the grain in which they were created, traverse a pore, and penetrate another grain form the basis for the indirect-recoil fraction. They must then migrate out of the pocket created by their passage to enter a pore. The diffusion fraction refers to radon atoms that begin and end their recoil within a single grain, then migrate to the pore through molecular diffusion.

Analysis of the emanation process for uniformly distributed radium in undamaged soil grains leads to much lower emanation coefficients than are generally observed. Consider first the maximum recoil fraction. Only radium atoms within the recoil range of the surface generate radon atoms that have any possibility of escaping the grain. Andrews and Wood (49) and Bossus (47) computed the escape probability for radon atoms generated within the recoil range of the surface of a spherical particle and obtained 23.5 and 25%, respectively. If we then consider a spherical particle, with diameter 20 μm (corresponding to a medium-coarse silt), having a radon recoil range of 0.035 μm, this model predicts that only 0.25% of the radon atoms generated in the grain leave it during recoil. An analysis of the

TABLE 2.6 Measurements of ^{222}Rn and ^{220}Rn Emanation Coefficients

Material	No. samples	Moisture content	Isotope	Emanation coef.[a]	Ref.
Rock (crushed)	58	Unknown	^{222}Rn	0.084 ± 0.086 (0.005–0.40)	52
Soil	21	Unknown	^{222}Rn	0.30 ± 0.16 (0.03–0.55)	52
Soil[b]	1	Dried, 105°C, 24 h 20% of dry wt	^{222}Rn	0.25	50
Soil[c]	1	Dried, 200°C, 90 h	^{222}Rn	0.68 0.09	56
Soil	1	Air-dry[d]	^{222}Rn	0.41	2
Soil	2	13–20% of dry wt	^{222}Rn	0.27 (0.22–0.32)	92
Soil	1	4% of dry wt	^{222}Rn	0.38 ± 0.08	100
Various soils (Hawaiian)					53
Lava fields		Unknown	^{222}Rn	0.02	
Thin organic soils		Unknown	^{222}Rn	0.55	
Deep agricultural soils		Unknown	^{222}Rn	0.70	
Various soils					118
Sand	7	Unknown	^{222}Rn	0.14 (0.06–0.18)	
Sandy loam	7	Unknown	^{222}Rn	0.21 (0.10–0.36)	
Silty loam	7	Unknown	^{222}Rn	0.24 (0.18–0.40)	

Material	n	Condition	Nuclide	Value	Ref.
[Heavy] loam	12	Unknown	^{222}Rn	0.20 (0.17–0.23)	
Clay	5	Unknown	^{222}Rn	0.28 (0.18–0.40)	
Various soils (Danish)	70	0–70% of dry wt	^{222}Rn	0.22 ± 0.13 (0.02–0.7)	119
Soil	2	Dried, 105°C, 24 h	^{220}Rn	0.09–0.10[e], 0.12–0.15	50
Sand	1	Saturated	^{222}Rn	0.243	49
Uranium Ore	6	Saturated	^{222}Rn	0.19 ± 0.10 (0.06–0.26)	55
		Dried, 110°C[f]		0.05 ± 0.03 (0.014–0.07)	
Uranium Ore (crushed)	17	Moist, saturated	^{222}Rn	0.28 ± 0.16 (0.055–0.55)	54
		Vacuum-dried		0.14 ± 0.11 (0.023–0.36)	
Tailings	2	Saturated	^{222}Rn	0.29, 0.31	55
		Dried, 110°C[f]		0.067, 0.072	

[a] Arithmetic mean ± one standard deviation (range of values).
[b] Sample sieved through 20 μm mesh.
[c] Sample of six giving highest reading.
[d] Exposed to laboratory air for several days.
[e] This sample, when moist, had an emanation coefficient for ^{220}Rn of 0.13.
[f] Dried to constant weight.

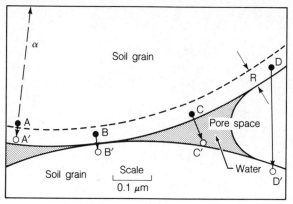

Figure 2.6. Schematic illustration of radon recoil trajectories in and between soil grains. Two spherical grains of 2-μm diameter (clay/silt) are in contact at point B. The stippled portion of the pore is water-filled. The recoil range, R, of the radon atoms is indicated by the dashed line. ^{226}Ra atoms, indicated by solid circles, decay, producing an alpha particle and a ^{222}Rn atom, which may end its recoil at the point indicated by the open circle. At A the radium atom is too deeply embedded within the grain for the radon atom to escape. At B and D the recoiling radon atom possesses sufficient energy after escaping the host grain to penetrate an adjacent grain. At C the radon atom terminates its recoil in the pore water. From Ref. 48, used by permission.

diffusion of radon in intact grains suggests that the diffusion fraction is entirely negligible: diffusion coefficients for argon in rock-forming minerals were measured to be 10^{-31}–10^{-69}m^2 s^{-1} (38); corresponding radon diffusion lengths are 10^{-13}–10^{-32} m.

Two hypotheses have been advanced to account for the large discrepancy between measured and theoretical emanation coefficients (38, 48). The first is that radium is not distributed uniformly but rather is concentrated in secondary crusts or films on the surfaces of the grains. The second hypothesis suggests that chemical corrosion and, particularly, radiation damage due to the decay of its precursors, damages the crystalline structure in the vicinity of the newly formed radon atom, thereby permitting it to migrate more readily than would otherwise be possible. These hypotheses are not mutually exclusive, and both are substantiated by experimental data.

The first hypothesis is supported by the results of two studies. In one, the ^{226}Ra and ^{224}Ra concentrations of two soil samples were measured as a function of grain size and found to decrease nearly monotonically as grain size increased (50). This trend would be expected if a portion of the radium content of each grain were contained in a surface layer. The second study measured ^{238}U and ^{232}Th series concentrations in 70 soil samples and found them to vary linearly with the fraction of the soil mass having particle diameter less than 20 μm (51). Tanner suggests that uranium and thorium are not compatible with the crystalline structure of major minerals and, hence, are commonly found in accessory minerals, adsorbed on the surface of clay particles, or are present in other coatings (48).

Data supporting the second hypothesis come from a study by Barretto of the effect of annealing rocks, sands, and minerals (52). Invariably, for the six samples studied the radon emanation coefficient dropped as the annealing temperature was increased. For heating to 1000°C, the average (± one standard deviation) of the emanation coefficient of the annealed sample, divided by its original emanation coefficient, was 0.23 (± 0.23).

Additional pertinent evidence is contained in the results of a study of radon emanation from the island of Hawaii (53). The ^{222}Rn emanation coefficient was found to be much smaller for samples from lava fields (average 0.02) than for samples from either thin organic soils (0.55) or deep agricultural soils (0.70). Being of recent origin, and formed by the rapid cooling of a molten solid, lavas would be expected to have relatively uniform distribution of ^{226}Ra and minimal radiation damage. Consequently, their much lower emanation coefficient is not surprising.

Moisture content has been demonstrated in several studies to have a large impact on the emanation coefficient (54–57). Data showing this effect for uranium ore tailings are presented in Figure 2.7. The explanation for this phenomenon appears to lie in the markedly lower recoil range for radon in water than in air. A radon atom entering a pore that is partially filled with water has a very high probability of terminating its recoil in the water. From there, it is readily transferred to the air in the pore. At equilibrium, the partitioning between air and water is described by Henry's law (see Chapter 4). Mass transfer from water to air is rapid: an aqueous diffusion coefficient of order 10^{-9} m^2 s^{-1} (58) and a water layer thick-

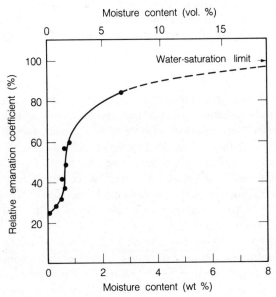

Figure 2.7. Effect of moisture content on ^{222}Rn emanation coefficient for a sample of uranium mill tailings. From Ref. 55. Reproduced from *Health Physics*, Vol. 42, p. 30, by permission of the Health Physics Society.

ness of order 10 μm suggest a characteristic time for transport to the air of 0.1 s; thus equilibrium is achieved rapidly.

The characteristic pore dimension of a soil is related to its grain-size distribution. For a soil having a narrow distribution of grain sizes, the characteristic pore size is the same order as the characteristic grain size. Hence, even for clayey soils, for which the characteristic grain size is of order 1 μm, the pore dimensions are much larger than the radon recoil range in water. Consequently, one would expect the dependence of emanation coefficient on moisture content in most soils to show the general trend indicated in Figure 2.7. As a soil is dried from saturation, the emanation coefficient drops slowly at first as the gravitational water is removed. Once the large pores are drained and capillary water begins to be affected, the emanation coefficient drops substantially, Finally, when only adsorbed water remains, there is little effect of further drying of the soil. This layer is too thin to be very effective in stopping the recoiling radon atoms.

In combination with the discussion in previous sections, this suggests that radon release from soil, combining emanation and transport, is maximal when the soil is moist. Having the small pores filled with water results in a high radon emanation coefficient, but—as most transport takes place through the larger pores—only reduces radon transport to a small degree. When dry, the soil has slightly enhanced transport, but a greatly reduced emanation coefficient. When wet, the emanation coefficient is slightly higher, but the diffusivity and permeability are greatly reduced. This intermediate level of moisture, corresponding approximately to the range between the wilting point and field capacity, is the most common state of natural soils.

To account for the moisture dependence of the emanation coefficient of radon from 17 samples of crushed ore, Thamer et al. proposed the following model (54). The ore was assumed to consist of radioactively inert rock grains held together by a porous cementing material. The pores were treated as cylinders with diameters varying according to a measured pore-size distribution. The radium in the sample was assumed to be uniformly distributed within an annular region of constant thickness around each pore. Finally, moisture was assumed to occur in layers of equal thickness on the inner surface of the radium-bearing annulus.

Two parameters were allowed to vary to fit the data: the inert rock fraction determined the magnitude of the dry emanation coefficient, and the thickness of the radium-bearing annular regions determined the ratio of saturated to dry emanation. With this model, the researchers were successful in matching the dependence of the emanation coefficient on moisture in most cases. Their model yielded values of 0.78 ± 0.11 for the inert rock fraction and 0.025 ± 0.011 μm for the thickness of the radium-bearing regions.

Temperature has also been found to be a factor in determining the radon emanation coefficient, although over the range of temperatures common for surface soils this effect is of minor importance. Stranden et al. (56) found that the radon exhalation rate for a soil sample increased by 55% when the temperature was increased from 5 to 50°C. They suggested that the increase with temperature may be due to a reduction in physical adsorption. Barretto (52) found a much smaller temperature dependence for the emanation coefficient of a granite sample: 0.106

at 265°C to 0.081 at −20°C. He found though that when the sample was cooled to −80°C, the emanation coefficient decreased markedly to 0.028. On the other hand, Tanner (59) found the rate of emanation of radon from a natural, uranium-mineralized, very permeable sandstone core to decrease with increasing temperature over the range of 24–100°C. The results were reversible, indicating that the observed effect was probably not due to changes in moisture content.

Radon condenses at temperatures much lower than those found in the environment. For a pure sample at standard pressure, the boiling point and melting point are −62°C and −71°C, respectively (60). At very low partial pressures, i.e., under all environmental conditions, radon condenses on surfaces at approximately −150°C (61). Common experimental techniques used to concentrate radon from an airstream involve collecting the radon on activated charcoal cooled to the temperature of solid CO_2 (−78.5°C) (62) or on glass wool cooled to the temperature of liquid N_2 (−196°C) (63).

4 BUILDING CHARACTERISTICS

Two aspects of building design and operation play key roles in influencing radon entry from soil. One is the design and operation of the ventilation system, which may affect the pressures that drive bulk airflow through the soil. The second is the design and construction of the building substructure, which controls the degree of movement between the air in the soil and the air in the building.

In addition to these factors, the very presence of a house may influence the spatial distribution of soil moisture and, thereby, the emanation and migration of radon. Except for one anecdotal report (64), such effects have not been documented; however, they seem reasonable to expect based on common experience. For example, a house serves as an umbrella to precipitation such that the soil underlying it tends to be drier than the surrounding uncovered soil. As we have seen, the moisture content of soil is an important factor influencing radon emanation, effective diffusion coefficient, and soil permeability.

A comprehensive treatment of building practices that influence radon entry is beyond the scope of this book. Even within a single country, relevant construction practices vary widely, depending principally on the purpose of the building, the climate, and the structural and drainage characteristics of the local soil. In the United States, construction practices are governed for the most part by municipal codes, rather than by federal or state guidelines. The discussion in this chapter covers only some of the key features of building practice pertaining to radon entry and focuses on single-family residential structures, which have been the most extensively studied. Further discussion may be found in Chapter 10.

4.1 Ventilation

Ventilation refers to the total supply rate of outdoor air into a building, whether intentional or not. It serves the purpose of controlling odors, maintaining a proper balance of metabolic gases, and diluting pollutants generated by indoor sources.

The most important aspect of ventilation for radon entry from soil is its relationship to the pressure difference between the base of the outside walls and the building's substructure openings. This relationship is discussed explicitly in Section 6.2. Here, our objective is to provide a brief introduction to building ventilation. This discussion complements Section 8.2 of Chapter 1.

The ventilation rate has three components. Infiltration refers to the uncontrolled leakage of air into the building through cracks and holes in the building shell. Natural ventilation is the flow of air into the building through open doors and windows. Mechanical ventilation is the provision or removal of air by means of blowers or fans.

In most single-family dwellings in the United States, at times when the outdoor air must be heated or cooled for thermal comfort, infiltration is the predominant component of ventilation. The forces that drive infiltration arise from wind and buoyancy; these are discussed quantitatively in a later section of this chapter. Models have been developed that predict infiltration on the basis of the wind speed (including corrections for local shielding), temperature difference, and leakiness of the structure (see Chapter 1, Section 8.2) (65). Data on infiltration rates in U.S. housing are presented in Chapter 4.

At times when the outdoor air temperature is in the approximate range of 15–25°C, depending on the habits of the building occupants, the rate of natural ventilation may become very large, and the indoor-outdoor pressure differences very small. Concentrations of radon and its progeny inside a residence with open doors and windows are typically close to the outdoor levels.

A major difficulty with the use of infiltration as the principal means of ventilating a building is the lack of control. A building with a relatively large leakage area may be uncomfortably drafty when weather conditions are severe. Rising energy prices beginning in 1973 led to financial pressures to reduce infiltration rates. But during mild weather, the infiltration rate of a "tight" building may be so low that moisture, odor, or other indoor air quality problems result. Consequently, there is considerable interest in the use of mechanical ventilation systems in residential buildings.

A balanced mechanical ventilation system is designed to operate with equal amounts of supply and exhaust air, often passed through a heat-recovery device to reduce energy costs (66). In this case, its effect on the pressure distribution across the base of the building walls is probably negligible. Alternatively, in an unbalanced system, either exhaust or supply ventilation is provided in excess. For example, in a supply-only system, the pressure inside the building is increased, and air flows out either through designed penetrations or through leaks in the building shell. This approach should in principle have the beneficial side effect of reducing radon entry by lowering, or even reversing, the pressure gradient in the surrounding soil. Caution must be exercised to avoid material damage in cold climates owing to the freezing condensation of moisture in exfiltrating air.

Mechanical systems provide the ventilation in most commercial buildings, although small ones may be ventilated like residences. Common commercial design specifies a higher rate of fresh-air supply than exhaust, so that the building is operated at a pressure slightly higher than ambient.

Intermittent activities of the building occupants may influence radon entry by altering the indoor-outdoor pressure differences. Fireplace operation can, because of the large rate of airflow out of the chimney, lower the pressure in a house and significantly increase the air-exchange rate (67). In the only case studied, a concomitant increase in the rate of radon entry was observed that nearly compensated for the increased ventilation rate (2). This result suggests that the use of exhaust fans for local (or general) ventilation may have the undesirable side effect of increasing radon entry rates. Recent modeling of this situation suggests that exhaust ventilation may be a suitable, but not optimal, method of providing air exchange for crawl-space houses and for basement houses surrounded by low-permeability ($<10^{-12}$ m^2) soil (120). Exhaust ventilation is not recommended for basement houses with highly permeable soil unless measures are taken to impede soil gas entry.

4.2 Substructure

Single-family dwellings in the United States are most commonly built with the lowest floor made either of poured concrete and in direct contact with the underlying soil, or of wood and suspended above the soil. In the former case, the floor may lie below the soil grade; this is designated a basement substructure. Alternatively, the floor may be built to the same level as the soil surface, a substructure type often called "slab-on-grade." The substructure for a house having a suspended wood floor is known as a crawl space.

Each type has unique characteristics that influence radon entry, with the greatest differences occurring between crawl-space substructures and the others. Among the three types, radon entry into basements has received most of the research and remedial attention (1–3, 68–70), but entry into slab-on-grade (71) and crawl-space houses (64) has been studied as well.

The influence of the building substructure on radon entry can be separated into two factors: the degree of coupling between indoor air and soil air, and the size and location of openings and penetrations through the substructure.

Consider first the degree of coupling. The interior of a slab-on-grade or a basement house is potentially well-coupled to the nearby soil. Recommended construction practice calls for the concrete slab to be underlaid by a layer of gravel or crushed stone that, in turn, lies on the subsoil (72). An intermediate plastic membrane may be present, depending on the normal moisture conditions of the surrounding soil. Any penetrations through the concrete and plastic sheeting, if present, constitute a link between the underlying soil and the indoor air that is distributed by means of the gravel layer to the entire area beneath the floor. If the pressure inside the house is reduced with respect to the pressure at the base of the outside walls, that pressure differential is effectively applied across the underlying soil. If the soil is sufficiently permeable, a large radon entry rate can result. Even in the absence of a gravel layer, a basement or slab-on-grade house is closely coupled to the soil.

A house with a crawl-space substructure may be well-coupled to the underlying soil or not, depending on whether the crawl space is vented. The venting generally required to prevent moisture damage, e.g., 0.67 m^2 of vent area per 100 m^2 of floor area (73), is sufficient in principle to uncouple the indoor air from the soil: essentially all air flowing through the floor of the living space enters the crawl space through the vents, rather than through the soil. Consequently, very high radon entry rates due to elevated soil gas influx, as sometimes found in houses with a basement, are not expected in houses having a vented crawl space.

On the other hand, if the crawl space is unvented and the underlying soil exposed, then the house is well-coupled to the soil, and the radon entry rate may be large. One study conducted in Illinois found that in 9 of 22 such houses indoor radon concentrations exceeded 180 Bq m^{-3} and in six of these the concentration was greater than 370 Bq m^{-3} (74).

Penetrations in the building shell that are most important for radon entry are those through the floor and, in the case of a house with a basement, those through the wall below soil grade. Common routes of entry and means of sealing them are discussed thoroughly in Chapter 10. We note here only a few points in this regard.

Penetrations in the floor of a slab-on-grade or basement house are commonly found at the floor-wall joint, around service entrances (particularly for water supply pipes and the sanitary sewer lines), and in association with floor drains or perimeter drainage systems. The size of these penetrations is almost invariably great enough so that the principal resistance to airflow through the soil and building substructure is in the soil. Hence, for radon entry into concrete-floored houses, the absolute size of penetrations, unless unusually small, is relatively unimportant. The relative size among penetrations and their position may be important. By influencing the length of the path that air must traverse through soil before entering the substructure, these latter factors play a role in determining the volume of soil that may contribute its radon to the indoor air.

In a crawl-space house, penetrations may be found along the foundation sill plate, and around plumbing and sewer pipes, electrical wiring, and heating and air-conditioning ducts where they pass throug the floor. As suggested by the previous discussion, if the crawl space is vented, these penetrations probably have little effect on radon migration through the nearby soil. Their total size does, however, influence radon entry by affecting the proportion of radon entering the crawl space from the soil that enters the house, rather than exiting to the outside air.

5   RADON MIGRATION IN SOIL

In this section, we develop a mathematical formulation describing the radon concentration in the pore air of a differential volume of soil. The equation accounts for the transport of radon by molecular diffusion and forced convection and the production and removal of radon by radioactive decay. In addition to the variables described in earlier sections, application of this equation to the problem of radon entry into buildings requires specifying the pressures at the surface of the soil and inside the building and the building geometry. Analytical solutions to this equation do not exist, except for the simplest geometries. Consequently, a complete treatment requires the use of a numerical model, an undertaking that has only recently been started (7, 75–77, 109, 120, 121). Dimensional analysis permits one to identify circumstances under which one or more of the terms of the governing equation become negligible and, consequently, may be ignored, thereby simplifying the detailed quantitative analysis.

We begin with discussions of the Fick's law and Darcy's law, which, respectively, underlie the description of transport due to molecular diffusion and forced convection. A general differential transport equation is then presented. By the use of scaling arguments, conditions are identified under which the problem of analyzing radon migration in soil near a building may be simplified.

5.1 Diffusive Transport—Fick's Law

To begin, we consider a gas made up of two species, A and B. The molar flux of A relative to stationary coordinates may be expressed (58) as

$$\mathbf{N_A} = x_A(\mathbf{N_A} + \mathbf{N_B}) - cD_o\nabla x_A \tag{8}$$

where $\mathbf{N_A}$ and $\mathbf{N_B}$ are the fluxes of A and B, respectively, with respect to fixed coordinates (moles $m^{-2}\,s^{-1}$), x_A is the molar fraction of A in the mixture, c is the molar concentration of the gas (moles m^{-3}), D_o is the diffusion coefficient ($m^2\,s^{-1}$) (see Section 2.3), and ∇ is the three-dimensional gradient operator. The first term on the right-hand side of Equation 8 represents the flux density of A due to convection, and the second term gives the diffusional flux density relative to the mean convective velocity. This expression embodies Fick's first law, which states that the diffusional flux density is proportional to the concentration gradient. Fick's law is based on experimental observations and is consistent with the postulates of kinetic theory for an ideal gas. Other physical conditions that may lead to a diffusive flux, in particular temperature gradients, pressure gradients, and external forces (e.g., due to an imposed electric field), are neglected in this expression. They are usually unimportant relative to the concentration gradient.

For the case of radon in air, we can make major simplifications in Equation 8. First, since the mole fraction of radon in air is always vanishingly small (40,000 Bq m^{-3}, a typical concentration in soil air, is equivalent to a mole fraction of ^{222}Rn of 7.6×10^{-16} at 20°C), the molecular diffusion of radon may be neglected as a source of convection of the mixture. That is, we may neglect the term $x_A\mathbf{N_A}$ as small compared to $\mathbf{N_A}$. A further simplification results from approximating the molar concentration of air as a constant. Hence,

$$\mathbf{N}_{Rn} = x_{Rn}\mathbf{N} - D_o\nabla c_{Rn} \tag{9}$$

where $\mathbf{N}$ is now the molar flux density of air relative to stationary coordinates and $c_{Rn} = cx_{Rn}$ is the molar concentration of radon. It is convenient to multiply this equation by Avogadro's number and the decay constant of radon so that

$$\mathbf{J}_{Rn} = I_{Rn}\mathbf{V} - D_o \nabla I_{Rn} \tag{10}$$

where I_{Rn} is the activity concentration of radon (Bq m^{-3}), $\mathbf{J}_{Rn}$ is the activity flux density (Bq m^{-2} s^{-1}), and $\mathbf{V} = \mathbf{N}/c$ is the net air velocity (m s^{-1}). The discussion in this section focuses on the implications of the diffusive flux ($-D_o \nabla I_{Rn}$). The convective flux ($I_{Rn}\mathbf{V}$) is discussed in the following section.

Before proceeding, it is worthwhile to note a potentially important assumption implicit in Equations 8–10. We have treated radon in air as an effectively binary mixture. This means that we neglect any transport of radon that may result from the diffusion of another species in air (except as that diffusion causes convection of the mixture). Whether multicomponent diffusion effects are important for radon migration in soil is not known. A case that may prove to be significant is radon migration due to the diffusion of water vapor. Further discussion of multicomponent diffusion may be found in Ref. 58.

Thus far in this section, we have assumed the radon to be migrating in open air. Considering the diffusion of radon in soil, we need to adjust our description to account for two effects of the solid matrix: the area through which radon may diffuse is reduced and the average path length that radon must traverse to reach one point from another is increased. These factors are embodied in the replacement of the binary diffusion coefficient, D_o, with an effective diffusion coefficient, D_e, so that

$$\mathbf{J}_{Rn}^d = -D_e \nabla I_{Rn} \tag{11}$$

In this equation, $\mathbf{J}_{Rn}^d$ represents the diffusive flux density of radon activity per unit of pore area of the soil. The relationships among D_e, D (the bulk diffusion coefficient), and D_o were discussed in Section 2.3.

Two implicit approximations remain in the description of diffusive flux given in Equation 11. It is worthwhile to examine them briefly before continuing. First, we have assumed that, as in open air, all the kinetic interactions of the radon atoms occur with gas molecules. This is a reasonable approximation so long as the pores are large relative to the mean free path of the radon atoms, which is comparable with that for the major constituents of air, 0.065 μm at 25°C. Pore dimensions are of the same order as grain size; hence, for all soils larger than clays, this assumption is good. For smaller pores, the molecular transport process is termed Knudsen diffusion. The flux density remains proportional to the concentration gradient; however, the diffusivity is proportional to the pore radius and thus is a strong function of position within the pores (78).

The second approximation is that all radon in the soil exists in one of two states: within the air contained in the soil or within the solid soil grains. This approximation embodies at least three simplifications. First, we are treating the pore size distribution as unimodal, or, in the parlance of Currie (39), we are treating the soil as solid grained, rather than crumbly. Alternatively, we are assuming that the characteristic time for transport out of the small pores of a grain into the major pores of the soil matrix is small relative to the transport time through the major pore.

The second simplification neglects the fraction of radon that is present in soil water. At 20°C, the coefficient of solubility, defined as the ratio of concentrations at equilibrium, for radon between water and air is 0.25 (79). If the moisture saturation is 50% and the temperature is 20°C, the amount of radon in the gas phase of the pores is 4 times as large as that in the water phase. This effect will be considered explicitly below. Finally, we neglect any possible adsorption of radon on the surfaces of the soil grains. As radon is an inert gas, and its condensation temperature is much lower than environmental temperatures, this would seem to be a good assumption. Experimental evidence of the effect of adsorption on radon release from geological materials has been reviewed by Tanner (48). He concluded that the studies were insufficient to determine whether this is an important factor.

For a dry, solid-grained soil through which radon migrates only by diffusion, the activity concentration in the pores is described by the following conservation-of-mass equation:

$$\frac{\partial I_{Rn}}{\partial t} = D_e \nabla^2 I_{Rn} - \lambda_{Rn} I_{Rn} + G \tag{12}$$

where λ_{Rn} is the decay constant of radon (2.1×10^{-6} s^{-1} for ^{222}Rn and 0.0125 s^{-1} for ^{220}Rn), and G is the volumetric radon generation rate in the soil pores (Bq m^{-3} s^{-1}). We have assumed that the diffusion coefficient is constant. The generation rate may be determined from parameters already introduced:

$$G = f \rho_s A_{Ra} \lambda_{Rn} \frac{1 - \epsilon}{\epsilon} \tag{13}$$

where f is the emanation fraction, ρ_s is the density of the soil grains [commonly 2.65×10^3 kg m^{-3} and rarely not in the range $(2.6–2.8) \times 10^3$ (9)], A_{Ra} is the radium activity concentration in the soil (Bq kg^{-1}), and ϵ is the porosity.

Considering the case of uncovered soil of infinite depth and extent, and assuming the radon concentration to be zero at the soil surface, the steady-state solution to the one-dimensional form of Equation 12 yields the radon activity concentration in the soil pores at a depth z below the surface:

$$I_{Rn}(z) = I_\infty (1 - e^{-z/l}) \tag{14}$$

where $I_\infty = G / \lambda_{Rn}$ is the activity concentration of radon in the pores at large depths and $l = (D_e / \lambda_{Rn})^{1/2}$ is known as the diffusion length. For ^{222}Rn, a typical value of l is 1 meter or less.

The flux density of radon from uncovered soil due entirely to diffusion is given by multiplying Equation 11 by ϵ so that the flux is determined per unit geometric area. Substituting Equation 14, we obtain the result

$$J_{Rn}^d = \epsilon \lambda_{Rn} l I_\infty = (D_e \lambda_{Rn})^{1/2} \rho_s f A_{Ra} (1 - \epsilon) \tag{15}$$

Taking as typical values for ^{222}Rn, $D_e = 2 \times 10^{-6}$ m^2 s^{-1}, $\rho_s = 2.65 \times 10^3$ kg m^{-3}, $f = 0.2$, $A_{Ra} = 30$ Bq kg^{-1}, and $\epsilon = 0.5$, we obtain $J_{Rn}^d = 0.016$ Bq m^{-2} s^{-1}. By comparison, Wilkening et al. (28) estimated the mean worldwide flux of ^{222}Rn to be approximately 0.015 Bq m^{-2} s^{-1}.

Because of its much larger decay constant, the activity flux of ^{220}Rn should generally be larger than that of ^{222}Rn, although the molar flux should be substantially less (see Chapter 1, Section 8.4). Flux of ^{220}Rn from dry, uncovered soil measured at six sites in New Mexico was found to be 1.6 ± 0.3 Bq m^{-2} s^{-1} (80), 100 times larger than the typical value for ^{222}Rn cited above, but, in molar terms, 60 times less.

The diffusion of radon from soil through concrete slabs and into houses has been analyzed theoretically (81–84). The results show that a structurally intact slab is an effective barrier against radon entry: a reduction in flux to approximately 5% or less of the value for uncovered soil is expected for a typical case (82, 85). Experimental measurements of flux through concrete slabs confirm that the diffusion of radon through concrete is much less than needed to account for radon in houses (1). If the slab is cracked, the diffusional flux may be greatly increased. Landman (83) determined that 25% of the flux from uncovered soil would penetrate the slab if a 1-cm gap existed for every 1 m of slab. Even for relatively large penetrations, however, the resulting diffusive flux is still much smaller than the observed entry rates in most houses.

In addition to affecting the emanating fraction and the diffusion coefficient, the presence of water in the soil pores alters the diffusive transport equation. If we assume that radon is partitioned between water and air according to Henry's law, and that diffusion of radon within the water can be neglected, then the transport equation can be written

$$\frac{1}{\epsilon} \frac{\partial (I_a \epsilon_a + I_w \epsilon_w)}{\partial t} = D_e' \nabla^2 I_a - \frac{1}{\epsilon} \lambda_{Rn} (I_a \epsilon_a + I_w \epsilon_w) + G' \qquad (16)$$

where I_a is the radon concentration in the air volume, I_w is the radon concentration in the water volume, and ϵ_a and ϵ_w are the air and water porosities, respectively, so that $\epsilon_a + \epsilon_w = \epsilon$. The radon concentrations in the two phases are related by $I_w = \kappa I_a$, where κ is the coefficient of solubility of radon in water. The solution to the steady-state problem for a semiinfinite soil is analogous to Equations 14 and 15 with modified diffusion length, infinite depth concentration, and surface flux.

$$l = \left[\frac{\epsilon}{\epsilon_a + \kappa \epsilon_w} \right]^{1/2} \left[\frac{D_e'}{\lambda_{Rn}} \right]^{1/2}$$

$$I_\infty = \frac{G' \epsilon}{\lambda_{Rn} (\epsilon_a + \kappa \epsilon_w)}$$

$$J_{Rn}^d = (D_e' \lambda_{Rn})^{1/2} \rho_s f' A_{Ra} (1 - \epsilon) \left[\frac{\epsilon_a}{(\epsilon_a + \kappa \epsilon_w) \epsilon} \right]^{1/2} \qquad (17)$$

For $\epsilon_a = \epsilon_w = 0.25$ and $\kappa = 0.25$, and assuming that moisture has no effect on D_e and f, l is increased by 26%, I_∞ is increased by 60%, and J_{Rn}^d is decreased by 37%. Of course, in general, the change in moisture has a substantial effect on both D_e and f. For example, the results presented in Figures 2.4 and 2.7 indicate that for the respective samples, the effective diffusion coefficient is decreased by a factor of 5, and the emanation coefficient is increased by a factor of 4, for the wet case relative to the dry case.

5.2   Convective Transport—Darcy's Law

In the middle of the nineteenth century, H. Darcy conducted experiments on the flow of water through sand columns. His results showed that for a given column the volumetric flow rate, Q, was proportional to the difference of the fluid heads at the inlet and outlet of the column, Δh, and to its cross-sectional area, A, and inversely proportional to the length of the column, L:

$$Q = \frac{c_1 \Delta h A}{L} \tag{18}$$

where c_1 is a constant dependent on the sand. Muskat (13) argued theoretically that the relationship

$$v = \frac{Q}{A} = \frac{c_2 d^2}{\mu} \frac{\Delta p}{\Delta L} \tag{19}$$

should hold under restricted conditions. In this expression, c_2 is a constant, d is a length scale related to the soil grain size or pore diameter, μ is the viscosity of the fluid, and $\Delta p / \Delta L$ represents the pressure drop per column length. The derivation of this equation follows from dimensional analysis and the postulate that, for sufficiently low Reynolds numbers (Re $= dv_i \rho / \mu$, where v_i is the interstitial fluid velocity and ρ is the fluid density), the flow through a porous material should be analogous to viscous flow through a pipe, as described by Poiseuille's law (58). In deriving Equation 19 and throughout the discussion that follows, the effects of gravity are neglected.

Equation 19 can be converted to differential form by allowing ΔL to become infinitesimal. Then, if the soil permeability is constant and isotropic, Darcy's law may be written

$$\mathbf{v} = -\frac{k}{\mu} \nabla P \tag{20}$$

where $\mathbf{v}$ is the superficial velocity vector, i.e., the flow per unit geometrical area defined over a region large relative to individual pores but small relative to the overall dimensions of the soil; k is the intrinsic permeability as discussed in Section

2.2; and ∇P is the pressure gradient. This expression appears to be valid even if the permeability is not constant.

If the soil permeability is not isotropic, the permeability coefficient is replaced with a 3×3 permeability matrix, $\mathbf{K}$, and Darcy's law becomes (9, 12, 24)

$$\mathbf{v} = -\frac{1}{\mu} \mathbf{K} \cdot \nabla P \tag{21}$$

Given the superficial air velocity through soil, the radon activity flux per unit pore area due to convective flow is expressed by

$$\mathbf{J}_{Rn}^c = \frac{I_{Rn}\mathbf{v}}{\epsilon} \tag{22}$$

Darcy's law has been observed to break down as the Reynolds number increases. In contrast to viscous flow in pipes, for which Poiseuille's law remains valid for $Re < 2000$, experimental evidence has shown deviations from Darcy's law for Reynolds numbers in the range of 0.1–75 (12). In the case of pipe flow, the deviations are associated with the onset of turbulence. Deviations from Darcy's law with increasing Reynolds numbers are sometimes attributed to turbulence (86). It is more likely, however, that the flow remains laminar and that this effect is due to the emerging importance of the inertial term in the Navier-Stokes equation as the Reynolds number increases through order 1 (12, 58, 87, 88).

Under most circumstances, for the problem of radon entry into buildings, Darcy's law would be expected to hold in the soil. For a typical pressure gradient of 5 Pa m^{-1}, the Reynolds number is less than one for all soils having a permeability less than approximately 10^{-9} m^2, i.e., for all soils finer than gravel.

A second assumption in the development of Darcy's law is, as in the case of applying Fick's law to porous media, that the pores are large relative to the mean free path of the gas. Corrections are possible if this assumption is not true (12); however, determining the fluid velocity analytically becomes more difficult. It seems probable that this refinement is not of great importance in the problem at hand as the pores of soils through which convective flow is likely to be important are generally large relative to the mean free path.

If we assume that Darcy's law holds, we may combine Equation 20 or 21 with a continuity equation and an equation of state to obtain a governing equation for the pressure in the soil. By solving the governing equation for a specified geometry subject to appropriate boundary conditions on the pressure and/or the velocity, we may determine the convective velocity field in the soil, or , alternatively, the volume flow rate, e.g., into a building substructure. The velocity field is needed as input to analysis of the full transport equation, as discussed in the next section. The volume flow rate into the building, combined with an estimate of the radon concentration in the entering air, can be used to compute the radon entry rate attributable to convective flow.

For the remainder of the discussion in this section, we assume Darcy's law accurately describes airflow through soil, and that the soil is homogeneous and isotropic with respect to the permeability. It can be shown that, under these constraints, and for the problem of radon migration in soil, air in the soil may be treated as incompressible and, in steady state, the pressure satisfies the Laplace equation:

$$\nabla^2 P = 0 \qquad (23)$$

This is a classic equation in applied physics which arises in connection with problems other than fluid flow in porous media, including electrical potential in the vicinity of charged bodies (89), fluid flow at high Reynolds number outside the boundary layer (87), and heat conduction in solids (90). Consequently, there is a considerable literature on methods of solving Laplace's equation. Analytical solution methods include conformal mapping and separation of variables through a coordinate transformation (91). The latter approach can be valuable for radon entry if the building being investigated has, or can be approximated as having, certain symmetry (2, 92). A graphical technique called flow-net sketching is useful if the problem can be treated as two-dimensional and the pressure at the surface of the soil is assumed to be constant (9, 10). It yields the fluid streamlines and isopotential lines and can be used to estimate the velocity field and the total flow rate. Similar results with similar constraints can be obtained from an experimental technique using the electrical analog to the fluid flow problem (9). The most powerful and flexible technique is numerical modeling using a finite-element method (93). It is also the most costly to develop and implement.

Several workers have reported on investigations of aspects of convective radon migration in soil for applications other than radon entry into buildings (49, 94–100). Of particular interest are the results of the studies in New Mexico of radon exhalation from uncovered soil. Clements and Wilkening (98) found that barometric pressure changes of 1000–2000 Pa over a period of 1–2 days produced convective velocities of order 10^{-6} m s^{-1} at the surface of a soil with permeability of 10^{-12} m^2. The radon flux from the surface was thereby changed by 20–60% compared to the rate associated with molecular diffusion alone. We shall see that this is a small effect for a large change in pressure relative to the effects of pressure differences on radon entry into buildings.

In a later study in gravelly sandy loam in the same area, Schery et al. (100) concluded that among the possible environmental influences leading to temporal variation in radon exhalation, atmospheric pressure changes and rainfall were the most important. Effects due to temperature and wind were either comparatively small or undetectable. The time-averaged radon flux from the uncovered soil surface was close to that expected for pure molecular diffusion. Based on an observed inconsistency between the near-surface radon concentration profile and the measured flux density, the investigators suggested that a contribution to the exhalation rate may have resulted from direct flow through inhomogeneities.

These studies suggest that molecular diffusion dominates convection as a process by which radon enters the atmosphere from uncovered soil. As is discussed in more detail in subsequent sections, the reverse is often true for buildings. There are two major differences between these cases. First, a building's substructure shell is an effective barrier to molecular diffusion, thereby reducing its importance. Second, the geometry of a building and its operation lead to sustained pressure differences which may induce small, yet persistent, airflows into a building through the soil. Such sustained flows generally do not exist for horizontal surfaces of uncovered soil.

5.3 General Transport Equation

Following the discussion of the previous two sections, we may combine the effects of diffusion and convection into a general transport equation for radon migration in soil. For soil with negligible moisture content, the result is

$$\frac{\partial I_{Rn}}{\partial t} = \nabla \cdot D_e \nabla I_{Rn} - \nabla \cdot I_{Rn} \frac{\mathbf{v}}{\epsilon} + f \rho_s \frac{1-\epsilon}{\epsilon} A_{Ra} \lambda_{Rn} - \lambda_{Rn} I_{Rn} \qquad (24)$$

If the moisture content of the soil is large enough for a significant fraction of the radon in the pores to be dissolved in the liquid, the transport equation is written

$$\frac{1}{\epsilon} \frac{\partial (I_a \epsilon_a + I_w \epsilon_w)}{\partial t} = \nabla \cdot D'_e \nabla I_a - \nabla \cdot I_a \frac{\mathbf{v}'}{\epsilon_a}$$

$$+ f' \rho_s \frac{1-\epsilon}{\epsilon} A_{Ra} \lambda_{Rn} - \frac{1}{\epsilon} \lambda_{Rn} (I_a \epsilon_a + I_w \epsilon_w) \qquad (25)$$

where the primes indicate new values accounting for the moisture content and where we have neglected any moisture migration and any migration of radon within the water.

As previously noted, these equations have not been solved analytically, except for the simplest geometry (98, 100). Consequently, to make much progress, we are left with two approaches: approximate analysis and numerical modeling. In the remainder of this subsection, we discuss aspects of approximate analysis. In Section 6.3, recent research on modeling radon entry into buildings, a task that is still in its early stages of development, is briefly discussed.

The most significant simplification possible in this problem is to be able to neglect one of the transport processes—molecular diffusion or convection—as negligible compared with the other. To compare the relative importance of the two processes, we make some simplifying assumptions to Equation 24, then make the equation dimensionless. The simplifying assumptions are that (i) the superficial velocity is described by Darcy's law; (ii) the soil is isotropic and homogeneous with respect to the diffusion coefficient, permeability, porosity, emanating fraction, radium content, and bulk density; and (iii) for the range of pressures of interest, air may be treated as incompressible. Then we may write

$$\frac{\partial I_{Rn}}{\partial t} = D_e \nabla^2 I_{Rn} + \frac{k}{\epsilon\mu} \nabla P \cdot \nabla I_{Rn} + G - \lambda_{Rn} I_{Rn} \qquad (26)$$

where G is defined by Equation 13.

To make the equation dimensionless (see, e.g., Ref. 58), we multiply and divide each variable by a unqiue combination of a characteristic time λ_{Rn}^{-1}, length L, and pressure difference ΔP_o, as needed to make each dimensionless. Having done so, we may write Equation 26 as

$$\frac{1}{N_\tau} \frac{\partial I_{Rn}^*}{\partial t^*} = \frac{1}{Pe_p} \nabla^{*2} I_{Rn}^* + \nabla^* P^* \cdot \nabla^* I_{Rn}^* + \frac{1}{N_\tau}(G^* - I^*) \qquad (27)$$

where the asterisks denote dimensionless quantities. This equation has two dimensionless groups

$$Pe_p = k\epsilon\Delta P_o(\mu D_e)^{-1} \qquad (27a)$$

and

$$N_\tau = \Delta P_o k(\mu\epsilon L^2 \lambda_{Rn})^{-1} \qquad (27b)$$

The dimensionless groups are important variables: Pe_p, effectively a Péclet number for mass transfer in a porous medium, characterizes the relative importance of convective transport with respect to diffusive transport, and N_τ characterizes the relative importance of radioactive decay with respect to convective flow as a means of removing radon from the soil pores.

Based on the values of these groups, we may simplify the problem as follows. First, if $Pe_p \gg 1$, diffusion may be neglected compared with convective flow as a transport process, and the governing equation in dimensional form becomes

$$\frac{\partial I_{Rn}}{\partial t} = \frac{k}{\epsilon\mu} \nabla P \cdot \nabla I_{Rn} + G - \lambda_{Rn} I_{Rn} \qquad (28)$$

If $Pe_p \gg 1$ and $N_\tau \gg 1$, the problem may be treated in steady state and radioactive decay neglected. The resulting equation is analogous to the convective heat transfer problem with internal sources in which conduction and viscous dissipation may be neglected (90).

If $Pe_p \ll 1$, convective transport may be neglected. The concentration is governed by the diffusion equation (Equation 12). Finally, if $Pe_p \ll 1$ and $N_\tau \gg Pe_p$, the problem reduces to Poisson's equation:

$$\nabla^2 I_{Rn} + \frac{G}{D_e} = 0 \tag{29}$$

Soil permeability is the most important parameter in determining which, if any, of these conditions is satisfied. Choosing typical values of $\Delta P_o = 3$ Pa, $\epsilon = 0.5$, $\mu = 17 \times 10^{-6}$ kg m^{-1} s^{-1}, and $D_e = 2 \times 10^{-6}$ m^2 s^{-1}, then $Pe_p = 1$ if $k = 2.3 \times 10^{-11}$ m^2. Assuming these typical values apply, then for soils with much larger permeabilities, i.e., coarse sands and gravels, transport by molecular diffusion can be neglected. For soils with much smaller permeabilities, i.e., silts and clays not having significant structural permeability, convective transport can be neglected. If we further take $L = 3$ m as the scale of soil length through which transport must be considered, then the permeability at which $N_\tau = 1$ is 5×10^{-11} m^2.

6 RADON ENTRY INTO BUILDINGS

6.1 Pressure-Generating Mechanisms

6.1.1 Wind. Consider the wind blowing directly on the side of a house. In the simplest model, if we neglect the shear stress between the wind and the ground, the change in momentum from the free-stream velocity must equal the increase in pressure at the wall where the velocity falls to zero. Hence

$$\Delta P_o = \tfrac{1}{2} \rho v^2 \tag{30}$$

where ρ is the air density, v is the velocity, and ΔP_o is the pressure at the wall minus the free-stream pressure. This equation may readily be derived from the one-dimensional, steady-state form of the Navier-Stokes equation, i.e., from a momentum balance, assuming the Reynolds number is much greater than one, a condition that for the case at hand is always satisfied.

Actual wind-induced pressures across the walls of a house are moderated from this simple calculation by several factors. Winds generally strike a house obliquely, reducing pressures. The height of a typical house is small enough that the effect of the ground on reducing wind speed is significant. Furthermore, houses are often shielded by other structures and vegetation. In accounting for these effects, wind engineers write Equation 30 as

$$\Delta P = C_d \left(\tfrac{1}{2} \rho v^2 \right) \tag{31}$$

where C_d is called the drag or pressure coefficient. It is determined empirically, often from wind tunnel studies. It is found to be relatively independent of wind speed, but greatly dependent on small details of shape, orientation, and shielding (101). In one study, ground-level data for an impermeable cube in a boundary-layer velocity profile indicated an average drag coefficient of 0.56 on the windward side, −0.49 on the side walls, and −0.15 on the leeward side (102).

These data apply only at the base of the walls, whereas for the problem of radon entry, we are interested in the pressures at the ground surface at distances up to several meters from the walls. A wind tunnel investigation of this matter was recently conducted (77). The results, reproduced in Figure 2.8, show drag coefficients on the windward side of 0.2–0.5 extending distances comparable to the house dimensions.

Taking 0.4 and 3 m s^{-1} as representative values of the windward drag coefficient and wind speed, respectively, and assuming the pressure inside the house is the same as the free-stream conditions, we obtain a pressure difference across the soil and substructure on the windward side of approximately 2 Pa. Note that the pressure difference varies as the square of the wind speed, so that considerably larger pressure differences are possible.

Pressures induced by winds can fluctuate rapidly; so it is important to consider how rapidly pressure fluctuations at the surface of the soil are transmitted through it. This question has been addressed theoretically by Fukuda (103), who obtained

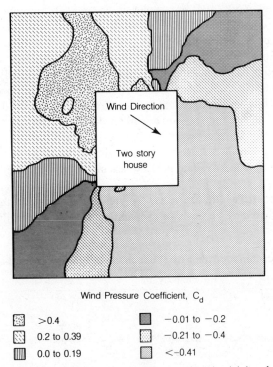

Wind Pressure Coefficient, C_d

>0.4		−0.01 to −0.2	
0.2 to 0.39		−0.21 to −0.4	
0.0 to 0.19		<−0.41	

Figure 2.8. Wind pressure coefficient, C_d, at ground surface in vicinity of a model two-story house. Measurements were conducted in a wind tunnel. From Ref. 77. Illustration after A. G. Scott, used by permission.

the following governing equation for the pressure fluctuations, φ, assuming them to be much smaller than the atmospheric pressure, P_a:

$$\frac{\partial \varphi}{\partial t} = \frac{k}{\epsilon \mu} P_a \nabla^2 \varphi \qquad (32)$$

where the symbols are as previously defined. This is the diffusion equation; the term $D_p = kP_a(\mu\epsilon)^{-1}$ is a "diffusion coefficient" for pressure disturbances. If, for simplicity, we consider a one-dimensional case, then the characteristic time for a pressure disturbance to propagate through a distance L_p is given by

$$\tau_p = \frac{L_p^2}{D_p} \qquad (33)$$

Values of τ_p for $L_p = 1$ m and 5 m for different soil types are given in Table 2.7. For sandy and gravelly soils, propagation times are minutes or less, whereas for clayey soils, pressure disturbances can take many days to propagate.

Van der Hoven analyzed the spectral distribution of the wind speed at 100 m at Brookhaven, New York (104). As shown in Figure 2.9, reproduced from his results, the wind energy distribution is roughly bimodal, with the low-frequency mode having a peak corresponding to a period of 4 days and the high-frequency mode having a peak at a frequency of about 1 minute. A large spectral gap for periods from about 10 minutes to 2 hours is believed to be generally present. From these data we can conclude that for soils with sufficiently high permeabilities for pressure-driven flow to be important, a large fraction of the wind power is sufficiently sustained so that the pressure disturbance is completely propagated through the soil and a steady-state pressure distribution may be assumed. However, a significant portion of the wind energy occurs with fluctuations at sufficiently high frequency so that the steady-state pressure assumption is not strictly valid.

6.1.2 Temperature Differences. A pressure differential that varies with height exists across any vertical wall separating air masses of different tempera-

TABLE 2.7 Characteristic Times for Propagation of Pressure Disturbances in Soil[a]

Soil type	Permeability (m^2)	τ_p ($L_p = 1$ m)	τ_p ($L_p = 5$ m)
Clay	10^{-16}	10 d	250 d
Sandy clay	5×10^{-15}	5 h	5 d
Silt	5×10^{-14}	30 min	12 h
Sandy silt and gravel	5×10^{-13}	3 min	75 min
Fine sand	5×10^{-12}	18 s	450 s
Medium sand	10^{-10}	0.9 s	23 s
Gravel	10^{-8}	0.01 s	0.2 s

[a]$\tau_p = (L_p^2 \mu\epsilon)(P_a k)^{-1}$; $\mu = 17.5 \times 10^{-6}$ kg m^{-1} s^{-1}, $\epsilon = 0.5$, $P_a = 1.01 \times 10^5$ Pa.

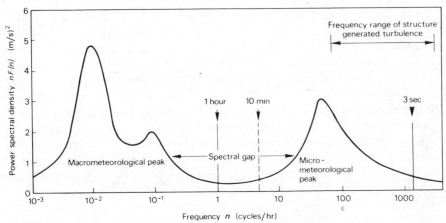

Figure 2.9. Horizontal wind-speed frequency spectrum measured at approximately 100 m height at Brookhaven, NY. From I. Van der Hoven (1957), *Journal of Meteorology,* **14**, 160. By permission of the American Meteorological Society.

tures. Otherwise known as the "stack effect," this pressure difference arises because air is a compressible fluid, whose density varies with temperature, and which is acted upon by gravity.

Consider a wall of height H separating air masses of temperature T_i and T_o. If we assume that the ideal gas law applies and that the temperature on either side of the wall is constant, then the conditions of fluid statics require that the pressure vary with height on either side of the wall according to

$$P = P_o e^{-mgz/RT} \qquad (34)$$

where P_o is the pressure at reference height $z = 0$; m is the molar weight of air (0.029 kg mol^{-1}); g is the acceleration of gravity (9.8 m s^{-2}); R is the universal gas constant (8.31 J mol^{-1} K^{-1}); and T is temperature. If we now define z_o as the height at which the pressures on either side of the wall are equal, then we find that the pressure difference across the walls is

$$\Delta P(z) \approx \alpha \left[\frac{1}{T_i} - \frac{1}{T_o} \right] (z - z_o) \qquad (35)$$

where $\alpha = 3454$ Pa m^{-1} K. In deriving Equation 35 we have made the approximation $e^{-x} \approx 1 - x$, valid for $x \ll 1$. As with wind-induced pressure differences, a positive ΔP implies a net inward pressure.

A representative situation has $T_i = 293$ K, $T_o = 273$ K, and $z_o = 3$ m, so that $\Delta P(0) = 2.6$ Pa. Since $|T_o - T_i| \ll T_o$ or T_i for any situation involving an occupied building, the pressure difference due to the stack effect is approximately proportional to the temperature difference.

6.1.3   Other Processes. Several other processes can, in principle, lead to convective flow of soil air into or through building substructures. Here we shall consider two factors: barometric pressure changes and precipitation. These processes are complex, and relatively little work pertaining to them has been reported. Consequently, our discussion will be brief and qualitative.

Compared with the pressure changes associated with winds and temperature differences, the magnitude of barometric pressure changes is large, with excursions from the long-term average routinely exceeding 100 Pa. However, these pressure changes can be effective in inducing the flow of soil air into a building only if they lead to a sustained difference in pressure between the indoor air and the pore air of the nearby soil. An inverse correlation between indoor radon concentration and the rate of change of barometric pressure was observed in the basement of a house in Princeton, New Jersey, during the late spring (69). The authors inferred that the short-term variation in radon entry rate exceeded an order of magnitude for rates of change in pressure from -76 to 45 Pa h^{-1} (-0.75 to 0.44 mbar h^{-1}). In another study, no correlation between radon entry rate into a house with a basement and rate of barometric pressure change was apparent (2).

Although there has been no experimental verification, one might expect to find the influence of barometric pressure changes to be substantial for a house with a basement in relatively permeable soil at a time when the surface of the soil was frozen. Under such circumstances, barometric pressure changes could lead to a flow of soil gas that is ''funneled'' through the basement as a result of the reduced permeability at the surface of the surrounding soil. A similar situation might exist for buildings with any type of substructure immediately following a heavy rain. Still another case where radon entry rate may be strongly correlated with barometric pressure changes is one in which landscaping has resulted in a low permeability cap over a relatively highly permeable soil.

One expects that the effect of barometric pressure changes on radon entry rate would also depend on the depth of the soil to an impermeable zone. If the air reservoir in the soil were restricted to a small depth below the foundation and above a low permeability layer (e.g., clay or water table), barometric pressure changes should be relatively ineffective in inducing flow.

Through a pistonlike displacement of soil air, a heavy rainfall could potentially lead to a short-term increase in radon entry rate independent of the barometric pressure. At such a time, the permeability of the wet soil surrounding the house is considerably smaller than that of the dry soil beneath it; hence, radon-bearing soil gas could be forced through penetrations in the substructure. Evidence that such an effect might occur is shown in Figure 2.10. During the two-day period of March 29–30, 1983, coincident with a heavy rainfall, radon concentrations indoors and in the crawl space rose to their highest values for the entire 5-week monitoring period. The investigators could not rule out the possibility that the increased concentrations were due to a reduction in permeability of the surrounding soil combined with the concurrent drop in barometric pressure (64).

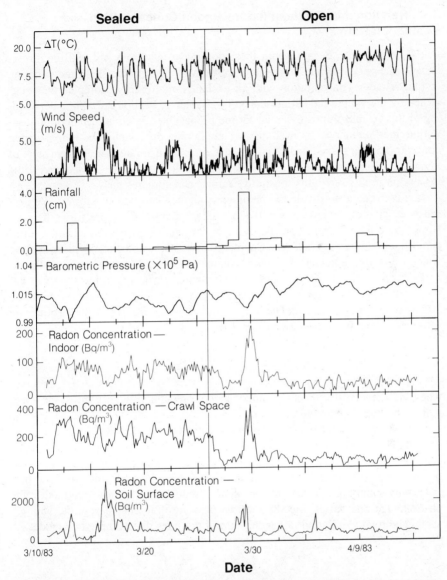

Figure 2.10. ^{222}Rn and meteorological measurements made over a 5-week period at a house with a crawl space in Portland, Oregon. The crawl-space vents were sealed during the first two weeks and open during the final 3 weeks. An episode of enhanced radon flux into the crawl space and house on March 29–30 corresponds to a period of heavy rainfall coupled with a modest drop in barometric pressure. ΔT represents the indoor-outdoor temperature difference. Reproduced from Ref. 64.

6.2 Relationship Between Indoor Radon Concentration and Ventilation Rate

6.2.1 Analysis. Because both the radon entry rate from soil and the air-exchange rate vary with pressure differences across the building shell, the variation of indoor radon concentration with air-exchange rate is more complex than suggested by the simple model introduced in Chapter 1, Section 2.2. An understanding of this relationship is essential for the proper interpretation of indoor concentration measurements, as well as for predicting the change in indoor radon concentration for a specified change in the air-exchange rate. The present state of knowledge is not sufficient to address all possible situations. Consequently, the discussion in this section is illustrative rather than comprehensive.

It is convenient to divide the radon entry modes into two categories. We designate as "passive" those modes that act independently of the pressure difference across the building shell. Specific examples of passive entry are molecular diffusion from building materials (see Chapter 3) and release associated with household water use (see Chapter 4). By contrast, modes that are limited by the rate of pressure-driven flow through the building substructure are designated as "active" entry mechanisms. High rates of radon entry from soil into residential basements are largely due to active modes. The total radon entry rate may be written as the sum of contributions from these two modes:

$$S_v = S_p + S_a(\Delta P_f) \tag{36}$$

where ΔP_f denotes the effective outdoor-indoor pressure difference across the lower part of the building structure.

It is likewise useful to distinguish two ventilation modes. In "balanced" systems the air-exchange rate is effectively independent of the pressure difference across the building shell. A mechanical ventilation system that provides equal supply and exhaust flows is balanced. Infiltration and mechanical ventilation that provides only supply or exhaust are considered "unbalanced" ventilation modes: the air-exchange rate varies directly with the pressure difference across the building shell. The total ventilation rate is the sum of the rates due to these two modes:

$$\lambda_v = \lambda_{v,b} + \lambda_{v,u}(\Delta P) \tag{37}$$

where ΔP is a characteristic pressure difference, such as the mean of the absolute value, across the building envelope.

The unbalanced ventilation component is related to the average pressure difference across the building shell by a power-law relationship (105):

$$\lambda_{v,u} = \frac{E}{V}(\Delta P)^n \qquad 0.5 < n < 1.0 \tag{38}$$

where E is the permeability coefficient of the building envelope (with dimensions $L^{3+n} T^{2n-1} M^{-n}$) and V is the interior volume. E is equal to the product $A_o(2/\rho)^n$, where A_o is the effective leakage area of the envelope (105).

The characteristic pressure difference can be estimated as the sum of three components—those due to temperature differences, wind, and unbalanced mechanical ventilation. (Flow from a chimney would be considered in the last of these categories.)

$$\Delta P = (\rho/2) f_s^2 \left| T_o - T_i \right| + (\rho/2) f_w^2 v^2 + \left| \Delta P_{mv,u} \right| \tag{39}$$

where ρ is the air density, and f_s and f_w are stack and wind parameters (see Chapter 1, Section 8.2 and Ref. 105).

The value of the exponent in Equation 38 is determined by the relative importance of two energy-loss mechanisms as air flows through the penetrations in the building shell. For penetrations that have relatively large width and short length, energy loss is largely due to the inertia of the air at the outlet of the crack. If this is the dominant situation for the structure, the value of the exponent approaches 0.5 for reasons that are analogous to the square-root dependence of the pressure difference with wind speed (see Equation 30). The other limiting case is fully developed laminar flow in the cracks. This case occurs if the cracks are long and narrow and if the flow has a small Reynolds number. In this case, viscous dissipation is the dominant energy loss mechanism. This flow regime is analogous to the flow through soil described by Darcy's law (Equation 20); the exponent in Equation 38 approaches 1.0 in the limit in which this mode dominates. Measurements of n yield values in the range 0.5–0.75 (106, 107). The value $n = 0.5$ has been adopted in a commonly used infiltration model (105).

The variation of the active component of the radon entry rate with pressure difference depends on both the mode of entry and the details of the building-soil air coupling. To be specific, we consider the common example of a house with a basement that has a perimeter penetration such as a crack at the floor-wall joint or a drain tile connected through an untrapped pipe to a basement sump (see also Chapter 10). For small source rates, the concentration of radon in the entering soil gas is independent of the flow rate and, consequently, independent of pressure difference. In this case, assuming that the effective pressure at the base of one or more of the walls is inward (i.e., ΔP_f is positive), $S_a \propto (\Delta P_f)$. On the other hand, if the source rate is large, the soil gas is depleted, and the influence of changes in pressure difference on radon entry is diminished. A theoretical analysis of this situation has shown that $S_a \propto (\Delta P_f)^{0.66}$ in this case, again assuming $\Delta P_f > 0$ (108). If ΔP_f is negative, i.e., the pressure across the building substructure is outward, we expect $S_a \cong 0$. These conditions are summarized by

$$S_a = \begin{cases} 0, & \Delta P_f < 0 \\ \beta(\Delta P_f)^m & \Delta P_f > 0, \quad 0.66 < m < 1.0 \end{cases} \tag{40}$$

where the coefficient β depends on the radium content and emanation coefficient of the soil, on the permeability of the soil, and on the coupling between the building interior and the soil air.

In analogy with Equation 39, ΔP_f can be expressed as the sum of three components (109):

$$\Delta P_f = \rho g (z - z_o) \frac{T_o - T_i}{T_o} + c_f \rho \frac{v^2}{2} + \Delta P_{mv,u} \tag{41}$$

where the thermal effect is an approximation of Equation 35 and c_f is an average pressure coefficient for the lower part of the structure (cf. Equation 31).

We may now write a general expression for the indoor radon concentration for this case. We may rewrite Equation 1 from Chapter 1 as

$$I - I_o = S_v / \lambda_v \tag{42}$$

where we have assumed $\lambda_v \gg d$, the radon decay constant (denoted λ_{Rn} elsewhere in this chapter). Substituting Equations 36, 40, and 41 for S_v and Equations 37–39 for λ_v, and assuming that $\Delta P_f > 0$, we obtain

$$I - I_o = \frac{S_p + \beta \left(\rho g (z - z_o) \dfrac{T_o - T_i}{T_o} + c_f \rho \dfrac{v^2}{2} + \Delta P_{mv,u} \right)^m}{\lambda_{v,b} + \dfrac{D}{V} \left[\rho \dfrac{f_s^2}{2} \left| T_o - T_i \right| + \rho f_w^2 \dfrac{v^2}{2} + \left| \Delta P_{mv,u} \right| \right]^n} \tag{43}$$

It is instructive to consider two limiting cases. In case a, we assume that the active entry rate is zero. In this case, $I - I_o = S_p / \lambda_v$, and we recover the simple result presented in Chapter 1. In case b, we assume first that $S_p = 0$ and $\lambda_{v,b} = 0$. We also assume that the ratios $\Delta T : v^2 : \Delta P_{mv,u}$ remain constant. The latter assumption would hold, for example, if one of the three terms greatly dominated the other two for both ΔP and ΔP_f. In this case, $I - I_o \propto (\Delta P)^{m-n}$. And, since $\lambda_v \propto (\Delta P)^n$, we obtain the result

$$I - I_o \propto \lambda_v^{[(m-n)/n]} \tag{44}$$

These results are presented in Figure 2.11. For much of case b, the indoor radon concentration is expected to increase with ventilation rate. Note, however, that many assumptions went into this analysis. For example, we implicitly assumed that a single pressure difference ΔP_f could be used to represent the entire base of the building. Although this is reasonable for the thermal and unbalanced mechanical ventilation components, wind pressures are highly directional. A more thorough analysis would treat the walls separately. In addition, the assumption that the pressures due to thermal effects, wind, and unbalanced ventilation remain in con-

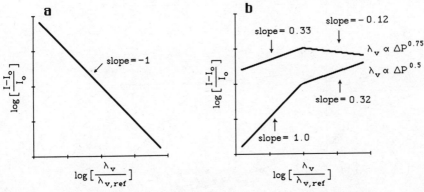

Figure 2.11. Relationship between radon concentration and air-exchange rate for a single structure. In case *a* it is assumed that either the ventilation system is entirely balanced or the radon entry mode is entirely passive. Case *b* represents the other extreme: the entry mode is active and the ventilation mode is unbalanced. In addition, the relative contributions of temperature difference, wind, and mechanical ventilation to the pressure difference are assumed to remain constant for case *b*. $\lambda_{v,ref}$ is an arbitrary, constant air-exchange rate.

stant proportion limits the applicability of this result. Mowris, in analyzing the effect of adding exhaust ventilation to houses, found consistent reduction of indoor radon concentration (109). In any case, it is clear that the relationship between indoor radon concentration and air-exchange rate is a complex one that varies considerably with the particular circumstances of a house.

6.2.2 *Experimental Results.*

The relationship between indoor radon concentration and air-exchange rate in a single house has been examined in detail in two studies. In the first, the ventilation rate in a house with a very low infiltration rate (<0.1 h^{-1}) was varied by means of a balanced mechanical ventilation system (110). As expected, the radon concentration varied as predicted by Equation 42.

In the second study, indoor radon concentration and air-exchange rate were monitored continuously in a house with a basement over a 5-month period (2). In this case, the changes in air-exchange rate were due to a combination of changing weather conditions, the intermittent use of a fireplace and exhaust fans, and the opening of doors and windows. A confounding feature of this experiment in the present context was the bimodal nature of the radon entry rate. It appeared that major pathways for radon entry could be either opened or closed, perhaps owing to changing moisture levels in the nearby soil.

The variation of radon concentration with air-exchange rate from this study is presented in Figure 2.12. In the case of high entry rate (open triangles), the variation is similar to the prediction of Equation 44 with $n = 0.75$ (cf. Fig. 2.11b). For the low-entry-rate case, the behavior is more complex, perhaps indicating that neither passive or active entry modes are dominant.

The curves plotted in Figure 2.12 reflect the predictions of two models. The

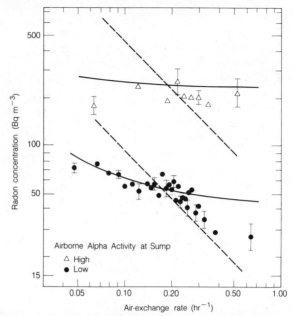

Figure 2.12. Scatter plot of ^{222}Rn concentration versus air-exchange rate averaged over three-hour periods. Measurements were made continuously at a house with a basement in Chicago over a 5-month period. Data were sorted into two groups according to radon concentration above a sump in the basement: the concentration at this point during the "high" periods averaged greater than 10,000 Bq m^{-3}; for "low" periods the average was less than 500 Bq m^{-3}. Each data point gives the geometric mean radon concentration of 19–21 measurements that have been grouped according to air-exchange rate. Error bars represent one geometric standard deviation of the mean. The dashed lines represent the expected relationship if the radon entry rate is independent of air-exchange rate. The solid lines reflect a model in which radon entry is presumed to have two components—one (diffusive) being constant, the other (convective) being proportional to air-exchange rate. Reproduced from Ref. 2.

dashed line corresponds to Equation 42 with $I \gg I_o$. The solid line reflects a simplified two-component entry model. In particular, the active entry component is assumed to be proportional to the infiltration rate. This would be expected if the exponent in Equation 38 was $n = 1$, and if the source rate was small. D'Ottavio and Dietz showed, by extending the formulation of this model to incorporate radon entering from outdoor air and the variability of radon concentration in soil air, that a better fit to a portion of the data could be obtained (111).

6.3 Modeling Radon Entry

The complexities associated with the production and migration of radon in soil, and its entry into buildings point to the need for detailed mathematical models to develop a complete understanding of the effects of the many factors involved. The development of such a model has been undertaken (7, 75–77). In this work, a finite-element approach is used, with the soil comprising 1780 variable-sized elements. The model has thus far been restricted to examining uniform and isotropic soils, houses with basements, radon transport due to convective flow, and pressure gradients arising from temperature differences and wind. Nevertheless, some interesting and useful results have been obtained: for one case, an increase in permeability from 10^{-11} to 10^{-10} m^2 led to an increase in radon entry rate by a factor of 4.5 (7); variations in wind speed and direction can lead to substantial changes in radon entry rate in the absence of other factors (77); for a typical Canadian house with surrounding soil having a radium content of 59 Bq kg^{-1} and permeability 5 $\times$ 10^{-11} m^2, the average radon entry rate and radon concentration would be 4 $\times$ 10^7 Bq h^{-1}, and approximately 200 Bq m^{-3}, respectively (77).

Recently, a finite difference model and a simplified analytical model were developed for computing soil gas entry rates into crawl space and basement houses (109, 120). The models have been used to examine the effect of exhaust ventilation on radon entry rates and indoor concentrations. They clearly have broader application.

Loureiro has developed perhaps the most general model of radon entry to date (121). Based again on a finite-difference method, the model simulates radon migration by both diffusion and convection in the vicinity of a basement having a floor–wall gap. An aggregate layer adjacent to the basement may be specified to have distinct characteristics from the remainder of the soil.

7 GEOGRAPHICAL CHARACTERIZATION

The importance of soil as a source of indoor radon, combined with the increasing evidence of unacceptably high radon concentrations in a significant fraction of houses, has raised the question of whether one might predict on a geographical basis where high indoor radon levels are likely to be found. If a method to achieve this were developed and validated, the cost of identifying houses with elevated levels could be considerably reduced. The case that such an effort could succeed is strengthened by the direct observation that there is a substantial variance in the mean indoor radon concentration among different areas (8). (See also Chapters 1 and 12, especially Figure 12.4.)

Several pertinent sources of information may be useful in a geographical characterization effort. From the discussion in this chapter, we may say that the potential for high radon entry rates depends on several factors: the radium content of the soil; the temporal state of the soil, particularly its moisture content; the soil permeability; and the weather—particularly temperature, wind, and rainfall. In the United States, information on these variables is available from the Department of Energy's National Uranium Resource Evaluation program (results distributed by the U.S. Geological Survey), the Department of Agriculture's Soil Conservation Service reports, and the Department of Commerce's National Climatic Center reports. The present state of knowledge concerning the relevance of these data to estimating radon source potential on a geographical basis is reported in a recent paper (112).

An important factor that is not completely understood is the extent to which some of these parameters vary over relevant spatial scales. The uncertainty is most evident with respect to permeability, which, because of the broad range of values it may have, is perhaps the most important of the determining variables. For geographical characterization to be useful, variations in permeability over a scale at least as large as a substantial fraction of a community must be of a comparable size to variations on a house-to-house basis.

One approach to geographical characterization that has been proposed is the development of a radon index number (RIN) that would combine the major factors determining radon entry into a single variable (76, 77). The proposed formulations have considered weather effects to be constant for a given area and, hence, do not incorporate them into the RIN. Building ventilation rates have been explicitly incorporated into one proposal, however. The two forms are given below.

$$\text{RIN} = \frac{hA_{Ra}}{-\log k} \tag{45}$$

where h is the inverse average air-exchange rate, A_{Ra} is the radium activity concentration of the soil, and k is the permeability (76).

$$\text{RIN} = \log A_{Ra} + 0.45 \log k \tag{46}$$

where the factor 0.45 was based on numerical modeling of radon entry as previously described (77).

Several other studies have addressed the topic of geographical characterization. In Sweden, "GEO-radiation" maps have been produced from airborne radiometric surveys, ground measurements of gamma radiation, and geological mapping (113, 114). The purpose of these maps is to document areas and rock types with gamma emission levels exceeding $7.7 \times 10^{-9} \text{ C kg}^{-1} \text{ h}^{-1}$ (30 μR h^{-1}), with the intention of identifying areas at risk for high indoor radon levels due to entry from soil. Kothari and Han (115) have shown a correlation for nine U.S. communities between the geometric mean indoor radon concentration and the geometric mean equivalent uranium (eU) concentration of the soil, as determined from an aerial radiometric survey. Figure 2.13, based on their results, shows that the order-of-magnitude range in eU is associated with roughly a factor-of-five range in indoor radon concentrations. Moed et al. (40) examined the aerial radiometric data from the NURE program for the western U.S., and produced the map of surface ^{226}Ra concentrations shown in Figure 2.5. They also showed that the variations in the aerial data corresponded to differences in radium content, radon flux, and gamma emission rate measured at the ground. Duval (116) has developed a technique of producing composite color images from the NURE data that may prove to be a useful tool in geographical characterization of radon source potential.

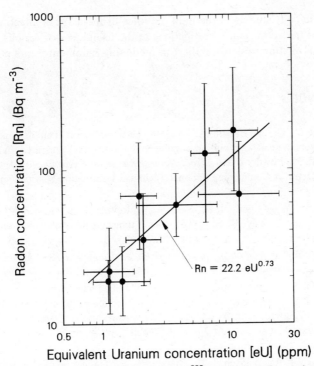

Figure 2.13. Scatter plot of geometric mean indoor ^{222}Rn concentration and soil equivalent uranium concentration for nine U.S. communities. Error bars indicate one geometric standard deviation. Each point represents radon measurements in 8–69 houses. Equivalent uranium concentration was determined from an analysis of airborne radiometric (NARR) data. 1 ppm equivalent uranium equals 12.4 Bq kg^{-1}. Data from Ref. 115.

8   CONCLUSIONS

Within the past decade the consensus concerning the nature and extent of the problem of radon in indoor air has been radically revised. Rather than being a problem that arises due to molecular diffusion of radon from industrially contaminated building materials or fill materials, we now recognize that the vast majority of structures with elevated indoor concentrations are unexceptional in other regards. In most cases, radon enters predominantly via the substructure through the combined effects of molecular diffusion and convective flow. The importance of the convective flow process is seen in the considerable success of control measures directed at blocking entry pathways or reversing the ordinary direction of flow, as discussed in Chapter 10.

Despite our considerable progress, much work remains before we can, first, confidently assert that we understand the sources of indoor radon and, second, fully exploit that understanding in reducing exposures. Key areas requiring further work include continued development of numerical models of the process of radon migration in soil, studies of the multiple roles of moisture in affecting radon emanation and transport, and investigations of the usefulness of various data, particularly those relating to permeability, in predicting radon entry rate potential.

REFERENCES

1. George, A. C., and Breslin, A. J. (1980). The distribution of ambient radon and radon daughters in residential buildings in the New Jersey–New York area. In T. F., Gesell, and W. M. Lowder (eds.), *Proc. Natural Radiation Environment III*, Conf-780422, U.S. Dept. of Commerce, National Technical Information Service, Springfield, VA p. 1272.

2. Nazaroff, W. W., Feustel, H., Nero, A. V., Revzan, K. L. Grimsrud, D. T., Essling, M. A., and Toohey, R. E. (1985). Radon transport into a detached one-story house with a basement, *Atmos. Environ.*, **19**, 31.

3. *Proc. Third Workshop on Radon and Radon Daughters Associated with Uranium Mining and Processing* (1980). Atomic Energy Control Board, Ottawa, Canada.

4. Ericson, S. O., and Schmied, H. (1984). Modified technology in new constructions, and cost effective remedial action in existing structures, to prevent infiltration of soil gas carrying radon. In B. Berglund, T. Lindvall, and J. Sundell (eds.), *Indoor Air: Buildings, Ventilation and Thermal Climate*, vol. 5, Swedish Council for Building Research, Stockholm, p. 153.

5. Nitschke, I. A., Wadach, J. B., Clarke, W. A., Traynor, G. W., Adams, G. P., and Rizzuto, J. E. (1984). A detailed study of inexpensive radon control techniques in New York State houses. In B. Berglund, T. Lindvall, and J. Sundell (eds.), *Indoor Air: Buildings, Ventilation and Thermal Climate*, vol. 5, Swedish Council for Building Research, Stockholm, p. 111.

6. Bruno, R. C. (1983). Sources of indoor radon in houses: A review, *J. Air Pollut. Contr. Assoc.*, **33**, 105.

7. DSMA Atcon, Ltd. (1983). Review of existing instrumentation and evaluation of possibilities for research and development of instrumentation to determine future levels of radon at a proposed building site, report INFO-0096, Atomic Energy Control Board, Ottawa.

8. Nero, A. V., Schwehr, M. B., Nazaroff, W. W., and Revzan, K. L. (1986). Distribution of airborne radon-222 concentrations in U.S. homes, *Science*, **234**, 992.

9. Scott, R. F., (1963). *Principles of Soil Mechanics*, Addison-Wesley, Reading, MA.

10. Terzaghi, K., and Peck, R. B. (1967). *Soil Mechanics in Engineering Practice*, 2nd ed., Wiley, New York.

11. Baver, L. D. (1940). *Soil Physics*, Wiley, New York.

12. Scheidegger, A. E. (1960). *The Physics of Flow Through Porous Media*, 2nd ed., Macmillan, New York.

13. Muskat, M. (1946). *The Flow of Homogeneous Fluids Through Porous Media*, Edwards, Ann Arbor, MI.

14. Collins, R. E. (1961). *Flow of Fluids Through Porous Materials*, Reinhold, New York.

15. *Symp. on Flow Through Porous Media* (1969). American Chemical Society Publications, Washington, DC.

16. Childs, E. C. (1969). *An Introduction to the Physical Basis of Soil Water Phenomena*, Wiley, London.

17. Marshall, T. J. and Holmes, J. W. (1979). *Soil Physics*, Cambridge University Press, London, p. 12.

18. Corey, A. T. (1957). Measurement of water and air permeability in unsaturated soil, *Soil Sci. Soc. Am. Proc.*, **21**, 7.

19. Botset, H. G. (1940). Flow of gas-liquid mixtures through consolidated sand, *Am. Inst. Mining Eng. Trans.*, **136,** 91.

20. Osaba, J. S., Richardson, J. G., Kerver, J. K., Hafford, J. A., and Blair, P. M. (1951). Laboratory measurements of relative permeability, *Am. Inst. Mining Eng. Trans.*, **192,** 47.

21. Mitchell, T. K., Hooper, D. R., and Campanella, R. G. (1965). Permeability of compacted clay, *Am. Soc. Civil Eng. Proc.*, **SM4,** 41.

22. Barden, L., and Pavlakis, G. (1971). Air and water permeability of compacted unsaturated cohesive soil, *J. Soil Sci.*, **22,** 302.

23. Garcia-Bengochea, I., Lovell, C. W., and Altschaeffl, A. G. (1979). Pore distribution and permeability of silty clays, *Proc. ASCE*, **105,** 839.

24. Rice, P. A., Fontugne, D. J., Latini, R. G., and Barduhn, A. J. (1969). Anisotropic permeability in porous media. In *Symp. on Flow Through Porous Media*, American Chemical Society Publications, Washington, DC. p. 48.

25. Bowles, J. E. (1979). *Physical and Geotechnical Properties of Soils*, McGraw-Hill, New York, p. 213.

26. Topp, G. C., Zabcuk, W. D., and Dumanski, J. (1980). The variation of in-situ measured soil water properties within soil map units, *Can J. Soil Sci.*, **60,** 497.

27. McKeague, J. A., Wang, C., and Topp, G. C. (1982). Estimating saturated hydraulic conductivity from soil morphology, *Soil Sci. Soc. Am. J.*, **46,** 1239.

28. Wilkening, M. H., Clements, W. E., and Stanley, D. (1972). Radon-222 flux measurements in widely separated regions. In J. A. S. Adams, W. M. Lowder, and T. F. Gesell (eds.), *Proc. Natural Radiation Environment II*, Conf-720805, U.S. Dept. of Commerce, National Technical Information Service, Springfield, VA, p. 717.

29. Pearson, J. E., and Jones, G. E. (1965). Emanation of radon 222 from soils and its use as a tracer, *J. Geophys. Res.*, **70,** 5279.

30. Fleischer, R. L., and Mogro-Campero, A. (1980). Techniques and principles for mapping integrated radon emanation within the earth. In T. F. Gesell and W. M. Lowder (eds.), *Natural Radiation Environment III*, Conf-780422, U.S. Dept. of Commerce, National Technical Information Service, Springfield, VA, p. 57.

31. Silker, W. B., and Kalkwarf, D. R. (1983). Radon diffusion in candidate soils for covering uranium mill tailings, report NUREG/CR-2924, PNL-4434, Pacific Northwest Laboratory, Richland, WA.

32. Strong, K. P., Levins, D. M., and Fane, A. G. (1981). Radon diffusion through uranium tailings and earth cover. In M. Gomez (ed.), *Radiation Hazards in Mining: Control, Measurement and Medical Aspects*, Society of Mining Engineers, New York, p. 713.

33. King, C. Y. (ed.) (1984/1985). Earthquake hydrology and chemistry, special issue of *J. Appl. Geophys.*, **122**, 294.

34. Hirst, W, and Harrison, G. E., (1939). The diffusion of radon gas mixtures, *Proc. Roy. Soc. London (A)*, **169**, 573.

35. Buckingham, E. (1904). Contributions to our knowledge of the aeration of soils, bulletin No. 25, US Dept. of Agriculture, Bureau of Soils, Washington, DC.

36. Penman, H. L. (1940). Gas and vapour movements in soil: The diffusion of vapours through porous solid, *J. Agr. Sci.*, **30**, 437.

37. Currie, J. A. (1960). Gaseous diffusion in porous media. Part 2—Dry granular materials, *Br. J. Appl. Phys.*, **11**, 318.

38. Tanner, A. B. (1964). Radon migration in the ground: A review, In J. A. S. Adams and W. M. Lowder (eds.), *Natural Radiation Environment*, University of Chicago Press, Chicago, p. 161.

39. Currie, J. A. (1961). Gaseous diffusion in porous media. Part 3—Wet granular materials, *Br. J. Appl. Phys.*, **12**, 275.

40. Moed, B. A., Nazaroff, W. W., Nero, A. V., Schwehr, M. B., and Van Heuvelen, A. (1984). Identifying areas with potential for high indoor radon levels: Analysis of the National Airborne Radiometric Reconnaissance Data for California and the Pacific Northwest, report LBL-16955, Lawrence Berkeley Laboratory, Berkeley, CA.

41. Kirkegaard, P., and Lovborg, L. (1980). Transport of terrestrial gamma radiation in plane semi-infinite geometry, *J. Comp. Phys.*, **36**, 20.

42. Myrick, T. E., Berven, B. A., and Haywood, F. F. (1983). Determination of concentrations of selected radionuclides in surface soil in the U.S., *Health Phys.*, **45**, 631.

43. Wollenberg, H. A. (1984). Naturally occurring radioelements and terrestrial gamma-ray exposure rates: An assessment based on recent geochemical data, report LBL-18714, Lawrence Berkeley Laboratory, Berkeley, CA.

44. Powers, R. P., Turnage, N. E., and Kanipe, L. G. (1980). Determination of radium-226 in environmental samples. In T. F. Gesell and W. M. Lowder (eds.), *Natural Radiation Environment III*, Conf-780422, US Dept. of Commerce, National Technical Information Service, Springfield, VA, p. 640.

45. Iyengar, M. A. R., and Markose, P. M. (1982). An investigation into the distribution of uranium and daughters in the environment of a uranium ore processing facility. Cited in Raghavayya, M., Khan, A. H., Padmanabhan, N., and Srivastava, G. K., Exhalation of Rn-222 from soil: Some aspects of variation. In K. G. Vohra, U. C. Mishra, K. C. Pillai, and S. Sadasivan (eds.), *Natural Radiation Environment*, Wiley Eastern, New Delhi, p. 584.

46. Kalin, M., and Sharma, H. D. (1981). Radium-226 and other group two elements in abandoned uranium mill tailings in two mining areas in south central Ontario. In M. Gomez (ed.), *Radiation Hazards in Mining: Control, Measurement and Medical Aspects*, Society of Mining Engineers, New York, p. 707.

47. Bossus, D. A. W. (1984). Emanating power and specific surface area, *Radiat. Prot. Dosim.*, **7**, 73.

48. Tanner, A. B. (1980). Radon migration in the ground: a supplementary review. In T. F. Gesell and W. M. Lowder (eds.), *Proc. Natural Radiation Environment III*, Conf-780422, US Dept. of Commerce, National Technical Information Service, Springfield, VA, p. 5.

49. Andrews, J. N., and Wood, D. F. (1972). Mechanism of radon release in rock matrices and entry into groundwaters, *Trans. Inst. Min. Metall. Sec. B*, **81**, 198.

50. Megumi, K., and Mamuro, T. (1974). Emanation and exhalation of radon and thoron gases from soil particles, *J. Geophys. Res.*, **79**, 3357.

51. Jasinska, M., Niewiadomski, T., and Schwabenthan, J. (1982). Correlation between soil parameters and natural radioactivity. In K. G. Vohra, U. C. Mishra, K. C. Pillai, and S. Sadasivan (eds.), *Natural Radiation Environment*, Wiley Eastern, New Delhi, p. 206.

52. Barretto, P. M. C., (1973). Emanation characteristics of terrestrial and lunar materials and the radon-222 loss effect on the uranium-lead system discordance, Ph.D. thesis, Rice University, Houston.

53. Wilkening, M. H. (1974). Radon-222 from the island of Hawaii: Deep soils are more important than lava fields or volcanoes, *Science*, **183**, 413.

54. Thamer, B. J., Nielson, K. K., and Felthauser, K. (1981). The effects of moisture on radon emanation including the effects on diffusion, report BuMines OFR 184-82, PB83-136358, US Dept. of Commerce, National Technical Information Service, Springfield, VA.

55. Strong, K. P., and Levins, D. M. (1982). Effect of moisture content on radon emanation from uranium ore and tailings, *Health Phys.*, **42**, 27.

56. Stranden, E., Kolstad, A. K., and Lind, B. (1984). The influence of moisture and temperature on radon exhalation, *Radiat. Prot. Dosim*, **7**, 55.

57. Ingersoll, J. G. (1983). A survey of radionuclide contents and radon emanation rates in building materials used in the U.S., *Health Phys.*, **45**, 363.

58. Bird, R. B., Stewart, W. E., and Lightfoot, E. N. (1960). *Transport Phenomena*, Wiley, New York.

59. Tanner, A. B. (1985). US Geological Survey National Center, Reston, VA, personal communication.

60. Gray, R. W., and Ramsay, W. (1909). Some physical properties of radium emanation, *J. Chem. Soc. (London) Trans.*, **95**, 1073.

61. Rutherford, E., and Soddy, F. (1903). Condensation of radioactive emanations, *Phil. Mag. Ser. 6*, **5**, 561.

62. Lucas, H. F. (1957). Improved low-level alpha scintillation counter for radon, *Rev. Sci. Instrum.*, **28**, 680.

63. Ingersoll, J. G., Stitt, B. D., and Zapalac, G. H. (1983). A fast and accurate method for measuring radon exhalation rates from building materials, *Health Phys.*, **45**, 550.

64. Nazaroff, W. W., and Doyle, S. M. (1985). Radon entry into houses having a crawl space, *Health Phys.*, **48**, 265.

65. Liddament, M., and Allen, C. (1983). The validation and comparison of mathematical models of air infiltration, technical note AIC-11, Air Infiltration Centre, Berkshire, England.

66. Fisk, W. J., and Turiel, I. (1983). Residential air-to-air heat exchangers: Performance, energy savings and economics, *Energy and Buildings*, **5**, 197.

67. Modera, M. P., and Sonderegger, R. C. (1980). Determination of the *in-situ* performance of fireplaces, report LBL-10701, Lawrence Berkeley Laboratory, Berkeley, CA.

68. Hernandez, T. L., and Ring, J. W. (1982). Indoor radon source fluxes: experimental tests of a two-chamber model, *Environ. Int.*, **8**, 45.

69. Hernandez, T. L., Ring, J. W., and Sachs, H. (1984). The variation of basement radon concentration with barometric pressure, *Health Phys.*, **46**, 440.

70. Holub, R. F., Droullard, R. F., Borak, T. B., Inkret, W. C., Morse, J. G., and Baxter, J. F. (1985). Radon-222 and ^{222}Rn progeny concentrations in an energy-efficient house equipped with a heat exchanger, *Health Phys.*, **49**, 267.

71. Scott, A. G., and Findlay, W. O. (1983). Demonstration of remedial techniques against radon in houses on Florida phosphate lands, report EPA 520/5-83-009, US Environmental Protection Agency, Eastern Environmental Radiation Facility, Montgomery, AL.

72. Crane, T. (1947). *Architectural Construction: The Choice of Membrane Materials*, Wiley, New York.

73. *Uniform Building Code* (1982). International Conference of Building Officials, Whittier, CA.

74. Rundo, J., Markun, F., and Plondke, N. J. (1979). Observation of high concentrations of radon in certain houses, *Health Phys.*, **36**, 729.

75. Scott, A. G. (1983). Computer modelling of radon movement. In A. C. George, W. Lowder, I. Fisenne, E. O. Knutson, and L. Hinchcliffe (eds.), *EML Indoor Radon Workshop, 1982*, report EML-416, Environmental Measurements Laboratory, New York, p. 82.

76. Eaton, R. S., and Scott, A. G. (1984). Understanding radon transport into houses, *Radiat. Prot. Dosim.* **7**, 251.

77. DSMA Atcon, Ltd. (1985). A computer study of soil gas movement into buildings, report 1389/1333, Department of Health and Welfare, Ottawa.

78. Youngquist, G. R. (1969). Diffusion and flow of gases in porous solids. In *Symp. on Flow Through Porous Media*, American Chemical Society Publications, Washington, DC, p. 58.

79. Boyle, R. W. (1911). The solubility of radium emanation. Application of Henry's law at low partial pressures, *Phil. Mag.*, **22**, 840.

80. Crozier, W. D. (1969). Direct measurements of radon-220 (thoron) exhalation from the ground, *J. Geophys. Res.*, **74**, 4199.

81. Culot, M. V. J., Olson, H. G., and Schiager, K. J. (1976). Effective diffusion coefficient of radon in concrete, theory and method for field measurements, *Health Phys.*, **30**, 263.

82. Collé, R., Rubin, R. J., Knab, L. I., and Hutchinson, J. M. R. (1981). Radon transport through and exhalation from building materials: A review and assessment, NBS technical note 1139, US Government Printing Office, Washington, DC.

83. Landman, K. A. (1982). Diffusion of radon through cracks in a concrete slab, *Health Phys.*, **43**, 65.

84. Landman, K. A., and Cohen, D. S. (1983). Transport of radon through cracks in a concrete slab, *Health Phys.*, **44**, 249.

85. Nero, A. V., and Nazaroff, W. W. (1984). Characterising the source of radon indoors, *Radiat. Prot. Dosim.*, **7**, 23.

86. Burmister, D. M. (1954). Principles of permeability testing of soils. In *Symp. on Permeability of Soils*, ASTM Special Technical Publication no. 163, American Society for Testing Materials, Philadelphia, p. 3.

87. Schlichting, H. (1979). *Boundary-Layer Theory*, 7th ed., McGraw-Hill, New York.

88. Whitaker, S. (1984). *Introduction to Fluid Mechanics*, reprint ed., R. E. Krieger Publishing Co., Malabar, FL.

89. Lorrain, P., and Corson, D. (1970). *Electromagnetic Fields and Waves*, 2nd ed., Freeman, San Francisco, Chap. 2.

90. Carslaw, H. S., and Jaeger, J. C. (1959, reprinted 1984). *Conduction of Heat in Solids*, 2nd ed., Oxford University Press, New York.

91. Morse, P. M., and Feshbach, H. (1953). *Methods of Theoretical Physics*, 2 vol., McGraw-Hill, New York, Chap. 10.

92. Nazaroff, W. W., Lewis, S. R., Doyle, S. M., Moed, B. A., and Nero, A. V. (1987). Experiments on pollutant transport from soil into residential basements by pressure-driven airflow, *Environ. Sci. Technol.*, **21**, 459.

93. Desai, C. S., and Abel, J. F. (1972). *Introduction to the Finite Element Method: A Numerical Method for Engineering Analysis*, Van Nostrand Reinhold, New York.

94. Bates, R. C., and Edwards, J. C. (1981). The effectiveness of overpressure ventilation: a mathematical study. In M. Gomez (ed.), *Radiation Hazards in Mining: Control, Measurement and Medical Aspects*, Society of Mining Engineers, New York, p. 149.

95. Israelsson, S. (1980). Meteorological influences on atmospheric radioactivity and its effects on the electrical environment. In T. F. Gesell and W. M. Lowder (eds.), *Natural Radiation Environment III*, Conf-780422, US Dept. of Commerce, National Technical Information Service, Springfield, VA, p. 210.

96. Kraner, H. W., Schroeder, G. L., and Evans, R. D. (1964). Measurements of the effects of atmospheric variables on radon-222 flux and soil-gas concentrations. In J. A. S. Adams and W. M. Lowder (eds.), *Natural Radiation Environment*, University of Chicago Press, Chicago, p. 191.

97. Rogers, V. C., Nielson, K. K., Merrell, G. B., and Kalkwarf, D. R. (1983). The effects of advection on radon transport through earthen materials, report NUREG/CR-3409, PNL-4789, RAE-18-4, US Nuclear Regulatory Commission, Washington, DC.

98. Clements, W. E., and Wilkening, M. H. (1974). Atmospheric pressure effects on ^{222}Rn transport across the earth-air interface, *J. Geophys. Res.*, **79**, 5025.

99. Schery, S. D., Gaeddert, D. H., and Wilkening, M. H. (1982). Transport of radon from fractured rock, *J. Geophys. Res.*, **87**, 2969.

100. Schery, S. D., Gaeddert, D. H., and Wilkening, M. H. (1984). Factors affecting exhalation of radon from a gravelly sandy loam, *J. Geophys. Res.*, **89**, 7299.

101. Sachs, P. (1972). *Wind Forces in Engineering*, Pergamon Press, Oxford.

102. Simiu, E., and Scanlan, R. H. (1978). *Wind Effects on Structures: An Introduction to Wind Engineering*, Wiley, New York.

103. Fukuda, H. (1955). Air and vapor movement in soil due to wind gustiness, *Soil Sci.*, **79**, 249.

104. Van der Hoven, I. (1957). Power spectrum of horizontal wind speed in the frequency range from 0.0007 to 900 cycles per hour, *J. Meteor.*, **14**, 160.

105. Sherman, M. H. (1980). Air infiltration in buildings, Ph.D. thesis, University of California, Berkeley.

106. Blomsterberg, A. K., Sherman, M. H., and Grimsrud, D. T. (1979). A model correlating air tightness and air infiltration in houses, report LBL-9625, Lawrence Berkeley Laboratory, Berkeley, CA.

107. Modera, M. P., Sherman, M. H., and Levin, P. A., (1983). A detailed examination of the LBL infiltration model using the mobile infiltration test unit, report LBL-15636, Lawrence Berkeley Laboratory, Berkeley, CA.

108. Nazaroff, W. W., and Sextro, R. G. (1987). Analysis of a technique for measuring the indoor radon-222 source potential of soil, submitted to *Environ. Sci. Technol.*

109. Mowris, R. J. (1986). Analytical and numerical models for estimating the effect of exhaust ventilation on radon entry in houses with basements or crawl spaces, M.S. thesis, University of Colorado (also issued as report LBL-22067, Lawrence Berkeley Laboratory, Berkeley, CA).

110. Nazaroff, W. W., Boegel, M. L., Hollowell, C. D., and Roseme, G. D. (1981). The use of mechanical ventilation with heat recovery for controlling radon and radon-daughter concentrations in houses, *Atmos. Environ.*, **15**, 263.

111. D'Ottavio, T. W., and Dietz, R. N. (1986). Discussion of 'Radon transport into a detached one-story house with a basement', *Atmos. Environ.*, **20**, 1065.

112. Nazaroff, W. W., Moed, B. A., Sextro, R. G., Revzan, K. L., and Nero, A. V. (1987). Factors influencing soil as a source of indoor radon: A framework for geographically assessing radon source potentials, report LBL-20645, Lawrence Berkeley Laboratory, Berkeley, CA.

113. Åkerblom, G., and Wilson, C. (1982). Radon—Geological aspects of an environmental problem, rapporter och meddalanden nr 30, Sveriges Geologiska Undersökning, Luleå, Sweden.

114. Wilson, C. (1984). Mapping the radon risk of our environment. In B. Berglund, T. Lindvall, and J. Sundell (eds.), *Indoor Air: Radon, Passive Smoking, Particulates and Housing Epidemiology*, vol. 2, Swedish Council for Building Research, Stockholm, p. 85.

115. Kothari, B. K., and Han, Y. (1984). Association of indoor radon concentrations with airborne surveys of uranium in surficial material, *Northeastern Environ. Sci.*, **3**, 30.

116. Duval, J. S. (1983). Composite color images of aerial gamma-ray spectrometric data, *Geophysics*, **48**, 722.

117. Marshall, T. J. (1985). A relation between permeability and size distribution of soil pores, *J. Soil Sci.*, **9**, 1.

118. Sisigina, T. I. (1974). Assessment of radon emanation from the surface of extensive territories. In *Nuclear Meteorology*, Israeli Program of Scientific Translations, Jerusalem, p. 239.

119. Damkjær, A., and Korsbech, U. (1985). Measurement of the emanation of radon-222 from Danish soils, *Sci. Total Environ.*, **45**, 343.

120. Mowris, R. J., and Fisk, W. J. (1987). Modeling the effects of exhaust ventilation on radon entry rates and indoor radon concentrations, report LBL–22939, Lawrence Berkeley Laboratory, Berkeley, CA, submitted to *Health Phys.*

121. Loureiro, C. (1987). Simulation of the steady-state transport of radon from soil into houses with basements under constant negative pressure, Ph.D. Thesis, University of Michigan, Ann Arbor.

3

Building Materials as a Source of Indoor Radon

ERLING STRANDEN

National Institute of Radiation Hygiene, Østerås, Norway

1 INTRODUCTION

In many cases, such as single-family residences in the Nordic countries and the United States, the soil and bedrock beneath houses are the main sources of indoor radon (1–4). In larger structures, the building materials may contribute a greater share to the indoor concentration, but the absolute contribution is usually small. However, certain materials have been found to constitute unusually large sources of radon, and in such cases, the building materials may be the source of unacceptably high indoor radon concentrations.

As early as the 1950s, Hultqvist reported high ^{226}Ra concentrations in certain building materials used in Sweden, especially a type of concrete based on alum shale (5). The use of alum shale-based concrete in Sweden was later banned, but still about 10% of Swedish houses have this kind of concrete as the main building material. Other building materials of natural origin containing enhanced levels of ^{226}Ra include granites, some clay bricks, and tuff (6–9).

In recent years, wastes from different industries have been used in the building industry. Fly ash from coal-fired power plants is used as an additive in cement, and by-product gypsum from the phosphate industry is utilized in plasterboards and in concrete (10–12). These wastes contain a higher-than-average concentration of ^{226}Ra, and in some cases, such building materials are a significant source of indoor radon.

New methods of heat conservation, such as thermal energy storage using rock or concrete in solar-heated houses, may also introduce relatively large masses of radon-producing materials into houses (13, 14).

Even though building materials usually contribute fairly little to the total indoor radon concentration, this source is more readily controllable than the other radon sources (especially soil). New building materials could be controlled by purely administrative measures, by specifying limits for the ^{226}Ra concentration or radon exhalation rate. In certain cases, where the building material constitutes a source

113

of high levels of indoor radon, future exposures may be reduced by banning materials in current use.

To be able to correctly assess building materials as the radon source, there is a need for knowledge of the radon transport mechanisms and application of the proper experimental techniques.

In this chapter, a review of the most important features of building materials as a radon source is therefore presented.

2   RADON TRANSPORT THROUGH BUILDING MATERIALS

In Chapter 2, the production and transport of radon through soil is discussed in detail. Many of the qualitative aspects of radon migration in the ground, described in Chapter 2 and in the reviews by Tanner, are transferable to the discussion of transport of radon in building materials, and we shall not discuss the different models for radon diffusion and active transport in detail in this chapter (15, 16).

The transport of radon in building materials can be classified as follows:

1. flow, where the fluid (liquid water, air, or water vapor) within the interstitial pore spaces of the material entrains the radon and acts as a carrier; and
2. diffusion, where the radon moves relative to the fluid in the internal pores of the material.

When radon is transported by either flow or diffusion, the transport takes place in the interstitial pores of the material. The fraction of radon produced that enters the interstitial pores is therefore a vital parameter in both processes. This parameter is often referred to as the emanation coefficient, emanation fraction, or emanation power. The emanation coefficient depends on factors such as grain size, pore size, and moisture content in the pores (15–18). Several authors have demonstrated that the direct recoil fraction of the emanation coefficient increases rapidly when the moisture content of the interstitial pores increases (17–20).

The active flow of radon is driven by a gradient in either moisture content, pressure, or temperature, whereas the diffusion depends on the radon concentration gradient in the material (21).

Fick's law, as discussed in Chapter 2, describes transport by diffusion. The diffusion coefficient is of vital importance for diffusion in building materials, as is the porosity of the material. The diffusion coefficient depends on the internal geometry of the material, the temperature, and the moisture content.

The solution of the transport equation depends on the situation studied, and this must be taken into account when experimental data are interpreted. In a review by the U.S. Department of Commerce, solutions for Fick's law are given for a number of cases, and the influence of convective flow is studied theoretically for a constant pressure gradient throughout the material (21). Often when building materials are assessed, only transport by pure diffusion is considered: it is believed that the active transport of radon produced in the material is of less importance because most materials that produce radon have a very low permeability. An exception to this general rule is the stone magazine often used for heat storage. The magazine contains a large number of stones. Diffusion may dominate the transport of radon out of the individual stones into the air space of the magazine. But, within these large pores, forced convection is the dominant transport mechanism.

A simple solution of the diffusion equation for building materials is discussed below:

The production rate of radon in the interstitial volume of the material per unit air volume may be written as

$$f = \frac{1}{\epsilon} \lambda I \rho \eta \tag{1}$$

where f = radon production rate $(\text{Bq h}^{-1}\text{m}^{-3})$
I = ^{226}Ra concentration (Bq kg^{-1})
λ = decay constant of ^{222}Rn (h^{-1})
ρ = density of the material (kg m^{-3})
ϵ = porosity of the material
η = emanation coefficient

For a free wall with thickness d, the solution giving the exhalation rate by diffusion into the room is (22)

$$E_d = \epsilon f L \tanh (d/2L) \tag{2}$$

where E_d = exhalation rate per unit area $(\text{Bq m}^{-2}\text{h}^{-1})$
L = diffusion length (m)
    = $\sqrt{(D_e/\lambda)}$ where D_e is the effective diffusion coefficient $(\text{m}^2\text{h}^{-1})$

This solution is valid only when both wall surfaces are free to exhale into a radon-free space. If the diffusion length is large compared to the wall thickness, Equation 2 may be approximated by

$$E_d = \epsilon f \frac{d}{2} = I \lambda \rho \eta \frac{d}{2} \tag{3}$$

3 EXPERIMENTAL METHODS FOR ASSESSMENT OF EXHALATION RATE

Several parameters could be measured in assessing the radon exhalation rate. The first step is often to measure the ^{226}Ra content of the material; if this concentration is low, no further steps are needed to conclude that the radon exhalation rate is fairly low. ^{226}Ra measurements are most often done by enclosing material samples in sealed containers and measuring the gamma rays from ^{214}Bi built up in the container. As ^{214}Bi is a radon decay product, it is necessary to store the container for a period of a few weeks to ensure equilibrium between ^{226}Ra and radon. The container must therefore be radon-tight. Calibrations should be done using standard samples with known ^{226}Ra contents.

The emanation coefficient, η, is frequently measured for assessment of the radon exhalation rate (10, 23). The exhalation rate could then be assessed from formulas like Equations 2 and 3 in this chapter.

The diffusion coefficient and porosity of building materials have also been investigated for some materials (23, 24, 27, 47). These parameters are necessary for theoretical calculation of exhalation rates and for assessing the microscopic processes that influence radon transport.

The most direct way of assessing the exhalation rate of building materials is to measure the radon exhalation directly from samples of finished building materials of typical size, from slabs of the building materials, or from walls (11, 22, 27, 28). Assessments of the exhalation rate have also been performed by continuously measuring radon concentration and ventilation rate in room air when the main source is believed to be the building materials (29).

The measurements of exhalation rate, diffusion coefficient, and emanation coefficient each involve assessment of the amount of radon released from a sample or surface of the material per unit time. In the following section, some methods are described and the main difficulties discussed.

3.1 Measurements on Enclosed Samples

The most common way to assess the exhalation rate or the emanation coefficient of a building material is to enclose a sample in a sealed container and measure the radon concentration in the air volume of the container after a given growth time. Ideally, the activity of radon is described by the following equation:

$$A = \frac{E}{\lambda}\left(1 - e^{-\lambda t}\right) \tag{4}$$

where A = total radon activity (Bq) in the container air at the end of a growth time, t (h)

$\quad\quad\;\; E$ = total exhalation rate (Bq h^{-1})

Equation 4 is valid only if (i) there is no leakage of radon out of the container and (ii) the activity concentration in the container air is low compared to the activity concentration in the pore air of the sample. When the radon concentration in the container air starts to approach that of the air in the sample, radon has a significant probability of diffusing back into the sample, so-called "back diffusion" (30, 37).

Equation 4 may thus be valid only for short growth periods. In Figure 3.1, the effects of back diffusion and leakage are illustrated (31). To be able to overcome this problem, the radon concentrations in the container should be followed during the growth period either by continuous measurements or by frequent grab sampling. Practical approaches to overcoming the difficulties of back diffusion and leakage are (i) to use short growth times and to assume that the radon growth follows Equation 4, or (ii) to determine a growth curve similar to those shown in Figure 3.1. From such growth curves, an "effective decay constant," λ^*, can be fitted, and Equation 4 is transformed:

$$A = \frac{E}{\lambda^*}\,(1 - e^{-\lambda^* t}) \tag{5}$$

where λ^* = $\lambda + \lambda_{b,1}$
$\lambda_{b,1}$ = a "decay" constant correcting for first-order removal of radon by back diffusion and leakage

Another method that could be used, especially for measurement of the emanation coefficient of small samples, is to fill a radon-tight container with the sample, flush the sample with radon-free air, and then enclose the sample for a 3-week period. By measuring the growth of ^{214}Bi by a gamma count of the sample, the radon released from an exposed sample may be assessed.

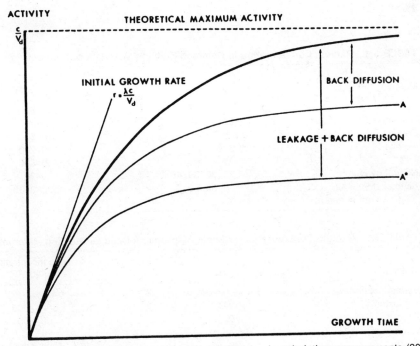

Figure 3.1. Effects of radon leakage and back diffusion in exhalation measurements (30). Reproduced from *Health Physics*, **45**, 370, by permission of the Health Physics Society.

3.2   Measurements on Slabs or Walls

The most common technique for such measurements is to seal a container to a part of the exhaling area and measure the radon growth in the container. In this method, the difficulties with back diffusion and leakage are even more important than for enclosed samples, and it is necessary to do frequent measurements to determine the radon growth curve.

Another method that could be used for measurements on slabs or wall surfaces is to seal a container with activated charcoal to the exhaling surface. The charcoal adsorbs virtually all the radon entering the container, and thus the back-diffusion problem should be reduced by this method. The radon accumulated on the charcoal may be determined by counting gamma emissions from the container after the end of the growth period (32, 33). Another method utilizing activated charcoal is to place a thermoluminescent dosimeter (TLD) in the middle of the charcoal. The adsorbed radon irradiates the TLD during the whole growth period, and the exhalation rate may then be determined from the integrated dose (34).

4   REVIEW OF EXPERIMENTAL DATA

In this section, some of the most interesting data relevant to radon exhalation from building materials are reviewed. An earlier review can be found in Nero and Nazaroff (42).

TABLE 3.1   Radium Concentration in Common Building Materials of Natural Origin

Material	Ref.	Radium concentration (Bq kg^{-1})
Concrete	35–39, 46	10–80
Clay brick	35–39, 46	20–200
Cement	35–39, 46	10–50
Granite	6, 7	100–200
Tuff	9	100–600
Natural gypsum	23, 36, 39, 46	5–20
Alum shale-based lightweight concrete	35, 36, 39	300–2500

TABLE 3.2   Radium Concentration of Some By-products Used as Building Materials

Material	Ref.	^{226}Ra concentration (Bq kg^{-1})
By-product gypsum	12, 40, 41	500–2000
Fly ash	10, 11, 46	50–300
Calcium silicate slag	39	1000–2000

4.1   Radium Concentrations in Building Materials

In Table 3.1 values of the radium concentration in different building materials of natural origin are summarized. In Table 3.2 the radium concentrations of some industrial by-products frequently used in the building industry are shown.

4.2   Emanation Coefficient and Diffusion Length

In Table 3.3, the emanation coefficient and diffusion length of some building materials are shown. The experimental data are not easily comparable, owing to differences in method, sample preparation, and other factors, but the table may give an idea of the expected range of values of these parameters.

4.3   Exhalation Rates

Measurements of exhalation rate have been performed in a number of studies. The most common procedure is to measure an enclosed sample of the building material, but measurements on walls and slabs have also been reported. In Tables 3.4 and 3.5 such data are summarized.

TABLE 3.3   Emanation Coefficient and Diffusion Length of ^{222}Rn in Some Building Materials

Material	Emanation coefficient	Diffusion length (m)
Concrete	0.1–0.4	0.06–0.2
Brick	0.02–0.1	0.2–0.4
Gypsum	0.03–0.2	0.8–1.3
Cement	0.02–0.05	—
Fly ash	0.002–0.02	—

Source: Refs. 10, 11, 23, 25–27, 46, 47.

TABLE 3.4   Radon Exhalation from Samples of Building Materials in the Nordic Countries

Material	Exhalation rate per unit mass (Bq h^{-1} kg^{-1})
Concrete	0.002–0.1
Brick	0.001–0.05
Alum shale concrete	2–3
Natural gypsum	0.002–0.02

Source: Ref. 29.

TABLE 3.5   Radon Exhalation from Walls or Slabs of Building Materials in the Nordic Countries

Material	Radon exhalation rate $(Bq\ h^{-1}\ m^{-2})$
Concrete	2–30
By-product gypsum	5–40
Alum shale concrete	50–200
Lightweight concrete	1–3
Brick	2–5

Source: Ref. 29.

4.4   Influencing Factors

The environmental factors that have the largest influence on radon exhalation from building materials are atmospheric pressure and humidity.

It is well documented that a sudden pressure drop results in increased radon exhalation from building materials during the time period over which the pressure drop occurs (43). In a study by McLaughlin and Jonassen, a strong correlation between pressure drop and exhalation rate was found, as seen in Figure 3.2 (43).

Studies on the effect of moisture content of concrete show that the radon exhalation rate may vary by a factor of 20 depending on the moisture content of the material. In Figure 3.3, this is illustrated (17–19).

Even the temperature of the material may influence the radon exhalation rate. Stranden, Kolstad, and Lind found a significant increase in radon exhalation from concrete samples with increasing temperature (17, 18).

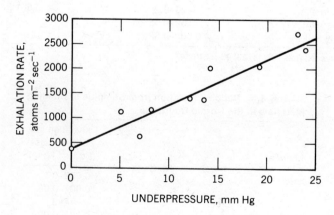

Figure 3.2. Effects of pressure drops on radon exhalation from walls (43).

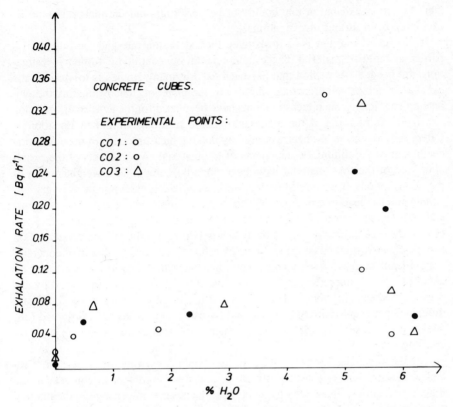

Figure 3.3. Effect of the moisture content of concrete on radon exhalation (18). Reproduced from *Health Physics*, **47**, 483, by permission of the Health Physics Society.

5 INTERPRETATION OF EXPERIMENTAL DATA

Even when experiments are carefully performed and experimental problems such as back diffusion and leakage have been taken into consideration, there are great difficulties in interpreting the experimental findings. The main problem is to scale-up measurements on samples to the dimensions of a wall.

The first question is "What should be measured and how?" As seen from the review of experimental data, there are several possibilities, and many of these measurements could be used in assessments of building materials as radon sources. It is, however, important that the measurements performed are the best means for the aim of the measurements.

For instance, if the aim of the measurements is to screen out materials that will not cause any radon problems, measurements of the radium contents could be the most easy and feasible way. If the radium concentration of the material is low, then the radon exhalation rate could not be very high and the material could be exempted from further investigations.

If, however, the aim is to investigate the exhalation rate and the impact of a particular building material on the indoor radon concentration, further investigations are needed. A method that has been used in many studies is to measure the exhalation rate of small crushed samples of the material, thus evaluating the emanation coefficient. Such measurements have been used for the assessment of radon exhalation from walls of the material by using formulas similar to Equation 3. Often, the exhalation has been assessed by making measurements of the emanation coefficient of the different components of the material. Assessments of the exhalation rate of the final material have been done by computing a weighted sum of the contributions from the different components. Such assessments are very uncertain and can lead to erroneous decisions. An example where such measurements and assessments can lead to serious errors is the use of fly ash in cement. Even though the emanation coefficient of fly ash is fairly low, the radium concentration is high. In assessing the contribution of fly ash to the radon exhalation of concrete, a significant increase is predicted. Yet when measurements have been made on cubes of fly ash concrete, some authors have actually found that the added fly ash causes a decrease in radon exhalation (11, 19, 20). In other cases, no significant difference between ordinary concrete and fly-ash concrete has been observed (28, 44). In a few cases, fly-ash concretes exhale somewhat more radon than ordinary concrete (45).

The discrepancies in these studies are probably caused by differences in ^{226}Ra concentration, porosity, surface structure, and fly-ash content in concrete in the different countries. The added fly ash probably causes some change in the internal structure of the concrete, so that the diffusion length and/or emanation coefficient is reduced. The effect of this reduction will depend on the amount of added fly ash and the structure of the ordinary concrete. The differences in these studies are probably real, but no detailed explanation for these findings has been published.

Obviously, the best way to assess the radon exhalation rate is to measure the exhalation rate of finished samples of the building materials or of walls or slabs.

The experimental setup is easier and less uncertain in sample measurements, but when such measurements are performed, the shape and dimensions of the sample should be such that it simulates the finished walls in the best way. Furthermore, owing to the large variations in radon exhalation with moisture content, the materials should be mature before the measurements are made. Concrete, for instance, has a high moisture content when it is prepared. For several months, the moisture content gradually decreases until it reaches a steady state. If we look at Figure 3.3, it is obvious that the result of the measurement will depend strongly on the age of the concrete.

One way to assess the radon exhalation from concrete samples is to use cubes of the material. The total exhalation rate from the cubes may be determined, or by sealing off the four sides of the cube, the exhalation rate of two opposite sides could be assessed (11, 28).

Stranden used cubes of dimensions $10 \times 10 \times 10$ cm^3 and measured the total exhalation rate from the cubes (11). The results of these measurements could be used in the assessment of the exhalation rate of 20-cm-thick walls. When the cubes are part of one side of such a wall, the total exhalation rate from each of these cubes will be the maximum exhalation rate out of the one side facing the room. In an area of 1 m^2 of the wall, 100 cubes will be present, and the exhalation rate from a unit area of the wall could be determined as $100 \times E_T$, where E_T is the total exhalation rate from one cube (Bq h^{-1}).

In the procedure of Mustonen, only two opposite areas of a 20-cm-thick cube are permitted to exhale (28). In this case, the exhalation rate from one side of a 20-cm-thick wall is assessed as the exhalation rate of the sample, divided by the area of the two opposite sides of the sample.

These approaches to sample preparation could also be applied to other types of materials. The dimensions of the samples should, however, reflect consideration of the actual uses of the material. An alternative approach is to measure the emanation characteristics of thin samples of the material (46) and combine this with independent knowledge of diffusion coefficients (47) to calculate the emanation rate expected from an arbitrary configuration.

In summary, the interpretation of experimental results should be done carefully, and it is important that the conclusions drawn are not more far-reaching than the experimental results permit. For quantitative assessments of building materials as a radon source, the following main rules should be considered: The building material should be in its final state and the sample be of a size and shape that can be used for simulating the exhalation rate of a wall. It is of extreme importance that the moisture content of the material is about the same as is expected in the final use of the materials.

In traditional building materials, the impact of the material as a radon source may be assessed by considering the diffusion process as expressed in measured exhalation rates. Heat accumulation in stone magazines is an example of new technology where this method does not apply. In this case, air is circulated through the stone magazine, and the main transport force is due to the airflow. For assessment of materials used for this application, the stone samples should be representative in size and shape of the stone material actually used in magazines. For such assessments, the total exhalation rate per mass of stone material should be measured. The contribution to indoor air radon could be assessed from the total mass of the stone magazine and the design of the heating system. In this case, however, it is important to note that the stones are heated in the magazine. Investigations have shown that the radon exhalation increases with increasing temperature, and some assessments of this effect should therefore be performed in this case (17, 18).

6 THE IMPACT OF BUILDING MATERIALS ON INDOOR RADON CONCENTRATIONS

As seen from the experimental data, there are large variations in the radon exhalation properties of different building materials. Furthermore, the actual use of the materials varies. For instance, concrete is used as the main building material in blocks of apartments. Ceramic tiles, on the other hand, are used in only small quantities in a dwelling. The importance of a building material will thus depend not only on the specific exhalation rate of the material, but also on the actual use of the material.

Some building materials, such as alum shale concrete in Sweden, have very high radium concentrations and radon exhalation rates. It is estimated that radon concentrations as high as 800 Bq m^{-3} can be caused by such a building material when it is the main material used in construction.

Even though the stone materials in thermal magazines studied by Stranden and by Nyblom were "normal," the stone magazines contributed significantly to the indoor radon concentration in several of the houses investigated (13, 14). This is due to the fact that the mass of stones is large in such magazines, and that radon is transported out of the stone magazine by the flow of air.

The contribution to indoor radon concentration from different building materials might be assessed by using the following formula:

$$C = \frac{E}{V} \frac{S}{\lambda_v} \qquad (6)$$

where C = radon concentration (Bq m^{-3})
  E = exhalation rate per unit area (Bq h^{-1} m^{-2})
  S = exhaling area (m^2)
  V = room volume (m^3)
  λ_v = air-exchange rate (h^{-1})

In a study by Krisiuk et al., the maximum radon concentration from a building material was assessed by assuming the room as a cavity with $S/V = 1.8$ m^{-1} (8). In Table 3.6 we have used the experimental data from Table 3.5 to evaluate the

TABLE 3.6   Assessment of the Radon Concentration in Air Due to Different Types of Building Materials

Material	Assumed exhalation rate (Bq h^{-1} m^{-2})	Radon concentration (Bq m^{-3}) Maximum[a]	Realistic value
Concrete	10	40	20[b]
Lightweight concrete	2	7	4[b]
Alum shale concrete	200	700	400[b]
Clay brick	4	15	5[c]
By-product gypsum	20	70	10[d]

[a]$S/V = 2.0$ m^{-1}.
[b]$S/V = 1.0$ m^{-1}.
[c]$S/V = 0.6$ m^{-1}.
[d]$S/V = 0.3$ m^{-1}.

radon concentration in indoor air due to different building materials. We have assumed an air-exhange rate of 0.5 h^{-1} and calculated the maximum radon concentration and the realistic radon concentration due to typical use of a given material.

As seen from this table, building materials usually contribute relatively little compared with soil to the indoor radon concentration. However, building materials such as alum shale concrete in Sweden may be the source of very high indoor radon concentrations.

Stone magazines used for heat accumulation may also be a significant source of indoor radon. In studies in Sweden and Norway, the stone magazine contributed to, on average, about 40 Bq m^{-3} in indoor air in the houses investigated (13, 14). If granite is used as stone material, the radon concentration due to the stone magazine could be more than 100 Bq m^{-3}.

7 PREVENTIVE MEASURES

Building materials that are intended to be used in the future should be investigated on the basis of their properties as radon sources. The preventive measures, in the case of new materials that would cause an unacceptable increase in the indoor radon concentration, could be purely administrative and legal. The production of certain materials could, for instance, be banned, or their future use restricted on the basis of national legislation. The criteria for such countermeasures should be stricter than for existing materials.

The International Committee on Radiological Protection (ICRP) recommends that an upper bound for the doses in future houses should be applied (48). Building materials should contribute only a fraction to this upper bound, and exemption levels or investigation levels should be based on such upper bounds. To be able to screen out materials that need no further assessment, it is feasible to use an exemption level based on the ^{226}Ra concentration. This exemption level should be such that even when the emanation coefficient is high and the material is used as the main building material, the calculated indoor radon concentration would not exceed a given fraction of the upper bound. Materials with radium concentration below the limit should be exempted from further investigation, and they could be used freely as building materials.

In cases where the radium concentration is higher than the exemption level, the radon exhalation rates and the impact on radon in indoor air should be assessed as realistically as possible. On the basis of such assessments, the material could be banned or its use restricted.

Even existing materials could be banned for further production if the material is proven to cause a significantly enhanced radiation dose to the population. In Sweden, alum shale concrete has been taken out of production solely on the basis of radiological assessments.

In existing houses where the building materials cause high radon concentrations, remedial actions have been tried with varying results. The principal means of reducing the radon transport from building materials to the building interior is to apply sealants to the exhaling walls. Radon exhalation from materials sealed with epoxies or other coatings may be reduced by up to 90% (49–51). Sealing surfaces or stopping transport via plastic or other barriers has proved effective in some cases that require remedial action, but this approch requires integrity of the barrier for long-term effectiveness. The general applicability and effectiveness of these measures as long-term passive controls are not known. It should be noted that the application of diffusion barriers results in a buildup of radon decay products in the building material, with a resulting increase in gamma radiation. This effect is small, however, compared to the effect of reduced radon exhalation.

In cases where only a portion of the structure is made of high activity materials, it is possible to replace the material. In cases where the main structure consists of high-activity material, the remedial action of replacing the material would be very expensive and seldom practical.

8   DISCUSSION AND CONCLUSIONS

Building materials usually contribute a relatively small fraction of the indoor radon concentration, at least in single-family houses, and when there are extremely high indoor radon concentrations, the main source is most often the soil and bedrock. Nevertheless, radon decay products in houses constitute the dominant mode of exposure for the populations in most developed countries, and even a relatively small contribution from building materials causes an increment in population dose that is significant compared to many other modes of exposure. Furthermore, building materials causing high concentrations have been used in several countries. In some cases these are materials of natural origin (i.e., granite or alum shale concrete), and in other cases they are by-products from different industries (by-product gypsum, waste rock from mining).

Both when collective doses and individual doses are considered, it is important to limit the use of building materials that cause a significant increase in indoor radon concentrations.

To be able to assess the building materials as radon sources, the experimental techniques must be chosen properly, and due attention must be given to the experimental difficulties involved. Furthermore, the interpretation of the experimental findings has to be done with care owing to the many factors that influence the radon transport from building material to room air.

Building materials of natural origin reflect the geological conditions at the site of production, and there are large regional differences even within the same country (37). The differences between countries may be even larger. Studies in the Nordic countries have shown that even the radon exhalation per unit radium activity concentration in a single type of building material varies from country to country (29). It is, therefore, not feasible to use values for radon exhalation or diffusion length from a given material obtained in another country.

The mechanisms of radon transport are complex, and many variables have to be taken into account, but the problems with building materials as a source of radon are far less complex than in the case of soil or bedrock. After all, the building materials are of finite size and a given material is used in specified applications.

By using the proper experimental techniques and applying the proper interpretation of the results, it is therefore possible to assess the source strength of building materials by relatively simple means. Furthermore, the introduction of highly active building materials in the future may be prevented by purely administrative and legal measures.

In some existing houses, high radon concentrations are caused by the building materials. The occurrence of such houses may be assessed by gamma measurements or by questionnaires administered to individuals or to local authorities. Preventive measures in such houses have been tried with varying results, and the long-term effects of sealants and diffusion barriers are not fully documented. Further research on such preventive measures is of great importance, because it is the only feasible way to reduce the source strength of the building materials. Furthermore, research on sealants and diffusion barriers is also important as a method for reducing the radon influx from the subsoil and bedrock.

REFERENCES

1. Stranden, E., Kolstad, A. K., and Lind, B. (1984). National Institute of Radiation Hygiene, Norway, working document, p. 5.
2. Swedjemark, G. A., and Mjønes, L. (1984). Radon and radon daughter concentrations in Swedish houses. *Radiat. Prot. Dosim.*, **7**, 341.
3. Castrén, O., Winqvist, K., Mäkeläinen, I., and Voutilainen, A. (1984). Radon measurements in Finnish houses. *Radiat. Prot. Dosim.*, **7**, 333.
4. Nero, A. V., Hollowell, C. D., Ingersoll, J. G., and Nazaroff, W. W. (1983). Radon concentrations and infiltration rates measured in conventional and energy-efficient houses. *Health Phys.*, **45**, 401.
5. Hultqvist, B. (1956). Studies on naturally occurring ionizing radiations. Kungl. Svenska Vetenskapsakademiens Handlingar, 4. serien, Band 6, Nr. 3, Stockholm, Almqvist & Wiksells Boktryckeri AB.
6. Kolb, W. (1974). Influence of building materials on the radiation dose to the population, *Kernenegie Offentlichkeit*, **4**, 18.
7. Soratin, H., and Steger, F. (1984). Natural radioactivity of building materias in Austria, *Radiat. Prot. Dosim.*, **7**, 59.
8. Krisiuk, E. M., Tarasov, S. I., Shamov, V. P., Shalak, N. I., Lisachenko, E. P., and Gomelsky, L. G. (1974). A study of radioactivity in building materials, National Committee on the Utilization of Atomic Energy, Leningrad.
9. Sciochetti, G., Clemente, G. F., Ingrao, G., and Scacco, F. (1983). Results of a survey on radioactivity of building materials in Italy, *Health Phys.*, **45**, 385.
10. Pensko, J., Stpiczynska, Z., and Blaton-Albricka, K. (1980). Emanating power of radon-222 measured in building materials. In T. F. Gesell and W. M. Lowder (eds.), *Natural Radiation Environment III*, US Dept of Energy, rep CONF-780422, p. 1407.

11. Stranden, E. (1983). Assessment of the radiological impact of using fly ash in cement. *Health Phys.*, **44**, 145.

12. O'Riordan, M. C., Duggan, M. J., Rose, W. B., and Bradford, G. F. (1972). The radiological implications of using by-product gypsum as building material, National Radiological Protection Board, report 7, Harwell, Didcot, England.

13. Stranden, E. (1981). Radon in houses utilizing stone magazines for heat accumulation, *Health Phys.*, **41**, 29.

14. Nyblom, L. (1980). Radon in the air in buildings where heat is accumulated in stone magazines. Nordic Society for Radiation Protection Meeting, Geilo, Norway (in Swedish).

15. Tanner, A. B. (1964). Radon migration in the ground: A review. In J. A. S. Adams and W. M. Lowder (eds.), *Natural Radiation Environment*, University of Chicago Press, Chicago, p. 161.

16. Tanner, A. B. (1980). Radon migration in the ground: A supplemental review. In T. F. Gesell and W. M. Lowder (eds.), *Natural Radiation Environment III*, US Dept of Energy, rep CONF-780422, p. 5.

17. Stranden, E., Kolstad, A. K., and Lind, B. (1984). The influence of moisture and temperature on radon exhalation, *Radiat. Prot. Dosim.*, **7**, 55.

18. Stranden, E., Kolstad, A. K., and Lind, B. (1984). Radon exhalation: Moisture and temperature dependence, *Health Phys.*, **47**, 480.

19. Pettersson, H., Hildingson, O., Samuelsson, C., and Hedvall, R. R. (1982). Radon exhalation from building materials, Statens Provningsanstalt Tekn. rapport SP-Rapp 1982:32, Borås, Sweden.

20. van der Lugt, G., and Scholten, L. C. (1985). Radon emanation from concrete and the influence of using fly ash in cement, *Sci. Total Environ.*, **45**, 143.

21. U.S. Dept of Commerce (1981). Radon transport through and exhalation from building materials: A review and assessment, NBS technical note 1139, Washington, DC.

22. Jonassen, N., and McLaughlin, J. P. (1980). Exhalation of radon-222 from building materials and walls. In T. F. Gesell and W. M. Lowder (eds.), *Natural Radiation Environment III*, US Dept of Energy CONF-780422, p. 1211.

23. Folkerts, K. H., Keller, G., and Muth, H. (1984). Experimental investigations on diffusion and exhalation of Rn-222 and Rn-220 from building materials, *Radiat. Prot. Dosim.*, **7**, 41.

24. Culot, M. V. J., Olson, H. G., and Schiager, K. J. (1973). Radon progeny control in buildings, final report to the Environmental Protection Agency, Colorado State University, Fort Collins.

25. Culot, M. V. J., Olson, H. G., and Schiager, K. J. (1976). Effective diffusion coefficient of radon in concrete: Theory and method for field measurements, *Health Phys.*, **30**, 263.

26. Jonassen, N., and McLaughlin, J. P. (1976). Radon in indoor air, research report 6, Lab. of Applied Physics I, Technical University of Denmark, Lyngby.

27. Stranden, E., and Berteig, L. (1980). Radon in dwellings and influencing factors, *Health Phys.*, **39**, 275.

28. Mustonen, R. (1984). Methods for evaluation of radiation from building materials, *Radiat. Prot. Dosim.*, **7**, 235.

29. The Radiation Protection Institute in Denmark, Finland, Iceland, Norway and Sweden (1982). Naturally occurring radiation in the Nordic countries-Levels, ISBN 82-90362-04-8.

30. Jonassen, N. (1983). On the determination of exhalation rates, *Health Phys.*, **45**, 369.

31. Jonassen, N. (1981). Radon exhaling properties of building materials. Presented at 2nd European Conference on Building Materials, Glasgow, Scotland.

32. Countess, R. J. (1976). Rn-222 flux measurements with a charcoal canister, *Health Phys.*, **31**, 455.

33. Countess, R. J. (1977). Measurements of Rn-222 flux with charcoal canisters, report HASL-325, Health and Safety Laboratory, New York.

34. Stranden, E. and Kolstad, A. K. (1985). Radon exhalation from the ground: Method of measurements and preliminary results, *Sci. Total Environ.*, **45**, 165.

35. Swedish National Institute of Radiation Protection (1981). Communication, Stockholm.

36. Ulbak, K. (1980). Natural radioactivity in building materials in Denmark. In Seminar on the Radiological Burden of Man from Natural Radioactivity in the Countries of the European Community, CEC doc. C/2408/80.

37. Stranden, E. (1979). Radioactivity of building materials and the gamma radiation in dwellings, *Phys. Med. Biol.*, **24**, 921.

38. Mustonen, R. (1979). Activity concentration of building materials in Finland. Nordic Radiation Protection Society, Meeting, Visby Sweden (in Swedish).

39. United Nations Scientific Committee on the Effects of Atomic Radiation (1982). Sources and effects of ionizing radiation, 1982 report to the General Assembly, UN, New York.

40. Hamilton, E. I. (1972). The relative radioactivity of building materials, *Am. Ind. Hyg. Assoc. J.*, **32**, 398.

41. Guimond, R. J., and Windham, S. T. (1975). Radioactivity distribution in phosphate products, by-products, effluents and wastes, report ORP/CSD-75-3, Office of Radiation Programs, U.S. Environmental Protection Agency, Washington, DC.

42. Nero, A. V., and Nazaroff, W. W. (1984). Characterising the source of radon indoors, *Radiat. Prot. Dosim.*, **7**, 23.

43. McLaughlin, J. P., and Jonassen, N. (1980). The effect of pressure drops on radon exhalation from walls. In T. F. Gesell and W. M. Lowder (eds.), *Natural Radiation Environment III*, US Dept. of Energy, CONF-780422, p. 1225.

44. Ulbak, K., Jonassen, N., and Bækmann, K. (1984). Radon exhalation from samples of concrete with different porosities and fly ash additives, *Radiat. Prot. Dosim.*, **7**, 45.

45. Siotis, I., and Wrixon, A. D. (1984). Radiological consequences of the use of fly ash in building materials in Greece, Radiat. Prot. Dosim., **7**, 101.

46. Ingersoll, J. G. (1983). A survey of radionuclide contents and radon emanation rates in building materials used in the U.S., *Health Phys.*, **45**, 363.

47. Zapalac, G. H. (1983). A time-dependent method for characterizing the diffusion of ^{222}Rn in concrete, *Health Phys.*, **45**, 377.

48. International Committee on Radiological Protection, ICRP (1984). Publication 39, Pergamon Press, Oxford.

49. Atomic Energy Control Board, Canada (1978). Workshop on radon and radon daugh-

ters in urban communities associated with uranium mining and processing, Elliot Lake, Ontario.

50. Atomic Energy Control Board, Canada (1979). 2nd Workshop on radon and radon daughters in urban communities associated with uranium mining and processing, Bancroft, Ontario.

51. Atomic Energy Control Board, Canada (1980). 3rd Workshop on radon and radon daughters in urban communities associated with uranium mining and processing, Port Hope, Ontario.

▬ 4

Radon Entry via Potable Water

WILLIAM W. NAZAROFF

Environmental Engineering Science, California Institute of Technology, Pasadena, California

Indoor Environment Program, Lawrence Berkeley Laboratory, University of California, Berkeley, California

SUZANNE M. DOYLE, ANTHONY V. NERO, Jr., and RICHARD G. SEXTRO

Indoor Environment Program, Lawrence Berkeley Laboratory, University of California, Berkeley, California

1 INTRODUCTION

High radon concentrations in potable water were first observed in Maine in the late 1950s (1). Initially, concern about radiation hygiene as a consequence of these observations focused on ingestion of radon-rich water, and researchers identified the stomach as the organ receiving the greatest dose (2–6). Later, Gesell and Prichard speculated that the inhalation exposure to radon progeny arising from the release of radon from domestic water use may be of greater significance than the ingestion exposure (7). More recent studies, comparing the expected lung and stomach doses resulting from radon-rich water, have concluded that the former is 3–12 times the latter (8–10). (See Ref. 66 for a review of the health effects of [222]Rn in drinking water.)

Several investigations in the past decade have addressed aspects of potable water as a source of airborne radon indoors. Key efforts in the United States include these: the development of an inexpensive technique for measuring radon in water (11); studies of the transfer of radon from water to air during different household uses (12–14); measurements of the indoor airborne radon concentration resulting from water use in different residences (13, 14); estimation of the population dose resulting from radon in potable water supplies in Houston, Texas (10); and surveys of radon concentrations in groundwater supplies (15–17). In addition, numerous investigations have been conducted in Finland, where groundwater radon concentrations are particularly high (9, 18–20).

In this chapter we review the state of knowledge of domestic water as a source of indoor airborne radon. Available data on residence volumes, air-exchange rates,

131

in-house water-use rates, and water-to-air transfer coefficients are combined to determine the distribution of incremental indoor radon concentrations in air that can be expected to result from a specified concentration in water. Data on the distribution of radon concentrations in U.S. water supplies are discussed, and the contribution of potable water to indoor radon concentrations is estimated. Technical measures for reducing radon concentrations in water supplies are presented.

The data used for analysis in this chapter are restricted to the United States; however, the methods of analysis are general and could be equally applied to the housing stock of other countries.

2 PREDICTING THE INDOOR RADON CONCENTRATION RESULTING FROM WATER USE

2.1 Long-Term-Average Single-Cell Model

From conservation of mass, the incremental average increase in indoor radon concentration resulting from water use can be estimated from the following equation (see Section 7):

$$C_a = \frac{C_w We}{V \lambda_v} \qquad (1)$$

where C_w is the radon concentration in water entering the residence ($Bq\ m^{-3}$)
W is the water-use rate per resident ($m^3\ person^{-1}\ h^{-1}$)
e is the use-weighted average transfer efficiency of radon from water to air (dimensionless)
V is the volume per resident of the dwelling ($m^3\ person^{-1}$) and
λ_v is the air-exchange rate of the residence (h^{-1}), assumed to be much greater than the decay constant for radon ($0.0076\ h^{-1}$)

An important question in assessing impact of radon in water on exposure to radiation is this: given a concentration of radon in water, C_w, what is the expected increase in the concentration in air, C_a, that results from water use? From Equation 1, the answer may be expressed in terms of a transfer factor, f:

$$C_a = f C_w \qquad (2)$$

where

$$f = \frac{We}{V \lambda_v} \qquad (3)$$

There are two distinct approaches for determining f. The first, which we shall use in this chapter, evaluates e, W, V, and λ_v from an examination of literature, then calculates the distribution of f by combining these parameters mathematically. The second approach determines C_a and C_w experimentally in a sample of houses and then evaluates f directly from Equation 2. In using the former approach, previous studies have specified one or more typical values of V and λ_v, combined them with limited data on W and e, and calculated f (12, 13, 21). These studies have concluded that the most typical value of f is in the vicinity of 10^{-4} and that the value for a specific residence can be an order of magnitude smaller or larger.

Two studies in the United States have evaluated f using the experimental approach. In the first of these, radon was monitored continuously for several days in each of four residences (13). The difference between average radon concentrations for the periods 0800–2400 and 0000–0800 was assumed to be due to radon liberated by water use. In the second study, identifiable peaks in indoor radon concentration in 13 houses were used to assess the contribution to indoor concentration from dishwashing, showering, and laundering (14). The contribution of other water uses—toilets, baths, and sinks—was based on estimated transfer coefficients and water use rates. The results of these studies are discussed in Section 2.6.

The results of measurements in 17 houses in two small regions are not sufficient to precisely estimate the distribution of f in the U.S. housing stock. Yet, determining f in a large number of houses using experimental techniques such as these poses substantial difficulties. The radon contribution by water use must be separated from that due to other sources. Thus, the small fraction of houses in which water is the predominant source are best suited as study sites. Even in these cases, contributions from other sources, particularly soil and outdoor air, must be accounted for—a necessity that is complicated by the potential for large temporal variability in entry rates from these sources. (See, for example, Chapter 2.) The approach presented here, mathematically combining data on the contributing factors to determine the distribution of f, constitutes a feasible alternative for obtaining statistically robust results. A closely related experimental approach is to measure W, e, V, and λ_v in a randomly selected set of houses and evaluate f for each from Equation 3. Although this approach appears to offer advantages over the other experimental technique, particularly in avoiding interference from radon sources other than water, it has not yet been used.

2.2 Water-Use Rates

The results from several studies giving residential in-house water-use rates per occupant for specific functions are listed in Table 4.1. Four of these studies report results from 29 individual residences (22–25). Two additional studies, not included in Table 4.1, give the total in-house consumption rate for 18 houses in Louisville, Kentucky (26), and for 43 homes in Wheatland and Laramie, Wyoming (27). Total in-house use rates per person for these 90 residences are plotted as a cumulative probability distribution in Figure 4.1. The data are well fitted by a lognormal distribution with a geometric mean of 7.9×10^{-3} m^3 person^{-1} h^{-1} (0.189 m^3 person^{-1} d^{-1}) and a geometric standard deviation of 1.57. The null hypothesis that the parent distribution is lognormal cannot be rejected, even at a significance level

134

TABLE 4.1 In-House Water Use Rates, by Function ($\times 10^{-3}$) (m^3 person^{-1} day^{-1})

Investigator[a]	Ref.	Dish-washing	Shower/bath	Toilet	Laundry	Other	Total
Cohen (8)	22	68.0	23.8	65.0	39.7		197
1			14.0	34.4	69.0		145
2			36.0	104	34.8		384
3			10.8	41.0			157
4			16.6	72.5			220
5			40.2	113			263
6			28.4	44.8	37.8		190
7			24.9	42.1	31.4		143
8			20.8	69.8	26.5		179
Ligman	57						
(35 rural)		11.6	41.9	68.2	51.9		174
(10 urban)		13.9	37.9	68.2	41.4		161
Laak (5)	23	13.6	32.1	74.8	28.0	7.9	156
A		12.1	58.2	112	54	11.3	246
B		34.4	20.0	138	7.9	12.2	212
C		12.9	22.3	42.3	16.3	5.7	99
D		7.9	18.9	51.8	29.9	3.8	112
E		7.9	37.8	49.9	17.0	10.2	123
Bennett (5)	24	14.0	32.9	55.6	43.8	21.9	168
1		4.6	13.1	68.7	55.4	38.5	180

2		1.3	31.8	38.8	26.8	17.8	117
3		7.3	61.7	89.9	20.9	49.7	230
4			29.6	108.4	59.8	93.0	291
5		3.7	40.9	37.8	34.3	19.1	136
Milne	58	27	80	121	27	10	265
Reid[b]	59	14	76	91	32	10	223
EPA (11)[c]	25	19	38	35	40	20	152
A		18.9	51.0	34.4	47.6	62.3	214
B		10.2	30.2	32.9	8.3	15.1	96
C		13.2	27.6	21.2	49.5	35.5	147
D		18.9	50.3	31.8	28.7	25.7	155
E		10.6	32.8	31.0	52.9	29.9	157
F		18.9	21.5	23.4	48.0	15.5	127
G		14.0	32.9	24.6	15.9	25.4	113
H		11.0	22.3	34.8	42.3	77.8	188
I		23.0	26.8	29.9	61.2	16.6	158
J		20.8	46.1	52.2	35.9	15.9	170
K		26.8	44.2	41.2	49.1	53.7	215
Partridge	12, 29	30–38	76–152	76–152	15–23	76–114	197–327

[a]Number of houses indicated in parentheses. For each study, the first line gives summary results; subsequent lines, where present, give average results for specific households. Study sites: Cohen—Connecticut (4), Rhode Island (2), California (2); Ligman—Wisconsin; Laak—probably Connecticut; Bennett—Boulder, Colorado; Milne—estimated; Reid—estimated; EPA—Wisconsin; Partridge—estimated.

[b]Cited in Ref. 60; apparently the basis for the analyses in Refs. 10, 13.

[c]The basis for the analysis in Ref 14.

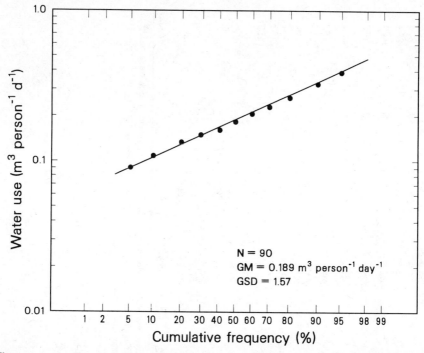

Figure 4.1. Cumulative frequency distribution of the average per capita in-house water use rate, *W*, in 90 U.S. residences. The straight line represents the lognormal distribution that best fits the data, using minimum variance unbiased estimators of the geometric mean and geometric standard deviation.

of 0.2, according to the Kolmogorov-Smirnov test (28). Three previous studies of indoor radon from potable water have cited water-use rates of 0.152 (14), 0.223 (13), and 0.262 (12, 29) m^3 person^{-1} d^{-1}, each of these values is within one geometric standard deviation of the geometric mean determined here.

2.3 Transfer Efficiency

Radon is relatively insoluble in water. Boyle measured the solubility coefficient as a function of temperature and found values of 0.51, 0.25, and 0.16 at 0.0, 20.0, and 39.1°C, respectively (30). As an example of the significance of these data, consider a toilet tank holding 0.02 m^3 of water at 20°C in a closed bathroom of 15 m^3. At equilibrium, assuming the initial concentration in air is zero, 99.97% of the radon originally in the water has been released. Measurements have shown that the actual fraction released in residences is generally much smaller, indicating that equilibrium is not attained. A complete theoretical analysis of the transfer of radon from water to air in households has not been undertaken; instead, researchers have measured the fraction released by different uses experimentally.

Transfer coefficients have been determined for major household water uses in three studies (12–14). In each case, concentrations of radon in the inlet and effluent streams were measured. In one study, transfer coefficients for some uses were estimated from laboratory investigations of the dependence of the liberated fraction on agitation and on the surface-to-volume ratio of the water reservoir (14). The results from these studies are summarized in Table 4.2, which shows good agreement among them.

To determine a use-weighted mean transfer efficiency, we have applied mean coefficients by use (the last column in Table 4.2) to average water use by function for the 21 houses for which use by function was comprehensively monitored (23–25). The results are plotted as a cumulative frequency distribution in Figure 4.2, which shows a geometric mean of 0.55 and a geometric standard deviation of 1.12. The range for the 21 houses considered was small (0.44–0.68), leading to the conclusion, as discussed below, that variability in the transfer efficiency is likely to be a small factor in the overall variability of f.

2.4 House Volume

In a study conducted for the U.S. Department of Energy, the floor area of the heated portion of 6051 randomly selected residences was measured (31). The report tabulates the number of residences in each of seven building-size classes for six categories corresponding to the number of household members. After assuming a fixed ceiling height of 2.4 m, we applied a least-squares analysis to the cumulative frequency plots of these volume data to derive lognormal statistics for volume per resident as a function of the number of residents per household. (See Figure 4.3.) These statistics were then combined mathematically, with weighting factors proportional to the number of people in each class, to obtain 99 m^3 person^{-1} and 1.90 as the geometric mean and geometric standard deviation, respectively, for the U.S. population. This distribution is plotted as the bold line in Figure 4.3 and is seen to agree well with the points enclosed by circles, which were determined by graphically aggregating the results from the other six curves.

TABLE 4.2   Transfer Coefficient for the Release of Radon from Water to Air, by Use

	Fraction of radon liberated			
Type of use	Ref. 12	Ref. 13	Ref. 14	Mean
Dishwasher	0.98	0.9	0.98	0.95
Shower	0.71	0.63	0.65	0.66
Bath	0.5	0.47	0.3[a]	0.42
Toilet	0.29	0.3	0.3[a]	0.3
Laundry	0.95	0.9	0.9[a]	0.92
Drinking and cleaning	0.28	0.45	0.1–0.5[a]	0.34

[a]Estimated in the reference.

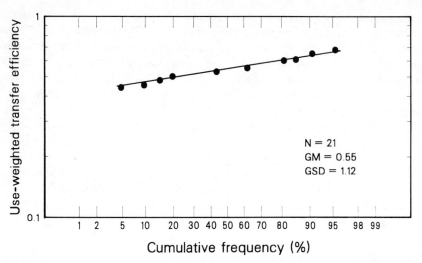

Figure 4.2. Cumulative frequency distribution of use-weighted transfer efficiency, e, for radon from water to air. Each of the 21 values was determined by summing the products of the use-specific transfer coefficients (Table 4.2, ''Mean'') and the fractional use rates for individual houses (Table 4.1).

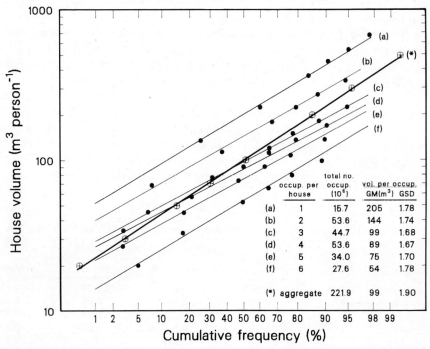

Figure 4.3. Cumulative frequency distribution of per capita household volume, V, for U.S. residences (31). Only heated volume is considered. Six curves, a–f, give distributions for specified numbers of residents per household; the bold line gives the aggregate distribution, representative of the entire U.S. population.

2.5   Air-Exchange Rate

Two studies have been published that give air-exchange rate data for a large number of U.S. residences. In the first of these, 1048 tracer-gas decay measurements, each giving the air-exchange rate over a few hours, were made in 266 dwellings occupied by low-income families and located in 14 cities spanning the major U.S. climatic zones (32). The individual measurement results are plotted as cumulative frequency curve a in Figure 4.4 and are fitted by a lognormal distribution whose geometric mean and geometric standard deviation are 0.9 h^{-1} and 2.13, respectively.

The second study evaluated average infiltration rates for the November–March heating season in 312 residences (33). In contrast to the first study, in which the median house age was 45 years, the houses in this investigation tended to be fairly new, with a median age of less than 10 years. Furthermore, these houses did not represent the distribution across U.S. climate zones: most were located in Wash-

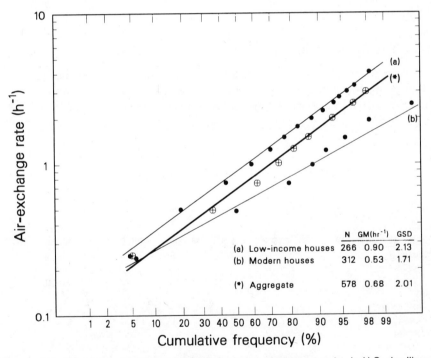

Figure 4.4. Cumulative frequency distribution of air-exchange rates, λ_v, in U.S. dwellings. The study of low-income houses measured air-exchange rates over intervals of a few hours (32); the distribution was determined from 1048 individual measurements in 266 houses (and therefore has a higher variance than it would if the average measurement in each house had been used). The study of modern houses determined average infiltration rates for a heating season (33). The studies were aggregated with weights proportional to the number of houses studied.

ington, California, Colorado, New York, and Ontario, Canada. The cumulative probability distribution of infiltration rates for these houses is plotted as curve *b* in Figure 4.4. The Kolmogorov-Smirnov test for goodness-of-fit indicates that the hypothesis that the parent distribution is lognormal can be rejected at a significance level of 0.05, although not at a significance level of 0.01.

As these two studies concentrated respectively on low-income houses, which are probably leakier than average, and on modern houses, which are probably tighter than average, we expect that the distribution for all U.S. housing lies between the two. We have estimated the parameters of the true distribution by aggregating the two sample distributions weighted proportionally to the number of houses. The resulting geometric mean is 0.68 h^{-1} and the geometric standard deviation is 2.01.

A caution must be noted in using these results: the measurements apply for the most part only to infiltration and only during the heating season. In many cases air-exchange rates at other times of the year are higher due to windows being open. If windows and doors are closed, however, the air-exchange rate may be lower because the milder weather conditions lead to reduced driving forces for infiltration.

2.6 The Distribution of *f*

A variable derived as the sum of independent, normally distributed parameters is itself normally distributed with a mean value given by the sum of the means and a variance given by the sum of the variances (34). Similarly, a variable that is the product of independent, lognormally distributed parameters is itself lognormally

TABLE 4.3 Summary of Lognormal Parameters for Variables Used in the Determination of *f*

Variable	N	GM	GSD	% Var[a]	GSE[b]	Units
Water-use rate (*W*)	90	7.9×10^{-3}	1.57	18	1.05	m^3 (person − h)$^{-1}$
House volume (*V*)	6051	98.7	1.90	37	1.01	m^3 person^{-1}
Air-exchange rate (λ_v)	578	0.68	2.01	44	1.03	h^{-1}
Transfer coefficient (*e*)	21	0.55	1.12	1	1.03	
Air-to-water ratio (*f*)		0.65×10^{-4}	2.88		1.063	

[a]Percent of variance in ln (*f*) that can be attributed to given parameter.
[b]Geometric standard error: GSE = exp (ln(GSD)/$N^{1/2}$). For *f* the GSE was determined as:

$$GSE_f = \exp \left[\{ \ln^2 (GSE_W) + \ln^2 (GSE_V) + \ln^2 (GSE_{\lambda_v}) + \ln^2 (GSE_e) \}^{1/2} \right]$$

distributed. Thus, given the lognormal statistics for W, e, V, and λ_v, as summarized in Table 4.3, the lognormal statistics for f can be determined as follows:

$$GM_f = \frac{GM_W GM_e}{GM_V GM_{\lambda_v}} \tag{4}$$

$$GSD_f = \exp\left[\left\{\left(\ln\left(GSD_W\right)\right)^2 + \left(\ln\left(GSD_e\right)\right)^2 + \left(\ln\left(GSD_V\right)\right)^2 + \left(\ln\left(GSD_{\lambda_v}\right)\right)^2\right\}^{1/2}\right]* \tag{5}$$

In these expressions GM_i represents a geometric mean, GSD_i represents a geometric standard deviation, and the subscripts designate a parameter. Using this approach to derive the parameters of the lognormal distribution for f yields a geometric mean of 0.65×10^{-4} with a geometric standard deviation of 2.88.

There are two methods of comparing this result with those of other studies. First, we can calculate the arithmetic mean of f from the following equation (applicable only for a lognormal distribution):

$$AM = GM \exp\left[\left(\ln\left(GSD\right)\right)^2/2\right]^\dagger \tag{6}$$

The resulting value, 1.14×10^{-4}, agrees well with the typically cited value of 1×10^{-4}. The second approach compares this distribution with that resulting from direct measurements of C_a/C_w. For this comparison we have constructed a plot, shown in Figure 4.5, of the cumulative frequency distribution derived from data for 13 houses in which C_a/C_w was directly measured and in which the radon concentration in water exceeded 40,000 Bq m^{-3} (13, 14). In four other houses in which such measurements were made, the waterborne radon concentrations were so small that the expected contributions to radon in air were small compared even with outdoor concentrations and therefore extremely difficult to measure. Considering the widely different means of determining f, the agreement between our computed distribution and the results of direct measurements is reasonably good: 12 of the 13 measurements lie between 5% and 95% contours of the computed distribution.

The fifth column in Table 4.3 (labeled ''% var.'') indicates the relative contributions of the various factors to the range of the distribution of f. These data indicate that differences among houses in volume per resident and air-exchange rate are more important than differences in water-use rate and transfer efficiency in accounting for the differences in f among the housing stock.

---

*The validity of assuming that the variables on the right-hand side of this equation are independent is examined in Section 5.3.
†The minimum variance unbiased estimator of AM is given by a somewhat more complex formula, which depends on the number of samples as well as the geometric mean and geometric standard deviation (35). For a large number of samples the expression converges to Equation 6. Taking $n = 21$ for the current case (corresponding to the number of determinations of e), the arithmetic mean determined by the more complex formula is 1.10×10^{-4}.

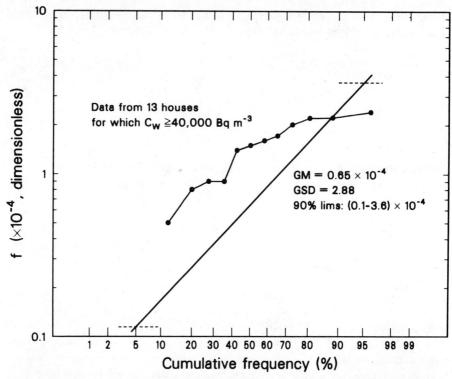

Figure 4.5. Cumulative frequency distribution of f, the airborne radon concentration in U.S. dwellings that can be ascribed to a specified waterborne concentration. The straight line represents the results of the analysis in this chapter. The 12 points plotted represent results of measurements of f in 12 of 13 houses for which the waterborne concentration exceeded 40×10^3 Bq m^{-3} (13, 14). For the thirteenth house, a negative value, not plotted, was determined for f. For three of the houses, the reference reports C_a as less than a limit. For this figure, we have plotted f for these houses at the corresponding limits, which are $(0.8, 0.9,$ and $1.7) \times 10^{-4}$, respectively.

In interpreting the results of this analysis, one must recognize the distinction between the variance associated with the distribution of a parameter and the uncertainty in the estimate of its mean. The former, reflected by the column labeled "GSD" in Table 4.3, provides information on the range of actual values in the parent distribution. The latter, reflected by the column labeled "GSE," indicates the degree to which the data are adequate in number to determine the mean of the parent distribution. Thus, a GSD of 2.88 for f suggests that the value of f for 68% of the housing stock is contained within the range $(0.23–1.87) \times 10^{-4}$—i.e., within a factor of 2.88 of the geometric mean. On the other hand, a GSE of 1.063 for f indicates that the 90% confidence limits on its geometric mean (assuming the sampling to be representative) are 0.58×10^{-4} and 0.73×10^{-4}. The data in the GSE column also indicate that the water-use rate contributes the greatest amount of the four factors to the uncertainty in GM$_f$, suggesting that additional experimental work to improve the estimate of f be directed at assessing W for a larger number of households.

From these results we can also determine the number of households needed to estimate GM_f by direct experimental measurement with a precision comparable to that of the present analysis. That number is given by

$$N = \left[\ln\left(GSD_f\right)/\ln\left(GSE_f\right)\right]^2 = 300 \qquad (7)$$

Thus, f would have to be measured in 300 residences to improve the statistical basis for estimating the parameters of the distribution. This analysis does not consider how well the data represent the U.S. housing stock. Because the sampling for each parameter except V cannot be considered random, the uncertainty in our estimate of the geometric mean of f is larger than that indicated by the GSE. However, an approach to improving the estimate of the distribution of f that uses direct experimental measurements would also experience difficulties in selecting a representative sample.

3 RADON CONCENTRATIONS IN POTABLE WATER SUPPLIES

Radon concentrations in water have been observed to range over an extremely large range, from effectively zero to more than 10^6 Bq m^{-3}. Surface waters, which serve 49.5% of the U.S. population (36), have the lowest concentrations. Private wells, serving 18.3% of the population, generally have the highest concentrations, whereas public groundwater supplies, which serve the remaining 32.2%, have intermediate concentrations. In assessing the data on radon in water supplies, we consider these three sources separately.

Considerable work has recently been undertaken by the U.S. Environmental Protection Agency (EPA) to measure radon concentrations in public groundwater supplies in the United States (16, 17). Using these data, along with other results from the literature, we have computed lognormal statistics for the 41 states for which data exist. (See Table 4.4.) In computing these statistics, the logarithm of each concentration measurement was weighted by the inverse of the logarithm of the variance due to counting uncertainty. The analysis was complicated by two features of the data: (i) due to background count rates and statistical variability, some of the measurement results were negative; and (ii) in early reports, measurements below the detection limit of approximately 600 Bq m^{-3} were reported as "not detectable." Consequently, the parameters of the distributions could not be determined from the first and second moments of complete sets of log-transformed data. Instead, for each state we estimated the geometric mean as the median of the entire set of data and determined the geometric standard deviation by calculating the second moment (about the median) of the measurements whose value exceeded the median.

To estimate the distribution of radon concentration in public groundwater supplies for the entire country, two approaches were used. First, the parameters of

TABLE 4.4 Radon Concentrations in Public Groundwater Supplies in the United States

State	Population served (1000s)	No. samples	Rn-222 conc. (10^3 Bq m^{-3}) GM	GSD	Ref.
Alabama	1200	104	3.29	3.10	41, 64
Arizona	1490	64	10.9	2.40	65
Arkansas	880	43	1.70	4.39	15, 40
Colorado	320	37	9.31	2.49	64
Delaware	254	36	3.56	1.88	61
Florida	6800	165	3.03	3.02	61
Georgia	1320	61	3.87	3.93	17
Idaho	592	85	8.30	2.41	62
Illinois	4050	158	4.95	2.09	65
Indiana	1920	117	2.51	2.83	15, 63
Iowa	1600	58	4.37	3.23	15, 40
Kansas	903	7	2.66	3.11	17
Kentucky	375	50	3.46	2.46	62
Louisiana	1850	22	3.44	2.54	15
Maine	101	68	37.4	2.38	39
Massachussetts	1550	100	26.8	1.76	64
Minnesota	1910	124	6.72	2.17	15, 64
Mississippi	1800	53	2.10	2.61	64
Montana	184	33	14.0	2.17	62
Nebraska	961	21	6.59	3.68	15
Nevada	329	26	13.3	2.28	61
New Hampshire	392	31	32.1	2.45	42, 62
New Jersey	3420	19	13.5	3.21	42
New Mexico	798	89	7.50	2.32	15, 63
New York	3510	150	4.06	2.87	40
North Carolina	474	181	4.87	9.42	39, 63
North Dakota	258	67	4.49	2.33	61
Ohio	2950	84	4.43	2.38	62
Oklahoma	662	56	4.82	1.97	15, 42
Oregon	344	65	8.44	2.03	62
Pennsylvania	2180	89	14.2	3.22	63
Rhode Island	142	92	65.6	5.90	65
South Carolina	541	185	5.03	6.28	42
South Dakota	321	79	9.83	2.57	61
Tennessee	1450	50	1.24	5.64	65
Texas	5030	278	4.85	2.70	15
Utah	662	98	10.6	1.95	64
Vermont	113	11	23.1	1.48	65
Virginia	707	101	8.37	3.69	65
Wisconsin	1620	143	7.43	2.78	63
Wyoming	122	18	12.7	2.67	65
Total	56,085[a]	3318	5.18[b]	3.53[b]	

[a]Includes 76% of population served by public groundwater supplies (36).
[b]Population-weighted statistics.

the lognormal distribution for each state were combined with weights proportional to the population using public groundwater (36). The result is a geometric mean of 5.2×10^3 Bq m^{-3} and a geometric standard deviation of 3.53. The data were also combined using a nonparametric approach: witht the assistance of a computer program, 5000 values were randomly selected from the set of individual EPA measurements and used to construct a cumulative probability distribution. The program was designed so that the probability of any given measurement being selected was proportional to the number of people using public groundwater in that state and inversely proportional to the number of measurements taken there.

Results from these two approaches are represented as case *a* in Figure 4.6, with the line representing the presumed lognormal distribution and the points resulting from the nonparametric analysis. The agreement is seen to be quite good, reinforcing the postulate that the parent distribution is well-represented by a lognormal. Using Equation 6 and the lognormal parameters for the country, the arith-

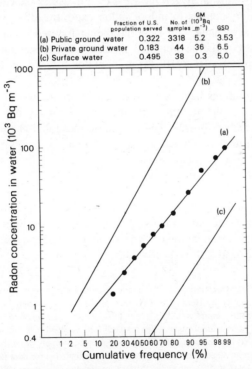

	Fraction of U.S. population served	No. of samples	GM $(10^3$Bq m$^{-3})$	GSD
(a) Public ground water	0.322	3318	5.2	3.53
(b) Private ground water	0.183	44	36	6.5
(c) Surface water	0.495	38	0.3	5.0

Figure 4.6. Cumulative frequency distributions of radon concentrations in potable water supplies in the United States. Distributions for surface water, public groundwater, and private groundwater supplies are plotted separately. For case *a*, the points shown were determined by a stochastic process from individual data; the line represents an analytical evaluation of the parameters of the distribution, assuming it to be lognormal.

metic mean radon concentration in public groundwater supplies is estimated to be 11.5×10^3 Bq m^{-3}.

A few cautions should be noted in interpreting these results. First, the data may be slightly positively biased by the fact that some sampling was done at distribution sites, rather than at household taps. A more important concern is potential sampling bias. In the entire EPA study, the supplies that were to be sampled were chosen by state officials with no randomness criteria specified by EPA. Furthermore, for most of the study, sampling was limited to supplies serving 1000 or more people. Although 86% of the U.S. population that is served by public groundwater is accounted for within these criteria, limited data show concentrations as much as an order of magnitude greater in smaller supplies (37) and perhaps three times as great on average (38). Horton has computed the arithmetic mean both with and without population-weighting according to supply size (17). He found a population-weighted mean of 8.6×10^3 Bq m^{-3} when size of individual supplies was considered compared with 13.0×10^3 Bq m^{-3} when it was not. Cothern et al. have also analyzed the EPA data to assess the contribution of U.S. public groundwater supplies to indoor radon exposure (38). After attempting to remove the bias associated with sampling being focused on large supplies, they concluded that the population-weighted average radon concentration in U.S. public groundwater supplies is 16×10^3 Bq m^{-3}, about 40% higher than the value obtained here.

Higher concentrations have been observed in private wells, although the data are quite limited. For the present work, the assessment was based on 44 measurements from nine states (39–42). The geometric mean and geometric standard deviation using an equal-weight calculation were found to be 36×10^3 Bq m^{-3} and 6.5, respectively. The dominant uncertainty in these results is due to unrepresentative sampling; hence, a more rigorous analysis of the data is unwarranted.

Information on radon concentrations in surface water supplies was derived from the same set of reports. Using a linear regression to the cumulative frequency plot of the 13 of 38 measurements that exceeded the detection limit of 0.6×10^3 Bq m^{-3}, the geometric mean and geometric standard deviation were estimated to be 0.3×10^3 Bq m^{-3} and 5.0, respectively.*

*Geometric mean ^{222}Rn concentrations for the three types of water supply, based largely on the same data, were recently reported by Hess et al. (37). For private wells and public groundwater supplies, the geometric means for the entire country agree within 10% of those reported here. Values for public groundwater supplies in individual states differ markedly, however. These differences appear to result from several factors: (i) duplicate samples from a single water supply were averaged in the present work, whereas Hess et al. treated the two values as independent; (ii) for data falling below the minimum detection limit, Hess et al. assigned an arbitrary small value ($\sim$4 Bq m^{-3}) for those data reported as not detectable or having negative values; and (iii) for some states Hess et al. incorporate into their analyses early data not included in the published EPA reports. In some cases these early data may have been collected as part of an effort to look for high concentrations of radon in water supplies, rather than to ascertain the actual concentration distribution (43). The aggregate geometric mean reported by Hess et al. for surface water supplies is almost an order of magnitude smaller than the value we have determined. For either case, however, the conclusion remains that compared with other sources, surface water supplies are a negligible factor in contributing to indoor radon.

By combining the distributions of C_w with the distribution of f, one obtains an estimate of the parameters of the distribution of C_a, the incremental airborne radon concentration in residences attributable to water. Following the approach used in deriving Equations 4–6, the distribution parameters were determined for the three types of water supply, as shown in Table 4.5. Also shown in the table are the fraction of houses in which the incremental indoor radon concentration due to the use of potable water exceeds two benchmark values. The lower number, 9.3 Bq m^{-3}, corresponds to the typical concentration entering residences from the outdoor air (44). The higher value, 33 Bq m^{-3}, corresponds to the estimated geometric mean radon concentration in U.S. residences (45). In only a small fraction of houses served by public groundwater supplies is water a major source of indoor radon. On the other hand, the limited data on radon concentrations in private wells suggests that a substantial fraction of these may constitute important sources of indoor radon.

These results also indicate that public groundwater supplies cause about 0.8% of the radon progeny exposure for the total U.S. population*; the total exposure is estimated to cause an average individual lifetime risk of lung cancer of about 0.2% (45–47). (See Chapters 1 and 12.) Thus the *average* individual lifetime risk due to radon from public water supplies is in the vicinity of 10^{-5} (0.008×0.002), equal to the *limiting* risk commonly used by governmental agencies for regulation of water and airborne environmental agents. Considering the broad distribution of C_a, a significant number of people are exposed to airborne radon from public water supplies at levels corresponding to risks of 10^{-4} to 10^{-3}, or even higher.[†] Given this observation, it is ironic that even if these supplies were controlled to the extent that they contributed nothing to indoor radon concentrations, the average public risk from exposure to airborne radon progeny would be essentially unchanged. These seemingly inconsistent features arise because, although 99% of indoor radon originates in sources other than public groundwater supplies, estimates suggest that the health risks associated with typical indoor radon levels are unusually high relative to those associated with other environmental pollutants.

Overall, considering all supply types, the mean contribution of potable water to indoor ^{222}Rn concentrations in U.S. housing is estimated to be 4.8 Bq m^{-3}. By comparison, corresponding estimates for Finland (9) and the Swiss Central Alps (67) are 5.6 Bq m^{-3} and 23 Bq m^{-3}, respectively. For Switzerland, the higher number results mainly from much smaller building volumes, 30 m^3 per occupant (67). In Denmark, ^{222}Rn concentrations in potable water were undetectable ($< 10^3$ Bq m^{-3}), except on the island of Bornholm (68).

---

*Estimates in Nero et al. (45) indicate an AM of 55 Bq m^{-3} for the annual average radon concentration in U.S. houses. The AM for radon from public groundwater (Table 4.5) is 1.3 Bq m^{-3}, applicable to 0.322 of the U.S. population. Thus, the average contribution of U.S. public groundwater supplies to indoor radon levels is $(0.322)(1.3)/55 = 0.0076$, or about 0.8%.

[†]The parameters of the lognormal distribution in Table 4.5 suggest that the fractions of the U.S. population exposed to an average C_a due to public water supplies exceeding 1.9 Bq m^{-3} and 19 Bq m^{-3}, respectively, are 0.05 and 0.002. These concentrations correspond to estimated lifetime risks of lung cancer, following the work cited above, of 10^{-4} and 10^{-3}, respectively.

TABLE 4.5   Estimated Contributions to U.S. Indoor Airborne ^{222}Rn Concentration for Three Types of Water Service

Type	Fraction of U.S. pop. served	C_a (Bq m^{-3})			Fraction exceeding:	
		GM	GSD	AM	9.3 Bq m^{-3}	33 Bq m^{-3}
Surface Public	0.495	0.020	6.86	0.13	0.0007	0.0001
groundwater	0.322	0.34	5.19	1.3	0.022	0.0027
Private wells	0.183	2.3	8.59	24.	0.26	0.11
Aggregate	1.0			4.8	0.055	0.021

4   CONTROLLING RADON CONCENTRATIONS IN POTABLE WATER

In cases where potable water is a source of unacceptably high radon concentrations, there are straightforward technical measures that can be applied to reduce exposures. In comparison with the many studies of radon exposure due to water use, relatively little attention has been devoted to controlling such exposures (48–51). Consequently, this discussion will be brief.

The first principle that must be recognized is that—given f of order 10^{-4}—it is advantageous to apply the control measure to the water itself, rather than to the air in the house. Given this principle, the available approaches are to extract the radon from the water using granular activated carbon (GAC) or an alternative solid sorbent; to transfer the radon to outdoor air by bubble or spray aeration; and to allow radon to decay by storing the water out of contact with the aquifer. Among these approaches, the last, requiring a large storage vessel, is the least practical. For example, applying it at a household scale might typically require a 10-m^3 storage tank (for in-house water use only) to achieve 90% reduction for a family of four. Fortunately, the other two approaches do appear practical.

Radon adsorption on GAC is well documented: for example, it is used as an analytical technique for extracting radon from an air sample (52), and, more recently, as a collection medium for a passive radon sampler (53). The effectiveness of GAC for continuous use in removing radon from drinking water has recently been evaluated (49–51). It was determined that for a capital investment of $850 and minor operating expense, units are available that can provide in excess of 99% removal efficiency for single-family households. The required volume of GAC is in the range of 0.03–0.07 m^3. Some attention must be given to the potential gamma-radiation hazard from the filter unit. Disposal of the spent carbon is another potential concern; however, comparing the expected specific activity of the carbon bed due, for example, to ^{210}Pb with the ^{210}Pb activity of ordinary soil suggests that this is at most a minor problem. The effective lifetime of such units is not known, but appears to be at least several years.

The aeration techniques take advantage of the relative insolubility of radon in water that leads to the problem in the first place. Diffused (bubble) aerators, with removal efficiency exceeding 99%, have a capital cost of approximately $2000

(51). Spray aeration units are more expensive ($3000) and have been found to be less effective (about 90% removal efficiency) (51).

5 LIMITATIONS OF THE CURRENT ANALYSIS

This section focuses on the uncertainties associated with estimating the parameters of the distribution of f. Limitations associated with the radon concentration data were discussed above and are also considered by Horton (17).

5.1 Use of the Lognormal Distribution

Throughout this chapter we have assumed that the parent distribution for various parameters is lognormal. This hypothesis is used for three purposes: (i) to combine the distributions of the four contributing factors to determine the distribution of f according to Equations 4 and 5; (ii) to determine the arithmetic means of the distributions of f and C_a according to Equation 6; and (iii) to estimate the fraction of households in which benchmark values of C_a are exceeded (Table 4.5). It cannot be *proven* that the parent distributions are lognormal: statistical tests can only evaluate the hypothesis that a sample distribution is *consistent* with a postulated form of the parent distribution. And even if the hypothesis is rejected by the statistical test, the data may still be sufficiently well approximated by a lognormal distribution that results based on that hypothesis constitute good estimates.

Considerable evidence supports the appropriateness of the lognormal distribution for representing f and C_w. Cumulative probability plots of the factors contributing to f suggest that the lognormal distribution is appropriate. The objective Kolmogorov-Smirnov test demonstrates for the water-use rates and air-exchange rate that the hypothesis that the parent distribution is lognormal cannot be rejected at a very high level of significance. The stochastic generation of a cumulative probability distribution for radon concentration in public groundwater supplies yields results that are consistent with a lognormal distribution (Fig. 4.6). In addition, it can be demonstrated on theoretical grounds that the random multiplicative combination of independent factors yields a lognormal distribution in the limit of a large number of factors, regardless of the distribution of each factor. And finally, a previous study of radon in water found that the distributions by state were better fitted by lognormal than by normal distributions (15).

5.2 Adequacy and Representativeness of the Data

Of the four factors needed to determine f, only the distribution of house volumes was obtained from a large random sample that may be considered representative of the U.S. housing stock. Of the remaining factors, we believe it is most important to improve information on in-house water use rates. Even though the current data show only moderate dispersion, we are not assured that the limited sample of 90 residences is representative of the entire country. The second priority for increasing the amount of data should be directed at the air-exchange rate. We are reasonably assured that no other large data sets currently exist; however, because of the recent development of infiltration models (54) and an integrating ventilation monitor (55), a systematic study of air-exchange rates in U.S. residences is now possible. The remaining factor, the use-weighted transfer coefficient, does not need much further consideration. Because any residence uses water in a mix of applications, some with high transfer efficiencies and others with low values, the use-weighted coefficient for any house will necessarily be intermediate between the minimum and maximum use-specific values of 0.3 and 1.0. The very narrow range for e observed, even for the limited data set considered here, combined with the good agreement among investigators on use-specific values, suggests that further refinements in determining the distribution of e are unlikely to substantially affect the estimates of f.

Note that we have effectively taken the perspective that this fundamental approach—based on data on four contributing factors—provides sounder information on f than direct experimental measurement of airborne and waterborne radon concentrations. The limited data of the latter kind have an average and range consistent with those resulting from the analytical approach taken here. Improvements in the statistical representation of direct experimental determinations of f by measuring C_a and C_w are subject to considerable difficulties in terms of the measurements themselves, and formidable problems in choosing a sample where the water contribution is dominant, yet which is also representative of the housing stock.

In terms of estimating risk associated with water use, the dominant uncertainties appear to be associated with the distribution of C_w rather than f. The problem is that radon concentrations in water from small public supplies and private wells are largely unknown. Yet the limited data that are available suggest that among water sources these make the dominant contribution to radon exposure.

5.3 Correlation Among Factors

In deriving Equation 1, it was assumed that the air-exchange rate, λ_v, and the incremental airborne radon concentration due to water use, C_a, were not correlated. No data exist to test the validity of this assumption. However, it is reasonable to expect, given the high proportion of water use in bathrooms and the common presence there of an exhaust fan or an open window, that these variables are correlated to a degree. Experiments would be needed to determine the importance of this possible correlation.

In determining the variance in f, we further assumed that the several contributing factors were independent (see Equation 5). This assumption, although a reasonable approximation, is not strictly valid. For example, one study showed that water-use rates are positively correlated with house value (56); hence, they probably are positively correlated with house volume. Data in another study show a negative correlation between house volume and air-exchange rate (33).

The complete form of Equation 5, accounting for correlation among factors, would include six additional terms, one for each pair of factors. The sign of each term can be plus or minus, depending on whether the correlation is positive or negative, and whether one factor multiplies or divides the other in determining f. The only available data for estimating the magnitude of these terms are the measurements of house volume and air-exchange rate in 312 houses (33). We computed the variance of the sum of the logarithms of these two factors, first assuming them to be independent, and then including the effects of cross-correlation. The cross-correlation term reduced the standard deviation of the sum by 11%. Since, in determining the variance of f, both negative and positive contributions from the cross-correlation terms are to be expected, the error in GSD_f due to assuming the factors to be uncorrelated is probably of order 10%. (Note that Equation 4 for the geometric mean does not depend on the factors being independent.)

5.4 Limitations of the Model

In assessing population exposures using the long-term-average single-cell model, two additional elements must be considered. First, although the model assumes a uniform indoor concentration, water use is highly localized and so the incremental radon concentration associated with water use should vary spatially. As a result, in some cases the single-cell model may not effectively describe the spatially averaged indoor concentration. For example, a bathroom exhaust fan may effectively prevent much of the radon released from a shower from reaching other rooms of the residence, even though it has a small impact on the air-exchange rate of the entire house. On the other hand, because of spatial association between occupants and the site of water use, the exposure to radon liberated by water is somewhat greater than the household average concentration. However, the effect of spatial variations on exposure is diminished by the mixing that occurs during the time over which the radon progeny concentrations increase to secular equilibrium. Prichard and Gesell, in considering these effects, concluded that the *average* indoor concentration arising from water use resulted in considerably greater exposure than did locally elevated concentrations associated with episodic emission (10).

The second factor to consider is the temporal association between occupancy and water use: most of the water use in a household occurs when people are present. As a result, the average exposure to radon progeny arising from the use of potable water is greater than the estimate obtained by multiplying the average incremental indoor concentration due to this source by the fraction of time a person occupies the dwelling. The upper bound on exposure, considering this factor alone, is obtained by assuming the same average concentration and 100% occupancy.

6 SUMMARY AND CONCLUSIONS

The incremental concentration of radon in indoor air in U.S. housing resulting from a specified concentration of radon in water has been determined using a long-term average, single-cell model and available data on house volumes, air-exchange rates, water-use rates, and water-to-air transfer coefficients. The ratio of airborne to waterborne concentration so determined is represented by a lognormal distribution with a geometric mean and geometric standard deviation of 0.65×10^{-4}

and 2.88, respectively. The statistical uncertainty in the geometric mean arising from limited sample size is 6%. This distribution is consistent with the results of direct measurements previously made in 13 houses.

Surface supplies of potable water do not contribute significantly to indoor radon concentrations. Groundwater supplies, which serve about 50% of the U.S. population, can in some circumstances constitute an important source. Public supplies derived from groundwater and serving 1000 or more persons have been extensively investigated; these are estimated to contribute 0.8% to the overall mean indoor concentration for all housing, or an average of 2% to the mean indoor radon concentration in houses using these sources. Private groundwater supplies appear to constitute a somewhat greater source; however, the data are fragmentary. Further sampling studies are warranted.

7 APPENDIX: DERIVATION OF EQUATION 1

We seek the average contribution, C_a, of potable water to the indoor airborne radon concentration. By treating the interior of a residence as a single, well-mixed volume, the rate of change of the total indoor radon concentration, C_i, may be described by the first-order differential equation

$$\frac{dC_i}{dt} = C_o \lambda_v^* + S - C_i \lambda_v^* + \frac{C_w W^* e^*}{V} \tag{8}$$

where C_o is the outdoor radon concentration
S is the entry rate per unit volume for all sources other than water (i.e., building materials and soil)
λ_v^* is the instantaneous air-exchange rate
C_w is the concentration of radon in water
W^* is the instantaneous water-use rate
V is the volume of the residence
e^* is the instantaneous use-weighted transfer efficiency of radon from water to air

We have neglected radioactive decay as a removal term as it is small relative to the air-exchange rate.

If Equation 8 is integrated over a long period and divided by the length of the period, the left-hand side tends to zero, and we obtain the equation

$$\frac{1}{T} \int_0^T C_i \lambda_v^* \, dt = \frac{1}{T} \int_0^T (C_o \lambda_v^* + S) \, dt + \frac{1}{T} \int_0^T \frac{C_w W^* e^*}{V} \, dt \tag{9}$$

Let $C_i = C + C_a^*$, where C is the indoor radon concentration in the absence of water use and C_a^* is the instantaneous concentration increase due to water. Then

$$\frac{1}{T} \int_0^T C\lambda_v^* \, dt = \frac{1}{T} \int_0^T (C_o \lambda_v^* + S) \, dt \tag{10}$$

and

$$\frac{1}{T} \int_0^T C_a^* \, dt = \frac{1}{\lambda_v' T} \int_0^T \frac{C_w W^* e^*}{V} \, dt \tag{11}$$

where

$$\lambda_v' = \frac{\int_0^T C_a^* \lambda_v^* \, dt}{\int_0^T C_a^* \, dt} \tag{12}$$

We define the time-average values, C_a, W, and e, by the relations

$$C_a = \frac{1}{T} \int_0^T C_a^* \, dt \tag{13}$$

$$W = \frac{1}{T} \int_0^T W^* \, dt \tag{14}$$

$$e = \frac{\int_0^T W^* e^* \, dt}{\int_0^T W^* \, dt} \tag{15}$$

Making the assumption that C_w and V are constant, we obtain from Equation 11

$$C_a = \frac{C_w W e}{\lambda_v' V} \tag{16}$$

In Equation 1, we have replaced λ_v' by λ_v. This is equivalent to assuming that the air-exchange rate is not correlated with C_a. Alternatively, this assumes that $W^* e^*$ and the air-exchange rate are not correlated.

REFERENCES

1. Smith, B. M., Grune, W. N., Higgins, F. B., Jr., and Terrill, J. G., Jr. (1961). Natural radioactivity in ground water supplies in Maine and New Hampshire, *J. Am. Water Works Assoc.*, **53**, 75.

2. Turner, R. C., Radley, J. M., and Mayneord, W. V. (1961). Naturally occurring alpha-activity of drinking waters, *Nature*, **189**, 348.

3. Von Dobeln, W., and Lindell, B. (1964). Some aspects of radon contamination following ingestion, *Ark. Fys.*, **27**, 531.

4. Hursh, J. B., Morken, D. A. Davis, T. P., and Lovaas, A. (1965). The fate of radon ingested by man, *Health Phys.*, **11**, 465.

5. Hems, G. (1966). Acceptable concentration of radon in drinking water, *Int. J. Air Water Pollution*, **10**, 769.

6. Suomela, M., Kahlos, H. (1972). Studies on the elimination rate and radiation exposure following ingestion of ^{222}Rn rich water, *Health Phys.*, **23**, 641.

7. Gesell, T. F., and Prichard, H. M. (1975). The technologically enhanced natural radiation environment, *Health Phys.*, **28**, 361.

8. Duncan, D. L., Gesell, T. F., and Johnson, R. H., Jr. (1976). Radon-222 in potable water. In *Proc. Health Physics Soc. Tenth Mid-Year Symposium: Natural Radioactivity in Man's Environment*, conf-761031, Rensselaer Polytechnic Institute Press, Troy, NY, p. 340.

9. Kahlos, H., and Asikainen, M. (1980). Internal radiation doses from radioactivity of drinking water in Finland, *Health Phys.*, **39**, 108.

10. Prichard, H. M., and Gesell, T. F. (1981). An estimate of population exposures due to radon in public water supplies in the area of Houston, Texas, *Health Phys.*, **41**, 599.

11. Prichard, H. M., and Gesell, T. F. (1977). Rapid measurements of ^{222}Rn concentrations in water with a commercial liquid scintillation counter, *Health Phys.*, **33**, 577.

12. Partridge, J. E., Horton, T. R., and Sensintaffer, E. L. (1979). A study of radon-222 released from water during typical household activities, U.S. Environmental Protection Agency technical note ORP/EERF-79-1, Eastern Environmental Radiation Facility, Montgomery, AL.

13. Gesell, T. F., and Prichard, H. M. (1980). The contribution of radon in tap water to indoor radon concentrations. In T. F. Gesell and W. M. Lowder (eds.), *Natural Radiation Environment III*, conf-780422, U.S. Dept. of Commerce, National Technical Information Service, Springfield, VA, p. 1347.

14. Hess, C. T., Weiffenbach, C. V., and Norton, S. A. (1982). Variations of airborne and waterborne Rn-222 in houses in Maine, *Environ. Int.*, **8**, 59.

15. Prichard, H. M., and Gesell, T. F. (1983). Radon-222 in municipal water supplies in the Central United States, *Health Phys.*, **45**, 991.

16. Horton, T. R. (1983). Methods and results of EPA's study of radon in drinking water, Environmental Protection Agency report EPA 520/5-83-027, Eastern Environmental Radiation Facility, Montgomery, AL.

17. Horton, T. R. (1985). Nationwide occurrence of radon and other natural radioactivity in public water supplies, Environmental Protection Agency report EPA 520/5-85-008, Eastern Environmental Radiation Facility, Montgomery, AL.

18. Asikainen, M. and Kahlos, H. (1979). Anomalously high concentrations of uranium, radium, and radon in water from drilled wells in the Helsinki region, *Geochim. Cosmochim. Acta*, **43**, 1681.

19. Asikainen, M., and Kahlos, H. (1980). Natural radioactivity of drinking water in Finland, *Health Phys.*, **39**, 77.

20. Castrén, O. (1980). The contribution of bored wells to respiratory radon daughter exposure in Finland. In T. F. Gesell and W. M. Lowder (eds.), *Natural Radiation Environment III*, conf-780422, U.S. Dept. of Commerce, National Technical Information Service, Springfield, VA, p. 1364.

21. Becker, A. P., III, and Lachajczyk, T. M. (1984). Evaluation of waterborne radon impact on indoor air quality and assessment of control options, Envirodyne Engineers, Inc., United States Environmental Protection Agency, Industrial Environmental Research Laboratory, Research Triangle Park, NC.

22. Cohen, S., and Wallman, H. (1974). Demonstration of waste flow reduction from households, Environmental Protection Agency report EPA 670/2-74-071, Cincinnati, OH.

23. Laak, R. (1974). Relative pollution strengths of undiluted waste materials discharged in households and the dilution waters used for each. In J. H. T. Winneberger (ed.), *Manual of Grey Water Treatment Practice*, Ann Arbor Science, Ann Arbor, MI, p. 68.

24. Bennett, E. R., and Linstedt, K. D. (1975). Individual home wastewater characterization and treatment, Completion Report Series no. 66, Environmental Resources Center, Colorado State University, Fort Collins, NTIS publication PB 245 259.

25. Small Scale Waste Management Project (1978). Management of small waste flows, Environmental Protection Agency report EPA 600/2-78-173, Municipal Environmental Research Laboratory, Cincinnati, OH.

26. Anderson, J. S., and Watson, J. S. (1967). Patterns of household usage, *J. Am. Water Works Assoc.*, **59**, 1228.

27. Barnes, J., Borrelli, J., and Pochop, L. (1979). Optimum lawn watering rates for esthetics and conservation, *J. Am. Water Works Assoc.*, **71**, 204.

28. Afifi, A. A., and Azen, S. P. (1972). *Statistical Analysis: A Computer-Oriented Approach*, Academic Press, New York.

29. Horton, T. R. (1984). Eastern Environmental Radiation Facility, Montgomery, AL, personal communication.

30. Boyle, R. W. (1911). The solubility of radium emanation. Application of Henry's law at low partial pressures, *Phil. Mag.*, **22**, 840.

31. Residential Energy Consumption Survey (1982). *Housing Characteristics, 1980*, Energy Information Administration, US Department of Energy report DOE/EIA-0314, Washington, DC.

32. Grot, R. A., and Clark, R. E. (1981). Air leakage characteristics and weatherization techniques for low-income housing, paper presented at the ASHRAE conference, *Thermal Performance of Exterior Envelopes of Buildings*, Orlando, FL.

33. Grimsrud, D. T., Modera, M. P., and Sonderegger, R. C. (1983). Calculating infiltration: Implications for a construction quality standard, paper presented at the ASHRAE conference, *Thermal Performance of Exterior Envelopes of Buildings II*, Las Vegas, NV, report LBL-9416, Lawrence Berkeley Laboratory, Berkeley, CA.

34. Hines, W. W., and Montgomery, D. C. (1980). *Probability and Statistics in Engineering and Management Science*, 2nd. ed., Wiley, New York.

35. Aitchison, J., and Brown, J. A. C. (1957). *The Lognormal Distribution*, University Press, Cambridge, England.

36. Solley, W. B., Chase, E. B., and Mann, W. B., IV (1983). Estimated use of water in

the United States in 1980, US Geological Survey Circular 1001, Department of the Interior.

37. Hess, C. T., Michel, J., Horton, T. R., Prichard, H. M., and Coniglio, W. A. (1985). The occurrence of radioactivity in public water supplies in the United States, *Health Phys.*, **48**, 553.

38. Cothern, C. R., Lappenbusch, W. L., and Michel, J. (1986). Drinking-water contribution to natural background radiation, *Health Phys.*, **50**, 33.

39. Environmental Protection Agency (1979). Environmental radiation data: report 16, USEPA Office of Radiation Programs, Washington, DC.

40. Environmental Protection Agency (1979). Environmental radiation data: report 17, USEPA Office of Radiation Programs, Washington, DC.

41. Environmental Protection Agency (1979). Environmental radiation data: report 18, USEPA Office of Radiation Programs, Washington, DC.

42. Environmental Protection Agency (1980). Environmental radiation data: report 19-20, USEPA Office of Radiation Programs, Washington, DC.

43. Horton, T. R. (1985). Eastern Environmental Radiation Facility, Montgomery, AL, personal communication.

44. Gesell, T. F. (1983). Background atmospheric ^{222}Rn concentrations outdoors and indoors: a review, *Health Phys.*, **45**, 289.

45. Nero, A. V., Schwehr, M. B., Nazaroff, W. W., and Revzan, K. L. (1986). Distribution of airborne ^{222}Rn concentrations in U.S. homes, *Science*, **234**, 992.

46. Jacobi, W. (1984). Possible lung cancer risk from indoor exposure to radon daughters, *Radiat. Prot. Dosim.*, **7**, 395.

47. James, A. C. (1984). Dosimetric approaches to risk assessment for indoor exposure to radon daughters, *Radiat. Prot. Dosim.*, **7**, 353.

48. Reid, G. W., Lassovszky, P., and Hathaway, S. (1985). Treatment, waste management and cost for removal of radioactivity from drinking water, *Health Phys.*, **48**, 671.

49. Lowry, J. D., and Brandow, J. E. (1981). Removal of radon from groundwater supplies using granular activated carbon or diffused aeration, University of Maine, Department of Civil Engineering, Orono, ME.

50. Lowry, J. D., and Brandow, J. E. (1985). Removal of radon from water supplies, *J. Environ. Eng.*, **111**, 511.

51. Lowry, J. D., (1986). University of Maine, personal communication.

52. Lucas, H. F. (1957). Improved low-level alpha scintillation counter for radon, *Rev. Sci. Instrum.*, **28**, 680.

53. Cohen, B. L., and Nason, R. (1986). A diffusion barrier charcoal adsorption collector for measuring Rn concentrations in indoor air, *Health Phys.*, **50**, 457.

54. Grimsrud, D. T., Modera, M. P., and Sherman, M. H. (1982). A predictive infiltration model—Long-term field test validation, *ASHRAE Trans.*, **88** (Part I), 1351.

55. Dietz, R. N., and Cote, E. A. (1982). Air infiltration measurements in a home using a convenient perfluorocarbon tracer technique, *Environ. Int.*, **8**, 419.

56. Linaweaver, F. P., Jr., Geyer, J. C., and Wolff, J. B. (1967). Summary report on the residential water use research project, *J. Am. Water Works Assoc.*, **59**, 267.

57. Ligman, K., Hutzler, N., and Boyle, W. C. (1974). Household wastewater characterization, *J. Environ. Eng.*, **100**, 201.

58. Milne, M. (1976). Residential water conservation, California Water Resources Center report No. 35, University of California, Davis.

59. Reid, G. W. (1965). Projection of future municipal water requirements, *Southwest Water Works J.*, March, p. 18.

60. U.S. Water Resources Council (1978). *The Nation's Water Resources, Part III: Functional Water Uses*, The Second National Water Assessment, Washington, DC.

61. Environmental Protection Agency (1981). Environmental radiation data: report 25–26, EPA Report 520/5-82-015, USEPA Office of Radiation Programs, Washington, DC.

62. Environmental Protection Agency (1981). Environmental radiation data: report 27, EPA Report 520/5-82-016, USEPA Office of Radiation Programs, Washington, DC.

63. Environmental Protection Agency (1982). Environmental radiation data: report 28, EPA Report 520/1-83-002, USEPA Office of Radiation Programs, Washington, DC.

64. Environmental Protection Agency (1982). Environmental radiation data: report 30, EPA Report 520/5-6-83-006, USEPA Office of Radiation Programs, Washington, DC.

65. Environmental Protection Agency (1983). Environmental radiation data: report 34, EPA Report 520/5-83-028, USEPA Office of Radiation Programs, Washington, DC.

66. Cross, F.T., Harley, N.H., and Hofmann, W. (1985). Health effects and risks from ^{222}Rn in drinking water, *Health Phys.*, **48,** 649.

67. Buchli, R., and Burkart, W. (1985). Main sources of indoor radon in the Swiss Central Alps, *Sci. Total Environ.*, **45,** 425.

68. Ulbak, K., and Klinder, O. (1984). Radium and radon in Danish drinking water, *Radiat. Prot. Dosim.* **7,** 87.

PART TWO

CHARACTERISTICS AND BEHAVIOR OF RADON DECAY PRODUCTS

5

Modeling Indoor Concentrations of Radon's Decay Products

EARL O. KNUTSON

Aerosol Studies Division, Environmental Measurements Laboratory, U.S. Department of Energy, New York, New York

1 INTRODUCTION

In 1972, Jacobi published a very useful mathematical model for predicting the concentration of airborne radon progeny influenced by various sources and sinks (1). Jacobi's main concern was uranium mine air, but the same processes and principles are at work in ordinary living spaces. Porstendörfer et al. (2) refined the model and used it to show the range of radon progeny concentrations that might be encountered in dwellings.

The need for a mathematical model of the type developed by Jacobi has increased substantially in the 1980s owing to the unhealthful levels of radon and its progeny discovered in many dwellings. Many scientists have responded to this need, particularly in North America and Europe. Their independent work, involving a variety of experimental and theoretical methods, has resulted in a series of scientific papers.

Our goal in this chapter is to present the model, which we henceforth call the Jacobi model, in sufficient detail to bring out the underlying physical principles. In the process, we shall critically review and compare recently published results to make the model as accurate as possible based on current knowledge.

The Jacobi model has several useful applications: estimation of population exposure to radon progeny based on measurements of radon alone; identification of the key parameters or variables needing measurement in a more thorough population exposure study; exploring radon progeny control and mitigation strategies— such as ventilation or air cleaning—on paper before they are tried in practice.

2 SOURCES, SINKS, AND CONVERSION PROCESSES

The Jacobi model can be described as consisting of 11 "cells" with a number of interconnecting paths, illustrated in Figure 5.1, adapted from Bruno (3). The three

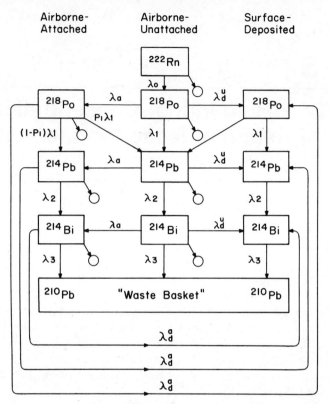

Figure 5.1. Cell diagram for indoor radon and radon progeny. Adapted from Ref. 3.

main rows in Figure 5.1 correspond to the three radionuclides (^{218}Po, ^{214}Pb, and ^{214}Bi) that need to be tracked in order to assess the healthfulness of indoor air. The fourth row (at the bottom) depicts ^{210}Pb, which is not considered to be a health concern and so terminates the diagram. The three columns correspond to the three physical states available to each nuclide, i.e., airborne-attached, airborne-unattached, and surface-deposited. We shall define the two airborne states later.

All downward-pointing arrows in Figure 5.1 depict movement of material by radioactive decay. Right-pointing arrows, including those around the bottom of the diagram, represent a deposition process that removes material from the air onto surfaces. Left-pointing arrows represent the attachment process. The slanting arrows that terminate on circles represent removal of airborne products by ventilation and filtration. The two remaining slanting arrows represent recoil processes.

An alternative diagram is given in Figure 5.2, from Porstendörfer (4). This diagram clearly shows that the main physical processes are decay, attachment, deposition, and recoil. These processes will be discussed in the balance of this section.

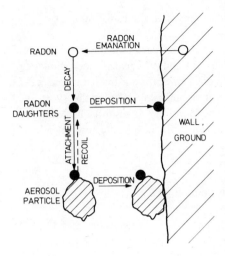

Figure 5.2. The basic processes influencing the activity balance of radon (^{222}Rn) and thoron (^{220}Rn) decay products. Reprinted, with permission of Nuclear Technology Publishing, from J. Porstendörfer (1984), *Radiat. Prot. Dosim.*, **7**, 107 (Ref. 4).

2.1 The Source Term and the Assumption of Complete Mixing

The pathways and mechanisms of radon entry into houses were discussed in Chapters 2 through 4. In this chapter our concern is with the movement and mixing of radon throughout the house and its accumulation indoors. Even more important, this chapter is concerned with the concentration and physical characteristics of radon progeny indoors.

As discussed in Chapter 2, minute flows of air allow radon to enter into a house from below ground level. The radon is then spread throughout the house by air currents, the intensity of which depend on the type of heating or cooling system used in the house and on such factors as localized heating by the sun. Houses with a forced-air heating system will have a high degree of mixing during the heating season. Even in houses with hot-water baseboard heaters, the air is normally very well mixed throughout the heated area (5). In solar-heated houses, convective airflow is usually an integral part of the design.

In many cases, this mixing is sufficiently fast and complete so that the concentration of radon is essentially uniform, at least within a given room or floor of the house. This is called the uniform-mixing hypothesis, or well-stirred hypothesis. By using this hypothesis in modeling, we do not need to account for each crack and radon entry point. Instead, the total input is used and treated as though the radon comes from a source distributed throughout the volume of the given room or floor.

Although it is usually found that the air is well mixed throughout a given floor of the house, there is ample evidence that mixing between floors is usually not complete. This can be seen from the fact that the radon concentration in the first floor of a house is commonly about 0.3–0.5 times that in the basement (6). Because of this weak mixing between floors, models based on a single well-mixed compartment cannot usually be applied to a whole house. One way around this is to use a "two-compartment" model in which there is limited airflow between two contiguous well-mixed compartments.

In this chapter, we shall use mainly a single-compartment model. Two-compartment or multicompartment models are useful and practical if radon alone is of concern. In contrast, our task in this chapter is to outline a mathematical model that will be useful in predicting concentrations and properties of the short-lived decay products of radon, as well as the concentration of radon itself. Multicompartment models describing both radon and its progeny become too unwieldy to be useful.

To summarize, the source term we will be using is

$$\text{the entry rate per unit volume} = S_r V^{-1}$$

where S_r = the total rate of entry of radon into the compartment and V = the volume of the compartment. Normally we will use atoms per hour as the unit for S_r and meters cubed as the unit of V.

As indicated in Figure 5.1, once radon has entered a compartment there are only two mechanisms or pathways by which it can leave: infiltration-exfiltration (some of the radon-laden indoor air is replaced by outdoor air), and radioactive decay (radon "leaves," but is replaced by other nuclides, namely radon progeny).

2.2   The Radioactive Transmutation Terms

In essence, the Jacobi model is based on an interrelated set of so-called "first-order processes," in which the rate of progress of each process is proportional to the concentration of the parent species for that process. In this model, all the essential information is contained in the set of proportionality constants, or rate constants. The first of these constants to be considered are the radioactive decay rates for ^{222}Rn, ^{218}Po, ^{214}Pb, ^{214}Bi, and ^{214}Po, shown in Table 5.1. The value given for the half-life of ^{218}Po is from the recent experiments of Van Hise et al. (7). We believe this is more accurate than the value 3.05 minutes, which it replaces. The remaining values are from Lederer and Shirley (8).

The radioactive decay constants are by far the most accurately known of the rate constants involved in the model. Moreover, they are true physical constants whose values do not change with circumstances. We use the notation λ_i, with $i =$

TABLE 5.1   Radon Progeny Decay Constants

Nuclide	Half-life	Decay constant	
		h^{-1}	s^{-1}
^{222}Rn	3.824 d	0.00755	2.10×10^{-6}
^{218}Po	3.11 min	13.37	0.00371
^{214}Pb	26.8 min	1.552	0.000431
^{214}Bi	19.7 min	2.111	0.000586
^{214}Po	164 μs	1.52×10^7	4.23×10^3

0, 1, 2, 3 corresponding to ^{222}Rn, ^{218}Po, ^{214}Pb, ^{214}Bi, respectively, for these decay constants.

2.3 Removal by Ventilation

Ventilation is the process whereby indoor air is gradually replaced by outdoor air. The terms infiltration and exfiltration are often used in this connection to emphasize that ventilation is in fact two simultaneous processes—outdoor air infiltrating the house through one set of cracks and openings, and an equal amount of indoor air exfiltrating through another set of cracks and openings. Ventilation is driven by pressure differences caused by the wind or by differences in air density between indoors and outdoors (the stack effect). As discussed in Chapter 2, these same forces may cause inflow of air from below ground level, thereby affecting the radon input term as well.

The complete-mixing hypothesis discussed for sources in Section 2.1 applies also to infiltration and exfiltration. For example, although outdoor air enters at discrete points, it is assumed to mix quickly so that, in effect, it appears instantly throughout the volume of the given space. Thus, the exact location of the leaks is not important, and infiltration is completely specified by its airflow rate, Q. The same is true of exfiltration, which, since air may be treated as incompressible for the small pressure differences of interest, entails the same airflow rate.

The rate of radon and progeny removal by exfiltration is QC_i. Thus:

$$\text{the volume-distributed ventilation sink} = QC_i V^{-1}$$

$$= \lambda_v C_i$$

where $\lambda_v = QV^{-1}$ is the rate constant for removal by ventilation and C_i is the concentration of the radon or progeny species of interest. We will usually use m^3 h^{-1} as the unit for Q, and m^3 as the unit for V. Thus λ_v has the unit h^{-1}. This is identical to "air changes per hour," a term commonly used in quantifying the ventilation rate.

Although many writers include terms in the Jacobi model to account for radon and progeny brought in by the infiltrating outdoor air, we prefer not to. As indicated in the recent review by Gesell (9), outdoor concentrations are usually low. The gain in accuracy of the model does not justify the additional complexity. In any case, the effect of outdoor radon is easy to gauge because its concentration simply adds to the calculated indoor value. The effect is more complicated for the progeny.

For years, there was a rule of thumb that the ventilation rate in residential houses was about 1 h^{-1}. A 1973 literature review by Handley and Barton (10) indicated that construction practices prior to 1973 resulted in infiltration rates of about 0.5– 1.5 h^{-1}, supporting this rule of thumb.

Recently, Grot and Clark (11) reported the results of measurements in 266 older houses, and Grimsrud et al. (12) reported on heating-season measurements in 312 newer residences. The geometric mean ventilation rate in these two studies was 0.90 and 0.53 h^{-1}, respectively, and the respective geometric standard deviations were 2.13 and 1.71 (see Figure 4.4). It is logical to expect that ventilation rates will decrease as construction practices and life-styles change in response to the increased cost of heating fuel. The two studies above may be evidence of this.

Weatherization of older houses also tends to reduce the ventilation rate. Lamb et al. (13) described detailed measurements in 10 houses, yielding preweatherization ventilation rates of 0.3–1.0 h^{-1} and an average reduction of 16% following weatherization. The authors also give evidence that the rate is different in different parts of the house, and that the number of door openings and closing is a key factor in ventilation.

In summary, it will be necessary in the model to consider ventilation rates ranging from about 0.2 to 1.5 h^{-1}.

2.4   Attachment of Radon Progeny to Aerosol Particles

2.4.1   *The Role of Indoor Aerosols.*   Air normally contains copious numbers of small solid or liquid particles called aerosol particles or aerosols. These particles range in size from almost atomic dimensions up to several micrometers in diameter. Cooking and smoking are prominent sources of indoor aerosols, but there are many other sources as well. Aerosols play an important role in the behavior of radon progeny indoors.

Radon progeny are formed throughout the volume of the compartment by the radioactive decay of radon gas. Like radon, the progeny can leave by exfiltration and by decay. Unlike radon, the progeny can attach themselves to aerosol particles, and the result is so different that it is best to treat it as a separate species. The terms "unattached" and "attached" are commonly used to distinguish between these two states of radon progeny. The properties of unattached progeny are discussed in Chapter 6. In Chapter 5, we are concerned with the attachment process, and with the properties of the resulting attached progeny.

The attachment process is described by a first-order term:

$$\text{rate of attachment of nuclide } i \text{ to aerosol particles} = \lambda_a C_i^u$$

where λ_a is the attachment rate constant and C_i^u is the concentration of unattached atoms of nuclide i. Allowed values for the subscript i are 1, 2, and 3, corresponding to ^{218}Po, ^{214}Pb, and ^{214}Bi, respectively. Normally, we will use the units h^{-1} for λ_a and atoms per meter cubed (m^{-3}) for C_i^u. The rate will then be given in units of "events" per meter cubed per hour.

The attachment rate constant varies widely, from 5 to 500 h^{-1}. To better understand the reasons for this broad range, it is necessary to discuss at some length the properties of the indoor aerosol.

2.4.2   *Properties of the Indoor Aerosol.*   For our purposes, the most important characteristic of an *individual* aerosol particle is its size, which we denote

by x. Many indoor particles are spherical, and x is taken to be the diameter of the sphere. Dust particles and particles formed in an open flame are not spherical, but it is common to assign an equivalent spherical diameter. This assignment normally occurs through the functioning of a particular type of measuring equipment.

An aerosol will usually involve millions of particles, with various sizes. One important characteristic of the aerosol is its concentration, N:

$$N = \text{the number of aerosol particles per unit volume}$$

Another important characteristic of the particle ensemble is its differential size distribution, $f(x)$:

$$f(x)\, dx = \text{the fractional number of particles in the ensemble that have particle sizes between } x \text{ and } x + dx$$

The differential distribution $f(x)$ has the property that its integral from $x = 0$ to $x = $ infinity is unity.

Knowledge about the concentration and size of typical indoor aerosols was increased substantially by three articles in the proceedings of an international seminar held in 1983 at Anacapri, Italy. Measurement results were reported for two houses in Belgium (14), 11 houses in Sweden (15), and three houses in the Netherlands (16). Figure 5.3, from the Netherlands study, shows the particle size distributions resulting from common indoor activities. Table 5.2, from the same source, identifies the activity for the curves in Figure 5.3 and lists three descriptive statistics for each aerosol measured. The quantity plotted on the vertical axis in Figure 5.3 is $dN/d(\log x)$ rather than $f(x)$. This is an alternate way of presenting aerosol size distributions related to $f(x)$ as follows:

$$dN/d(\log x) = Nxf(x) \ln 10$$

where $\ln 10$ is the natural log of 10.

Stoute et al. (16) draw four conclusions from their study:

1. No great significant differences were found between spectra of several houses, measured under the same conditions, e.g., walking, cooking and smoking. The mean particle concentrations in dwellings without activities were about 2×10^4 particles cm^{-3}.

2. Cooking or smoking leads to number concentrations that are one or two orders of magnitude higher than otherwise occur. Smoking gives relatively large particles, while cooking, walking, and vacuum cleaning give much smaller particles.

3. The aerosol spectra change slowly in time, when a specific action has ceased; small particles will coagulate and large particles will plate out; after 3–4 hours the size distribution stabilizes.

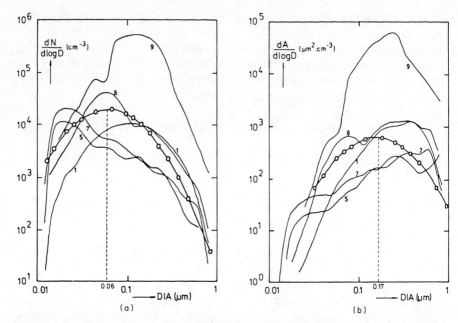

Figure 5.3. Measured indoor aerosol size distributions. (*a*) Number-weighted distributions; (*b*) area-weighted distributions. For further information, see Table 5.2. Reprinted, with permission of Nuclear Technology Publishing, from J.R.D. Stoute et al. (1984), *Radiat. Prot. Dosim.*, **7**, 159 (Ref. 16).

TABLE 5.2   Summary Data for Aerosol Distributions in Figure 5.3

NR	Activity	House	CMD (μm)	AMD (μm)	σ_g
1	No activity	1	0.11	0.32	2.08
2	No activity	2	0.08	0.29	2.22
3	No activity	3	0.10	0.24	1.93
4	Walking	1	0.05	0.16	2.16
5	Walking	2	0.04	0.17	2.35
6	Walking	3	0.06	0.15	1.97
7	Vacuum cleaning	1	0.03	0.09	2.09
8	Cooking	1	0.07	0.17	1.94
9	Smoking	1	0.13	0.23	1.70
10	Smoking	2	0.12	0.40	2.17
11	"Average"		0.06	0.17	

CMD = count median diameter
AMD = area median diameter
Source: Reprinted with permission from Ref. 16.

168

4. The average value of the count median diameter (CMD) was around 0.06 μm and the area median diameter was around 0.17 μm.

These conclusions should be viewed with caution owing to the small number of houses represented. Measurements in more houses would probably give a broader range of concentrations. Also, if the cooking includes frying, it is likely that larger particles similar to those from smoking would be produced. The production of aerosols—especially fine particles—by walking is surprising. The production of small particles by vacuum cleaning is plausible, owing to the arcing that generally occurs at the brushes of the motor.

The Swedish study (15) concurs with the conclusion regarding the importance of cooking and smoking on the resulting particle sizes, but finds more variation between dwellings. In the Belgian study (14), it was found that the aerosol concentration outdoors was usually higher than that indoors. The indoor concentration tended to track the outdoor, suggesting some infiltration, but the highest indoor concentrations were due to indoor activity.

Shown in Figures 5.4 and 5.5 are the additional particle-size distributions from a recent study of two houses in New Jersey (17). The size distribution and amounts of aerosol resulting from common indoor activities are shown in Figure 5.4. It is seen that cigarette smoking and frying eggs and meat produce larger particles, and that cooking soup produces small particles. (The small particles are probably from the gas flame. The probable reason for the difference between frying and cooking is that the former produces large particles that efficiently collect the small particles.) The evolution of the spectrum of particle sizes from burning an unvented

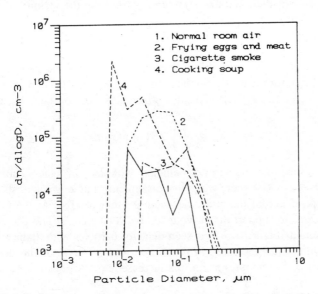

Figure 5.4. Indoor number-weighted aerosol size distributions as affected by common indoor activities. From Ref. 17.

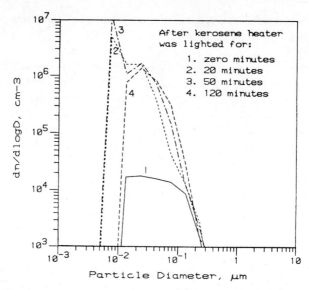

Figure 5.5. Effect of unvented kerosene heater on indoor number-weighted aerosol size distributions. From Ref. 17.

kerosene heater is shown in Figure 5.5. For the first 50 minutes, the aerosol is characterized by a very high concentration of very small particles. During the second hour, coagulation has apparently taken hold, consuming small particles and producing larger ones. After 120 minutes of burning, the small particle population has nearly disappeared, and the number of particles in the vicinity of 0.1 μm has increased greatly.

Attachment is the process whereby an unattached radon progeny atom or cluster, which undergoes random motion like any gas molecule, strikes and sticks to an aerosol particle. The probability that this will happen within a given time increment is proportional to the number of targets, N, and also depends strongly on the size of the particles, $f(x)$. Thus the attachment rate constant, λ_a, is given by:

$$\lambda_a = N \int_0^\infty \beta(x) f(x) \, dx \qquad (1)$$

where $\beta(x)$ is the attachment rate coefficient with units of meters cubed per hour.

As recently as 1979, there was some disagreement among scientists concerning the size dependence of the attachment rate coefficient (18). At the present time, evidence seems to support the curve given by Porstendörfer and Mercer (19), reproduced here as Figure 5.6. It is seen that, for particles with diameters less than about 0.1 μm, $\beta(x)$ increases in proportion to the square of the diameter. For particles larger than about 0.5 μm, the increase is proportional to the diameter to the first power.

Figure 5.6 is based on experiment. Junge (20) indicates that the theory of the process was first clearly stated by Lassen in 1960–1961. More recently, Porstendörfer et al. (21) have reexamined the theory in light of all data accumulated since

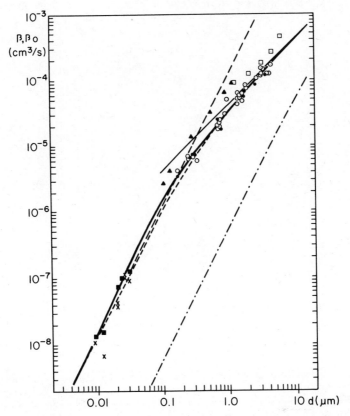

Figure 5.6. Attachment rate coefficient vs. particle diameter: theory and experiment. Experimental results: ▲ Porstendörfer (1968); □ Kruger and Andrews (1976); ■ Ref. 19, [212]Pb ions; × Ref. 19, [212]Pb atoms; ● Ref. 21, [212]Pb ions; ○ Ref. 21, [212]Pb atoms. Theory: ▬▬ Diffusion theory, atoms ($D = 0.068$ cm^2 s^{-1}; $S = 1$);---Diffusion theory, ions ($D = 0.068$ cm^2 s^{-1}; $S = 1$); ·—· Diffusion theory, iodine ($D = 0.076$ cm^2 s^{-1}; $S = 0.005$); ——— $2\pi Dd$; --Kinetic theory, $\frac{1}{4}\bar{v}d^2 S$ ($S = 1$). Reprinted, with permission, from *J. Aerosol Sci.*, vol. 10, J. Porstendörfer, G. Roebig, and A. Ahmed, Experimental determination of the attachment coefficients of atoms and ions on monodisperse aerosols, Copyright 1979, Pergamon Press, Ltd.

1960 and found that an expression derived by Bricard and others provides a good fit.

Figure 5.7 shows the result of one aerosol measurement in the Belgian study. The left curve is the number-weighted size distribution, $dN/(d \log x)$, and the right curve is the "attachment rate spectrum," obtained by multiplying $dN/(d \log x)$ with the attachment rate constant (from Figure 5.6). It is seen that the maximum attachment rate is in the particle size range 0.1–0.2 μm diameter. By integrating curves like this, Raes et al. (14) found that attachment rate constants varying from about 3 h^{-1} to 600 h^{-1}. This broad range is due to a combination of variations in the size distribution and variations in aerosol number concentration.

Aerosol measurements like those in Figure 5.7 are expensive and time-consum-

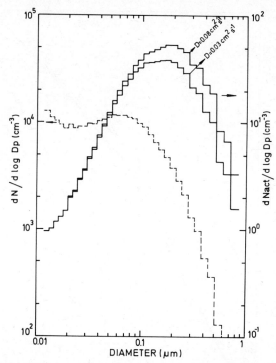

Figure 5.7. Indoor aerosol size distributions. *Dashed curve:* number-weighted distribution; *solid curves:* corresponding attachment rate spectra for two assumed [218]Po diffusion coefficients. Reprinted, with permission of Nuclear Technology Publishing, from F. Raes et al. (1984), *Radiat. Prot. Dosim.*, **7**, 127 (Ref. 14).

ing and therefore would not be done except in research projects. On the other hand, measurements of the aerosol concentration, N, can be made quite easily and inexpensively with a portable condensation nucleus counter. Given in Table 5.3, from Porstendörfer (4), are the average attachment coefficients, which can be multiplied by N to estimate the attachment rate constant.

The right curve in Figure 5.7 suggests that most of the radon progeny activity will be found attached to particles in the size range 0.1–0.2 μm in diameter, and direct measurements confirm this. The exact size of attached radon progeny is not a critical issue in the Jacobi model; so no further discussion is needed here. However, we shall return to the size question later because it is important in calculating the lung deposition of radon progeny, which is described in Chapter 7.

2.5 Removal by Deposition on Walls and Other Surfaces

Radon progeny, whether attached or unattached, tend to deposit on and stick to surfaces exposed to the air. Since material removed from the air is no longer available to be breathed, surface deposition supplements ventilation as a means of reducing human exposure to radon progeny. The term "plateout" is often used for

TABLE 5.3 Average Attachment Rate Coefficients

Author	$\bar{\beta}$ (cm^3 h^{-1})	Comments
Mohnen	5.1×10^{-3}	Room aerosol $Z \approx 3 \times 10^4$ cm^{-3}
Porstendörfer	1.8×10^{-3}	Outdoor aerosol $Z \approx 5 \times 10^4$ cm^{-3}
Kawano et al.	7.4×10^{-3} 8.3×10^{-3}	Outdoor aerosol $Z = 1.3 \times 10^3$ cm^{-3} $Z = 3.2 \times 10^4$ cm^{-3}
Ikebe et al.	6.8×10^{-3}	Outdoor aerosol $Z = (1–5) \times 10^4$ cm^{-3}
Porstendörfer and Mercer	2.2×10^{-3}	Outdoor aerosol $Z = (3–5) \times 10^4$ cm^{-3}
Porstendörfer and Mercer	4.3×10^{-3}	Room aerosol $Z = (0.7–1.4) \times 10^4$ cm^{-3}
Porstendörfer and Mercer	4.7×10^{-3}	Room aerosol plus cigarette smoke $Z = (5–10) \times 10^4$ cm^{-3}

Source: Reprinted with permission from Ref. 4.

surface deposition of radon progeny, although some authors prefer to reserve the term plateout only for the unattached radon progeny.

Bruno (3) gave a simple calculation which is a useful point of departure for discussing radon progeny plateout. Consider a room in which there is no ventilation or other air motion, and no aerosol. ^{218}Po is formed at a uniform rate, $\lambda_0 C_0$, throughout the volume (C_0 = radon concentration, atoms m^{-3}), and its only loss pathways are radioactive decay and deposition. The sink term due to decay is $\lambda_1 C_1^u$ (C_1^u = concentration of unattached ^{218}Po, atoms m^{-3}). Since there is no air motion, deposition can only occur by molecular diffusion. If we consider an area of the wall far from any corner, then the steady-state concentration of ^{218}Po is governed by a one-dimensional diffusion equation:

$$-D^u \frac{d^2 C_1^u}{dz^2} = \lambda_0 C_0 - \lambda_1 C_1^u \tag{2}$$

D^u is the diffusion coefficient of the unattached ^{218}Po, for which (following Bruno) we take the classical value 0.022 m^2 h^{-1} (0.06 cm^2 s^{-1}).

The solution to the diffusion equation is shown in Figure 5.8. C_1^u is zero at the wall, increasing to $\lambda_0 C_0 \lambda_1^{-1}$ at about 10 cm from the wall. Fick's law applied to the gradient at the wall shows that there is a flux to the wall, given by:

$$\text{flux} = \lambda_0 C_0 \lambda_1^{-1} (D^u \lambda_1)^{0.5}$$

$$\text{(units: atoms m}^2 \text{ h}^{-1})$$

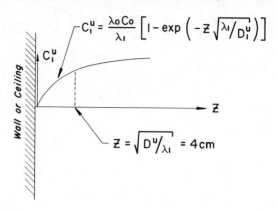

Figure 5.8. Concentration gradient for diffusion of ^{218}Po to a surface in dead-calm air. (In a real situation, air mixing would reduce the boundary layer thickness from 4 cm to a few millimeters.)

It is seen that the flux is proportional to the concentration of ^{218}Po at a point well away from the wall. The proportionality constant, $(D^u \lambda_1)^{0.5}$, has units m h^{-1} and is called the deposition velocity.

$$\text{deposition velocity, } v_d^u = (D^u \lambda_1)^{0.5} = 0.54 \text{ m h}^{-1}$$

This should serve to introduce the concept of deposition velocity, and also to indicate a possible value for it.

In the real situation, air mixing will keep the radon progeny concentration uniform to a point much closer to the wall than indicated in Figure 5.8. This will increase the deposition velocity from the value given above, but accurate prediction of the value is beyond the present state of the art. Reasoning by analogy with results from fluid mechanics, Bruno (3) suggests deposition velocities in the range of 7 to 22 m h^{-1}, depending on the intensity of air motion. However, these values need to be tested by experiment.

The model now requires an extension to the well-mixed hypothesis: we assume that all surface area in the room is equally effective in removing radon progeny from the air. Thus,

the rate of removal of unattached radon progeny nuclide i by plateout $= v_d^u S C_i^u$

where S is the total area of the surface exposed to the room air. S includes the area of the walls, floor, and ceiling, and furniture in the room. Referring again to the well-mixed hypothesis, this removal is felt instantaneously throughout the volume of the chamber, so that the above equation may be divided by V:

equivalent volume-distributed sink term for loss
of unattached nuclide i by plateout $= \lambda_d^u C_i^u$

where the plateout rate constant λ_d^u is given by $v_d^u S V^{-1}$. There is an analogous expression for the attached progeny:

$$\text{equivalent volume-distributed sink term for loss}$$
$$\text{of attached nuclide } i \text{ by plateout} = \lambda_d^a C_i^a$$

where the superscript a, referring to attached, has replaced the superscript u. Deposition velocities for attached progeny are much smaller than those for the unattached species.

Much effort has been invested since 1980 in an attempt to obtain experimental values of the deposition velocities v_d^u and v_d^a. Tests have been done in small chambers where it is practical to exclude aerosols so that the progeny are entirely unattached, and in large chambers where attachment has to be taken into account. Results from large-chamber tests on deposition of reactive gases or aerosols are also useful.

2.5.1 Small-Chamber Radon Progeny Tests, Aerosols Excluded.

Perhaps the most clear-cut experiment is that reported by McLaughlin and O'Byrne (22). As a chamber, they used an airtight 50-L cylindrical drum in which was mounted a surface-barrier, alpha-particle detector. The experiment started by filling this drum with particle-free, radon-laden air. When the steady state was reached, as indicated by a stable count rate, the air was quickly pumped out and replaced with radon-free air. From then on only the nuclides deposited on the detector contributed to the count rate. The deposit of ^{218}Po, distinguished by its alpha-particle energy, was measured and decay-corrected back to its value just before the radon was pumped out.

From the deposit on the 450-mm^2 detector, the authors estimated the total deposit by assuming it was uniform over the internal surface. Also, since the drum was airtight, the sum of the deposited and airborne ^{218}Po activity was assumed to be equal to the activity of the parent, radon, which had been measured. In this way, the partition between deposited and airborne ^{218}Po was determined. Since the deposited ^{218}Po activity had only one source (deposition) and one sink (decay), it was relatively easy to extract the deposition velocity from the data. The series of experiments yielded deposition velocities ranging from 1.2 to 1.7 m h^{-1}, with a mean value of 1.44 m h^{-1}. McLaughlin and O'Byrne also attempted to measure the deposition velocity of attached ^{218}Po. Here they succeeded only in setting an upper limit of 0.09 m h^{-1}.

Although the McLaughlin and O'Byrne experiment was clear-cut, caution is advised when applying the results to larger chambers, which probably have more air motion.

Earlier, in an article on the wall loss of sulfur dioxide and ozone in small chambers, Cox and Penkett (23) also gave the results of a few tests with thoron (^{220}Rn) progeny. Thoron gas (half-life = 55.6 seconds) was admitted into a 1.0-m^3 aluminum chamber, along with about 1 ppm of nitric oxide, which prevented the formation of radiolytic aerosols. Filter samples were taken at prescribed intervals to track the concentration of the second decay product, ^{212}Pb (half-life = 10.6 h; the first decay product, ^{216}Po, is difficult to measure owing to its short half-life, 0.145 seconds). The measured deposition velocity for ^{212}Pb was 4.0 m h^{-1} (0.11 cm s^{-1}), and we should expect this to hold also for radon progeny. For comparison, the deposition velocity obtained for sulfur dioxide increased with increasing humidity, reaching 1.4 m h^{-1} at 86% relative humidity.

The deposition velocity obtained by Cox and Penkett for thoron progeny is higher than that obtained by McLaughlin and O'Byrne for radon progeny. The difference is probably due to air motion, since the Cox and Penkett chamber contained a large stirring paddle.

2.5.2 Large-Chamber Tests on Deposition of Radon Progeny and Reactive Gases.

There are three reports in the literature on experiments directly measuring deposition within larger rooms. In one, Scott (24) made measurements in a large, well-ventilated basement with elevated radon levels (1100–2600 Bq m^{-3}). At these concentrations the activity could be counted from radon progeny accumulating on the surface of an alpha-contamination probe. By mathematically analyzing the buildup and decay (observed by covering the probe) of surface activity, together with the measured air concentrations, Scott was able to derive deposition velocities for both the attached and unattached radon progeny. In the calculation, it was assumed that 20% of ^{218}Po was unattached and the ^{214}Bi was 100% attached. The values derived were 0.2 m h^{-1} for attached radon progeny and 6.1 m h^{-1} for unattached radon progeny. In further tests, Scott found that unattached deposition velocity varied from 3.6 to 18 m h^{-1}, for different surfaces in the room. Airflow measurements were made which provided plausible reasons for these variations.

The second significant report is that of Toohey et al. (25), who performed an experiment similar to Scott's. The buildup and decay of radon progeny activity depositing on the window of a gas flow proportional counter located in a utility room was analyzed. Assuming that 10% of the ^{218}Po was unattached, they arrived at a value of 16 m h^{-1} for the unattached deposition velocity. However, from their description of the circumstances, it seems likely that the unattached fraction was higher—perhaps 30–40%. The deposition velocity from their experiment would then be about 5 m h^{-1}.

It is clear that both experiments mentioned above could have benefited by a direct measurement of the unattached fraction of ^{218}Po.

The third report on measurement of radon progeny deposition velocity is that of Bigu (26), who also reported values for thoron progeny. Bigu included a measurement of the unattached fraction of ^{218}Po, ^{214}Pb, and ^{214}Bi, and of ^{212}Pb and ^{212}Bi. The experiments were done in a 26-m^3 chamber, with and without a circulating fan in operation. The technique was to mount disks of stainless steel or filter paper on the chamber's inside walls, allowing these disks to come into radioactive equilibrium, then remove and quickly alpha-count them. An equation was applied to determine the unattached deposition velocity from the measured air and surface activities. Since there is no reason to expect that ^{222}Rn progeny and ^{220}Rn progeny deposition velocities should differ, we can pool the results, yielding the range 2–19 m h^{-1}. The "fan-off" values were near the lower end of this range, and the "fan-on" values were near the upper end.

Deposition of reactive gases on walls is also of interest, since the physical mechanisms must be very similar to those for unattached radon progeny. Wilson (27) reports on the removal of sulfur dioxide by adsorption on the walls and other surfaces of a 47-m^3 room. Although the room had windows and two interior doors, it was reasonably airtight. The experiment consisted of charging the room with sulfur dioxide and helium and monitoring the rate of decrease of the concentration of both. The difference of the two rates was attributed to adsorption of sulfur dioxide on surfaces.

With normal walls and floor, the half-life for the decrease of sulfur dioxide concentrations due to adsorption was 40–60 min. By painting the walls and floor with a solution of sodium carbonate, the sulfur dioxide half-life dropped to 7 min, which is equivalent to a deposition velocity of 2.2 m h^{-1}. Separate tests indicated that the latter removal rate was limited by transport through the air, rather than by the adsorption capacity of the surface. The latter result should, therefore, apply approximately to unattached radon progeny as well.

Wilson also found that stirring the air with two fans decreased the sulfur dioxide half-life from 7 to 2.5 min, equivalent to 6.3 m h^{-1} deposition velocity. The air motion caused by the fans was quite intense (sufficient to move loose papers).

2.5.3 Large-Chamber Tests on Deposition of Aerosols.
There are also three or four reports in the literature on experiments which, although not involving radon progeny, give valuable information relative to deposition of attached radon progeny. Offermann et al. (28) describe an experiment on the loss rate of cigarette smoke particles in the Indoor Air Quality Research House at Lawrence Berkeley Laboratory. The experiment room was carefully sealed so that the ventilation rate was very low, about 0.05 h^{-1}. By tracking the particle-size distribution and correcting for the removal by ventilation, the authors determined the deposition rates for particles of various sizes in the range 0.1–1.3 μm. The curve has a minimum value, about 0.05 h^{-1}, located at 0.3 μm, and increases to about 0.13 h^{-1} at 0.1 μm. Using the nominal value of S/V for the experiment room (1.9 m^{-1}), these two rates correspond to deposition velocities of 0.026–0.07 m h^{-1}. In view of the particle sizes, the deposition velocity of attached radon progeny should fall within this range as well.

A second useful study not involving radon progeny is that of Sinclair et al. (29), who measured air concentration and surface accumulations of certain ionic species in two telephone-switching offices. Of interest here are the measurements on sulfates, which probably had a particle size around 0.5 μm. Surface accumulation was determined for certain structural surfaces of telephone-switching equipment frames, assuming that the surfaces had not been disturbed since their installation. The deposition velocities determined in two offices were 0.11 and 0.18 m h^{-1}, respectively. These values are probably too high for residential radon progeny, for two reasons: (i) the air recirculation rate was quite high in two offices, indicating the air velocities were probably also high; and (ii) the accumulation was measured on structural elements protruding into the airflow, thereby collecting more than the usual amount of deposition.

Harrison (30) described an experiment to measure the deposition of uniform-sized latex particles in a small (0.195 m^3) chamber. For 0.234-μm particles he found extremely small values, about 0.004 m h^{-1}, for the deposition velocity. We interpret this to mean that very small deposition velocities can occur if the air is nearly motionless.

2.5.4 *Summary of Deposition Velocity Results.*

The experiments cited above suggest quite strongly that the deposition velocity of the unattached radon progeny, averaged over the surface of a typical room, is in the range of 5–10 m h^{-1}. For exploratory calculations, we can safely use the value 8 m h^{-1}. It is logical to expect that the velocity will vary from surface to surface within a given room, and Scott (24) showed that this is the case, but the value 8 m h^{-1} appears to be a representative average.

There appears to be some conflict between results for unattached radon progeny and results for reactive gases, notably sulfur dioxide. If the surface is sufficiently adsorbing, sulfur dioxide should deposit faster than unattached radon progeny owing to the difference in molecular weights. Experiments, however, indicate the contrary—that unattached radon progeny deposit with about three times the velocity of sulfur dioxide. The conclusion to be drawn here is that the physics of the process is not well understood, and that the experiments are imprecise.

The experimental values for the deposition velocity of the attached radon progeny seem to be less consistent than those for the unattached, with possible values ranging from 0.03 to 0.2 m h^{-1}. Since this quantity is less important in the model than its unattached counterpart, we can safely take a value of 0.08 m h^{-1}, one-hundredth of the unattached value.

Although there are other reported experiments that can be considered, they are less clear-cut and are best considered after the model is given in its entirety. The full model is given in the next section.

3 THE STEADY-STATE JACOBI MODEL

In this section, we shall collect the mathematical source and sink terms that govern the contents of the compartments shown in Figure 5.1. Except for recoil, all the contributing processes (the arrows in Figure 5.1) have been discussed at some length in Section 2. It remains only to equate the appropriate source and sink terms. Table 5.4 shows the symbols and units that are used in the model.

We shall follow the usual practice and consider only the steady-state form of the equations. This is a simplification, since some of the rate "constants" (e.g., attachment rate, deposition velocity, ventilation rate) change quite often. We shall return to the question of changing parameters in Section 4.3. For the present, we assume that the steady-state model will reasonably describe the average effect over several days or weeks, if average values of the input parameters are used.

TABLE 5.4   Symbols and Units Used in the Model

Symbol	Unit	Meaning
S_r	atoms h^{-1}	Radon input rate
C_i^u	atoms m^{-3}	Concentration of airborne unattached nuclides (i = 0, 1, 2, 3 for radon and its first three progeny)
C_i^a	atoms m^{-3}	Concentration of airborne attached nuclides (i = 1, 2, 3)
C_i^s	atoms m^{-2}	Concentrations of surface-deposited nuclides (i = 1, 2, 3)
C_i^{s*}	atoms m^{-3}	Volume-equivalent concentration of surface-deposited nuclides (i = 1, 2, 3)
λ_i	h^{-1}	Radioactive decay constants (i = 0, 1, 2, 3)
A_i^u	Bq m^{-3}	Activity of airborne unattached progeny (i = 1, 2, 3)
A_i^a	Bq m^{-3}	Activity of airborne attached progeny (i = 1, 2, 3)
A_i^s	Bq m^{-2}	Activity of surface-deposited progeny (i = 1, 2, 3)
A_i^{s*}	Bq m^{-3}	Volume-equivalent activity of surface-deposited progeny (i = 1, 2, 3)
S	m^2	Surface area available for deposition
V	m^3	Volume of room or space being considered
λ_v	h^{-1}	Ventilation rate constant
λ_a	h^{-1}	Attachment rate constant
v_d^a	m h^{-1}	Deposition velocity for attached progeny
v_d^u	m h^{-1}	Deposition velocity for unattached progeny
p_1	—	Probability that the decay product will recoil (detach) from the aerosol particle when the attached ^{218}Po decays
λ_d^a	h^{-1}	Rate constant for deposition of attached progeny
λ_d^u	h^{-1}	Rate constant for deposition of unattached progeny

3.1   The Balance Equations in Terms of Concentration

3.1.1   Radon-222.
For radon gas, the input rate is S_r and the rate of loss to the two possible paths is $\lambda_0 C_0 V$ and QC_0, respectively. The volume is needed in the first loss term because we have to consider the total loss in the compartment, not the loss in a single cubic meter. After equating the source term to the loss terms, the equation is divided through by V to yield the "per unit volume" equation:

$$S_r V^{-1} = \lambda_0 C_0 + \lambda_v C_0 \tag{3}$$

where $\lambda_v = QV^{-1}$ is the ventilation rate.

3.1.2   Polonium-218.
For unattached ^{218}Po, the source term is the decay of radon gas and there are four possible loss paths. For loss by deposition, the total

rate considering all surfaces is $v_d^u S C_1^u$. After dividing through by V, this balance equation is:

$$\lambda_0 C_0 = (\lambda_1 + \lambda_v + \lambda_a + \lambda_d^u) C_1^u \tag{4}$$

where $\lambda_d^u = v_d^u S V^{-1}$.

For attached ^{218}Po the source term is $\lambda_a C_1^u$ and there are three loss paths. Thus:

$$\lambda_a C_1^u = (\lambda_1 + \lambda_v + \lambda_d^a) C_1^a \tag{5}$$

For deposited ^{218}Po the two source terms are $v_d^u C_1^u$ and $v_d^a C_1^a$, which give the rate of deposition on a unit area of surface. The one loss term is $\lambda_1 C_1^s$. After equating these, we multiply through by S and divide through by V. This puts all terms on a per-unit-volume basis, which facilitates comparison to the other equations. The result is:

$$\lambda_d^u C_1^u + \lambda_d^a C_1^a = \lambda_1 C_1^{S*} \tag{6}$$

where $C_1^{S*} = C_1^S S V^{-1}$.

The surface area S includes the areas of the floor, ceiling and walls, as well as area of other objects, such as furniture, with surfaces exposed to the air. Porstendörfer (4) has used an area about 2.5 times the nominal area in some of his calculations.

3.1.3 Lead-214.

For unattached ^{214}Pb there are three possible source terms: decay of unattached ^{218}Po, decay of attached ^{218}Po accompanied by recoil, and decay of surface-deposited ^{218}Po accompanied by recoil. The second of these occurs with a nonzero probability, p_1. The third is usually considered to have very low probability, and we will follow the usual practice of ignoring this source. The four loss terms are analogous to those for unattached ^{218}Po. Thus:

$$\lambda_1 C_1^u + p_1 \lambda_1 C_1^a = (\lambda_2 + \lambda_v + \lambda_a + \lambda_d^u) C_2^u \tag{7}$$

For attached ^{214}Pb there are also two source terms. Thus:

$$\lambda_a C_2^u + (1 - p_1) \lambda_1 C_1^a = (\lambda_2 + \lambda_v + \lambda_d^a) C_2^a \tag{8}$$

For the recoil probability p_1, Mercer (31) has advocated the value 0.83. This value has gained wide acceptance in the literature, and is recommended.

For surface-deposited ^{214}Pb there are three source terms, the first of which is decay of ^{218}Po previously deposited on the surface. The volume equivalent form is:

$$\lambda_1 C_1^{S*} + \lambda_d^u C_2^u + \lambda_d^a C_2^a = \lambda_2 C_2^{S*} \tag{9}$$

3.1.4 Bismuth-214. The three remaining equations, all for ^{214}Bi, are simpler because recoil is not a factor. They are:

$$\lambda_2 C_2^u = (\lambda_3 + \lambda_v + \lambda_a + \lambda_d^u) C_3^u \tag{10}$$

$$\lambda_2 C_2^a + \lambda_a C_3^u = (\lambda_3 + \lambda_v + \lambda_d^a) C_3^a \tag{11}$$

$$\lambda_2 C_2^{S*} + \lambda_d^u C_3^u + \lambda_d^a C_3^a = \lambda_3 C_3^{S*} \tag{12}$$

This completes the set of equations that can be used to predict the partitioning of radon progeny activity among its possible states.

3.2 The Balance Equations in Terms of Activities

The above equations were formulated in terms of atom concentration, because it is numbers of atoms that are conserved. For most calculations, however, activity concentrations are more convenient. Conversion of the equations to activities is straightforward: substitute $A_i^x \lambda_i^{-1}$ for each C_i^x and clear fractions. Thus:

$$\lambda_0 S_r V^{-1} = (\lambda_0 + \lambda_v) A_0 \tag{13}$$

$$\lambda_1 A_0 = (\lambda_1 + \lambda_v + \lambda_a + \lambda_d^u) A_1^u \tag{14}$$

$$\lambda_a A_1^u = (\lambda_1 + \lambda_v + \lambda_d^a) A_1^a \tag{15}$$

$$\lambda_d^u A_1^u + \lambda_d^a A_1^a = \lambda_1 A_1^{S*} \tag{16}$$

$$\lambda_2 A_1^u + p_1 \lambda_2 A_1^a = (\lambda_2 + \lambda_v + \lambda_a + \lambda_d^u) A_2^u \tag{17}$$

$$\lambda_a A_2^u + (1 - p_1) \lambda_2 A_1^a = (\lambda_2 + \lambda_v + \lambda_d^a) A_2^a \tag{18}$$

$$\lambda_2 A_1^{S*} + \lambda_d^u A_2^u + \lambda_d^a A_2^a = \lambda_2 A_2^{S*} \tag{19}$$

$$\lambda_3 A_2^u = (\lambda_3 + \lambda_v + \lambda_a + \lambda_d^u) A_3^u \tag{20}$$

$$\lambda_3 A_2^a + \lambda_a A_3^u = (\lambda_3 + \lambda_v + \lambda_d^a) A_3^a \tag{21}$$

$$\lambda_3 A_2^{S*} + \lambda_d^u A_3^u + \lambda_d^a A_3^a = \lambda_3 A_3^{S*} \tag{22}$$

3.3 Recapitulation of Parameters

Review of the equations just given will show that the following groups of rate constants appear frequently:

$$\lambda_i + \lambda_v + \lambda_a + \lambda_d^u$$

$$\lambda_i + \lambda_v + \lambda_d^a$$

TABLE 5.5   Typical Values of Key Rate Parameters

Parameter	Typical values, h^{-1}	
	Range	"Baseline"[a]
λ_1	13.37	13.37
λ_2	1.552	1.552
λ_3	2.111	2.111
λ_v	0.2–1.5	0.55
λ_a	5–500	50
λ_d^u	10–40[b]	20
λ_d^a	0.1–0.4	0.2

[a] The "baseline" values are the geometric midpoint of the intervals at left.
[b] For λ_d^u, we have assumed that v_d^u is in the range 5 to 10 m h^{-1} and $S\,V^{-1}$ is in the range 2 to 4 m^{-1}.

The relative magnitude of the terms in these groups is important because it shows the fate of the airborne nuclides. Table 5.5 compares the typical values of these terms. The radioactive decay constants are shown as a single value because they are true physical constants. The other parameters vary from one environment to another, as discussed above, and Table 5.5 shows the typical range of values.

For unattached radon progeny, it is seen in Table 5.5 that both attachment and deposition are fast processes. They are comparable, especially at low aerosol concentrations. For attached radon progeny the competitive processes are deposition and ventilation, and these are comparable especially at low ventilation rates.

Also shown in Table 5.5 are "baseline" values of the parameters, useful as a point of departure for calculations. As the baseline value we have simply taken the geometric mean of the two end points of the corresponding range.

4   PREDICTIONS OF INDOOR CONCENTRATIONS

4.1   Definitions—Potential Alpha-Energy Concentration, Unattached Fraction, Equilibrium Ratio

The potential alpha-energy concentration (PAEC) is an aggregated measure of the concentration of the short-lived progeny of radon. (See Chapter 1, Section 8.1). A definition is given in the equation below:

$$\text{PAEC}^x = 3690 A_1^x + 17830 A_2^x + 13120 A_3^x$$

$$\text{(unit: MeV m}^{-3}\text{, provided that } A_i^x \text{ is in Bq m}^{-3}\text{).} \qquad (23)$$

The superscript x, with the allowed values u and a, permits us to distinguish the contributions of the two important states of radon progeny—unattached and attached—to the PAEC. When we want to denote the total PAEC, this superscript will be omitted. Another, more common, unit for this quantity is the working level (WL), usually defined as 1.3×10^8 MeV m^{-3}. (There is an alternative definition which differs by about 2%.) The formal SI unit would be J m^{-3}, where 1 MeV = 1.602×10^{-13} J.

One of the important quantities related to health effects of radon progeny is the fraction of PAEC which is unattached, f_p:

$$f_p = PAEC^u (PAEC^u + PAEC^a)^{-1} \qquad (24)$$

One can also define the unattached fraction of each radon decay product separately:

$$f_i = A_i^u (A_i^u + A_i^a)^{-1} \qquad (25)$$

These two are superficially similar, but the values differ considerably (f_1 is typically 3 to 5 times f_p). Unfortunately, some articles in the literature do not make clear which unattached fraction is meant in a given case. Later we will see that all the unattached fractions are strongly dependent upon the attachment rate constant.

Since radon gas is more easily measured than the PAEC, whereas PAEC is the more significant from the perspective of health effects, the relationship between the two is of interest. At the steady state, the activity concentration of each radon decay product must be in the range 0 to A_0, where A_0 is the activity concentration of radon gas. Thus for a given A_0 (in Bq m^{-3}), the maximum PAEC (sum of attached and unattached PAEC) is 34,640 A_0 MeV m^{-3}. This leads to the definition of the equilibrium ratio, e_p:

$$\begin{aligned} e_p &= PAEC(34640A_0)^{-1} \\ &= (0.1065A_1 + 0.515A_2 + 0.379A_3)A_0^{-1} \end{aligned} \qquad (26)$$

Later we will find that this ratio depends on the rates of ventilation and plateout relative to the rate of radioactive decay.

4.2 Model Predictions for "Baseline" Values of the Parameters

At this point it is possible to exercise the Jacobi model. As a point of departure, Table 5.6 shows model predictions obtained using the baseline parameter values shown in Table 5.5. As the baseline value for the activity concentration for radon, we have taken 100 Bq m^{-3}, which is within the range typically observed indoors.

The value $A_0 = 100$ Bq m^{-3} in Table 5.6 represents the maximum value for the ^{218}Po, ^{214}Pb and ^{214}Bi entries in the detailed-results section of the table. It is seen that the sum of the free, attached, and deposited ^{218}Po is 97 Bq m^{-3}, which means that 97% of the ^{218}Po is accounted for, the balance being carried away by ventilation air. About 25% of the ^{218}Po, and nearly 50% of the ^{214}Pb and ^{214}Bi, is

TABLE 5.6 Jacobi Model Predictions for Partitioning of Radon Progeny Using Baseline Values of the Parameters

Parameters:

$$\lambda_d^u = 20.0 \ h^{-1} \qquad \lambda_d^a = 0.200 \ h^{-1}$$
$$\lambda_v = 0.55 \ h^{-1} \qquad \lambda_a = 50.0 \ h^{-1}$$
$$A_0 = 100.00 \ Bq \ m^{-3} \qquad p_1 = 0.830$$

Detailed Results:

	Free	Attached	Deposited	Total
^{218}Po	15.9	56.4	24.7	97.0 Bq m^{-3}
^{214}Pb	1.4	35.8	46.7	83.9 Bq m^{-3}
^{214}Bi	0.0	27.1	49.6	76.8 Bq m^{-3}
PAEC	83.4	1202.2	1574.9	2860.5 GeV m^{-3}

Key Results:

e_p, Eq-ratio   0.371
f_1, Free ^{218}Po 0.220
f_p, Free PAEC 0.065

TABLE 5.7 Sensitivity Analysis—Effect of Changing Parameter Values

Parameter (h^{-1})	Calculated variable	Values		
$\lambda_v =$		0.2	0.55	1.5
	f_1	22%	22%	23%
	f_p	5.4%	6.5%	9.3%
	e_p	45%	37%	25%
$\lambda_a =$		5.0	50	500
	f_1	74%	22%	2.8%
	f_p	42%	6.5%	0.7%
	e_p	12%	37%	57%
$\lambda_d^u =$		10	20	40
	f_1	22%	22%	22%
	f_p	6.2%	6.5%	7.1%
	e_p	47%	37%	26%
$\lambda_d^a =$		0.1	0.2	0.4
	f_1	22%	22%	22%
	f_p	6.2%	6.5%	7.1%
	e_p	39%	37%	34%

deposited on surfaces. Plateout is clearly a very important part of the activity balance for indoor radon progeny for these typical conditions.

The values for PAEC in Table 5.6 should be judged against its upper limit, 3464 GeV m^{-3}. It is seen that nearly one-half of this amount is tied up on surfaces in the room. The key-results part of the table shows that the airborne PAEC amounts to 37% of its upper limit.

4.3   Sensitivity to Changes in Parameters

Table 5.7 shows an analysis of the sensitivity of the calculated quantities f_1, f_p and e_p to variations in each of the four main parameters. In each block of the table, only one of these parameters is varied, the others being held at their baseline values.

It is seen in Table 5.7 that f_1 is virtually unaffected by any parameter other than λ_a; thus a measurement of either of these virtually determines the other. The variable f_p is determined mainly by λ_a, but is also affected by ventilation.

The table also shows that the parameter λ_d^a has very little effect on the three key variables. Many authors make use of this to simplify the balance equations by dropping the terms containing λ_d^a. We will retain these terms for the time being.

Finally, it is seen that the equilibrium ratio e_p is quite strongly affected by three of the four parameters. All three will have to be taken into account to properly predict e_p. Furthermore, comparison of measured and predicted values of e_p over a range of conditions constitutes a relatively sensitive test of the model.

5   COMPARISON OF MODEL TO DATA FROM CONTROLLED EXPERIMENTS

To test the validity of the model presented here, it is necessary to compare the predictions to data from controlled experiments. The sensitivity analysis in Table 5.7 shows that the ventilation rate, attachment rate, and unattached deposition rate are all influential and should be measured directly, if possible. The ventilation rate can be measured readily (although not trivially) by the tracer gas technique (32). The attachment rate can be estimated rather well from detailed measurements of the aerosol properties (see Section 2.4), or from a measurement of the unattached fraction of ^{218}Po (see Section 4.2).

Deposition, however, is difficult to measure directly. The deposit per unit area is so small that the measurement is possible only in areas of elevated radon concentration, such as those encountered by Scott (24) and by Toohey et al. (25). Even there, deposition has to be measured on a rather small and artificial surface, then extended to the entire surface by a broad extrapolation. A careful accounting of the surface is itself a considerable task, since furniture, draperies, persons, and clothing all contribute surface for deposition. As a consequence, most of the available deposition data were obtained in laboratory studies at elevated radon concentrations.

We will consider the chamber experiments of George et al. (33) and Rudnick et al. (34). Some results from houses will also be considered, where there were sufficient measurements of ventilation and aerosol properties to permit checking the model.

5.1 George et al. Chamber Experiments

George et al. (33) reported the results of 11 experiments using a 1.9-m^3 chamber and two experiments using a 20-m^3 chamber. These experiments included measurements of ventilation, radon, airborne radon progeny, and radon progeny deposited on circular "plateout disks" mounted in the chamber. Furthermore, the aerosols were carefully controlled and measured in these experiments. In each experiment, the measurements were made after a steady state had been reached. The attachment rate calculations were presented in a sequel article by Knutson et al. (35).

Table 5.8 shows the key results from the 13 tests, together with the calculations from the model just given. In the first 11 calculations the rate constant for unattached deposition was taken to be 40 h^{-1}, somewhat higher than the baseline value from Table 5.6 owing to the high surface-to-volume ratio of the small chamber ($S/V = 4.7$ m^{-1}). The baseline value, 20 h^{-1}, was used for tests P and Q in the large chamber, which had a more common S/V, 2.1 m^{-1}.

TABLE 5.8   Comparison of George et al. (33) Results to the Jacobi Model

	Experiment			Model[a]	
Test	Radon (Bq m^{-3})	Attachment rate (h^{-1})	Equilibrium ratio (%)	Equilibrium ratio (%)	Unattached PAEC (%)
C	11,400	3.8	10	4	68
D	13,100	10.4	12	6	43
F	13,100	3.8	9	4	68
G	12,200	2.5	11	4	77
H	17,000	9.4	28	8	34
I	14,400	2022	56	51	19
J	17,500	888	55	49	0.4
K	16,800	612	53	48	0.6
L	17,500	1866	55	51	0.2
M	16,100	458.4	53	46	0.8
N	16,300	270.6	50	42	1.4
P	1300	48	57	32	7.7
Q	3000	45.6	56	38	6.7

[a] These values were calculated using the "baseline" values of the parameters; they therefore differ from those given in the article by Knutson et al. (35).

The ventilation rate constants were: 2.33 h^{-1} for tests C–G; 0.63 h^{-1} for tests H–N; 0.84 h^{-1} for test P; and 0.43 h^{-1} for test Q. Unattached deposition rates were taken as 40 h^{-1} for tests C–N and 20 h^{-1} for tests P–Q. Attached deposition rates were taken as 0.01 times the unattached rate.

It is seen in Table 5.8 that the model with the present "consensus" values of the parameters predicts the equilibrium ratio quite well at high aerosol concentrations. At the lower aerosol concentrations, there was clearly less deposition than predicted by the present model. Knutson et al. (35) concluded that, overall, these data implied an unattached deposition velocity of 1.2–2.4 m h^{-1}, roughly fourfold smaller than the "consensus" values. These lower values were particularly needed to fit the measured surface deposition, not shown in Table 5.8.

5.2 Rudnick et al. Chamber Experiments

Rudnick et al. (34) did radon progeny activity-balance experiments in a 78-m^3 chamber, mainly to investigate the effect of air motion on the radon progeny concentration in air. The ventilation rate was varied over a wide range, 0.13–0.9 h^{-1}. From the information given, we estimate that the chamber had a low S/V (1.4 m^{-1}), and we, therefore, expect that the deposition rate constant should be at the low end of the "consensus" range (10 h^{-1}).

Table 5.9 shows experiment and model results. The experimental values were derived by reading points from Figure 2 of their article, combined with an assumed 100% yield from their radon source. Since test-by-test information was not available for the aerosol, we assumed the baseline value (50 h^{-1}) for the attachment rate constant. Table 5.9 shows that the model reasonably well reproduces the equilibrium ratio that was measured in the experiments. If anything, the model values are slightly lower than the experimental; i.e., the model overpredicts deposition.

Rudnick's experiment included tests of the effect of a 130-cm ceiling fan and a 51-cm box fan. When operated at high speed, both these fans reduced the equilibrium ratio by factors of two to four, depending on ventilation rate. Clearly, this means that the fans increase deposition. A test calculation (not shown) with the present model indicated that taking $\lambda_d^u = 40$ h^{-1} produces an approximate fit.

A word is in order about the difference between the model presented here and that presented by Rudnick et al. The latter model does not differentiate between attached and unattached deposition rates. Thus, the plateout factors given by Rud-

TABLE 5.9 Comparison of Model to Rudnick et al. (34) Results for Quiescent Air

		Experimental			Model	
		PAEC (GeV m^{-3})				
Ventilation (h^{-1})	Radon (Bq m^{-3})	Maximum	Actual	Equilibrium ratio (%)	Equilibrium ratio (%)	Unattached PAEC (%)
0.13	2610	90,400	57,200	63	64	4.6
0.23	1510	52,300	35,100	67	59	4.9
0.52	680	23,600	14,300	61	50	5.8
0.68	522	18,100	8,710	48	46	6.2
0.90	396	13,700	6,110	45	41	6.9

nick et al. are equivalent to a weighted average of the attached and unattached deposition rate constants given here.

5.3   EML-LBL Experiment at the LBL Indoor Air Quality Research House (36)

In May 1984, the Environmental Measurements Laboratory (EML) and Lawrence Berkeley Laboratory (LBL) conducted a plateout experiment at LBL's Indoor Air Quality Research House. The room in which the experiments were done has a volume of 36 m^3 and its nominal surface area is 68 m^2. The part of the house containing the room had been tightly sealed, so that the observed ventilation rate in the room during the experiment period was 0.062 h^{-1}. The protocol included a complete suite of measurements of the airborne materials: aerosol number concentration, radon and radon progeny activity concentration, radon progeny unattached fraction, and both number-weighted and activity-weighted size distributions of the aerosol. Plateout measurements were made using paper disks mounted on the walls and ceiling and on upward-facing surfaces. The ^{218}Po and PAEC unattached fractions were measured near the time each test was terminated.

The quality of data from the experiment can be judged from a budget of the measured activities. Since the ventilation rate constant in these tests was small compared to the radioactive decay constants, the room was essentially airtight and the sum of the airborne and deposited activity for each decay product should equal the activity of the parent, radon. (The deposited activity was estimated by extrapolating from the activity measured on five disks of 0.0073 m^2 each to the entire surface of the room.) It was found that the airborne plus deposited decay products showed deficits ranging from 10 to 40% relative to radon. This deficit probably reflects uncertainties in the extrapolation, and it was found that balances within 10% for all nuclides and all tests could be obtained by doubling the estimated deposition. Although arbitrary, this could be justified in part because the original estimate did not take into account the furniture in the room, which also presented surfaces for deposition. It is also possible that the average deposition velocity was higher than indicated by the five paper disks.

Three tests were done at three widely differing aerosol concentrations. In applying the model, the attachment rate constant was adjusted by trial and error to give the best fit to the unattached fraction measurements; this yielded the values 40, 5, and 700 h^{-1} for tests 1–3, respectively. The low attachment rate in test 2 was obtained by filtering the air in the room for about one hour, several hours before the above measurements were taken. The high value in test 3 was obtained by smoldering a cigarette in the room several hours prior to the measurements. For the attachment coefficients it would have been quite satisfactory to take the baseline, low, and high values that were discussed in Section 3.3.

Since the ventilation rate was very low, and since the room air was not being stirred, the deposition rate constant for unattached radon progeny was taken as 10 h^{-1}, at the low end of the usual range.

Table 5.10 compares the experimental results to the model predictions and shows

TABLE 5.10   Comparison of Model to Data from Three Plateout Tests in the LBL IAQRH

Test	Parameter	Experiment (%)	Model (%)
1	f_1	32	25
	f_p	5	5
	e_p	65	63
2	f_1	55	73
	f_p	42	30
	e_p	26	28
3	f_1	2	1.9
	f_p	0.1	0.3
	e_p	82	86

that this common-sense application of the model yields a good prediction of the equilibrium factor. Comparison of the predicted to the measured decay product deposits, not shown in Table 5.10, also yielded good agreement provided that the surface deposition estimate was doubled, as discussed above. However, the low value of the unattached deposition rate constant appears to be satisfactory in spite of the implied large surface-to-volume ratio.

5.4   Comparison of Model to Measurements in Houses

George and Breslin (6) reported annual-average data from 21 houses in New Jersey and New York, giving 0.5 and 0.07 for the average equilibrium ratio and the average unattached fraction of PAEC, respectively. The latter number closely matches the value in Table 5.6 for the baseline values of the present model. The former number, however, is substantially larger than in Table 5.6. Table 5.7 shows that such high values of the equilibrium ratio can occur, given a high attachment rate (500 h^{-1}), a low ventilation rate (0.2 h^{-1}), or a low unattached plateout rate (10 h^{-1}). Bruno (3) has also studied these data and has argued in favor of a high ventilation rate (1.0 h^{-1}) together with a low value (8 h^{-1}) for the deposition rate constant of the unattached progeny. (Bruno also assumed that the deposition rate for the attached progeny was negligibly small.) In any case, the model is nearly consistent with the data, except that the equilibrium factor is somewhat difficult to match.

Israeli (37) presented a summary of data obtained over a 1-year period in 20 houses in Butte, Montana. Radon concentration and PAEC were measured throughout the year in each house and reported as annual averages. The grand average equilibrium factor was 0.33, close to the baseline value listed in Table 5.6. Israeli analyzed these data in more detail making use of the monthly average values of radon concentration and PAEC, as well as the aerosol concentration and ventilation rate, which had been measured once (in winter) in each house. Israeli concluded that the deposition rate was 3–12 h^{-1} for unattached progeny and 0.3–2 h^{-1} for attached progeny. These results are surprising in that the ratio unattached/attached deposition rate is of order 10, which is much lower than the value

100 that was advocated in Section 2.5 of this chapter. The low value of this ratio seems questionable on physical grounds, and, therefore, Israeli's results do not dictate a change in the present model.

An important feature of Israeli's analysis is the result that deposition velocity changes with season. For both attached and unattached, the winter values were 3–7 times higher than in summer. As Israeli points out, the probable reason is that indoor air velocities are higher during the heating season than in summer (the houses were not air-conditioned).

Two recent papers describe experiments in actual houses, in which the primary objective was to test the model. (More precisely, the model was assumed to be correct and the measurements were used to pin down the values of the key parameters.) In one study, Vanmarcke et al. (38) made detailed measurements of radon progeny, aerosol properties, and ventilation rate over several winter days in each of three houses in Belgium. From the aerosol properties, they calculated the hour-by-hour attachment rate constant (yielding values of 20–$1000 \ h^{-1}$), and they inferred the deposition rate constant for the attached radon progeny (0.2–$0.6 \ h^{-1}$). From the radon progeny measurements they deduced the value $18 \ h^{-1}$ for the average deposition rate of the unattached radon progeny. These values are within the ranges suggested in Table 5.5, showing that the model works in a real-life situation. (The authors also made measurements in a laboratory basement, which yielded a lower value, $8 \ h^{-1}$, for the unattached deposition rate.)

The second paper, that of Porstendörfer et al. (39), reported measurements of radon, radon progeny, and unattached fractions in several houses in southern Germany. In the absense of aerosol sources, the equilibrium ratios were 0.3 ± 0.1. Ratios up to 0.5 could be reached with such aerosol sources as a smoky candle or a hot tiled stove. The unattached fraction of PAEC was found to be 0.06–0.15, with a mean of 0.1. These values are substantially the same as those in Table 5.6, which are derived from the present model.

Porstendörfer et al. presented a detailed analysis of their data. The unattached fraction measurements made it possible to deduce the attachment rates, yielding values of 20–$1000 \ h^{-1}$. Combining this information with the measured equilibrium ratio for ^{218}Po, the authors deduced unattached deposition rate constants ranging from 16 to $900 \ h^{-1}$. There is considerable overlap between these values and the ranges given in Table 5.5. (The highest values corresponded to an unusual, unrepresentative, aerosol condition.) Values from 0 to $0.47 \ h^{-1}$ were found for the attached deposition rate, and the average deposition rate constants were 40 and $0.2 \ h^{-1}$ for unattached and attached radon progeny, respectively.

Contrary to the present model, Porstendörfer et al. found that their data favored a recoil factor, p_1, of 0.5 rather than 0.83. However, the value of this parameter is not very critical in the model.

5.5 Summary

There is good evidence from a variety of experiments, done in different countries, in laboratory chambers and in houses, that the Jacobi model with the parameters given in Table 5.5 works quite well in predicting equilibrium factors and unattached fractions. The model shows that the aerosol properties, followed by the ventilation rate, are the most important parameters in applying the model.

6 ADVANCED TOPICS

In this section, we shall further explore the validity of the uniform mixing and steady-state assumptions, which are important parts of the Jacobi model as developed here. Also given are the results of direct measurements of the activity-weighted, aerosol-size distribution, data that are important in dosimetry calculations. Finally, we shall call attention to some recent studies aimed at developing a "first-principles" calculation of the deposition of atoms, ions, and aerosol particles onto surfaces.

6.1 Incomplete Mixing

It was assumed in Section 2 that the air in a given space is sufficiently mixed to keep the concentration of nuclides in air uniform throughout that space, except perhaps within a thin layer adjacent to surfaces. This was called the uniform-mixing hypothesis. In this section we consider this concept further.

The key question with regard to mixing is the rate at which air parcels travel throughout the space in question, relative to the rate of other physical processes. For example, in order to achieve complete mixing of thoron (^{220}Rn; half-life = 56 s), a given air parcel has to visit all parts of the space in question in a time of the order of 1 min; i.e., the air must recirculate about 60 times/h. Obviously, it would be unlikely to find thoron uniformly mixed, because its short half-life means that thoron atoms are likely to decay before moving far from their point of entry into a house.

For radon (half-life = 3.8 days), radioactive decay does not jeopardize complete mixing. There are, however, other limiting processes. For example, if outdoor (low-radon) air is infiltrating a given room at 1 m^3 h^{-1} around a window, nonuniform concentrations might occur unless there is a recirculating flow of about 10 m^3 h^{-1}.

For houses with central heating, it is likely that indoor radon will be uniformly mixed, at least during the heating season. A typical furnace has a maximum heat output of 100,000 Btu h^{-1} (105,600 kJ h^{-1}), which is used to heat the air in the house, either directly (forced-air system) or indirectly (hot-water system). Assuming in either case that the air temperature increases 40°F on passing through the heat exchanger, 100,000 Btu h^{-1} of heat input implies about 3500 m^3 h^{-1} of air movement. Since the heated volume in a typical house might be 300 m^3, we would expect an air turnover rate of 12 h^{-1} while the furnace is running. If the furnace duty cycle is 25–50%, the air turnover rate might be 3–6 h^{-1}, which should be sufficient to mix all but the draftiest houses. (Bruno (3) states that air turnover rates over 5 h^{-1} are uncomfortable and, therefore, rarely used.)

Clearly, a central forced-air heating system would be effective in mixing air throughout the heated part of a house. It is not obvious that hot-water systems are effective in promoting mixing. However, in one winter experiment in a house with a hot-water system (6), a tracer gas was found to mix throughout the main floor, provided that all the interior doors were left open. On the other hand, mixing between floors was poor, in spite of an open stairwell. (In this case, the lower floor, the basement, was several degrees colder than the upper floor.)

Examples of incomplete mixing can be found in the literature. Abu-Jarad (40) reports on measuring the decay of a tracer gas at four points in a given room, starting with an initially well-mixed tracer. All probes showed a decay rate implying about 2 h^{-1} air infiltration, and the probe near the window measured about 30% less tracer than the three other probes. We conclude that, even in a very drafty room, the concentration was reasonably uniform at the four points measured. The author did not specify whether the measurements were made in the heating season.

Traynor et al. (41) studied the interroom transport of pollution from unvented kerosene space heaters. Two heaters, one convective (7300 kJ h^{-1}) and one radiant (6400 kJ h^{-1}), were operated in a 31-m^3 bedroom, and the spread of pollution to the remainder of the house (205 m^3) was measured. Tests were done with both heaters, and with the bedroom door closed, open 2.5 cm, and wide open. The interroom flow averaged 6, 30, and over 300 m^3 h^{-1} for the three door positions. This indicates that if there is a local heat source and the interior doors are open, there will be intense mixing.

Related to uniform mixing, another assumption made in Section 2 was that of uniform deposition, so that all surfaces are equally effective in collecting radon progeny. In general, uniform deposition requires that two conditions are met: (i) the radon progeny are uniformly mixed in air; and (ii) the airflow characteristics are the same past all surfaces. The former condition (already discussed) is frequently met, but this is not true of the latter condition. The airflow conditions in a corner, for example, cannot be the same as on a broad wall.

Scott (24) studied the deposited activity on different surfaces in the room where he made the deposition measurements discussed in Section 2.5. The results were as follows (units, kBq m^{-2}): floor tiles, 240; Formica table top, 330; interior wood-paneled wall, 370; interior drywall, 460; exterior wood-paneled wall, 560. Abu-Jarad measured deposition at three points in each of several rooms. He found that in some rooms, all three detectors agreed, in others two agreed, and in still others no two detectors agreed.

Bigu and Frattini (42) tested the effect of surface material on deposition velocity. Materials, including metals, plastics, cloth, fiberglass, and filter papers, were exposed in a radon/thoron chamber two or three at a time, then counted for surface activity. The experiment did not permit ranking the materials on a common scale, but differences as large as 60% were found in the groups of two or three. On the other hand, George et al. (33) found no difference between paper and aluminum as deposition surfaces, or between the vertical and horizontal orientation.

The weight of the evidence shows that deposition can differ by factors of about two between different surfaces in the same room. Nonuniformity of deposition is not a serious problem in the model so long as there is good mixing in the air. All that is needed is to select a reasonable average deposition velocity. The physics of deposition is not yet fully understood.

6.2 Activity-Weighted Aerosol Size Distributions

One form of aerosol size distribution was discussed in Section 2.4, where the number-weighted size distribution was used in the calculation of the attachment rate. It was stated that the "attachment rate spectrum" (e.g., the right curve in Figure 5.7) should be a good predictor of the size of particles on which the radon progeny reside. In the present section we shall define the activity-weighted size distribution and discuss direct methods of measuring it.

It is instructive to consider the numbers. Using the conditions in Table 5.6 as an example, the attached ^{218}Po activity is 56.4 Bq m^{-3}, corresponding to approximately 15,000 atoms m^{-3}. The aerosol concentration for these conditions might be 15×10^9 particles m^{-3}, so that particles outnumber ^{218}Po atoms one million to one. Given this high ratio, the 15,000 atoms are most probably attached to 15,000 distinct particles. For radiological health purposes, it is desired to know the size distribution of these 15,000 particles, which is generally quite different from the size distribution of the 15×10^9 particles.

The size distributions of particles carrying ^{214}Pb or ^{214}Bi are also important for radiological health considerations, and they may differ slightly from that for ^{218}Po. Such differences may occur if there is coagulation or size-dependent loss of the aerosol between the time of attachment and the time of decay. This time, which is available for coagulation or loss, is different for the three nuclides, owing to their different half-lives. For the same reasons, the radon progeny size distribution may differ from the attachment rate spectrum discussed in Section 2.4.

Various terminology has emerged concerning size distributions. The phrase "size distribution of active particles," based on the fact that each active particle has exactly one attached radioactive atom, is often used and is often shortened to *active size distribution*. Disadvantages include the implication that all radon decay products atoms are equally important (not true from a health standpoint) and the implication that the "inactive" particles are unimportant (when, in fact, they may contain chemical toxicants). We prefer a more comprehensive term, *activity-weighted aerosol size distribution*, which works for the individual radon progeny nuclides and adapts easily to such aggregated measures as potential alpha-energy concentration. The type of weighting must be made clear in each situation.

Direct measurement of the activity-weighted size distribution can be accomplished by a sampler that segregates particles according to size, so that the activity of each size fraction can be determined separately. Several factors make this a difficult task: the activities, already low, become lower yet when segregating the particles into several groups; the activities are short-lived, dictating short sampling times; the peak of the spectrum falls in a size range that is particularly awkward to size-segregate. Owing to these difficulties, the direct measurement of the activity-weighted size distribution is a relatively recent development. Judging from the discusssion in Junge's book (43), no satisfactory measurement had been made prior to 1963. Even today, these measurements remain a specialty practiced only by a few experts.

The most appropriate current method for measurement of radon progeny particle size is the diffusion battery technique described by Sinclair et al. (44). Three designs are described, to cope with different activity levels, from occupational to outdoor. Results obtained with these batteries may be seen in various articles (6, 44–46).

Figure 5.9 shows three activity-weighted size distributions measured in houses under normal conditions of occupancy, expressed in terms of the PAEC in each size class (6). The major part of the PAEC is concentrated in a peak centered at 0.1–0.15 μm, with location and shape similar to those expected from the attachment rate spectrum. The smaller peak comprises 5–10% of the total PAEC and is thought to be the unattached fraction of PAEC. The size indicated (0.007–0.01 μm) is considerably larger than expected for atoms (about 0.001 μm), a matter still being studied (cf. Chapter 6).

Although very few direct measurements have been made in houses, it appears that the distributions in Figure 5.9 are the norm. Significant deviations from Figure 5.9 could occur, but only in unusual cases. Direct measurements made at the LBL

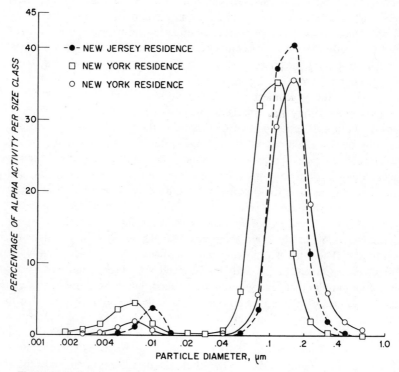

Figure 5.9. Activity-weighted particle size distributions measured indoors (6).

Indoor Air Quality Research House (radon levels were enhanced to make measurements more reliable) showed the main distribution peak varying from 0.07 μm to 0.3 μm for unusually clean and unusually smoky air, respectively.

Curves 2 and 3 of Figure 5.5 show a case where the peak of the activity-weighted size distribution might be expected to occur at very small particle size, since the attachment rate spectrum peaks at about 0.025 μm. However, in this situation there appears to be intense coagulation of aerosol particles. Thus, in the interim between attachment and decay, it is likely that the particles carrying the radon decay products will grow in size, shifting the activity-weighted size distribution in the direction of the curves in Figure 5.9. Because of the unknown extent of coagulation, direct measurements are necessary if accurate activity-weighted size distributions are desired.

In summary, curves like those in Figure 5.9 can be expected to apply, except in rare cases.

6.3 Response to Parameters That Vary with Time

In Section 3, attention was focused on the steady state that would result if all the parameters in the model remained constant for a sufficiently long time. However, many of the parameters will vary from day to night, and even from hour to hour. One example is the attachment coefficient, which must change from hour to hour because the indoor aerosol changes in response to activities such as cooking and smoking. In this section we shall address some of the consequences of changing parameters.

It is easy to construct the differential equations that predict the effect of changing parameters. The source and sink terms for each species were discussed in Section 3. The rate of change in air concentration of a given species is equal to the source terms minus the sink terms (all terms expressed on a per-unit-volume basis). Thus:

$$dA_0/dt = \lambda_0 S_r V^{-1} - (\lambda_0 + \lambda_v)A_0 \tag{27}$$

$$dA_1^u/dt = \lambda_1 A_0 - (\lambda_1 + \lambda_v + \lambda_a + \lambda_d^u)A_1^u \tag{28}$$

$$dA_1^a/dt = \lambda_a A_1^u - (\lambda_1 + \lambda_v + \lambda_d^a)A_1^a \tag{29}$$

$$dA_1^{S*}/dt = \lambda_d^u A_1^u + \lambda_d^a A_1^a - \lambda_1 A_1^{S*} \tag{30}$$

$$dA_2^u/dt = \lambda_2 A_1^u + p_1 \lambda_2 A_1^a - (\lambda_2 + \lambda_v + \lambda_a + \lambda_d^u)A_2^u \tag{31}$$

$$dA_2^a/dt = \lambda_a A_2^u + (1 - p_1)\lambda_2 A_1^a - (\lambda_2 + \lambda_v + \lambda_d^a)A_2^a \tag{32}$$

$$dA_2^{S*}/dt = \lambda_2 A_1^{S*} + \lambda_d^u A_2^u + \lambda_d^a A_2^a - \lambda_2 A_2^{S*} \tag{33}$$

$$dA_3^u/dt = \lambda_3 A_2^u - (\lambda_3 + \lambda_v + \lambda_a + \lambda_d^u)A_3^u \tag{34}$$

$$dA_3^a/dt = \lambda_3 A_2^a + \lambda_a A_3^u - (\lambda_3 + \lambda_v + \lambda_d^a)A_3^a \qquad (35)$$

$$dA_3^{S*}/dt = \lambda_3 A_2^{S*} + \lambda_d^u A_3^u + \lambda_d^a A_3^a - \lambda_3 A_3^{S*} \qquad (36)$$

To illustrate the effect of changing parameters, Figure 5.10 shows the effect of a sudden doubling of the attachment rate, starting from the steady state depicted in Table 5.6. A change of this magnitude could easily happen due to a sudden production of aerosol. The curves in Figure 5.10 were developed by a step-by-step integration of the above equations.

It is seen in Figure 5.10 that the change in concentration of unattached ^{218}Po is 95% complete in 0.03 h; the governing process is the attachment rate, 100 h^{-1}. The change in attached ^{218}Po takes longer, about 0.25 h; here the decay constant, 13.37 h^{-1}, governs. The succeeding decay products take longer to adjust. The changes in attached and surface deposited ^{214}Bi are only about 80% complete after 1.5 h.

The ventilation rate also changes. A report by Nazaroff et al. (47) gives results from 15 weeks of measurements during February to May in a single-family house near Chicago. The average ventilation rate was 0.22 h^{-1}, but use of the fireplace increased the rate to the range of 0.6–1.0 h^{-1}. However, the radon concentration (also measured) did not necessarily decrease during fireplace operation, indicating that there is a coupling between the ventilation rate and the radon source strength.

Experience with the time-dependent form of the Jacobi model is not sufficient as yet to determine its usefulness or accuracy. Applying the time-dependent model

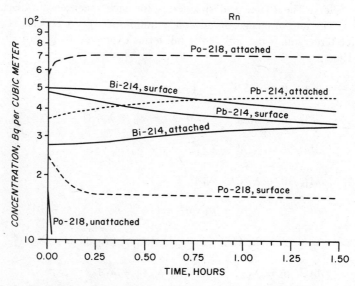

Figure 5.10. Predicted response of decay product concentrations to a change in attachment rate from 50 to 100 h^{-1}.

to data from continuous measurements might help to clarify coupling terms such as that between the ventilation rate and the source strength.

6.4   Developments in Atom, Ion, and Particle Deposition

In the Jacobi model, the removal of radon progeny from air by plateout is treated as a subject where experience is the best guide. In Section 2.5 it was stated that the range 5–10 m h^{-1} (0.14–0.28 cm s^{-1}) was a reasonable summary of experience regarding the unattached deposition velocity, which is the main parameter used to calculate plateout. In the present section, we shall call attention to some recent studies whose objective has been to develop a better understanding of the basic science of the deposition process.

A simple (and inadequate) discussion of the theory of deposition was given in Section 2.5 in connection with Figure 5.8. The key to the process is the shape of the radon decay product concentration profile, i.e., the breakdown of uniform mixing, near the surface. The two studies cited below are aimed at a more complete and accurate calculation of this profile in realistic situations.

6.4.1   Convective Transport Model. In a recent doctoral dissertation, Schiller (48) applied mass transfer theory to calculate the deposition rate in dead calm air and in three types of laminar airflow. A main feature of the thesis was a calculation of the complete airflow field within a room-shaped cavity, one wall of which was slightly heated while the opposite wall was slightly cooled. The calculation yielded the air velocity profiles near both these walls, as well as near the floor and ceiling.

Among the findings of the thesis were the following:

1. The presence of aerosol particles alters the near-surface concentration profile of unattached radon progeny. Thus, in addition to governing the fraction attached, the aerosol also affects the deposition velocity of the unattached fraction. The deposition velocity increases with aerosol concentration.

2. Air movement also increases deposition velocity.

3. The air movement and aerosol concentration effects interact, so that their combined effect is less than the sum of their independent effects.

4. In a realistic case, the maximum air velocity reached in the room-shaped cavity was 7 cm s^{-1} at 2 cm from the center of the warm wall. The maximum velocities near the floor and ceiling were about 0.4 cm s^{-1}, at 4–5 cm from the surface.

5. A realistic range for the deposition velocity of the unattached radon progeny is 0.7–2.8 m h^{-1} (0.02–0.08 cm s^{-1}).

6. The three short-lived decay products have different concentration profiles, and, therefore, different deposition velocities.

The Schiller calculation illuminates many features of the deposition process, but is restricted to laminar flow. It is probable that in real life, some turbulence develops within the layer of air next to walls and other surfaces. This would enhance deposition and may be the reason that the best measurements yield a range of values fourfold higher than those calculated above. Scott postulated turbulence in the boundary layer in order to account for the deposition velocity measured in his experiment.

6.4.2 Turbulent Boundary Layer Model.

To calculate deposition velocity, including the effects of turbulence, Holub (49) proposed to apply an equation developed by Crump and Seinfeld (50) to describe wall losses in aerosol chambers. In deriving this equation, Crump and Seinfeld assumed that the diffusion coefficient is the sum of two parts—the ordinary (molecular) diffusion coefficient and the turbulent diffusion coefficient. Drawing on experience in aerodynamics, the turbulent diffusion coefficient is assumed to increase with the square of the perpendicular distance from the surface. The Crump and Seinfeld equation also takes into account particle-settling velocity. A more recent form of the equation includes the effect of electrostatic charge (51).

The Crump and Seinfeld equation is compact and is solidly based on the physics of the deposition process. However, there is one parameter—the coefficient of eddy diffusivity—left to be determined by experiment. Experience thus far indicates that this parameter differs considerably from one situation to another (51, 52), and thus far there is no reliable method for estimating its value.

6.4.3 Thermophoresis and Electric Charge Effects.

In addition to diffusion (Section 2.5), van de Vate (53) has suggested that thermal effects and electrical effects can be significant in causing deposition of aerosol particles. Thermal deposition, called thermophoresis, occurs when the surface is substantially colder than the air—as with the perimeter walls during the heating season. Although van de Vate demonstrated this effect for small aerosol chambers with heat input, it is not clear how to estimate the magnitude of this effect as applied to rooms in houses. Also, it is not clear how it applies to unattached radon progeny.

Electrical effects occur when both the particles and the surfaces are electrically charged. As discussed in the next chapter, about 90% of freshly formed ^{218}Po is positively charged, and this charge may persist for a few seconds or minutes, depending on circumstances. Regarding the aerosol particles of most interest here, 0.1 μm and larger, more than half normally carry charge. Surfaces of materials with low electric conductivity are prone to develop and hold surface charge, for example by rubbing. Thus, it is conceivable that electrical effects can augment diffusion in causing deposition.

Electrical effects were studied by McMurry and Rader (51) in connection with aerosol chambers used to study the formation of photochemical smog. These chambers are made of a plastic film that is prone to surface charging. The authors calculated that the greatest effect—a 3- to 5-fold augmentation—should occur for particles of about 0.2 μm diameter. In houses, surface charges and, therefore, electrical deposition are probably less significant.

For unattached progeny, two opposing electrical effects can be envisioned. If there are surface charges, electrically charged progeny should deposit faster than uncharged. On the other hand, there is evidence (54) that charged progeny have a lower diffusion coefficient, which would impede their diffusional deposition. Porstendörfer et al. (39) suggested that charge neutralization was the cause of the very high unattached deposition velocities observed in a few of their tests.

6.4.4 Summary. The recent physics/mass transfer studies of plateout have contributed greatly to knowledge about the process, but thus far the equations developed are not adequate to predict deposition velocity in real situations. Experience remains the best guide in this matter. It is very likely that future studies, building on those outlined above, will provide the missing link and make these methods practical.

7 SUMMARY

In this chapter we have presented a model—a calculation technique—useful for predicting indoor concentrations of radon and its decay products. The sources, sinks, and conversion processes involved in the model have been examined individually. The main parameters of the model are ventilation rate, attachment rate, deposition rate of unattached progeny, deposition rate of attached progeny, and recoil factor.

The literature has been reviewed to determine the normal range of each parameter. From these, "baseline values" of each parameter were suggested as a starting point in calculations. The model itself consists of a set of mass balance equations, which are made very simple by the assumption of uniform mixing. Further simplification was achieved by focusing on the steady state. These two restrictions were examined in Section 6.

Using the baseline values of the parameters, the model predicts an equilibrium ratio of 37% and an unattached fraction of PAEC of 6.5%. A sensitivity analysis showed that the parameter most influential on the equilibrium ratio is the attachment rate. This is due mainly to the very broad range, 5–500 h^{-1}, found in the literature for the attachment rate. After attachment rate, deposition of the unattached progeny and ventilation were about equally important in influencing the equilibrium ratio.

The model hinges on a phenomenological approach to deposition, parameterized in terms of a deposition velocity. Attempts to provide a more solid scientific basis for deposition were reviewed in Section 6.4. Progress is being made, and the results to date will help to guide further research. However, the older, parametric model remains the best choice for estimating conditions in actual rooms.

REFERENCES

1. Jacobi, W. (1972). Activity and potential alpha energy of ^{222}Rn and ^{220}Rn daughters in different air atmospheres, *Health Phys.*, **22,** 441.

2. Porstendörfer, J., Wicke, A., and Schraub, A. (1978). The influence of exhalation, ventilation and deposition processes upon radon (^{222}Rn) and thoron (^{220}Rn) and their decay products in room air, *Health Phys.*, **34**, 465.

3. Bruno, R. C. (1983). Verifying a model of radon decay product behavior indoors, *Health Phys.*, **45**, 471.

4. Porstendörfer, J. (1984). Behaviour of radon daughter products in indoor air, *Radiat. Prot. Dosim.*, **7**, 107.

5. Knutson, E. O., unpublished data.

6. George, A. C., and Breslin, A. J. (1980). The distribution of ambient radon and radon daughters in residential buildings in the New Jersey–New York area. In T. F. Gesell and W. M. Lowder (eds.), *The Natural Radiation Environment III*, DOE report CONF-780422, US Department of Energy, p. 1272.

7. Van Hise, J. R., Martz, D. E., Jackson, R. A., Kunihira, D. Y., and Bolton, E. (1982). ^{218}Po half-life, *Phys. Rev. C*, **25**, 2802.

8. Lederer, C. M., and Shirley, V. S. (eds.) (1978). *Table of Isotopes*, 7th ed., Wiley, New York.

9. Gesell, T. F. (1983). Background atmospheric ^{222}Rn concentrations outdoors and indoors: A review, *Health Phys.*, **45**, 289.

10. Handley, T. H., and Barton, C. J. (1973). Home ventilation rates: A literature survey, AEC report ORNL-TM-4318.

11. Grot, R. A., and Clark, R. E. (1981). Air leakage characteristics and weatherization techniques for low-income housing, paper presented at the ASHRAE conference Thermal Performance of Exterior Envelopes of Buildings, Orlando, FL.

12. Grimsrud, D. T., Sherman, M. H., and Sonderegger, R. C. (1983). Calculating infiltration: implications for a construction quality standard, paper presented at the ASHRAE conference Thermal Performance of Exterior Envelopes of Buildings II, Las Vegas, NV.

13. Lamb, B., Westberg, H., Bryant, P., Dean, J., and Mullins, S. (1985). Air infiltration rates in pre- and post-weatherized houses, *J. Air Pollut. Control Assoc.*, **35**, 545.

14. Raes, F., Janssens, A., Declercq, A., and Vanmarcke, H. (1984). Investigation of the indoor aerosol and its effect on the attachment of radon daughters, *Radiat. Prot. Dosim.*, **7**, 127.

15. Johansson, G. I., Samuelsson, C., and Pettersson, H. (1984). Characterisation of the aerosol and the activity size distribution of radon daughters in indoor air, *Radiat. Prot. Dosim.*, **7**, 133.

16. Stoute, J. R. D., Groen, G. C. H., and deGroot, T. J. H. (1984). Characterisation of indoor atmospheres, *Radiat. Prot. Dosim.*, **7**, 159.

17. Tu, K. W., and Knutson, E. O. (1987). Indoor/outdoor aerosol measurements for two residential buildings in New Jersey, *Aerosol Sci. Technol.*, in press.

18. Ho., W. L. (1979). An experimental study of the attachment of radium A to monodispersed aerosols, Ph.D. thesis, University of Illinois, Urbana.

19. Porstendörfer, J., and Mercer, T. T. (1978). Adsorption probability of atoms and ions on particle surfaces in submicrometer size range, *J. Aerosol Sci.*, **9**, 469.

20. Junge, C. E. (1963). *Air Chemistry and Radioactivity*, Academic Press, New York, p. 222.

21. Porstendörfer, J., Roebig, G., and Ahmed, A. (1979). Experimental determination of

the attachment coefficients of atoms and ions on monodisperse aerosols, *J. Aerosol Sci.*, **10**, 21.

22. McLaughlin, J. P., and O'Byrne, F. D. (1984). The role of daughter product plateout in passive radon detection, *Radiat. Prot. Dosim.*, **7**, 115.

23. Cox, R. A., and Penkett, S. A. (1972). Effect of relative humidity on the disappearance of ozone and sulphur dioxide in contained systems, *Atmos. Environ.*, **6**, 365.

24. Scott, A. G. (1983). Radon daughter deposition velocities estimated from field measurements, *Health Phys.*, **45**, 481.

25. Toohey, R. E., Essling, M. A., Rundo, J., and Hengde, W. (1984). Measurements of the deposition rates of radon daughters on indoor surfaces, *Radiat. Prot. Dosim.*, **7**, 143.

26. Bigu, J. (1985). Radon daughter and thoron daughter deposition velocity and unattached fraction under laboratory-controlled conditions and in underground uranium mines, *J. Aerosol Sci.*, **16**, 157.

27. Wilson, M. J. G. (1968). Indoor air pollution, *Proc. Roy. Soc. A*, **300**, 215.

28. Offermann, F. J., Sextro, R. G., Fisk, W. J., Grimsrud, D. T., Nazaroff, W. W., Nero, A. V., Revzan, K. L., and Yater, J. (1985). Control of respirable particles in indoor air with portable air cleaners, *Atmos. Environ.*, **19**, 1761.

29. Sinclair, J. D., Psota-Kelty, L. A., and Weschler, C. J. (1985). Indoor/outdoor concentrations and indoor surface accumulations of ionic substances, *Atmos. Environ.*, **19**, 315.

30. Harrison, A. W. (1979). Quiescent boundary layer thickness in aerosol enclosures under convective stirring conditions, *J. Colloid Interface Sci.*, **69**, 563.

31. Mercer, T. T. (1976). The effect of particle size on the escape of recoiling RaB atoms from particulate surfaces, *Health Phys.*, **31**, 173.

32. Hunt, C. M. (1980). Air infiltration: A review of some existing measurement techniques and data. In C. M. Hunt, J. C. King, and H. R. Trechsel (eds.), *Building Air Change and Infiltration Measurements*, American Society for Testing and Materials, Philadelphia, p. 3.

33. George, A. C., Knutson, E. O., and Tu, K. W. (1983). Radon daughter plateout—I: measurements, *Health Phys.*, **45**, 439.

34. Rudnick, S. N., Hinds, W. C., Maher, E. F., and First, M. W. (1983). Effect of plateout, air motion and dust removal on radon decay product concentration in a simulated residence, *Health Phys.*, **45**, 463.

35. Knutson, E. O., George, A. C., Frey, J. J., and Koh, B. R. (1983). Radon daughter plateout—II: prediction model, *Health Phys.*, **45**, 445.

36. Knutson, E. O., unpublished data.

37. Israeli, M. (1985). Deposition rates of Rn progeny in houses, *Health Phys.*, **49**, 1069.

38. Vanmarcke, H., Janssens, A., Raes, F., Poffijn, A., Berkvens, P., and Van Dingenen, R. (1987). The behavior of radon daughters in the domestic environment: Effect on the effective dose equivalent. In P. K. Hopke, *Radon and Its Decay Products: Occurrence, Properties, and Health Effects*, ACS Symposium Series 331, American Chemical Society, Washington, DC, p. 301.

39. Porstendörfer, J., Reineking, A., and Becker, K. H. (1987). Free fractions, attachment rates, and plateout rates of radon daughters in houses. In P. K. Hopke, *Radon and Its*

Decay Products: Occurrence, Properties, and Health Effects, ACS Symposium Series 331, American Chemical Society, Washington, DC, p. 285.

40. Abu-Jarad, F. (1982). Variation in long-term radon and daughters concentrations with position inside a room, *Radiat. Prot. Dosim.*, **3**, 227.

41. Traynor, G. W., Apte, M. G., Carruthers, A. R., Dillworth, J. F., Grimsrud, D. T. and Thompson, W. T. (1984). Indoor air pollution and inter-room transport due to unvented kerosene-fired space heaters, report LBL-17600, Lawrence Berkeley Laboratory, Berkeley, CA.

42. Bigu, J., and Frattini, A., (1985). Radon progeny and thoron progeny plate-out on a variety of materials, Minerals Research Program Mining Research Laboratories Division report MRP/MRL 85-72 (TR), Canada Centre of Mineral and Energy Technology.

43. Junge, C. E., loc cit., p. 226.

44. Sinclair, D., George, A. C., and Knutson, E. O. (1978). Application of diffusion batteries to measurement of submicron radioactive aerosols. In D. Shaw (ed.), *Airborne Radioactivity*, American Nuclear Society, LaGrange Park, IL, p. 103.

45. Knutson, E. O., George, A. C., Knuth, R. H. and Koh, B. R. (1984). Measurements of radon daughter particle size, *Radiat. Prot. Dosim.*, **7**, 121.

46. George, A. C., Knutson, E. O., Sinclair, D., Wilkening, M. H., and Andrews, L. (1984). Measurements of radon and radon daughter aerosols in Socorro, New Mexico, *Aerosol Sci. Technol.*, **3**, 277.

47. Nazaroff, W. W., Feustel, H., Nero, A. V., Revzan, K. L., Grimsrud, D. T., Essling, M. A., and Toohey, R. E. (1985). Radon transport into a detached one-story house with a basement, *Atmos. Environ.*, **19**, 31.

48. Schiller, G. E. (1984). A theoretical convective transport model of indoor radon decay products, Ph.D. thesis, University of California, Berkeley.

49. Holub, R. F. (1984). Turbulent plateout of radon daughters, *Radiat. Prot. Dosim.*, **7**, 155.

50. Crump, J. G., and Seinfeld, J. H. (1981). Turbulent deposition and gravitational sedimentation of an aerosol in vessels of arbitrary shape, *J. Aerosol Sci.*, **12**, 405.

51. McMurry, P. H., and Rader, D. J. (1985). Aerosol wall losses in electrically charged chambers, *Aerosol Sci. Technol.*, **4**, 249.

52. Crump, J. G., Flagan, R. C., and Seinfeld, J. H. (1983). Particle wall losses in vessels, *Aerosol Sci. Technol.*, **2**, 303.

53. Vate, J. F. van de (1980). Investigation into the dynamics of aerosols in enclosures used for air pollution studies, research report ECN-86, Netherlands Energy Research Foundation.

54. Goldstein, S. D. (1984). The environmental properties of polonium-218, M.S. thesis, University of Illinois, Urbana.

6

The Nature and Determination of the Unattached Fraction of Radon and Thoron Progeny

COLIN R. PHILLIPS, ATIKA KHAN, and
HELEN M. Y. LEUNG

Department of Chemical Engineering and Applied Chemistry, University of
Toronto, Toronto, Ontario, Canada

1 THE IMPORTANCE OF THE UNATTACHED FRACTION OF RADON PROGENY

It is well known that in an atmosphere of radon and its progeny the major part of the radiation dose to the human lung comes from inhaled and subsequently deposited radon progeny. However, there is considerable uncertainty with respect to the exact mechanisms of deposition and transport of the radon progeny in the lung and delivery of the dose to the lung tissue.

At birth from its ^{222}Rn parent, ^{218}Po is a free, positive ion and is usually unattached to an aerosol particle. Subsequently, ^{218}Po may participate in one or more of the following processes, not necessarily in the order stated: (i) neutralization, (ii) reaction, including hydration followed by nucleation and growth, (iii) attachment to an aerosol particle. Each of these processes is discussed in detail later. The process of attachment is a result of the random movements of the progeny and the aerosol particles and may be considered to be a special case of aerosol coagulation. Following attachment, the behavior of the radon progeny is a function of the aerosol particle mechanics. The unattached fraction has a diffusivity of the same order as that of the parent gas, ^{222}Rn, much higher than that of the attached fraction, whose diffusivity is governed by the aerosol size distribution. Thus, in simplistic terms, the radon progeny activity size distribution may be thought of as bimodal, with a fairly sharp small-diameter mode near molecular size corresponding to the unattached fraction and a broader large-diameter mode corresponding to the attached fraction.

An understanding of the unattached fraction of radon progeny has only developed over the last three decades or so. In 1956, Chamberlain and Dyson (1) demonstrated the preferential deposition of unattached radon progeny in the human upper respiratory tract as a result of the large values of the diffusion coefficient of the unattached fraction. They reported that the average unattached fraction of the radon progeny in uranium mines was about 0.1. Since then special attention has been devoted to the unattached fraction of radon progeny in uranium mine air. In 1959, the ICRP (2) introduced an equation for calculating the maximum permissible air concentration of radon (MPC) as a function of the unattached fraction. Based on an unattached fraction of about 0.1, the MPC for radon was given as

$$\mathrm{MPC_{Rn}} = \frac{1.11 \times 10^5}{1 + 1000\,f} \left(\frac{\mathrm{Bq}}{\mathrm{m}^3}\right) \tag{1}$$

where f = the fraction of the equilibrium number of ^{218}Po atoms that are unattached to condensation nuclei. This ICRP equation considers only the unattached fraction of ^{218}Po atoms and does not take into account the radiation dose to the bronchial epithelium arising from any of the other unattached radon progeny or from the attached fraction. It should be noted that it is also possible for ^{214}Pb and ^{214}Bi atoms to exist in unattached form (3–5).

Models for calculating lung dose (bronchial basal cell dose, pulmonary dose, and total lung dose) are reviewed in ICRP publication 32 "Limits for Inhalation of Radon Daughters by Workers" (6). The equations used show that the unattached fraction is assigned a 6–38 times higher relative weighting (sievert per joule inhaled potential alpha energy) than the attached fraction for bronchial basal cell dose. Although a detailed discussion of dosimetric models is provided in Chapter 7, a short review of the subject is appropriate here for the purpose of understanding the role of the unattached fraction in dosimetry.

Palmer et al. (7) studied the lung deposition of radon progeny in humans using total body counting and, based on the measurements in both active and inactive uranium mines, concluded that nearly all the inhaled radon progeny were deposited in the respiratory tract, especially in the upper bronchial tree, where most carcinomas originate (8). George and Breslin (9) found that the nose removed more than 65% of the unattached progeny inhaled, but less than 2% of the attached progeny. Since lung carcinomas are known to occur in the tracheobronchial region of the lung, the unattached fraction, ordinarily small, would therefore not contribute a significant dose to this critical region. Others (10–13) have also demonstrated that the major part of the radiation dose to the lung arises from the attached, rather than the unattached, fraction.

ICRP 32 (6) now recognizes both attached and unattached fractions in lung models. In Jacobi and Eisfeld's (14) dosimetric model for the inhalation of ^{222}Rn and their short-lived progeny, the mean dose equivalent, $\overline{H}$, in sievert per joule inhaled potential α energy from ^{222}Rn progeny, is given as a function of the unattached fraction, f_p, as follows:

Bronchial basal cell layer: $\overline{H} = 18(1 + 9.4f_p)$ (2)

Pulmonary tissue: $\overline{H} = 5.2(1 - f_p)$ (3)

where f_p = unattached fraction of the total potential α energy of the radon progeny mixture. Jacobi and Eisfeld concluded that for typical mine atmospheres (f_p was assumed to be ≤ 0.05), the dose contribution from the unattached fraction is relatively small. However, it should be noted that the dose from the unattached fraction might be significant in well-ventilated mine areas with low dust production in which miners work over long periods of time. Unattached fractions in buildings and houses are usually higher than in mines because the aerosol concentration is usually lower. Use of air cleaners may further increase the unattached fraction.

The relative importance of the attached and unattached fractions must clearly depend on the nature of the unattached fraction since this affects the mechanism of attachment to aerosols. Depending on the size of the aerosol, two main mechanisms have been proposed for the attachment process, namely, a classical diffusion mechanism (15, 16) and a gas kinetic mechanism (17). Combinations or hybrids of these have also been proposed (18–20). Attachment models are described in Section 3.

Models for attachment rate require knowledge of the diffusion coefficient or the mean velocity of the unattached atoms and their state of charge. The relationship between the diffusion coefficient, D, and the mean velocity, $\overline{V}$, can be seen as follows:

From kinetic theory

$$\overline{V} = \left(\frac{8kT}{\pi m}\right)^{1/2}$$ (4)

From the Stokes-Einstein equation

$$D = \frac{kT}{f_c}$$ (5)

where k = Boltzmann's constant (1.38×10^{-16} erg/K)
$\quad\;\; T$ = temperature
$\quad\;\; m$ = atomic mass
$\quad\;\; f_c$ = friction coefficient = $3\pi\mu d/C$

where μ = gas viscosity
$\quad\;\; d$ = particle diameter
$\quad\;\; C$ = slip correction factor = $1 + (2l/d)\{A_1 + A_2 \exp[-A_3(d/l)]\}$

where l = mean free path (~ 0.065 μm), and A_1, A_2, A_3 are constants [1.257, 0.400, and 0.55 (21) or 1.246, 0.42, 0.435 (20)]. Therefore,

$$D = \frac{\pi m \overline{V}^2}{8 f_c}. \tag{6}$$

Experimental values usually used for the diffusion coefficient and mean velocity of unattached atoms are $D \approx 0.054$ cm^2 s^{-1} and $\overline{V} \approx 1.38 \times 10^4$ cm s^{-1}, respectively. These values obviously depend on whether and to what extent the progeny atom is encumbered by clustering and other factors. Thus, the major difficulty in the determination of absolute attachment rates lies in the fact that little is known about the nature of unattached radon progeny. The terms "free ions," "uncombined," and "unattached" radon progeny are widely used in referring to airborne radon progeny that are not attached to the ambient aerosol (1, 12, 22, 23). It is likely that unattached radon progeny are not a single chemical species, and that, therefore, a single value for the diffusion coefficient does not exist. Newly formed ions may become hydrated or react chemically with oxygen or trace gases in the atmosphere (24). A description of the system in terms of attached and unattached fractions—the latter normally including all airborne radon progeny charged or neutral, in any physicochemical form, that are not attached to the ambient aerosol—is less precise than a description in terms of a multimodal size distribution (normally two modes, the very small unattached mode and the larger attached mode). From physical and dosimetric points of view, however, the concept of an unattached fraction is useful and is retained as the vehicle for discussion here.

2   THE NATURE OF THE UNATTACHED FRACTION

2.1   Interactions During the Life History of the Unattached Radon Progeny

The nature of unattached radon progeny may be considered to be governed by atmospheric chemistry as much as by physics. Of the radon progeny, ^{218}Po is of particular interest because it is the first short-lived progeny in the chain, because little is known about its physicochemical nature, and because of its relatively short half-life.

At birth, ^{218}Po is positively charged as a result of the stripping of orbital electrons by the departing alpha particle or as a result of the recoil process (24). The recoil atom (^{218}Po) has an energy of about 101 keV and a range of about 50 μm in air or about 0.03 μm in a particle of density 2×10^3 kg m^{-3} (25). The amount of charge acquired by ^{218}Po during the recoil motion is not known but has been assumed to be a single positive charge (24). From the recoil energy (101 keV), the velocity of the recoil of ^{218}Po is about 3.0×10^7 cm/s, as follows:

$$V = (3.00 \times 10^{10} \text{ cm/s}) \sqrt{\frac{2E}{\left(931 \frac{\text{MeV}}{\text{amu}}\right) m}} \simeq 3.0 \times 10^7 \text{ cm/s} \qquad (7)$$

where E = energy of the atom (MeV)
m = mass of the atom in amu
V = velocity (cm/s)

Since the recoil range in air is about 50 μm, the stopping time can be estimated to be of order nanoseconds from the following equation (26):

$$T \simeq 1.2 \times 10^{-7} R_c \sqrt{\frac{m}{E}} \simeq 2.8 \times 10^{-10} \text{ s} \qquad (8)$$

where R_c = recoil range in meters
T = stopping time, s

After birth, the ^{218}Po atom undergoes about 1.0×10^{12} collisions until it thermalizes. After thermalization, the mean velocity of the atoms is about 1.4×10^4 cm/s and their collision frequency of the order of 1×10^9 collisions/s.

Over the recoil path, ^{218}Po atoms may remain charged because of the short time of travel. Whether the ^{218}Po atoms have a positive charge at the end of their recoil paths depends on the nature of the charge transfer process. Neutralization is complicated and may involve one or more processes, as described below, depending on the ionization potential of the ^{218}Po species or compound present, the ionization potential of the gas molecules, and the concentration, nature, and electron affinity of negative small ions present in the air.

2.1.1 Recombination with Negative Small Ions.
Polonium-218 atoms may recombine with small negative ions (including electrons). The half-life for neutralization of ^{218}Po ions, assuming a single positive charge, can be estimated from the equation of Gunn (27):

$$\tau_{1/2} = \frac{0.693 \epsilon_0}{NeB} \qquad (9)$$

where $\tau_{1/2}$ = the ion half-life for neutralization
N = the number concentration of negative ions in the air, m^{-3}
e = the electronic charge, 1.602×10^{-19} C
B = the mobility of the ions $\sim 1.6 \times 10^{-4}$ m^2 (Vs)$^{-1}$
ϵ_0 = permittivity of free space = 8.85×10^{-12} F/m

Raabe (24) estimated the half-life for neutralization of ^{218}Po ions by small negative ions to be 20 minutes at ground level when the negative small ion concentration is about 2×10^8 m^{-3}. The value of 20 minutes is much longer than the radioactive half-life of ^{218}Po, 3.11 min. For a mine, Raabe assumed the negative ion concentration to be proportional to the radon concentration; in a mine at 3700 Bq m^{-3} (100 pCi/L) of radon, he estimated the half-life for neutralization of ^{218}Po by small negative ions to be 1.2 seconds. It should be noted, however, that the exact relationship between the negative small ion concentration and the radon concentration is not known.

2.1.2 *Charge Transfer Process with Neutral Atoms.* Polonium-218 ions
may become neutralized by removing electrons from colliding neutral molecules. However, based on the arguments of Busigin et al. (28), this process is unlikely since the ionization potential of a polonium atom (8.43 eV) is lower than that of various gas molecules, unless there are hydrocarbons which have even lower ionization potentials. Instead, Busigin et al. (28) suggested that ^{218}Po$^+$ ions would be unstable and would react chemically with oxygen in an air environment to form ^{218}PoO$_2$$^+$, for which they estimated the ionization potential to be about 10 eV, that is, higher than that of ^{218}Po$^+$. Recently, Goldstein and Hopke (29) estimated the ionization potential of ^{218}PoO$_2$$^+$ to be in the range 10.3–10.53 eV. In such circumstances, PoO$_2$$^+$ ions can become neutralized by removing electrons from trace gases such as NO or NO$_2$. Other chemical reactions of Po$^+$ with atmospheric constituents are possible. In the presence of carbon monoxide, polonium carbonyl may form (30), which is likely to have a high enough ionization potential to become neutralized by removing electrons from colliding molecules.

Whichever neutralization mechanism is dominant probably depends on the degree of air ionization and the concentrations of trace gases and organic vapors in the atmosphere. Negative ion recombination depends on the ionization level, which, in turn, depends on the radon concentration in the gaseous environment. On the other hand, neither the charge transfer process nor the chemical reaction of Po$^+$ with O$_2$ or trace gases depends on the ionization level; rather they depend on the concentration of the relevant trace gas and, therefore, would be more rapid in polluted atmospheres. Radon progeny interactions may be complicated further by the clustering of polar molecules around the Po$^+$ ions to form stable complexes. Hawrynski (31) has postulated the existence of clusters of water molecules around ionized radon decay products and suggests that air humidity strongly influences the diameter of the cluster. Under normal conditions, the cluster diameters are estimated to be 1.3 nm for 1% relative humidity (RH) (40 water molecules forming the clusters) and 2.3 nm for 100% RH (220 water molecules in the cluster). The time for cluster formation is estimated as $< 10^{-3}$ s. Both the electric charge contained in the cluster and its diameter determine the value of the diffusion coefficient. The diffusion coefficient of the cluster was found to vary from 0.0096 cm^2/s for 100% RH to 0.0224 cm^2/s for 1% RH.

Raes et al. (32) studied the impact of ion clustering and growth under different environmental conditions. In the case of the clustering of pure H_2O around an ion at 100% RH, the formation of neutral H_2O clusters is thermodynamically impossible. Ions will grow spontaneously to an equilibrium size in a few microseconds. Equilibrium sizes were calculated as a function of the RH and relative acidity; the corresponding diffusion coefficients are shown in Figure 6.1. The relative acidity is defined as the ratio of the gas phase H_2SO_4 concentration to the gas phase H_2SO_4 concentration over a flat surface of pure liquid H_2SO_4. At zero relative acidity, values of the diffusion coefficient vary from about 0.14 (0% RH) to 0.08 cm^2/s (100% RH). In the case of the clustering of a binary solution of condensable species such as $H_2O-H_2SO_4$ around an ion, there are two possible situations. At low H_2O and H_2SO_4 concentrations in the gas phase (region I), stable clusters will

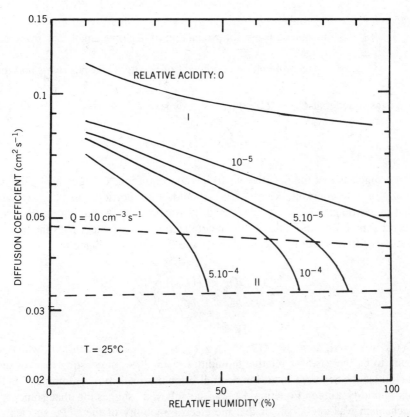

Figure 6.1. Diffusion coefficient of stable $H_2O-H_2SO_4$ ion clusters at different relative humidities and relative acidities. The relative acidity is defined as the ratio of the gas phase H_2SO_4 concentration to the gas phase H_2SO_4 concentration over a flat surface of pure liquid H_2SO_4. Region I contains the environmental conditions where only stable ion clusters will be formed, and region II the conditions where both stable and unstable ion clusters will be formed. Reproduced from *Health Phys.*, **49**, 1184, 1985, by permission of the Health Physics Society.

be formed spontaneously around the ion. At high H_2O or H_2SO_4 concentrations in the gas phase (region II), clusters will not be stable and will grow spontaneously. However, ions that are neutralized before reaching the critical size corresponding to the maximum in the ΔG vs size plot for neutral clusters may evaporate. Ions that grow larger than the critical size will not evaporate and will result in an ion-induced aerosol, thereby broadening the size distribution of the free ions.

Evidence was presented by Busigin et al. (33) to suggest that neutralization of charged $^{218}Po^+$ species by negative small ions may be significant at relative humidities >15–20%. This conclusion was based on a model described by

$$\frac{dC_-}{dt} = \xi C_{Rn} - \gamma C_+ C_-$$ (10)

where C_-, C_+ = concentrations of negative and positive small ions
       ξ = rate constant for production of negative small ions from radon gas
      γ = recombination coefficient of negative and positive small ions

If it is assumed that $C_- \approx C_+$, then at steady state

$$C_- = C_+ = (\xi C_{Rn}/\gamma)^{1/2}$$ (11)

which suggests that the negative small ion concentration, C_-, and hence the neutralization rate constant, K, of $^{218}Po^+$ should be proportional to $(C_{Rn})^{1/2}$ rather than proportional to C_{Rn}, as postulated by Raabe (24). Assuming no change in electrical mobility, the ratios of the neutralization rate constant K to the mobility B at two different radon concentrations 1 and 2 should be related by

$$\frac{(K/B)_1}{(K/B)_2} = \left(\frac{(C_{Rn})_1}{(C_{Rn})_2}\right)^{1/2}$$ (12)

If $(C_{Rn})_1$ is fixed, then $(K/B)_2[(C_{Rn})_1/(C_{Rn})_2]^{1/2}$ should be constant, which was found to be the case for relative humidities >15–20%, suggesting that for these humidities the negative small ion neutralization mechanism may dominate. Below this humidity range, Equation 12 was not obeyed, suggesting that some other mechanism was operative, or that the electric mobility of the ^{218}Po species was different at these low humidities. Because of limited data, these conclusions must be considered tentative.

Neutralized ^{218}Po atoms either decay directly to ^{214}Pb, or interact with aerosol particles, or become lost to the walls by collision. The most probable series of events experienced by a ^{218}Po recoil ion may be summarized as:

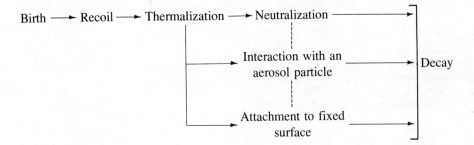

2.2   Physical Parameters Characterizing Unattached Radon Progeny

In order to understand the physical and chemical nature of radon progeny, knowledge of the following is required:

1. The diffusion coefficient, D, of the neutral unattached radon progeny.
2. The fraction born charged, f, which is defined as the fraction of unattached radon progeny possessing a positive charge at the end of the recoil path. (A single positive charge is assumed.)
3. The electrical mobility, B, of the charged, unattached radon progeny.
4. The neutralization rate constant, K, of the charged, unattached radon progeny.

These items are discussed in detail below.

2.2.1   The Diffusion Coefficient of Neutral Unattached Radon Progeny.   In early measurements of the diffusion coefficient, little distinction was made between charged and neutral species. Furthermore, the possibility of formation of clusters of molecules around the atom was not considered. Experimental values of the diffusion coefficient of ^{218}Po are summarized in Table 6.1. From kinetic theory, a single uncharged ^{218}Po atom in air would be expected (24) to have a diffusion coefficient of 0.14 cm^2 s^{-1}. Since the thermalization time for the recoil ^{218}Po atom is of the order of nsec, no simple measurement technique exists. Since for most measurements the age of ^{218}Po (from the time of "birth") is reported as "old," physical or chemical interaction may occur between the ^{218}Po atom and the surrounding gas molecules. Not surprisingly, therefore, values for the diffusion coefficients of the ^{218}Po atom fall into a wide range, 0.027–0.096 cm^2 s^{-1}, consistent with some form of molecular clustering around ^{218}Po. Raabe (24) proposed that six water molecules cluster around a ^{218}Po atom and obtained a diffusion coefficient of 0.054 cm^2 s^{-1}. Polar molecules, such as CO_2, are also known to form clusters around ions (34–36).

The effect of ventilation rate was studied by Raghunath and Kotrappa (37) and Kotrappa et al. (38). Kotrappa et al. (38) found that the value of D for ^{212}Pb changed from 0.006 to 0.056 cm^2 s^{-1} for a ventilation rate change from 5 to 90

TABLE 6.1 Summary of Experimental Results for the Diffusion Coefficient of Unattached ^{218}Po and ^{212}Pb

Ref.	D (cm^2 s^{-1})	Gas[a]	Species	Remarks[b]
Wellisch (45)	0.045	Dry air	^{218}Po	D applies to neutral ^{218}Po species only
Chamberlain and Dyson (1)	0.054	Air	^{212}Pb	
Madelaine (39)	0.005 0.060	Air	^{212}Pb	D decreased with the age of the air
Raabe (43)	0.047	Air, RH = 15%	^{218}Po	D applies to neutral ^{218}Po species only
	0.034	Air, RH = 35%	^{218}Po	Radon concentration was high (5.55 × 10^3 Bq/m^3)
Porstendörfer (41)	0.076	Air	^{212}Pb	D applies to neutral species only
	0.050	Air	^{212}Pb	D applies to charged species only
Fontan et al. (40)	0.020 0.090	Air	^{212}Pb	D applies to neutral species only; D decreased with the age of the air
Thomas and LeClare (46)	0.053 0.085	Very dry air Air, RH = 20%	^{218}Po ^{218}Po	The average age of ^{218}Po was 15–29 s
Billard et al. (47)	<0.05	Air	^{218}Po	It was observed that unattached ions grow; a value of about 4 times lower than 0.05 cm^2 s^{-1} was recommended for these ions
Kotrappa et al. (38)	0.0535 0.0524 0.0604 0.0540	Air, RH = 5–10% Air, RH = 10–20% Air, RH = 20–80% Air, RH = 80–90%	^{212}Pb ^{212}Pb ^{212}Pb ^{212}Pb	It was concluded that RH does not have a significant effect on D; ventilation rate about 90 air changes/h and thoron concentration about 3.7 × 10^5 Bq/m^3
		Air with varying ^{220}Rn (Bq/m^3)		Ventilation rate:
	0.006	6.29 × 10^6	^{212}Pb	5 air changes/h
	0.007	5.18 × 10^6	^{212}Pb	5 air changes/h
	0.007	1.11 × 10^6	^{212}Pb	5 air changes/h
	0.050	4.44 × 10^6	^{212}Pb	30 air changes/h
	0.049	3.55 × 10^6	^{212}Pb	30 air changes/h
	0.049	2.78 × 10^6	^{212}Pb	30 air changes/h
	0.048	5.92 × 10^5	^{212}Pb	30 air changes/h
	0.056	5.70 × 10^5	^{212}Pb	90 air changes/h
	0.054	3.77 × 10^5	^{212}Pb	90 air changes/h
	0.055	2.63 × 10^5	^{212}Pb	90 air changes/h
	0.056	6.66 × 10^4	^{212}Pb	90 air changes/h

TABLE 6.1 (*Continued*)

Ref.	D (cm^2 s^{-1})	Gas[a]	Species	Remarks[b]
Porstendörfer and Mercer (42)	0.024	Air, RH < 2%	^{212}Pb	D applies to positively charged species
	0.068	Air, RH = 30–90%	^{212}Pb	As above
	0.068	Air, all RHs	^{212}Pb	D applies to neutral species; water vapor had no influence on D
Raghunath and Kotrappa (37)				Ventilation rate was:
	0.0648	Air, RH = 10%	^{218}Po	6 air changes/h
	0.0436	Air, RH = 90%	^{218}Po	6 air changes/h
	0.0811	Air, RH = 10%	^{218}Po	60 air changes/h
	0.0803	Air, RH = 90%	^{218}Po	60 air changes/h
	0.0725	Ar, RH = 10%	^{218}Po	6 air changes/h
	0.0713	Ar, RH = 90%	^{218}Po	6 air changes/h
	0.0955	Ar, RH = 10%	^{218}Po	60 air changes/h
	0.0913	Ar, RH = 90%	^{218}Po	60 air changes/h
Frey et al. (48)	0.044	Dry N_2	^{218}Po	Diffusion tube
	0.031	97% O_2 (dry)	^{218}Po	measurements;
	0.031	10 ppm NO (dry)	^{218}Po	radon concen-
	0.072	10 ppm NO_2 (dry)	^{218}Po	trations were not
	0.079	8.3 ppm NO with 8% O_2	^{218}Po	reported; D applies to both
	0.052	N_2, RH = 20%	^{218}Po	neutral and
	0.079	N_2, RH = 80%	^{218}Po	charged ^{218}Po
	0.027	Dry air	^{218}Po	species
Busigin et al. (33)	0.10	Ar, RH = 0%	^{218}Po	D applies to neutral
	0.028	Ar, RH = 8%	^{218}Po	^{218}Po species; the
	0.043	Ar, RH = 15%	^{218}Po	radon concen-
	0.046	Ar, RH = 100%	^{218}Po	tration was not
	0.048	Air, RH = 0%	^{218}Po	held constant
	0.035	Air, RH = 8%	^{218}Po	
	0.065	Air, RH = 15%	^{218}Po	
	0.076	Air, RH = 100%	^{218}Po	
Goldstein and Hopke (29)	0.034	Dry N_2	^{218}Po	D applies to both
	0.031	Dry oxygen	^{218}Po	neutral and
	0.037	3.0 ppm of n-C_4C_{10} in dry O_2	^{218}Po	charged ^{218}Po species
	0.0375	5.0 ppm of isobutane in dry O_2	^{218}Po	
	0.0355	1.5 ppm of C_5H_{10} in dry N_2	^{218}Po	
	0.0375	1.5 ppm of C_5H_{10} in dry O_2	^{218}Po	
	0.0365	16 ppb of n-C_5H_{12} in dry N_2	^{218}Po	
	0.0700	40 ppb of n-C_5H_{12} in dry O_2	^{218}Po	
	0.0345	1.25 ppm of NH_3 in dry N_2	^{218}Po	
	0.0725	1.25 ppm of NH_3 in dry air	^{218}Po	

TABLE 6.1   *(Continued)*

Ref.	D (cm^2 s^{-1})	Gas^a	Species	Remarks^b
Goldstein and Hopke (29)	0.0730	100 ppb of NO$_2$ in dry O$_2$	^{218}Po	
	0.0715	50 ppb of NO$_2$ in dry O$_2$	^{218}Po	
	0.0320	10 ppm of NO in dry N$_2$	^{218}Po	
	0.0720	8.3 ppm of NO in dry O$_2$	^{218}Po	
	0.0670	50 ppb of NO in dry O$_2$	^{218}Po	

^{a}Gas at room temperature (20°C) and pressure.
^{b}Unless stated otherwise, no attempt was made to measure the diffusion coefficients of charged and neutral species separately.

air changes per hour. Thoron concentration did not have an effect on diffusion coefficients. These findings suggest that ^{218}Po or ^{212}Pb clusters grow with time. Madelaine (39) and Fontan et al. (40) also observed growth of ^{212}Po (ThB).

The diffusion coefficient of a charged atom is smaller than that of a neutral atom. Porstendörfer (41) reported that the diffusion coefficient of the charged ^{212}Pb species in air was 0.05 cm^2 s^{-1} and that of the neutral species, 0.076 cm^2 s^{-1}. For ^{218}Po in air, a diffusion coefficient of 0.024 cm^2 s^{-1} was found for the charged species and 0.068 cm^2 s^{-1} for the neutral species (42).

Goldstein and Hopke (29) determined the diffusion coefficient of unattached ^{218}Po in dry O$_2$ and N$_2$ in the presence of trace gases (n-C$_4$H$_{10}$, i-C$_4$H$_{10}$, C$_5$H$_{10}$, n-C$_5$H$_{12}$, NH$_3$, NO$_2$, and NO). The diffusion coefficient for ^{218}Po in a neutral state was found to be 0.072 cm^2/s and for a mixture of charged and neutral species, 0.037 cm^2/s.

Data on the effect of humidity on the diffusion coefficient are conflicting. There are two different theories. One theory is based on the clustering of water molecules and atoms. According to Raes et al. (32), under unsaturated conditions (< 100% RH), the formation of neutral H$_2$O clusters is thermodynamically impossible. Ions will grow to an equilibrium size in a few microseconds. Figure 6.1 shows the effect of humidity on the diffusion coefficient under different environmental conditions. As the relative humidity increases, the diffusion coefficient decreases. The second theory is based on neutralization of charged species to neutral species (29). The H$_2$O molecule is believed to enhance the neutralization process. Since the diffusion coefficient of the neutral species is larger than that of the charged species, the diffusion coefficient of the mixture (both charged and neutral species) is expected to increase with the extent of neutralization. Thus, the diffusion coefficient is expected to increase with increasing relative humidity. Most studies suggest that as the relative humidity increases, the diffusion coefficients of ^{218}Po and ^{212}Pb decrease owing to the clustering of water molecules (31, 32, 37, 43). In some studies, an increase in humidity has been found to increase the diffusion coefficient (29). Porstendörfer and Mercer (44) found that the diffusion coefficient of ^{212}Pb increased with humidity, resulting in an increased attachment rate of up to 100% over the range 30–80% RH. In other studies, no effect of humidity on the diffusion coefficient was found (38, 42).

It may be concluded that no single diffusion coefficient exists for ^{218}Po and ^{212}Pb, and that the diffusion coefficient depends on the age and charge state of the species, the level of humidity, the concentrations of trace gases, and the ionization level. Values of the diffusion coefficient of ^{218}Po and ^{212}Pb must therefore be regarded as particular values for a given set of conditions. Moreover, the size distribution of the free radioactive fraction may be broadened either by clustering or by attachment to the freshly formed nuclei. Use of a single diffusion coefficient may therefore not be appropriate in many situations.

2.2.2 *The Fraction of Unattached Radon Progeny Born with a Positive Charge.*

A distinction must be made between the charged fraction of radon progeny at birth and the charged fraction of unattached radon progeny at some later time. The fraction born charged is defined as the fraction of unattached radon progeny having positive charge at the end of the recoil path when ^{218}Po is very young (age of a few nsec); the charged fraction is defined as the fraction of unattached radon progeny remaining positively charged under the prevailing ambient conditions. Thus, the charged fraction depends on the age of the species. Table 6.2 summarizes the reported results for the fraction born charged and the charged fraction of unattached radon and thoron progeny.

In 1912–1914 Wellisch and Bronson (49) and Wellisch (45, 50) conducted a series of experiments on the deposition of radon decay products in an electric field using a cylindrical condenser into which radon and a gas were introduced. The relative amounts of activity on the central electrode and the cylinder wall were determined after equilibrium had been established for different positive potentials applied to the cylinder wall. At a small applied potential (+4 volts), the cathode activity (or the charged fraction) decreased owing to recombination of positively charged particles with negative ions and further decreased by the extra ionization produced by the X rays. At higher potentials of up to 4000 volts, the percent activity on the cathode increased with the applied potential and then leveled off. The maximum percent cathode activity was independent of the potential above a certain level and the pressure of the gas, but dependent on the nature of the gas.

Much later, Porstendörfer and Mercer (42) studied the influence of electric field and humidity on the diffusion coefficient of thoron (^{220}Rn) in a cylindrical condenser under laminar flow conditions. They found that the collection efficiency of the decay products increased with applied voltage and reached a constant value of 88% at an applied voltage of 500 V (an electric field of about 550 V/cm). The collection efficiency increased with increase in the relative humidity and decreased with increase in the thoron (^{220}Rn) concentration. Porstendörfer and Mercer (42) concluded that the fraction of ^{212}Pb born charged was 0.85–0.88, independent of the relative humidity and the thoron concentration.

TABLE 6.2 Reported Values of the Charged Fraction (and Fraction Born Charged)

Ref.	Electric field (V/cm)	Fraction of charged decay products	RH (%)	Gas	Species	Collection time	Remarks
Wellisch (45)		0.882^a 0.882^a 0.789^a 0^a	0 0 0 0	Air Hydrogen CO_2 Ethyl ether	Radon progeny		Cylindrical condenser; closed system
Porstendörfer and Mercer (42)	550 (av. electric field)	$0.85\text{–}0.88^a$	Independent	Air	^{212}Pb	Few msec	Cylindrical condenser; flow-through system with 5.5×10^{-6} m³/s flow rate; thoron concentration 10^9–10^{12} atoms/m³
Busigin et al. (33)	–50 to 50	0.513^a 0.353^a 0.298^a 0.298^a	0 8 15 100	Air	^{218}Po		Parallel plate condenser; closed system; steady-state model accounts for neutralization, diffusion, and electrostatic collection; low fraction born charged; neutralization postulated to occur before or at end of recoil path
		0.405^a 0.245^a 0.203^a 0.230^a	0 8 15 100	Argon	^{218}Po		
Dua et al. (51)	1.5	0.685 0.637 0.575	0–5 15–20 80–90	Air	Thoron progeny	0.7 s	Relatively low radon and thoron concentrations

	Value	%	Medium	Species	Time	Remarks
	9	0–5 15–20 80–90	Air	Thoron progeny	0.1 s	Parallel plate condenser with flow-through system; flow rate 3.8 × 10⁻² m/s
	2700	15–20	Air	Thoron progeny	0.4 msec	0.975^a
	1.5	0–5 15–20 80–90	Air	Radon progeny	0.7 s	0.544 0.412 0.106
	9	0–5 15–20 80–90	Air	Radon progeny	0.1 s	0.709 0.670 0.472
	32	0–5 15–20 80–90	Air	Radon progeny	0.03 s	0.841 0.811 0.604
	136	15–20 80–90	Air	Radon progeny	0.01 s	0.814 0.751
	1800	0–5 15–20 80–90	Air	Radon progeny	0.6 msec	0.823^a 0.820^a 0.844^a
Jonassen (52)			Indoor air	^{218}Po ^{214}Pb ^{214}Bi		0.19 0.76 0.15 — High negative voltage (few thousand volts) applied to a wire; nucleus concentration about 0.5 × 10¹⁰ m⁻³; radon concentration about 185–370 Bq m⁻³; indirect method

[a]Fraction born charged.

Busigin et al. (33) studied the electrostatic collection of ^{218}Po in air and argon using a parallel plate condenser. A steady-state model was used to account for neutralization, diffusion, and electrostatic collection of ^{218}Po atoms in the closed system. Values for the diffusion coefficient of neutral ^{218}Po atoms, the fraction born charged, and the ratio of the neutralization rate constant to the mobility were obtained for field strengths ranging from -50 V/cm to $+50$ V/cm. The fraction born charged was found to decrease with increasing relative humidity and was explained as being due to neutralization at or just before the end of the recoil path of the ^{218}Po ions.

Dua et al. (51) investigated how the charged fraction of the decay products of radon (^{222}Rn) and thoron (^{220}Rn) varied with the electric field and the relative humidity in a parallel plate condenser with a flow-through system. They concluded that the charged fraction of the decay products decreased with an increase in the relative humidity. The influence of relative humidity on charged fraction was smaller for thoron (^{220}Rn) decay products than for radon (^{222}Rn) decay products owing to the short half-life of ^{216}Po (0.16 s) and decreased progressively with an increase in the electric field strength. Jonassen (52) studied the effect of electric fields on ^{222}Rn decay products in indoor air. At radon concentrations in the range 185–370 Bq m^{-3} and low condensation nuclei concentrations (5,000–10,000 cm^{-3}), the charged fractions of ^{222}Rn progeny were found to be 0.19 for ^{218}Po, 0.76 for ^{214}Pb, and 0.15 for ^{214}Bi. (The value of 0.76 seems anomalous.) Jonassen (53) estimated the charged fraction of unattached airborne radon progeny to be about 0.1–0.2.

There remains the question of the possible existence of negatively charged ^{218}Po ions. Wellisch (49) concluded that there were no "negative carriers of activity" from his results showing an increase in cathode activity with an increase in the applied potential. He considered that the anode activity was due to the diffusion of neutral species. The work of Chamberlain et al. (54), Szucs and Delfosse (55), and Bricard et al. (56) confirms the dominance of positive charge on ^{218}Po and ^{214}Pb atoms. Duport (57) found that in an inactive uranium mine with the age of air about 8 minutes, the negatively charged fraction of ^{218}Po was $<0.5\%$. Dua et al. (58) found more than 90% of the thoron decay products to have a positive charge with a median of about one elementary unit of charge at 0.05 seconds after formation. A single positive charge has usually been assumed.

2.2.3 The Mobility of Unattached Radon and Thoron Progeny. In the atmosphere near the earth's surface, the concentration of ^{218}Po is estimated to be in the range 1–2 $\times$ 10^7 atoms/m^3 and the concentration of ^{212}Pb about 7.5 atoms/m^3 (56). Some of these atoms are neutral (20% in the case of ^{218}Po); the rest, which have a unit positive charge, constitute the small radioactive ions. The spectrum of mobility of small radioactive ions derived from ^{222}Rn and ^{220}Rn in natural, unfiltered air when artificially enriched with ^{222}Rn and ^{220}Rn progeny is shown in Figure 6.2 (56). Only a few percent of the ions have mobilities in the range 1.9–2.3 cm^2 s^{-1} V^{-1}, the remainder being in the range 0.3–1.2 cm^2 s^{-1}

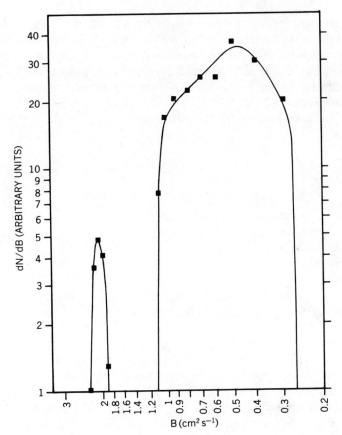

Figure 6.2. The mobility distribution of small radioactive ions derived from thoron and radon in unfiltered air when enriched with ^{222}Rn and ^{220}Rn progeny. From Ref. 56. Reproduced with permission from *Comptes rendus de l'Académie des Sciences de Paris*.

V^{-1}. The first range probably accounts for unattached ions and the second for attached or clustered ions. The distribution of mobilities, like the distribution of diffusivities, is therefore bimodal. Rutherford (59) obtained a mobility of 1.3 cm^2 s^{-1} V^{-1} for the recoil products from radium and thorium emanations in air. Franck (60) and Franck and Meitner (61) found mobilities for ^{208}Tl atoms of 1.56 cm^2 s^{-1} V^{-1} in air, 1.54 cm^2 s^{-1} V^{-1} in nitrogen, and 6.21 cm^2 s^{-1} V^{-1} in hydrogen.

Wilkening et al. (62) studied the mobilities and concentrations of the short-lived decay products of radon existing as positive small ions in the lower atmosphere. Most of the ions (75%) had mobilities greater than 0.67 cm^2 V^{-1} s^{-1}. From the activity deposited on an electrode in outdoor air, Jonassen and Wilkening (63) deduced that the ion mobilities were less than 1.7 cm^2 V^{-1} s^{-1}. Fontan et al. (40) measured the mobility distribution of the decay products of ^{220}Rn and ^{88}Kr in filtered air and obtained four groups of mobilities (2, 1.3, 0.95, and 0.55 cm^2 s^{-1} V^{-1}). As the age of the ions increased, the concentration of the ions in the highest group decreased the most. Chamberlain and Dyson (1) deduced by an indirect method that the mobility of ^{212}Pb was 2.2 cm^2 s^{-1} V^{-1}. Thomas and LeClare (46) suggested that ^{218}Po had a diffusion coefficient of 0.08 cm^2 s^{-1}, corresponding to an ion mobility of 3.2 cm^2 s^{-1} V^{-1}. The ion mobility was deduced from the diffusion coefficient through the Einstein equation

$$\frac{B}{D} = \frac{e}{kT} \tag{13}$$

where B = the mobility of the ion
D = the diffusion coefficient of the ion
e = the elementary charge
k = Boltzmann's constant
T = absolute temperature.

Jonassen and Hayes (64) found that the mobility distribution of ^{222}Rn progeny small ions in laboratory air ranged from 0.3 to 3 cm^2 s^{-1} V^{-1}, with a mean value of 0.9 cm^2 s^{-1} V^{-1}.

In the diffusion coefficient experiments of Porstendörfer and Mercer (42), the mobility of positively charged ^{212}Pb species in dry air (relative humidity <2%) was 0.96 cm^2 s^{-1} V^{-1} (deduced from the diffusion coefficient of 0.024 cm^2 s^{-1}); in moist air, the mobility was 2.72 cm^2 s^{-1} V^{-1} (deduced from the diffusion coefficient of 0.068 cm^2 s^{-1}). Jonassen (52) investigated the effect of electric fields on ^{222}Rn progeny in indoor air. At radon activities in the range 185–370 Bq m^{-3} and low condensation nuclei concentrations, the average mobility of the ^{218}Po ions was found to be about 10 times that of ^{214}Pb and ^{214}Bi. The above findings are summarized in Table 6.3.

2.2.4 Neutralization of Positively Charged Radon Progeny.
Very little research has been conducted on the rate of neutralization of charged radon progeny atoms. No absolute values for the neutralization rate constant, K, are available. The effect of neutralization can be inferred from either electrostatic collection measurements or diffusion coefficient measurements. In the case of electrostatic collection, as the rate of neutralization increases, the number of charged atoms decreases, and, therefore, the rate of collection decreases. In diffusion coefficient measurements, a high diffusion coefficient suggests a neutral species and a low diffusion coefficient suggests a charged species. The diffusion coefficient of neutral ^{218}Po has been found to be about 0.068 cm^2/s and that of charged ^{218}Po about 0.024 cm^2/s (42). The presence of charge on the atom results in increased interaction with surrounding ions and therefore a lower diffusivity. However, care must be taken to ensure that no clustering occurs in the measurement.

Busigin et al. (28) found that the rate of neutralization for $^{218}Po^+$ ion increased

TABLE 6.3 Mobilities of Radon and Thoron Progeny Ions

Ref.	Mobility ($cm^2\ s^{-1}\ V^{-1}$)	Species	Gas	Remarks
Rutherford (59)	1.3	Recoil products from radium and thorium emanation	Air	
Franck (60)	1.56	^{208}Tl	Air	
Franck and Meitner (61)	1.54	^{208}Tl	Nitrogen	
	6.21		Hydrogen	
Chamberlain and Dyson (1)	2.2	^{212}Pb	Air	Indirect method
Bricard et al. (56)	Only a few percent of the ions had mobilities in the range 1.9–2.3; the remainder were in the range 0.3–1.2	Small radioactive ions derived from thoron and radon	Natural unfiltered air	
Wilkening et al. (62)	75% > 0.67 in the range 0.25–1.5	Short-lived products of radon	Lower atmosphere	
Fontan et al. (40)	4 groups of mobilities: 2, 1.3, 0.95, and 0.55	Decay products of ^{220}Rn and ^{88}Kr	Filtered air	As the age of the ion increased, the relative concentration of ions with the highest mobility ($2.2\ cm^2\ V^{-1}\ s^{-1}$) decreased the most
Jonassen and Wilkening (63)	<1.7	Activity deposited on an electrode	Outdoor air	
Thomas and LeClare (46)	3.2	^{218}Po	Air	Deduced from diffusion coefficient of $0.08\ cm^2\ s^{-1}$

TABLE 6.3 (*Continued*)

Ref.	Mobility ($cm^2 s^{-1} V^{-1}$)	Species	Gas	Remarks
Jonassen and Hayes (64)	0.3–3 with a mean value of 0.9	^{222}Rn progeny small ions	Laboratory air	Free of condensation nuclei
Porstendörfer and Mercer (42)	0.96	Positively charged ^{212}Pb	Dry air (RH < 2%)	Deduced from diffusion coefficient of 0.024 $cm^2 s^{-1}$
	2.72	Positively charged ^{212}Pb	Moist air	Deduced from diffusion coefficient of 0.068 $cm^2 s^{-1}$
Jonassen (52)	No absolute values	^{222}Rn progeny	Indoor air	Rough estimation from the electric decay constants; radon concentration (185–370 Bq m^{-3}); mobility of the ^{218}Po ions is about 10 times higher than that of ^{214}Pb and ^{214}Bi; condensation nucleus concentration about (0.5–1) × 10^{10} m^{-3}

with decreasing ionization potential of the gaseous atmosphere (Figure 6.3). They suggested that ^{218}Po is not normally present as a single ^{218}Po$^+$ but reacts with other chemical species to form a chemical compound (normally the oxide, PoO$_2$) with a substantially higher ionization potential.

The effect of humidity on the neutralization rate can be observed in the results of George and Breslin (65). The neutralization rate for ^{218}Po$^+$ ion increases with increasing humidity. The effect of humidity on the neutralization rate is most important for relative humidities $< 15\%$ (Figure 6.4). Above 15%, the rate of neutralization was higher and varied little with humidity. Frey et al. (48) examined humidity effects on neutralization of ^{218}Po species. From diffusion coefficient measurements in N$_2$ they concluded that ^{218}Po is completely neutralized at and above 80% RH ($D = 0.079$ cm^2/s), partially neutralized at 20% RH ($D = 0.052$ cm^2/s), and not neutralized at 0% RH ($D = 0.044$ cm^2/s). They suggested that neutralization occurs by the scavenging of electrons from the recoil path of the polonium by water molecules. However, Goldstein and Hopke (29) point out that it cannot be the water molecule itself that is trapping the electrons. Radiolysis of the water molecules leads to formation of the OH radicals, which are good electron

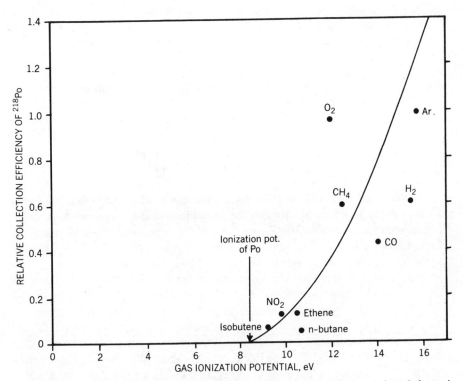

Figure 6.3. The dependence of the relative electrostatic collection efficiency of newly formed ^{218}Po on the ionization potential of the gaseous environment. From Ref. 28. Reproduced from *Health Phys.*, **40,** 341, 1981, by permission of the Health Physics Society.

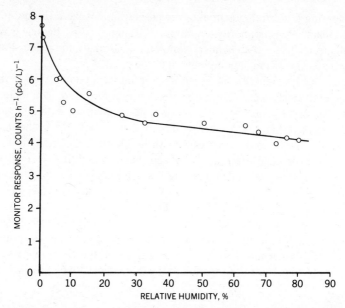

Figure 6.4. Variation of response with relative humidity of an integrating radon monitor based on the electrostatic collection of ^{218}Po (RaA). From Ref. 65. Reproduced by permission of the author.

acceptors. Work by Coghlan and Scott (66) demonstrates inhibition of condensation nuclei formation in the presence of OH radical scavengers such as methanol or ethanol, the trend in inhibition correlating well with the rate constant for reaction between the inhibiting compound and OH radicals. The formation of hydroxyl radicals therefore plays an important role both in the neutralization process for the polonium ion and in the reaction chemistry leading to the formation of radiolytic nuclei.

Porstendörfer and Mercer (42) studied the electrostatic collection of thoron (^{220}Rn) decay products. In dry air, the neutralization rate increased with an increase in thoron concentration (Figure 6.5). At the same thoron concentrations the neutralization rate was significantly greater in dry air than in moist air, contrary to the findings of George and Breslin (65) and Frey et al. (48).

Busigin et al. (33) studied the electrostatic collection of unattached ^{218}Po atoms in different gaseous environments. As noted previously, their results indicate that the ^{218}Po$^+$ ion combines with negative small ions at relative humidities above 15–20% (25°C). At lower humidities, neutralization may occur by some different mechanism. As estimated from the ratio of the neutralization rate constant, K, to the mobility, B, the neutralization rate constant is given in Table 6.4. The mobility of the ^{218}Po$^+$ ion was taken to be 2.17 cm^2 s^{-1} V^{-1} in air and 2.04 cm^2 s^{-1} V^{-1} in argon.

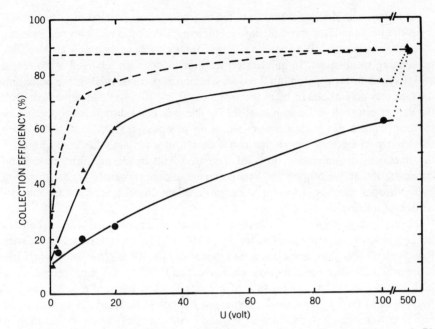

Figure 6.5. Collection of the positive thoron decay products in an electrical field -------- RH > 30% (22°C). ——— RH < 2% (22°C). ● $C°_{Tn} = (5-7) \times 10^4$ cm^{-3}. ▲ $C°_{Tn} = (1-5) \times 10^3$ cm^{-3}. From Ref. 42. Reproduced by permission of the Health Physics Society.

TABLE 6.4 ^{218}Po Neutralization Rate (33)

Gas	H_2O partial pressure (mm Hg)	K/B (V cm^{-2})	K^a (s^{-1})	C_{Rn} (atoms cm^{-3})
Argon (99.9995% minimum purity)	0	6.05	12.34	1.069×10^6
	2.02	6.03	12.30	3.802×10^6
	3.78	6.02	12.28	2.973×10^6
	25.21	4.93	10.06	1.430×10^6
Air	0	5.54	12.03	5.297×10^6
	2.02	7.45	16.17	4.453×10^6
	3.78	5.48	11.89	2.451×10^6
	25.21	3.71	8.05	1.657×10^6

^{a}Estimated from K/B where $B = 2.04$ cm^2 s^{-1} V^{-1} in argon and 2.17 cm^2 s^{-1} V^{-1} in air (B is calculated theoretically).

Goldstein and Hopke (29) inferred the degree of neutralization of ^{218}Po species from the magnitude of the diffusion coefficient. They proposed two mechanisms of neutralization of ^{218}Po ion, an electron transfer mechanism and an electron-scavenging mechanism. In an electron transfer mechanism, charged ^{218}Po reacts with oxygen to form polonium dioxide. The ionization potential of the polonium dioxide was determined to be in the range of 10.35–10.53 eV, in agreement with the earlier estimate of Busigin et al. (28). The polonium dioxide then accepts an electron from a gas with a lower ionization potential (28). Although the exact mechanism of electron scavenging is not known, it was found that in dry nitrogen the fractional neutralization of ^{218}Po increased with increasing nitrogen dioxide concentration above 50 ppb and was complete at concentrations greater than 700 ppb. Nitrogen dioxide is known to be an excellent electron acceptor for the formation of a negative ion.

Neutralization rates given in Table 6.4 indicate that the ion half-life is about 70 ms at a radon concentration of about 3.7×10^6 Bq/m^3, which is consistent with Raes' calculation (32). Raes calculated that at 3.7×10^6 Bq/m^3 the ion half life is about 0.1 s. Since the neutralization rate depends on the radon concentration, a high radon concentration implies a high neutralization rate and a small charged fraction of ^{218}Po. In Dua's work on charged fraction (51), relatively high charged fractions were reported, probably as a result of the relatively low concentration of thoron.

3 DETERMINATION OF THE UNATTACHED FRACTION OF RADON AND THORON PROGENY

3.1 Introduction

The significance of the unattached fraction of radon and thoron progeny in determining the dose to the lung (1, 13, 67–70) has already been discussed. The dose to the bronchial basal cells from unattached ^{218}Po may be 6–38 times that from attached radon progeny (71) (sievert per joule inhaled potential alpha energy), mainly because of the efficient deposition of unattached ^{218}Po in the upper bronchial tree.

Quantitative information on the unattached progeny of radon and thoron can be obtained by employing either theoretical or experimental procedures. Theoretical procedures have been developed to calculate the rate of attachment of radon and thoron progeny to aerosols (5, 16–20, 44, 72–85). As described below, the rate of attachment can subsequently be used to predict the unattached fraction in an atmosphere of known aerosol concentration and particle size. Experimental methods have also been developed for measuring the unattached fraction. The methods are largely based on diffusive collection of unattached atoms and electrical collection of unattached activity. The electrical methods rely on the assumption that the unattached fraction is the same as the charged fraction. There is, however, strong evidence (28, 53) to suggest that this assumption is not valid. The term *unattached fraction* should therefore be used strictly for the fraction of activity not attached to aerosols, in either a neutral or a charged state, whereas the term *charged fraction* should be used for the fraction of activity existing in a charged state regardless of whether it is attached to aerosols. Furthermore, collection of activity by electrical means may not allow calculation of the true charged fraction because in almost all commonly used geometries the electric field is nonuniform and may lead to collection of neutral particles by induced polarization. Only diffusion-based methods, as described below, can, therefore, be considered reliable for measuring unattached fractions. There are, however, many problems in measuring unattached activity. Results of such measurements should therefore be interpreted carefully. Important problems in measuring unattached fractions are discussed in Section 4.

3.2 Theoretical Procedures for Determination of the Unattached Fraction

The attachment of radon and thoron decay products to aerosols has been extensively studied (5, 16–20, 44, 72–85) but is still incompletely understood. The usual study objective is to determine the attachment coefficient, β, which then allows the rate of attachment, λ_s, of radon and thoron progeny to aerosols to be calculated from the relation

$$\lambda_s = \beta Z \tag{14}$$

where Z = the aerosol concentration. The sticking probability of decay products to aerosols is taken as unity.

In Equation 14 the attachment coefficient β is a function of the particle size. A single value of β is, therefore, valid only for monodisperse aerosols. In practice, real aerosols in houses, buildings, and mines are polydisperse. The attachment coefficient is therefore better represented as an average attachment coefficient $\overline{\beta}$ given by

$$\overline{\beta} = \frac{\displaystyle\int_0^\infty \beta(d_p)\, n(d_p)\, d(d_p)}{\displaystyle\int_0^\infty n(d_p)\, d(d_p)} \tag{15}$$

The normalized aerosol size distribution $n(d_p)$ may often be represented as lognormal. The size distribution function is then given by

$$n(d_p) = \frac{N}{d_p \sqrt{2\pi}\, \ln \sigma_g} \exp\left(-\frac{1}{2}\left(\frac{\ln d_p / \overline{d}_p}{\ln \sigma_g} \right)^2 \right) \tag{16}$$

where N is the total aerosol number concentration, $\overline{d}_p$ is the count median diameter and σ_g is the geometric standard deviation.

As demonstrated later, the attachment rate λ_s can be used in appropriate radio-active decay equations to predict the fraction of radon and thoron progeny in un-attached form. The success of this method, however, depends on the accuracy with which the attachment coefficient, $\bar{\beta}$, is known. Unfortunately, determination of $\bar{\beta}$ is not easy because of the complexity of the interactions between radon and thoron progeny and aerosols, as previously discussed. Theoretical attachment models available to date are listed in Table 6.5, together with the experimental conditions used for their testing. It is evident that conditions vary with respect to aerosol size and concentration, radon and thoron concentrations, temperature, relative humid-ity, and type of aerosols. Furthermore, discrimination between attached and un-attached decay products has been effected by different, sometimes imperfect, means. To date, the most authoritative version of the attachment coefficient seems to be that presented by Porstendörfer and co-workers (78, 84). Their experiments seem to confirm the following relationships for an assumed monodisperse aerosol:

for small particles (diameter, $2R \ll l$, where l is the mean free path of gas molecules in air ∼0.065 μm)

$$\beta(R) = \pi R^2 \bar{V} \tag{17}$$

and for large particles (diameter, $2R \gg l$)

$$\beta(R) = 4\pi RD \tag{18}$$

In Equation 17, $\bar{V}$ is the mean thermal velocity of the progeny, given by Equation 4, and in Equation 18, D is the diffusion coefficient of the unattached species. When the diameter of an aerosol particle is of the order of the mean free path of gas molecules ($2R \sim l$), the following attachment coefficient equation can be used (74):

$$\beta(R) = \frac{4\pi \bar{V} R^2 (R + l) D}{4D(R + l) + \bar{V} R^2} \tag{19}$$

The attachment coefficient equations (17), (18) and (19) are discussed in more detail in Section 4.

The values of $\bar{V}$ and D in Equations 17–19 need to be chosen carefully. The mean thermal velocity $\bar{V}$ for radon progeny has generally been taken as 1.38×10^4 cm/s (24, 71). Values of D are affected by the atmospheric conditions, as discussed in Section 2.2. The value of $\bar{V}$ itself is a function of temperature (Equa-tion 4).

If the size distribution and number concentration of the aerosol are known in the atmosphere in which information on the unattached fraction is desired, the attachment rate, λ_s, can readily be determined from Equation 14 using a value of the attachment coefficient, β, determined from Equation 17, 18, or 19, depending on whether the median particle diameter is less than, greater than, or approxi-

TABLE 6.5 Attachment Coefficient Studies Reported in the Literature

Attachment coefficient	Type of aerosols	Particle size range (radius in μm)	Aerosol concentrations	Other remarks	Ref.
$\beta \propto \dfrac{R^2}{1+hR}$ R = particle radius $h = \dfrac{V}{4D}$, where V = mean gas kinetic velocity D = diffusion coefficient	Monodisperse DOP and latex spheres mixed with ^{220}Rn	0.04–0.6	10^3–10^4/cm^3	Particle sizes separated by diffusion batteries; value of h found to be = 7×10^4/cm	19
$\beta \propto R$	Polydisperse wax particles mixed with ^{220}Rn	0.7–5	10^3–10^4/cm^3	Particle sizes separated by electrostatic precipitator	81
Theoretically derived:[a] $\beta = \dfrac{\pi R^2 V}{1 + \dfrac{VR}{4D} \cdot \dfrac{1}{1+\delta/R}}$ Theoretical mean for this work = 1.58×10^{-6} cm^3/s; experimental mean for this work = $(1.41 \pm 0.03) \times 10^{-6}$ cm^3/s	Natural—mixed with ^{220}Rn	0.06–0.1	3×10^4/cm^3	Attachment coefficient is for neutral decay products; a cylindrical capacitor used as a mobility analyzer	74
$\beta \propto \dfrac{R^2}{1+hR}$ where $h = \dfrac{V}{4D}$	Polystyrene latex mixed with ^{220}Rn	0.1–2	10^3–10^4/cm^3	^{220}Rn concentrations between 100 and 10^5 atoms/cm^3; deposition pattern of daughters measured in a diffusion tube; difficulties in measuring aerosol concentrations and producing monodisperse particles	82

TABLE 6.5 *(Continued)*

Attachment coefficient	Type of aerosols	Particle size range (radius in μm)	Aerosol concentrations	Other remarks	Ref.
$\beta \propto$ surface area of the particle	Polydisperse polystyrene	0.02–0.5	$10^4/cm^3$	^{222}Rn concentration was 2×10^{-8} Ci L^{-1}; aerosols analyzed by Goetz aerosol spectrometer	17
$\beta = \dfrac{\pi R^2 V(1 + \sqrt{\pi y})}{1 + \dfrac{RV}{4D}}$ where $y = q^2/2RKT$; T = absolute temp.; K = Boltzmann's constant; πR^2 = collision cross-section; $1 + \sqrt{\pi y}$ = electrostatic enhancement factor due to image forces	Aerosols generated by electrical heating of a coil of nichrome wire	0.01–0.08	10^2–$10^6/cm^3$	42.1-cm-long diffusion tube preceded the filter for complete collection of unattached decay products of ^{222}Rn; best fit to data found for 90% ^{218}Po as neutral and 10% as carrying a unit charge	5
$\beta = 2.4 \times 10^5 \, R^2$ cm^3/min with sticking probability $S = 0.08$	Monodisperse polystyrene	0.6–2.9	1–30/cm^3	^{212}Pb concentration was $\sim 4 \times 10^3$ atoms/cm^3; measurements made between 22 and 27°C with RH < 15%	77
$\beta \propto \dfrac{R^2}{1 + hR}$ same as in Equation (19)	Natural	0.02–0.06	1.3×10^3 – $5 \times 10^4/cm^3$	Measurements were aimed at positive small ions of ^{218}Po	75
$\beta = \pi V R^2 S$ with sticking probability, $S = 1$. Kinetic theory of attachment was found to be valid in this size range	Condensation aerosols with geometric SD = 1.3	Median particle diameter = 0.009–0.03	$\sim 10^6/cm^3$	^{220}Rn concentrations in the range 10^3–5×10^5 atoms/cm^3; diffusion tube used for measurements; loss to the walls of the tube estimated at 5–20%	78

$\beta = 4.1 \times 10^5 \, R^2$ cm^3/min Sticking probability = 0.13	0.6–2.65	1–67/cm^3	Monodisperse polystyrene	Experimental procedure of Ref. 77 was repeated in this case for ^{222}Rn; attachment mechanism found to be the same for ^{220}Rn and ^{222}Rn (kinetic collision theory) with larger sticking probability for ^{222}Rn	83
$\beta = 4\pi DR$ Sticking probability, $S = 1$	0.05–2.5	10^3–10^4/cm^3	Monodisperse DEHS (di-2-ethylhexyl silicate)	No difference found between the attachment coefficients of charged and neutral atoms	84
$\beta \propto R^b$ $b = 1$ for 0.25–1.35 μm $b = 1.34$ for 0.1–0.33 μm	0.1–1.35	10^5–10^6/cm^3	Polydisperse fluorescein (separated into different size groups by aerosol centrifuge)	Same as above	85
$\beta \propto$ particle cross-section area; sticking probability was found to decrease with increasing temp. and/or relative humidity	1–5	20–128/cm^3	Monodisperse uranine, methylene blue, and sodium chloride	Attachment coefficient was found to be insensitive to the surface composition of the particle; radon-222 concentration was 1000–6000 pCi/L	79

$^a\delta$ is a function of particle radius and mean free path of decay products.

mately equal to 0.065 μm. For polydisperse aerosols, an average attachment coefficient, $\bar{\beta}$, must be determined from Equation 15, as noted previously. Calculations based only on the average diameter or the count median diameter (and not including the standard deviation of the distribution) will in general be in error.

In order to calculate the unattached fraction, appropriate radioactive decay equations must be formulated and solved. Unattached ^{218}Po is formed from the decay of radon and thereafter either becomes attached to aerosols at a rate λ_s or decays while unattached. Upon decay of attached ^{218}Po, a certain fraction, α, of the recoiling ^{214}Pb atoms may become detached.

The recoil mechanism has been investigated experimentally and confirmed by many workers. Values of the recoil fraction, α, have been found to be 0.6 (12), 0.5 (24), 0.4 (83), and 0.81 (86). McLaughlin (5) and Mercer (87) suggest that this fraction depends on particle size. Mercer (87) argues that if an atom diffuses into the carrier aerosol, the value of the recoil fraction is smaller than the average of 0.81 predicted earlier (88). A recent NCRP publication (71) uses a recoil fraction of 0.81 and a mean diffusion velocity of 1.38×10^4 cm/s for calculation of the unattached fraction of radon progeny. A fraction of the ^{214}Bi can also become unattached on recoil; however, its recoil (β) energy is much smaller than that of ^{214}Pb, and no experimental evidence has been found to support the recoil detachment of ^{214}Bi (5, 23, 24, 87). The recoil formation term of unattached ^{214}Bi is therefore generally taken to be zero.

Unattached ^{214}Pb can be formed either from the decay of unattached ^{218}Po or from the decay of the recoil-detached fraction, α, of attached ^{218}Po. The removal of unattached ^{214}Pb can take place by attachment to aerosols at a rate λ_s, or by radioactive decay leading to the formation of ^{214}Bi. The net removal rate of unattached radon progeny (excluding radioactive decay) can be described by the coefficient λ_r, which includes removal by plateout on fixed surfaces, λ_p, and removal by ventilation, λ_v, in addition to removal by attachment to aerosols, λ_s:

$$\lambda_r = \lambda_s + \lambda_p + \lambda_v \tag{20}$$

Based on this model of modes of formation and removal of unattached radon progeny, the following equations can be written for the net formation rates of unattached ^{218}Po, ^{214}Pb, and ^{214}Bi:

$$\frac{dN_{2_f}}{dt} = \lambda_1 N_1 - (\lambda_r + \lambda_2)N_{2_f} \tag{21}$$

$$\frac{dN_{3_f}}{dt} = \lambda_2 N_{2_f} + \alpha\lambda_2(N_2 - N_{2_f}) - (\lambda_r + \lambda_3)N_{3_f} \tag{22}$$

$$\frac{dN_{4_f}}{dt} = \lambda_3 N_{3_f} - (\lambda_r + \lambda_4)N_{4_f} \tag{23}$$

In these equations, N_{2_f}, N_{3_f}, and N_{4_f} represent the number concentrations of unattached ^{218}Po, ^{214}Pb, and ^{214}Bi atoms, respectively. The λ_i are the radioactive decay constants, and the subscripts 1, 2, 3, and 4 refer to ^{222}Rn, ^{218}Po, ^{214}Pb, and ^{214}Bi, respectively. N_1, N_2, N_3, and N_4 represent the total number concentrations of ^{222}Rn, ^{218}Po, ^{214}Pb, and ^{214}Bi atoms, respectively.

Assuming the initial concentrations are zero, the solutions of Equations 21–23 are

$$N_{2_f} = \frac{\lambda_1 N_1}{\lambda_2 + \lambda_r}\left(1 - e^{-(\lambda_2 + \lambda_r)t}\right) \tag{24}$$

$$N_{3_f} = \frac{\lambda_1 N_1}{\lambda_3 + \lambda_r}\left[\frac{\lambda_2(1 - \alpha)}{\lambda_2 + \lambda_r} + \alpha\right]\left(1 - e^{-(\lambda_3 + \lambda_r)t}\right)$$

$$+ \frac{\lambda_1 N_1 \lambda_2(1 - \alpha)}{(\lambda_2 + \lambda_r)(\lambda_3 - \lambda_2)}\left(e^{-(\lambda_3 + \lambda_r)t} - e^{-(\lambda_2 + \lambda_r)t}\right)$$

$$+ \frac{\lambda_1 N_1 \alpha}{\lambda_3 - \lambda_2 + \lambda_r}\left(e^{-(\lambda_3 + \lambda_r)t} - e^{-\lambda_2 t}\right) \tag{25}$$

$$N_{4_f} = \frac{\lambda_1 N_1 \lambda_3}{(\lambda_4 + \lambda_r)(\lambda_3 + \lambda_r)}\left[\frac{\lambda_2(1 - \alpha)}{\lambda_2 + \lambda_r} + \alpha\right]\left(1 - e^{-(\lambda_4 + \lambda_r)t}\right)$$

$$+ \frac{\lambda_1 N_1 \lambda_3}{(\lambda_4 - \lambda_3)}\left[\frac{\alpha}{\lambda_3 - \lambda_2 + \lambda_r} + \frac{\lambda_2(1 - \alpha)}{(\lambda_2 + \lambda_r)(\lambda_3 - \lambda_2)}\right.$$

$$\left. - \frac{\lambda_2(1 - \alpha)}{(\lambda_2 + \lambda_r)(\lambda_r + \lambda_3)} - \frac{\alpha}{\lambda_3 + \lambda_r}\right]$$

$$\cdot \left(e^{-(\lambda_3 + \lambda_r)t} - e^{-(\lambda_4 + \lambda_r)t}\right) - \frac{\lambda_1 N_1 \lambda_2 \lambda_3(1 - \alpha)}{(\lambda_2 + \lambda_r)(\lambda_3 - \lambda_2)(\lambda_4 - \lambda_2)}$$

$$\cdot \left(e^{-(\lambda_2 + \lambda_r)t} - e^{-(\lambda_4 + \lambda_r)t}\right) - \frac{\lambda_1 N_1 \lambda_3 \alpha \left(e^{-\lambda_2 t} - e^{-(\lambda_4 + \lambda_r)t}\right)}{(\lambda_r + \lambda_4 - \lambda_2)(\lambda_3 - \lambda_2 + \lambda_r)} \tag{26}$$

The total number concentrations of ^{218}Po, ^{214}Pb, and ^{214}Bi (N_2, N_3, and N_4, respectively), again assuming initial concentrations to be zero, are given by

$$N_2 = \frac{\lambda_1 N_1}{\lambda_2}\left(1 - e^{-\lambda_2 t}\right) \tag{27}$$

$$N_3 = \frac{\lambda_1 N_1 \lambda_2}{\lambda_3(\lambda_2 - \lambda_3)}\left[\left(1 - e^{-\lambda_3 t}\right) - \frac{\lambda_3}{\lambda_2}\left(1 - e^{\lambda_2 t}\right)\right] \tag{28}$$

$$N_4 = \frac{\lambda_1 N_1}{\lambda_2 - \lambda_3}\left[-\frac{\lambda_3}{\lambda_4}\left(1 - e^{-\lambda_4 t}\right) + \frac{\lambda_2}{\lambda_4}\left(1 - e^{-\lambda_4 t}\right)\right.$$

$$\left. - \frac{\lambda_2}{\lambda_4 - \lambda_3}\left(e^{-\lambda_3 t} - e^{-\lambda_4 t}\right) + \frac{\lambda_3}{\lambda_4 - \lambda_2}\left(e^{-\lambda_2 t} - e^{-\lambda_4 t}\right)\right] \tag{29}$$

The unattached fractions of ^{218}Po, ^{214}Pb, and ^{214}Bi (f_2, f_3, and f_4, respectively) can be calculated as

$$f_2 = \frac{N_{2_f}}{N_2} \tag{30}$$

$$f_3 = \frac{N_{3_f}}{N_3} \tag{31}$$

$$f_4 = \frac{N_{4_f}}{N_4} \tag{32}$$

The parameter t can be used as an effective time according to the disequilibrium conditions of the radon progeny concentrations and can be determined conveniently from the tabulation of values of t for a wide range of disequilibrium conditions of radon progeny prepared by Evans (89). An approximate effective time can be used since the calculation procedure is not very sensitive to this parameter. As an example, for a concentration ratio of $1:1:0.6:0.3$ for ^{222}Rn: ^{218}Po: ^{214}Pb: ^{214}Bi, an effective time of either 30 or 40 min can be used. The most important part of the entire calculation is determination of the attachment rate, λ_s. Determination of the plateout rate constant, λ_p, and the ventilation rate constant, λ_v, is discussed in Chapter 5.

3.3   Methods for Measuring Unattached Radon and Thoron Progeny Activity

Most commonly used methods for measuring the unattached fractions of radon and thoron progeny are based on their diffusional properties. Because of their small size and mass, unattached decay products have higher diffusivities than attached decay products, and diffuse more readily to surfaces. In diffusion-based measurement methods, therefore, the preferential diffusive deposition of the unattached decay products is exploited. It is important to note, however, that in most methods the theoretical collection of attached decay products is not zero, nor is the theoretical collection of unattached decay products 100%. Geometries used for the preferential removal of the unattached fraction include the walls of a cylindrical tube, the wires of a wire screen, and the channel walls of a diffusion battery. The efficiency of such collection devices is directly related to the geometry and dimensions of the device and the flow velocity of the airstream. The main advantage of diffusion-based methods is that, presuming the apparatus remains uncharged, no assumption needs to be made about the charged state of the unattached fraction. Unattached neutral decay products, unattached ions, or their mixtures are measured only by virtue of their small mass and, consequently, high diffusivity. Available diffusion-based methods for measuring unattached activity are critically reviewed here.

3.3.1 Diffusion Tube Method. The method for determining unattached fractions using a long cylindrical tube originated from a technique developed by Townsend (90) for determining diffusion coefficients. The method consists of drawing an air sample through the tube and measuring the penetration fraction, that is, the fraction of the species transmitted. The penetration fraction is a function of the diffusivity of the particles, length of the tube, and flow rate through the tube. From a comparison of various mathematical representations of the penetration fraction through a cylindrical tube, Soderholm (91) has recommended the following form as the most accurate:

$$F_c = 0.81905 \exp\left(-11.488 \; \mu_c\right) + 0.09753 \exp\left(-70.072 \; \mu_c\right)$$

$$+ \; 0.03250 \exp\left(-178.95 \; \mu_c\right) + 0.01544 \exp\left(-338.10 \; \mu_c\right) \quad (33)$$

where $\mu_c = DL/Q$ and the equation holds for $\mu_c > 7.22 \times 10^{-3}$. In this equation, F_c is the penetration fraction, D is the diffusion coefficient of the diffusing species (cm^2/s), L is the length of the tube (cm), and Q is the flow rate through the tube (cm^3/s).

The diffusion tube method has been used both for measuring the diffusion coefficient of unattached ^{218}Po (1, 34) and ^{212}Pb (40) and for determining the unattached fraction of radon progeny (22, 57, 92, 93). McLaughlin (5) used a diffusion tube apparatus, first described by Nolan and O'Toole (94), consisting of a 42.1-cm-long diffusion tube and claimed that almost complete (>99%) collection of the unattached fraction occurred in the tube at a flow rate of 2.5 L/min.

The unattached fraction of radon and thoron progeny can be determined either from a measurement of the activity deposited on a filter at the exit of the tube or by counting the activity deposited on the tube walls directly, provided that the total concentration of the species under consideration in the airstream entering the tube is known (for example, from side-by-side sampling through a reference filter). Direct counting of the activity deposited on the tube walls can be achieved by lining the tube walls with filter papers which can be counted later for alpha activity. After aspiration of the sample through the tube, Fusamura et al. (92) inserted a 2-mm-diameter stainless-steel wire electrode into a 43-cm-long and 1.7-cm-inner-diameter diffusion tube and counted in the flow of a counting gas (1 part isobutane and 9 parts helium) in the proportional region. With an applied voltage of 1450 V, the counting efficiency for alpha particles was 0.359 and for beta particles, 2.5 $\times 10^{-5}$. The influence of sampling, waiting, and counting periods on the sampling and counting efficiencies was calculated from the decay equations.

Measurements of activity on a filter at the exit end of a diffusion tube or of activity on a filter lining the tube walls were made by Kruger and Andrews (77), Porstendörfer and Mercer (78), and Busigin et al. (28) in studies on attachment and diffusion coefficients of radon and/or thoron progeny.

Porstendörfer and Mercer (95) derived mathematical expressions for the flux distribution of free and attached radon and thoron decay products as a function of distance along a cylindrical tube in laminar airflow. The graphical representation of the flux distribution for thoron decay products inside a cylindrical tube is shown in Figure 6.6.

3.3.2 Diffusion Sampler.

Mercer and Stowe (96) first demonstrated that un-attached ^{218}Po and ^{212}Pb can be collected with up to 80% efficiency in a round-jet sampler. The sampler they designed consisted of two parallel circular disks, each 0.015 cm thick and 2.22 cm in diameter, held apart by a 0.20-cm-thick spacer ring. Air entered through a small hole (0.135 cm diameter) in the upper aluminum disk and left through openings in the spacer ring, depositing the unattached radon decay products on the disk surfaces in a deposition area of 2.8 cm^2 on each disk. A similar sampler with a thicker (0.35 cm) spacer ring and the lower disk replaced by a membrane filter was used as a reference. After simultaneous sampling through both samplers, the two disks from the sampler and the disk and the filter from the reference sampler were simultaneously counted in alpha counters. The deposition efficiency of unattached radon and thoron progeny was found to be a function of the flow rate and the inlet hole diameter. A schematic diagram of the sampler, now commonly known as the diffusion sampler, is shown in Figure 6.7.

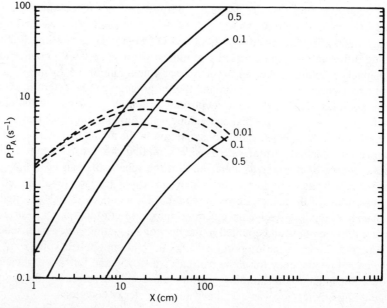

Figure 6.6. Flux distribution of free (P) and attached (P$_A$) thoron decay products as a function of distance, x, in a cylindrical tube. λ_s = the attachment rate; r_o = the radius of the tube; V = the linear air velocity; D = the diffusion coefficient; and q_o = the rate of formation of atoms per unit volume at $x = 0$. -------- P. ——— P$_A$. Parameter: λ_s (s^{-1}); $q_o = 1$ cm^{-3} s^{-1}; $D = 0.068$ cm^2 s^{-1}; $r_o = 0.91$ cm; $V = 2.1355$ cm s^{-1}. From Ref. 95. Reprinted with permission from *Journal of Aerosol Science*, **9**, J. Porstendörfer and T. T. Mercer, Concentration distribution of free and attached Rn and Tn decay products in laminar aerosol flow in a cylindrical tube. Copyright 1978, Pergamon Press, Ltd.

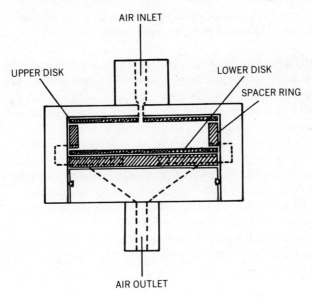

Figure 6.7. Mercer and Stowe's diffusion sampler. From Ref. 96.

Mercer and Mercer (97) worked out a detailed theory of diffusional deposition in such samplers. The most accurate form of the mathematical expressions for the penetration fraction, F_p, of particles at a distance r from the axis of the disk was shown by Soderholm (91) to be

$$F_p = 0.91035 \exp{(-7.5407\ \mu)} + 0.05414 \exp{(-85.726\ \mu)}$$
$$+ 0.01528 \exp{(-249.27\ \mu)} + 0.00681 \exp{(-498.15\ \mu)} \quad (34)$$

for $\mu > 2.66 \times 10^{-3}$, where $\mu = \pi D(R_0^2 - r^2)/Qh$, D is the diffusion coefficient of the particle (cm^2/s), R_0 is the radius of each circular disk (cm), Q is the volumetric flow rate, and h is the separation between plates.

George and Hinchliffe (98) built three diffusion samplers similar to Mercer's device (96) in principle, but of slightly different dimensions. The collection efficiencies of these devices for unattached progeny were demonstrated to be ~80–90% for a flow rate of 0.47 L/min. George and Hinchliffe carried out measurements of unattached radon progeny in mines using the most efficient device with collection efficiency of 91.2% at 0.47 L/min, 83.5% at 1 L/min, and 77.5% at 2 L/min. The diameter of each 0.03-cm-thick disk for this device was 2.2 cm, with spacer thickness of 0.216 cm and an inlet hole diameter of 0.155 cm.

The diffusion sampler built by Kotrappa et al. (99) for measuring diffusion coefficients and unattached fraction of radon and thoron progeny was reported to collect 65% of the unattached decay products of thoron at a sampling rate of 1.41 L/min. The diffusion sampler technique was also used by Bigu and Kirk (100),

Duport (57), and Harley and Pasternack (69) for determining unattached fractions of radon progeny and thoron progeny, respectively.

3.3.3 The Diffusion Battery Method.
Duggan and Howell (23) developed a method to measure unattached decay products of radon in which air was sampled through a pair of filters positioned side by side, with one filter preceded by a diffusion battery. The diffusion battery was designed to remove most of the unattached decay products of radon. The difference in activity of the two filters gave an estimate of the unattached fraction of radon progeny.

A diffusion battery generally consists of a number of rectangular plates or cylindrical channels. The deposition of unattached radon decay products in the walls or channels of a diffusion battery is determined by its dimensions, the sampling flow rate, and the diffusion coefficient of the diffusing species. The penetration fraction of a particle with diffusion coefficient D (cm^2/s) passing through a single channel of a cylindrical-type diffusion battery is given by Equation 33. For a rectangular-type diffusion battery the penetration fraction is given by Equation 34, where μ is now given by

$$\mu = DLW/Qh \qquad (35)$$

where L is the length and W is the width of each rectangular plate, h is the separation between two adjacent plates, and other symbols have the same meaning as in Equation 34.

Based on theoretical considerations, the dimensions of a rectangular-plate-type diffusion battery were optimized by Duggan and Howell (23). The diffusion battery consisted of 28 rectangular parallel plates each 5 cm wide and 20 cm long. The spacing between two adjacent plates was 0.07 cm, and a flow rate of 80 L/min was used for sampling. This geometry was theoretically capable of removing greater than 99% of the unattached radon decay products of diffusion coefficient 0.05 cm^2/s and only 2 and 13% of the attached radon decay products of diffusion coefficients 3×10^{-5} and 3×10^{-4} cm^2/s, respectively. However, such small attached fraction collection efficiencies may lead to significant errors if unattached fractions of ~10% or less are to be measured. Duport et al. (101) also used a diffusion battery of 24 rectangular channels ($1.1 \times 10 \times 35$ cm) at a flow rate of 30 L/min for measurement of the unattached fraction of radon progeny. A diffusion battery consisting of a cylindrical tube in which 400 smaller tubes (130 cm long and 6 mm inner diameter) were tightly packed was used by Kruger and Nöthling (83) for attachment studies on radon and thoron progeny.

Since diffusion batteries are widely employed for aerosol size distribution measurements, the theoretical and operational aspects of deposition in different types of diffusion batteries have been investigated by many workers (102–105). Multi-tube batteries, screen-type batteries, and reticulated vitreous carbon batteries have been used by Sinclair et al. (106) for measuring size distributions of submicron radioactive aerosols. Bimodal distributions were found in both indoor and outdoor air, the smaller mode being representative of unattached radon progeny. Such detailed size distributions therefore provide information on the unattached fraction. Table 6.6 summarizes the methods of measuring unattached fractions described so far.

3.3.4 The Wire Screen Method.
Wire screens have been demonstrated to possess excellent properties for removing unattached ^{212}Pb and ^{218}Po. Barry (107) developed the following semiempirical equation for the fractional collection efficiency of a wire screen:

$$E = 0.74 \, M_i D (\text{Re}^{0.78})(\text{Sc}^{0.75})/u \qquad (36)$$

where M_i = mesh size (no. of wires/in.)
  D = diffusion coefficient (cm^2/s)
  u = linear air velocity (cm/s)
  d = wire diameter (cm)
  Re = ud/v = Reynolds number
  Sc = v/D = Schmidt number
  v = kinematic viscosity (cm^2/s)

This equation, however, does not hold for very low air velocities or high diffusion coefficients. An improved semiempirical equation for the wire screen efficiency was developed by Thomas and Hinchliffe (108) by modeling the wire screen as an assemblage of very short (length = wire diameter × constant) rectangular diffusion tubes. The resulting equation is

$$E = 1 - (0.82e^{-0.233h} + 0.18e^{-16.7h}) \qquad (37)$$

where $h = 100 \, M_c^2 \, dD/u$, with M_c = no. of wires/cm, and other symbols are the same as defined in Equation 36. In spite of the utility of Thomas and Hinchliffe's equation, a short tube assemblage model must be considered to be a poor representation of screen geometry, which contains tapered crevices and square openings.

The wire screen method is perhaps the simplest of all available methods for measuring unattached fractions of radon and thoron progeny. The equipment consists of a reference filter placed in an open-face filter holder and a wire screen, with a backup filter separated from it by an O ring, contained in another open-face filter holder. The thickness of the O ring should be sufficient (~4 mm or larger) to prevent recoil-detached ^{214}Pb on the backup filter from reaching the wire screen.

In the first variant of the method, separate air samples are drawn through the two filter holders positioned side by side, and the activities on the reference and the backup filter are counted according to a suitable counting scheme. The unattached fraction, f, is given by

TABLE 6.6 Summary of Nonscreen Methods for Measuring the Unattached Fraction of Radon Progeny

Ref.	Method	Geometry	Flow rate (L/min)	Efficiency (%)
Fusamura et al. (92)	Diffusion tube	43 cm long, 1.7 cm inner dia., cylindrical tube	10	~36 for alphas; ~0.0025 for betas at applied voltage of 1450 V[a]
Porstendörfer and Mercer (78)	Diffusion tube	100 cm long, 1.82 cm diameter	0.333	≥97[a]
Kruger and Andrews (77)	Diffusion tube	14.5 cm long, 1 cm dia.	0.2	Transmission of unattached fraction small (no numbers were specified)[b]
McLaughlin (5)	Diffusion tube	42.1 cm long	2.5	>99
Mercer and Stowe (96)	Diffusion sampler	0.015 cm thick and 2.22 cm dia. parallel disks with 0.20 cm thick spacer ring; inlet hole dia. = 0.135 cm	0.27	~80[a]
George and Hinchliffe (98)	Diffusion sampler	0.03 cm thick, 2.2 cm dia. disk with 0.216 cm thick spacer; inlet hole dia. = 0.155 cm	2	77.5[a]
Kotrappa et al. (99)	Diffusion sampler	3.774 cm dia. disks; inlet hole dia. = 0.2 cm; spacer thickness = 0.226 cm	1.41	65[a]
Bigu and Kirk (100)	Diffusion sampler	Same as above	2	53[b]
Duggan and Howell (23)	Diffusion batteries	28 rectangular parallel plates, 5 × 20 cm with 0.07 cm spacing	80	>99[b]
Duport et al. (101)	Diffusion batteries	24 rectangular parallel plates, 10 × 35 cm; 1.1 cm spacing	30	70[b]

[a]Efficiency determined experimentally.
[b]Efficiency determined theoretically.

$$f = \frac{C_{ref} - C_{filter}}{E C_{ref}} \tag{38}$$

where C_{ref} and C_{filter} are the concentrations of the species under investigation on the reference and the backup filters, respectively, and E is the screen efficiency for the removal of unattached decay products of radon and thoron. The screen efficiency can be determined theoretically from Equation 37 or obtained experimentally in an aerosol-free environment in a laboratory radon/thoron chamber.

In the second variant of the method, the screen is counted directly, and the equation becomes

$$f = \frac{C_{ws}}{E(C_{ws} + C_{filter})} \tag{39}$$

where C_{ws} is the concentration of the species on the wire screen determined from counting of the wire screen. In this case, it is difficult to determine the absolute activity on the screen because of the complex geometry and the irregular deposition of activity on and between the wires. However, this variant of the method avoids the need to subtract two large counts and, since a single sampling pump can be used, avoids problems of flow stability between two pumps. In this variant, the screen and the filter behind it are both counted. On balance, this second variant of the method is preferred for unattached fractions of < 10%. The problems associated with determination of both the counting efficiency and deposition efficiency of wire screens are discussed further in the next section.

For unattached ^{218}Po measurements, James et al. (109) used a 200-mesh wire screen, held at a distance of 2 cm from the surface of a membrane filter. The collection efficiency of the screen was determined from gamma counting, using two 10-cm-diameter NaI crystals under 4π geometry. The efficiency was found to be more than 98% at a sampling flow rate of 10 L/min through a 4.2-cm-diameter screen (linear velocity of 12 cm/s). A simple diffusion tube model with tube length equal to the thickness of the screen was found to be suitable for theoretically describing the collection efficiency of the screen.

Using ambient condensation nuclei (~ 0.05 μm diameter) and silver particles (~ 0.01 μ diameter) in an atmosphere of radon, George (110) found that a 60-mesh/inch screen exhibits "zero" collection efficiency for both types of aerosols at a linear air velocity of 11.5 cm/s. At the same linear air velocity, using 1.9-cm-diameter screens, the average screen efficiency of a 60-mesh screen for collecting unattached decay products was found to be 77%. A comparison of wire screen measurement parameters used by different workers is shown in Table 6.7.

The wire screen method has also been used by Raghavayya and Jones (3), Stranden and Berteig (111), Bigu and Kirk (100), Harley and Pasternack (69), Duport (57), and Busigin et al. (112) for unattached radon and/or thoron progeny measurements.

TABLE 6.7 Summary of Screen Methods for Measuring the Unattached Fraction of Radon Progeny

Ref.	Wire screen mesh size (in.$^{-1}$)	Wire diameter (cm)	Linear air velocity (cm/s)	Screen efficiency (%)	Efficiency determination method
James et al. (109)	200	0.00508	12	100	α counting, plus 4π-γ counting of the wire screen
George (110)	60	0.018	11.5	77	Difference in reference and backup filter α activities
Stranden and Berteig (111)	174	0.0056	21	86	A backup screen was used in place of the backup filter; both screens were α-counted for efficiency determination
Raghavayya and Jones (3)	120	0.0094	12.2	92.6	Theoretical (Ref. 108)
Bigu and Kirk (100)	150	0.006	9.6	95	Theoretical (Ref. 108)
Thomas and Hinchliffe (108)					Theoretical (Equation 37)

4   UNCERTAINTIES IN THE DETERMINATION OF UNATTACHED FRACTIONS OF RADON AND THORON PROGENY

Determination of the unattached fraction of radon and thoron progeny is subject to uncertainties that must be considered in the interpretation and application of the data. These uncertainties are present in both theoretical and experimental methods and are particularly significant at low unattached fractions (< 10%). An estimate of uncertainties should, therefore, accompany unattached fraction data, a practice not often followed in the past. Known uncertainties, their sources and available methods for their estimation, are therefore reviewed here.

4.1   Uncertainties in the Theoretical Procedure

The success of any theoretical procedure for determining the unattached fraction of radon and thoron progeny depends on the validity of the attachment theory used for calculating the attachment rate. Theoretical calculations require values of two experimental parameters, the aerosol concentration and the particle radius R (or, better, the size distribution), the accuracy of which have an important effect on the overall accuracy of the estimate of the unattached fraction. Attachment coefficient calculations for polydisperse aerosols are complex but rigorous (if the particles are spherical). The simple procedure of approximating a polydisperse aerosol size distribution as monodisperse may lead to misleading results.

The choice of theoretical model for calculation of the attachment coefficient may have a significant effect on the calculated unattached fraction, especially for small particles ($R < 0.03\ \mu$m) and low aerosol concentrations ($Z < 40,000/\text{cm}^3$), as can be seen from Figure 6.8.

Equation 17 is based on the kinetic theory model for attachment of radon progeny to aerosols and assumes that random collisions occur between the unattached progeny, aerosol particles, and gas molecules. The attachment coefficient is, therefore, proportional to the collision cross-section, πR^2, and to the mean relative velocity, $\overline{V}$, between unattached decay products and aerosol (24). Usual assumptions are that (i) the size and mass of the unattached radon progeny are negligibly small compared to the size and mass of an aerosol, and (ii) the unattached radon progeny concentration is low enough that agglomeration of unattached progeny need not be taken into account.

Equation 18 is based on the diffusion theory model for the attachment of atoms to aerosols and originates from the theory of diffusional coagulation of spherical particles developed by Smoluchowski (15). In this theory, it is assumed that a diffusion gradient is established around the aerosol particle, which acts as a sink for the diffusing species. The concentration of the diffusing species at the surface of the aerosol particle is, therefore, assumed to be zero. Van Pelt (16) confirmed an attachment coefficient equation of the form given by Equation 18, in agreement with Raabe (24). Other assumptions include quasi-steady-state coagulation, a much greater concentration of unattached radon progeny than of aerosol, and the possi-

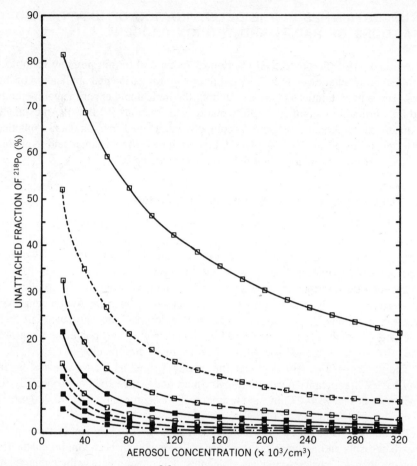

Figure 6.8. Unattached fraction of ^{218}Po versus the aerosol concentration calculated on the bases of diffusion theory (Equation 18) and kinetic theory (Equation 17). ——— $R = 0.01\ \mu$m. ----- $R = 0.02\ \mu$m. — — — $R = 0.03\ \mu$m. —·—· $R = 0.05\ \mu$m. ■ Diffusion theory. □ Kinetic theory.

bility that the aerosol itself does not coagulate. In particular, the second of these assumptions is not generally true, since radon progeny concentrations are often much lower than aerosol concentrations.

It should be noted that the diffusion theory requires knowledge of the diffusion coefficient of the unattached progeny in order to calculate the attachment coefficient. The diffusion coefficient of unattached radon or thoron progeny depends strongly on the environment in which the measurements are made, as discussed in Section 2.2. On the other hand, the thermal velocity $\overline{V}$ used in the kinetic theory varies with temperature. Variations in both the diffusion coefficient and the mean thermal velocity affect the attachment coefficient determined by Equation 19, which is a hybrid theory (74).

A further complication in the attachment rate determination arises from the fact that the effect of the charge of radon or thoron progeny on their attachment to aerosols is not usually included. In Table 6.5 only McLaughlin's (5) attachment model takes into account the state of charge of radon progeny. Using Keefe and Nolan's formula (113) for the effective ion-nucleus recombination coefficient, McLaughlin calculated the attachment coefficients of ^{218}Po to condensation nuclei as a function of the degree of neutralization of the ions and found a noticeable increase in the attachment rate with increasing charged fractions. However, Porstendörfer et al. (84) found no significant difference between the attachment coefficients of charged and neutral decay products. Interactions between charged radon progeny and charged aerosols which could also influence the attachment rate have not been studied in detail.

The sticking probability of unattached decay products to aerosols has been found to be unity by Porstendörfer and Mercer (78) and Porstendörfer et al. (84). However, Kruger and Andrews (77) found the sticking probability to be 0.08 for ^{212}Pb, and Kruger and Nöthling (83) found it to be 0.13 for radon progeny. Ho et al. (79) also found a value of sticking probability of less than unity. However, in the three latter studies, very low aerosol concentrations ($< 128/\text{cm}^3$) were used, in contrast to aerosol concentrations of 10^3–$10^6/\text{cm}^3$ for the other studies. The sticking probability may therefore be taken as unity for residences and mines in which aerosol concentrations are always greater than $10{,}000/\text{cm}^3$.

Based on the above discussion, it can be concluded that for approximate calculations of unattached fractions, the effect of charge can probably be ignored, the diffusion coefficient can be taken as $0.054 \text{ cm}^2/\text{s}$, and the sticking probability can be taken as unity.

The dependence of attachment coefficient on particle size for the kinetic theory (Equation 17), diffusion theory (Equation 18), hybrid theory (Equation 19), and Fuchs' theory (20) is shown in Figure 6.9 for an assumed radon progeny diffusivity of $0.054 \text{ cm}^2 \text{ s}^{-1}$. In Fuchs' model, this diffusivity corresponds to a radon progeny diameter of $0.00098 \text{ }\mu\text{m}$ and a radon progeny mass of 4.4×10^{-22} g. Results for Fuchs' model are also shown for an assumed radon progeny diameter of 0.002 μm. Fuchs' model is the most complete and takes into account the size and diffusion coefficient of both the unattached atom and the aerosol. Figure 6.9 shows that both the hybrid theory and Fuchs' theory reduce to the kinetic theory for particles much smaller than the mean free path of gas molecules in air ($R \ll 0.065 \text{ }\mu\text{m}$) and to the diffusion theory for larger particles. Either the hybrid theory (Equation 19) or Fuchs' model (20) may be used for the entire particle size range.

In order to compute the attachment rate, λ_s, the aerosol concentration and the particle size, or distribution of size, are also required. Uncertainties associated with measuring attachment rate and size should therefore be taken into account. The aerosol concentration is usually measured by a condensation nucleus counter, an electrostatic classifier, or an optical particle counter. The size of the smallest detectable particle, that is, the cutoff diameter, varies from instrument to instrument. For example, of the condensation nucleus counters, the Environment One (RICH 100 Model) has a cutoff diameter of $0.0025 \text{ }\mu\text{m}$, compared to $0.0005 \text{ }\mu\text{m}$

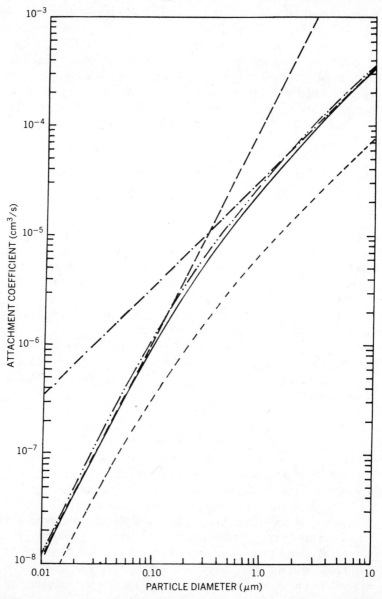

Figure 6.9. Dependence of the attachment coefficient of radon progeny on particle size according to various theories. — — — — Kinetic theory (Equation 17) (for $D = 0.054$ cm^2 s^{-1}). — · — · — · — Diffusion theory (Equation 18) (for $D = 0.054$ cm^2 s^{-1}). — · · — · · — · · — Hybrid theory (Equation 19) (for $D = 0.054$ cm^2 s^{-1}). ---------------- Fuchs' model (20) for a radon progeny clustered diameter of 0.002 μm. ———— Fuchs' model (for $D = 0.054$ cm^2 s^{-1}); this diffusivity corresponds to a radon progeny clustered diameter of 0.00098 μm and a mass of 4.4×10^{-22} g [calculated from the equations $D = kT/f_c$ (Equation 5) and $V = (8kT/\pi m)^{1/2}$].

for the General Electric condensation nucleus counter (114). Cooper and Langer (114) have discussed the limitations of condensation nucleus counters and recommend that data below 0.03 μm particle diameter be treated with caution. They also recommend frequent calibrations in order to obtain reliable data.

Frequently the median of a lognormal particle size distribution determined from diffusion battery measurements or mobility analysis is used for the particle radius, R, in the attachment coefficient computation. However, it must be realized, as mentioned in Section 3.2, that the practice of representing the size distribution of a polydisperse aerosol with a single value is an approximation. The further the geometric standard deviation for an aerosol size distribution is from unity, the greater is the degree of approximation.

4.2   Uncertainties in the Measurement of Unattached Activity

All measurement methods for unattached fractions are subject to fairly large uncertainties. An uncertainty common to all the diffusion-based methods described in Section 3.3 is that resulting from flow rate fluctuations during sampling. Portable pumps for sampling air through filters produce flow rates that are typically constant to $\pm 5\%$. Flow fluctuations considerably increase the overall uncertainty in measurement. Another source of uncertainty common to all filter-counting methods arises from the choice of the sampling and counting scheme. The modified Tsivoglou method (115) may be acceptable for high concentrations of radon and thoron progeny, such as those found in underground mines, but for low concentrations in indoor air the sampling and counting scheme must be optimized. Optimization is important in determining the unattached activity deposited by diffusion on a surface by direct counting and in determining the difference of activities between reference and backup filters. An example of the merits of such an optimization is shown in Table 6.8, where counting schemes for a typical underground mine situation [100 pCi/L (3.7 kBq/m^3) of ^{218}Po, 60 pCi/L (2.2 kBq/m^3) of ^{214}Pb, and 40 pCi/L (1.5 kBq/m^3) of ^{214}Bi] are shown together with the relative standard deviations of measurement for ^{218}Po, ^{214}Pb, and ^{214}Bi for both the total and the unattached (2% of the total) activity. The effects of fluctuations in both flow rate and concentration are demonstrated. The large increase in the measurement uncertainty for unattached activity is mainly due to poorer counting statistics. Optimized intervals show improved precision for both attached and unattached activity.

Because of the low activities of unattached radon and thoron progeny, small variations in the flow rates through the diffusion sampling device and its reference may result in a significant error in the measurement. The pump flow rates should be known accurately for the entire sampling period. Concentration fluctuations of $\sim 5\%$ or less do not influence results significantly and may be ignored. The efficiency of the counting system should be known accurately.

Individual methods for measuring unattached fractions have their own inherent

TABLE 6.8 Comparison of Uncertainties for Different Counting Schedules for Radon/Thoron Progeny Measurements[a]

Sampling time (min)	Counting scheme (min after sampling)	Ref.	Concentration mode[c]	$\Delta V^b = 0, \Delta C = 0$			$\Delta C = 0, \Delta V = 0.05$			$\Delta C = 0.05, \Delta V = 0.05$		
				RS1[d]	RS2	RS3	RS1	RS2	RS3	RS1	RS2	RS3
5	2–5, 6–20, 21–30	Thomas (115)	T	0.06	0.03	0.05	0.28	0.15	0.26	0.28	0.16	0.27
			U	0.44	0.22	0.36	0.51	0.27	0.44	0.52	0.27	0.44
5	2–5, 7–15, 25–30	Busigin and Phillips (116)	T	0.06	0.03	0.05	0.24	0.12	0.21	0.24	0.12	0.21
			U	0.44	0.23	0.36	0.49	0.26	0.41	0.49	0.26	0.41
5	2–5, 9–25, 40–70	This work	T	0.04	0.01	0.02	0.19	0.07	0.15	0.19	0.07	0.15
			U	0.28	0.07	0.16	0.34	0.10	0.22	0.34	0.10	0.22

[a] All relative standard deviations calculated for 10 L/min flow rate and 40% counting efficiency. Concentrations of ^{218}Po, ^{214}Pb, ^{214}Bi were taken as 100, 60, 40 pCi/L, respectively. The method of Busigin and Phillips (116) was followed for calculating these uncertainties.

[b] ΔV = fractional flow rate fluctuations; ΔC = fractional concentration fluctuation during sampling.

[c] T = measurement of total activity; U = measurement of 2% unattached activity.

[d] RS represents the relative standard deviation of measurement; the numbers 1, 2, and 3, represent ^{218}Po, ^{214}Pb, and ^{214}Bi, respectively.

errors. In samplers based on diffusion, some attached activity is almost always collected in addition to the unattached activity. The attached activity may deposit on the inner surfaces of the sampler as a result of inertial impaction or diffusion. The positive error in measurement of unattached ^{218}Po arising from this mechanism has been estimated by van der Vooren et al. (117) as $\sim 4\%$ for the diffusion battery method, $\sim 1.6\%$ for Kotrappa et al.'s (99) diffusion sampler, and $\sim 0.2\%$ for certain wire screens, based on collecting aerosol of median activity diameters of 0.065–0.19 μm and size distributions typical of underground uranium mines.

There are also sources of uncertainty associated with the efficiency calibration of devices for measuring unattached fractions. Since the equations for calculating the penetration fractions in each case are based on diffusion coefficients of the unattached atoms, all the uncertainties associated with the diffusion coefficient values for radon and thoron progeny, as discussed earlier, become associated with the calculation.

Each method has its own limitations. Smutek (118) and Davies (119) have discussed limitations of the equation for cylindrical diffusion channels. The solution of the equation for Mercer's diffusion sampler is based on assumptions (97) that may not all be valid in a practical situation. Calibration and use of diffusion batteries with ultrafine aerosols is discussed by Brown et al. (105). The calibration procedure of Cheng and Yeh (102) for a screen-type diffusion battery describes corrections both for penetration through the battery and for doubly charged particles. The calibration procedure may be applied to wire screens.

The wire screen method for measuring unattached fractions is the simplest, but is limited by difficulties in detecting the activity deposited on the screen. The wire screen has a complicated geometry made up of wires in a woven network. Measurements have been made of the fraction, α_{ws}, of alpha particles emerging from the screen in the direction of the detector with sufficient residual energy for their detection (4, 112). Mercer (4) found the value of α_{ws} to be 0.75, based on reinterpretation of Raghavayya and Jones' (3) experimental data for 120 mesh/inch wire screen at 12.2 cm/s linear air velocity. Stranden and Berteig (111) found values of α_{ws} between 0.60 and 0.78 in 15 measurements with a 174 mesh/inch wire screen, backup filter, and reference filter at a linear air velocity of 21 cm/s. However, this procedure for determining α_{ws} leads to similar uncertainties in the data as obtained by counting the reference and the backup filter and using Equation 38 for determining the unattached fraction. In determining the unattached fraction, counting of the screen and its backup filter would remove the flow rate uncertainty. The values of α_{ws} reported above seem high if it is true that the screen can be modeled as an assemblage of cylindrical tubes for calculation of deposition efficiency. Thomas and Hinchliffe (108) proposed such a model and successfully fitted it to experimental data, as subsequently Stranden and Berteig (111) did. In such a model, deposition is in a fictitious cylindrical tube located between the wires of the screen and would result in a lower value of α_{ws} than if deposition were uniform around each wire of the screen. Although the cylindrical tube model can describe experimental data, it cannot because of this alone be considered to be validated as an exact description of the deposition pattern. Preferential deposition on the front surface of the screen or in the wedge-shaped crevices between the overlapping screen wires may in fact occur. Determination of the absolute alpha activity deposited on the screen is, in fact, quite difficult.

In summary, the above discussion suggests that in determining unattached fractions calibration of experimental devices is difficult and that optimized sampling and counting schedules are required. For these reasons, it is necessary that estimates of uncertainties be provided with the data to aid in interpretation of the results.

5 SUMMARY

The term unattached fraction as applied to the progeny of radon and thoron refers to the fraction, whether charged or neutral, not attached to aerosol particles. According to this definition, progeny subject only to reaction and/or molecular clustering would be defined as unattached. It therefore follows that the properties of the unattached fraction, in particular electrical mobility and diffusivity, will not have unique values and will depend on the properties and composition of the gaseous environment. This fact of nonuniqueness has special significance when diffusivity is used to determine the unattached fraction and requires that the cutoff boundary demarcating unattached and attached values be chosen with care. Since normally the total size distribution is bimodal, with the two modes fully separated, an appropriate value can usually be chosen.

Because of the dependence of the diffusivity on the composition of the gaseous environment, and because of significant uncertainties with respect to geometric efficiencies and—especially for low unattached fractions—counting statistics, unattached fraction data may be subject to considerable uncertainty, particularly when the unattached fractions are calculated for individual radon or thoron progeny (isotopes), using the decay equations. Mathematical solution of the simultaneous decay equations amplifies the uncertainties for the unknowns, that is, the concentrations. Unattached fractions for progeny collected over specified time intervals, that is, without converting to isotope concentrations, are subject to less uncertainty.

As implied above, the unattached fraction is not necessarily the same as the charged fraction, and values of the latter should therefore not be included in the unattached data sets. Neutralization probably occurs by means of two main processes, namely, scavenging of electrons from trace gases (for example, nitrogen oxides, hydrocarbons) of lower ionization potential than the charged species (for example, Po^+ or PoO_2^+), and/or reaction with negative small ions.

Knowledge of the properties of the unattached fraction is of value in understanding the behavior of the progeny of radon and thoron in gaseous environments such as buildings and uranium mines and in estimating their delivered lung dose.

REFERENCES

1. Chamberlain, A. C., and Dyson, E. D. (1956). The dose to the trachea and bronchi from the decay products of radon and thoron, *Br. J. Radiol.*, **29**, 317.

2. ICRP publication 2 (1959). *Report of Committee II on Permissible Dose for Internal Radiation*, Pergamon Press, Oxford.

3. Raghavayya, M., and Jones, J. H. (1974). A wire screen filter paper combination for the measurement of fractions of unattached radon daughters in uranium mines, *Health Phys.*, **26**, 447.

4. Mercer, T. T. (1975). Unattached radon decay products in uranium mine air, *Health Phys.*, **28**, 158.

5. McLaughlin, J. P. (1972). The attachment of radon daughter products to condensation nuclei, *Proc. Royal Irish Acad.*, **72**(Sect. A.), 51.

6. ICRP publication 32 (1981). *Report of the International Commission on Radiological Protection on Limits for Inhalation of Radon Daughters by Workers*, Pergamon Press, Oxford.

7. Palmer, H. E., Perkins, R. W., and Stuart, B. O. (1964). The distribution and deposition of radon daughters attached to dust particles in the respiratory systems of humans exposed to uranium mine atmospheres, *Health Phys.*, **10**, 1129.

8. Ham, J. M. (Commissioner) (1976). Report of the Royal Commission on the Health and Safety of Workers in Mines, Ministry of the Attorney General, Province of Ontario, Toronto.

9. George, A. C., and Breslin, A. J. (1967). Deposition of natural radon daughters in human subjects, *Health Phys.*, **13**, 375.

10. Martin, D., and Jacobi, W. (1972). Diffusional deposition of small-sized particles in the bronchial tree, *Health Phys.*, **23**, 23.

11. Harley, N. H., and Pasternack, B. S. (1972). Alpha absorption measurement applied to lung dose from radon daughters, *Health Phys.*, **23**, 771.

12. Haque, A. K. M. M., and Collinson, A. J. L. (1967). Radiation dose to the respiratory system due to radon and its daughter products, *Health Phys.*, **13**, 431.

13. Altshuler, B., Nelson, N., and Kuschner, M. (1964). Estimation of lung tissue dose from the inhalation of radon and daughters, *Health Phys.*, **10**, 1137.

14. Jacobi, W., and Eisfeld, K. (1982). Internal dosimetry of inhaled radon daughters. In M. Gomez (ed.), *Proc. Int. Conf. on Radiation Hazards in Mining: Control, Measurement and Medical Aspects*, Soc. of Mining Engineers, New York, p. 31.

15. Smoluchowski, M. von (1916). Versuch einer Matematischer Theorie der Koagulationshinetik Kolloider Losungen, *Ztschr. Phys., Chem.*, **92**, 129.

16. Van Pelt, W. R. (1971). Attachment of radon-222 decay products to a natural aerosol as a function of aerosol particle size, Ph.D. thesis, New York University, New York.

17. Raabe, O. G. (1968). The adsorption of radon daughters to some polydisperse submicron polystyrene aerosols, *Health Phys.*, **14**, 397.

18. Arendt, P., and Kallmann, H. (1926). Uber den Mechanismus der Aufladung von Nebelteilchen, *Ztschr. Phys.*, **35**, 421.

19. Lassen, L., and Rau, G. (1960). The attachment of radioactive atoms to aerosols, *Ztschr. Phys.*, **160**, 504.

20. Fuchs, N. A. (1964). *The Mechanics of Aerosols*, Macmillan, New York.

21. Friedlander, S. K. (1977). *Smoke, Dust and Haze*, Wiley, New York.

22. Craft, B. F., Oser, J. L., and Norris, F. W. (1966). A method of determining relative amounts of combined and uncombined radon daughter activity in underground uranium mines, *Am. Ind. Hyg. Assoc. J.*, **27**, 154.

23. Duggan, M. J., and Howell, D. M. (1969). The measurement of the unattached fraction of airborne RaA, *Health Phys.*, **17**, 423.

24. Raabe, O. G. (1969). Concerning the interactions that occur between radon decay products and aerosols, *Health Phys.*, **17**, 177.

25. Jacobi, W. (1972). Activity and potential α-energy of ^{222}radon- and ^{220}radon-daughters in different air atmospheres, *Health Phys.*, **22**, 441.

26. Knoll, G. F. (1979). *Radiation Detection and Measurement*, Wiley, New York.

27. Gunn, R. (1954). Diffusion charging of atmospheric droplets by ions, and the resulting combination coefficients, *J. Met.*, **11**, 339.

28. Busigin, A., van der Vooren, A. W., Babcock, J. C., and Phillips, C. R. (1981). The nature of unattached RaA (^{218}Po) particles, *Health Phys.*, **40**, 333.

29. Goldstein, S. D., and Hopke, P. K. (1985). Environmental neutralization of polonium-218, *Environ. Sci. Technol.*, **19**, 146.

30. Bagnall, K. W. (1957). *Chemistry of the Rare Radionuclides*, Butterworths, London.

31. Hawrynski, M. J. (1984). The theory of clusters. In H. Stocker (ed.), *Proc. Int. Conf. on Occupational Radiation and Safety in Mining*, Canadian Nuclear Assoc., Toronto, Canada, p. 551.

32. Raes, F., Janssens, A., and Vanmarcke, H. (1985). A closer look at the behaviour of radioactive decay products in air, *Sci. Total Environ.*, **45**, 205.

33. Busigin, C., Busigin, A., and Phillips, C. R. (1982). The chemical fate of ^{218}Po in air. In M. Gomez (ed.), *Proc. Int. Conf. on Radiation Hazards in Mining: Control, Measurement and Medical Aspects*, Soc. of Mining Engineers, New York, p. 1043.

34. Tyndall, A. M. (1938). *The Mobility of Positive Ions in Gases*, Cambridge University Press, London, p. 36.

35. Bloom, J., and Margenau, H., (1952). Ion clustering, *Phys. Rev.*, **85**, 670.

36. Magee, J. L., and Funabashi, K. (1959). The clustering of ions in irradiated gases, *Radiat. Res.*, **10**, 622.

37. Raghunath, B., and Kotrappa, P. (1979). Diffusion coefficients of decay products of radon and thoron, *J. Aerosol Sci.*, **10**, 133.

38. Kotrappa, P., Bhanti, D. P., and Raghunath, B. (1976). Diffusion coefficients for unattached decay products of thoron—Dependence on ventilation and relative humidity, *Health Phys.*, **31**, 378.

39. Madelaine, G. (1966). Behavior of radon and thoron daughters in aerosol free air, *Tellus*, **18**(2), 593.

40. Fontan, J., Blanc, D., Huertas, M. L., and Marty, A. M. (1969). Mesure de la mobilité et du coefficient de diffusion des particles radioactives. In S. C. Coroniti, and J. Hughes (eds.), *Planetary Electrodynamics*, vol. 1, Gordon & Breach, New York.

41. Porstendörfer, J. (1968). The diffusion coefficients and mean free paths of the neutral and charged radon decay products in air, *Ztschr. Phys.*, **213**, 384.

42. Porstendörfer, J., and Mercer, T. T. (1979). Influence of electric charge and humidity upon the diffusion coefficient of radon decay products, *Health Phys.*, **37**, 191.

43. Raabe, O. G. (1968). Measurement of the diffusion coefficient of RaA, *Nature*, **217**, 1143.

44. Porstendörfer, J., and Mercer, T. T. (1980). Diffusion coefficients of radon decay products and their attachment rate to the atmospheric aerosols. In T. F. Gesell and W. M. Lowder (eds.), *Natural Radiation Environment III*, Conf-780422, US Dept. of Commerce, National Technical Information Service, Springfield, VA.

45. Wellisch, E. M. (1914). Experiments on the active deposit of radium, *Phil. Mag. S. 6*, **28**(166), 417.

46. Thomas, J. W., and LeClare, P. C. (1970). A study of the two-filter method for radon-222, *Health Phys.*, **18**, 113.

47. Billard, F., Madelaine, G., Chapuis, A., Fontan, J., and Lopez, A. (1971). Contribution to the study of air pollution in uranium mines, *Radioprotection*, **6**(1), 45.

48. Frey, G., Hopke, P. K., and Stukel, J. J. (1981). Effect of trace gases and water vapour on the diffusion coefficient of Po-218, *Science*, **211**, 480.

49. Wellisch, E. M. and Bronson, H. L. (1912). The distribution of the active deposit of radium in an electric field, *Phil. Mag. S. 6*, **23**(137), 714.

50. Wellisch, E. M. (1913). The distribution of the active deposit of radium in an electric field—II., *Phil. Mag. S. 6*, **26**(154), 623.

51. Dua, S. K., Kotrappa, P., and Gupta, P. C. (1983). Influence of relative humidity on the charged fraction of decay products of radon and thoron, *Health Phys.*, **45**, 152.

52. Jonassen, N. (1983). The effect of electric fields on ^{222}Rn daughter products in indoor air, *Health Phys.*, **45**, 487.

53. Jonassen, N. (1984). Electrical properties of radon daughters. In H. Stocker (ed.), *Conf. on Occupational Radiation Safety in Mining*, Can. Nuclear Assoc., Toronto, Canada, p. 561.

54. Chamberlain, A., Magan, W., and Wiffen, R. (1957). Role of condensation nuclei as carriers of radioactive particles, *Geofis. Pura. Appl.*, **36**, 233.

55. Szucs, S., and Delfosse, J. (1965). Charge spectrum of recoiling ^{216}Po in the decay of ^{220}Rn, *Phys. Rev. Lett.*, **15**(4), 163.

56. Bricard, J., Girod, P., and Pradel, J. (1965). Spectre de mobilité des petits ions radioactifs de l'air, *C. R. Acad. Sci., Paris*, **260**, 6587.

57. Duport, P. (1978). L'Aerage et les caracteristiques de l'atmosphere d'une mine d'uranium laboratorie, doctoral thesis, published as CEA-R-4927, a report by the Commissariat à l'Energie Atomique, France.

58. Dua, S. K., Kotrappa, P., and Bhanti, D. P. (1978). Electrostatic charge on decay products of thoron, *Am. Ind. Hyg. Assoc. J.*, **39**, 339.

59. Rutherford, E. (1903). Excited radioactivity and the method of its transmission, *Phil. Mag.*, **V**, 95.

60. Franck, J. (1909). Über die lonenbeweglichkeit der radioaktiven Restatome und die Masse des Gasions, *Verh. Deut. Phys. Gesell.*, **XI**, 397.

61. Franck, J., and Meitner, L. (1911). Über radioaktive Ionen, *Verh. Deut. Phys. Gesell.*, **XIII**, 671.

62. Wilkening, M. H., Kawano, M., and Lane, C. (1966). Radon daughter ions and their relation to some electrical properties of the atmosphere, *Tellus*, **18**(2), 679.

63. Jonassen, N., and Wilkening, M. H. (1970). Airborne measurements of radon 222 daughter ions in the atmosphere, *J. Geophys. Res.*, **75**(9), 1745.

64. Jonassen, N., and Hayes, E. I. (1972). Mobility distribution of radon-222 daughter small ions in laboratory air, *J. Geophys. Res.*, **77**(30), 587.

65. George, A. C., and Breslin, A. J. (1977). Measurements of environmental radon with integrating instruments, presented at Atomic Industrial Forum Uranium Mill Monitoring Workshop, Albuquerque, NM.

66. Coghlan, M., and Scott, J. A. (1983). A study of the formation of radiolytic condensation nuclei. In L. H. Ruhnke and J. Latham (eds.), *Proc. in Atmospheric Electricity*, A. Deepak Publishing, Hampton, VA.

67. Jacobi, W. (1964). The dose to the human respiratory tract by inhalation of short-lived ^{222}Rn decay products, *Health Phys.*, **10**, 1163.

68. James, A. C., Jacobi, W., and Steinhäusler, F. (1982). Respiratory tract dosimetry of radon and thoron daughters: The state of the art and implications for epidemiology and radiobiology. In M. Gomez (ed.), *Proc. Radiation Hazards in Mining: Control, Measurement and Medical Aspects*, Soc. of Mining Engineers, New York, p. 42.

69. Harley, N. H., and Pasternack, B. S. (1973). Experimental absorption applied to lung dose from thoron daughters, *Health Phys.*, **24**, 379.

70. George, A., and Breslin, A. J. (1969). Deposition of radon daughters in humans exposed to uranium mine atmospheres, *Health Phys.*, **17**, 115.

71. NCRP report no. 78 (1984). Evaluation of occupational and environmental exposures to radon and radon daughters in the United States, National Council on Radiation Protection and Measurements, Bethesda, MD.

72. Jacobi, W. (1961). The attachment to natural aerosols of naturally occurring radioactive aerosols, *Geofis. Pura Appl.*, **50**, 260.

73. Baust, E. (1966). The attachment of radioactive atoms and ions to spherical aerosol particles, *Ztschr. Phys.*, **199**, 187.

74. Mohnen, V. (1967). Investigation of the attachment of neutral and electrically charged emanation decay products to aerosols, AERE Trans. 1106 (doctoral thesis).

75. Kawano, M., Ikebe, Y., and Shimo, M. (1969). Measurement of the attachment coefficient of small ions and radioactive ions to condensation nuclei. In S. C. Coroniti and J. Hughes (eds.), *Planetary Electrodynamics*, Vol. 1, Gordon and Breach, New York.

76. Duggan, M. J., and Howell, D. M. (1969). Relationship between the unattached fraction of RaA and the concentration of condensation nuclei, *Nature*, **224**, 1190.

77. Kruger, J., and Andrews, M. (1976). Measurement of the attachment coefficients of Rn-220 decay products to monodisperse polystyrene aerosols, *J. Aerosol Sci.*, **7**, 21.

78. Porstendörfer, J., and Mercer, T. T. (1978). Adsorption probability of atoms and ions on particle surfaces in submicrometer size range, *J. Aerosol Sci.*, **9**, 469.

79. Ho, W. L., Hopke, P., and Stukel, J. J. (1982). The attachment of RaA (Po-218) to monodisperse aerosols, *Atmos. Environ.*, **16**, 825.

80. Raabe, O. G. (1977). Interaction between radon daughters and aerosols. In J. E.

Turner and C. F. Holoway (eds.), *Workshop on Dosimetry for Radon and Radon Daughters*, Technical Information Service, Springfield, VA.

81. Lassen, L., and Weicksel, H. (1961). Die Anlagerung radioaktiver Atome an Aerosole (Schebstoffe) in Grossenbereich 0.7-5 μ Radius, *Ztschr. Phys.*, **161**, 339.

82. Porstendörfer, J. (1968). Die experimentelle Bestimmung der Koeffizienten der Anlagerung der neutralen und electrisch geladenen Radon-Folgeprodukte an Aerosole, *Ztschr. Phys.*, **217**, 136.

83. Kruger, J., and Nöthling, J. F. (1979). A comparison of the attachment of the decay products of radon-220 and radon-222 to monodisperse aerosols, *J. Aerosol Sci.*, **10**, 571.

84. Porstendörfer, J., Röbig, G., and Ahmed, A. (1979). Experimental determination of the attachment coefficients of atoms and ions on monodisperse aerosols, *J. Aerosol Sci.*, **10**, 21.

85. Menon, V. B., Kotrappa, P., and Bhanti, D. P. (1980). A study of the attachment of thoron decay products to aerosols using an aerosol centrifuge, *J. Aerosol Sci.*, **11**, 87.

86. Kolerskii, S., Kusnetsov, Yu. V., Polev, N. M., and Ruzer, L. S. (1973). Effect of recoil nuclei being knocked off aerosol particles on free-atom concentrations of daughter emanation products, *Izmeritel'naya Tekhnika*, **16**(10), 57 (in Russian); *Meas. Tech.*, **16**, 1527 (English trans.).

87. Mercer, T. T. (1976). The effect of particle size on the escape of recoiling RaB atoms from particulate surfaces, *Health Phys.*, **31**, 173.

88. Mercer, T. T., and Stowe, W. A. (1971). Radioactive aerosols produced by radon in room air. In W. H. Walton (ed.), *Inhaled Particles*, Unwin, Old Woking, p. 839.

89. Evans, R. D. (1969). Engineers' guide to the elementary behaviour of radon daughters, *Health Phys.*, **17**, 229.

90. Townsend, J. S. (1900). The diffusion of ions into gases, *Phil. Trans. Roy. Soc. A*, **193**, 129.

91. Soderholm, S. C. (1979). Analysis of diffusion battery data, *J. Aerosol Sci.*, **10**, 163.

92. Fusamura, N., Kurosawa, R., and Maruyama, M. (1967). Determination of f-value in uranium mine air. In *Assessment of Airborne Radioactivity in Nuclear Operations*, IAEA, Vienna, p. 213.

93. Shimo, M., Asano, Y., Hayashi, K., and Ikebe, Y. (1985). On some properties of ^{222}Rn short-lived decay products in air, *Health Phys.*, **48**, 75.

94. Nolan, P. J., and O'Toole, C. P. J. (1959). The condensation nuclei produced by point discharge, *Geofis. Pura Appl.*, **42**, 117.

95. Porstendörfer, J., and Mercer, T. T. (1978). Concentration distribution of free and attached Rn and Tn decay products in laminar aerosol flow in a cylindrical tube, *J. Aerosol Sci.*, **9**, 283.

96. Mercer, T. T., and Stowe, W. A. (1969). Deposition of unattached radon decay products in an impactor stage, *Health Phys.*, **17**, 259.

97. Mercer, T. T., and Mercer, R. (1970). Diffusional deposition from a fluid flowing radially between concentric parallel circular plates, *J. Aerosol Sci.*, **1**, 279.

98. George, A. C., and Hinchliffe, L. (1972). Measurements of uncombined radon daughters in uranium mines, *Health Phys.*, **23**, 791.

99. Kotrappa, P., Bhanti, D. P., and Dhandayuthum, R. (1975). Diffusion sampler useful

for measuring diffusion coefficients and unattached fraction of radon and thoron decay products, *Health Phys.*, **29**, 155.

100. Bigu, J., and Kirk, B. (1980). Determination of the unattached radon daughter fractions in some Canadian uranium mines, CANMET Division report MRP/MRL 80-112 (OP), Canadian Centre for Mineral and Energy Technology, Elliot Lake.

101. Duport, P., Madelaine, G., and Renoux, A. (1975). Mesure de la fraction libre presente dans l'air d'une mine d'uranium laboratoire, *Chemosphere*, **5**, 283.

102. Cheng, Y. S., and Yeh, H. C. (1980). Theory of a screen-type diffusion battery, *J. Aerosol Sci.*, **11**, 313.

103. Cheng, Y. S., Keating, J. A., and Kanapilly, G. M. (1980). Theory and calibration of a screen-type diffusion battery, *J. Aerosol Sci.*, **11**, 549.

104. Brown, K., and Gentry, J. W. (1984). The sensitivity of the glass capillary array diffusion battery for particles under 30 nm, *J. Aerosol Sci.*, **15**, 252.

105. Brown, K. E., Beyer, J., and Gentry, J. W. (1984). Calibration and design of diffusion batteries for ultrafine aerosols, *J. Aerosol Sci.*, **15**, 133.

106. Sinclair, D., George, A. C., and Knutson, E. O. (1978). Application of diffusion batteries to measurement of submicron radioactive aerosols. In *Proc. Amer. Nucl. Soc. Series on Assessment of Airborne Radioactivity*, p. 103.

107. Barry, P. J., (1968). Sampling for airborne radioiodine by copper screens, *Health Phys.*, **15**, 243.

108. Thomas, J. W., and Hinchliffe, L. E. (1972). Filtration of 0.001 μm particles by wire screens, *Aerosol Sci.*, **3**, 387.

109. James, A. C., Bradford, G. F., and Howell, D. M. (1972). Collection of unattached RaA atoms using a wire gauze, *Aerosol Sci.*, **3**, 243.

110. George, A. C. (1972). Measurement of uncombined fraction of radon daughters with wire screens, *Health Phys.*, **23**, 390.

111. Stranden, E., and Berteig, L. (1982). Radon daughter equilibrium and unattached fraction in mine atmospheres, *Health Phys.*, **42**, 479.

112. Busigin, C. J., Busigin, A., and Phillips, C. R. (1983). Measurement of charged and unattached fractions of radon and thoron daughters in two Canadian uranium mines, *Health Phys.*, **44**, 165.

113. Keefe, D., and Nolan, P. J. (1962). Combination coefficients of ions and nuclei, *Proc. Roy. Irish Acad.*, **62**, 43.

114. Cooper, G., and Langer, G. (1978). Limitations of commercial condensation nucleus counters as absolute aerosol counters, *J. Aerosol Sci.*, **9**, 65.

115. Thomas, J. W. (1972). Measurement of radon daughters in air, *Health Phys.*, **23**, 783.

116. Busigin, A., and Phillips, C. R. (1980). Uncertainties in the measurement of airborne radon daughters, *Health Phys.*, **39**, 943.

117. van der Vooren, A. W., Busigin, A., and Phillips, C. R. (1982). An evaluation of unattached radon (and thoron) daughter measurement techniques, *Health Phys.*, **42**, 801.

118. Smutek, M. (1972). On the separation of air-borne particles by diffusion, *Aerosol Sci.*, **3**, 337.

119. Davies, C. N. (1973). Diffusion and sedimentation of aerosol particles from Poiseuille flow in pipes, *Aerosol Sci.*, **4**, 317.

PART THREE

THE BASIS FOR HEALTH CONCERNS

▬ 7

Lung Dosimetry

ANTHONY C. JAMES

Radiological Measurement Department, National Radiological Protection
Board, Chilton, Didcot, Oxfordshire, England

1 INTRODUCTION

The risk of lung cancer from exposure to radon progeny in homes can be estimated
by considering the radiation dose delivered to sensitive cells (1). This has been
done for radon progeny (2) and other inhaled radionuclides (3) by the International
Commission on Radiological Protection (ICRP). The procedure used was (i) to
evaluate doses absorbed by tissues for a given intake of a radionuclide; (ii) to
weight these doses according to standard estimates of risk from irradiating each
tissue; and (iii) to add up the total risk contributed by all irradiated tissues (4).
The composite reference quantity, related by ICRP to risk, is known as the "effective dose equivalent." Another approach employing dosimetry to estimate risk
(5) is to scale the excess rate of lung cancer incidence in uranium miners (Chapter
8) in proportion to the radiation doses received in mines and homes (6–8).

The dose to lung tissue from inhalation of radon progeny cannot be measured.
It must be calculated by modeling the sequence of events involved in inhalation,
deposition, clearance, and decay of radon progeny within the bronchial airways.
Various models, reviewed below, show that the dose for a given exposure depends
on environmental and personal factors, principally the aerosol size distribution,
breathing rate, and lung size. However, rather disparate assumptions have been
made by authors in modeling lung dose, leading to divergent estimates of risk.
Fortunately, some of the key assumptions can be refined. An improved understanding of the physical behavior and size distribution of radon progeny aerosols in
room air is emerging (9), supported by data from homes. Research has also progressed in the fields of measuring and modeling aerosol deposition in lung, the
clearance of radon progeny, and the identification of cells involved in the development of lung cancers. This chapter assembles this newer information and thus
reassesses the dose to lung from exposure to radon progeny.

Whereas rough estimates of the risk of lung cancer from exposure to radon
progeny can be made directly from epidemiological studies of mining populations,
there are no epidemiological data for people exposed to thoron progeny. In this

259

case, risk can only be estimated by considering the doses to various tissues; this is the standard procedure adopted by ICRP (2, 3).

2 LUNG CANCER

Cancer of the respiratory tract is the most common form of lethal cancer in most industrialized countries. Overall it accounts for about one-fifth of all cancer deaths. In some countries the proportion is even higher; in England and Wales almost half the fatal cancers in men between the ages of 45 and 64 are lung cancers (10), and in the United States the proportion is about one-third (11). Cancers occur in various parts of the respiratory tract, as shown in Table 7.1 (12), but mainly in the lung. Most of these cancers are associated with smoking (10–13).

Most lung cancers arise in the bronchial airways and are classified as bronchogenic. It is difficult to localize the origin of tumors to specific airways, since they are often large by the time of diagnosis. However, somewhat less than half are thought to occur in the central part of the lung, in the relatively large bronchi (14). The remainder occur in small airways deeper in the lung, with relatively few in the alveoli. There are different types of lung tumor, distinguished by the appearance of cells at histological examination (15). The four main categories (16) and their occurrence, estimated from a recent survey of 28,000 cancer cases in the general population of the United States (17), are given in Table 7.2

Epidermoid tumors and small cell carcinomas occur mainly in the large airways, whereas adenocarcinomas and large cell carcinomas are mainly peripheral in small airways (14). The occurrence of different types of tumor varies with age at which the cancer occurs. This makes it difficult to establish any dependence of tumor type on causative agent—cigarette smoking, exposure to radon progeny and other pollutants, or combinations of these factors. Early studies of lung cancer incidence in uranium miners from the Colorado Plateau in the United States (18) indicated that about two-thirds of the tumors were small cell carcinomas, a much higher proportion than found in the general population. However, most of the 50 cases were in men who started mining early in life, were exposed to high concentrations of radon progeny, and died relatively young. Subsequent follow-up of this mining

TABLE 7.1 Estimated Number of Cancer Cases by Type in the United States: 1972

Site	Males	Females
Lip	1,600	200
Tongue	2,000	800
Other oral	3,600	2,400
Pharynx	3,100	1,400
Larynx	6,000	800
Lung	62,000	14,000
Other respiratory	1,400	1,100

Data from Schneiderman et al. (Ref. 12).

TABLE 7.2   Distribution of Tumor Types in 28,000 Cases of Lung Cancer

Tumor type	Frequency (%)
Squamous cell carcinoma (epidermoid tumor)	32
Adenocarcinoma	26.5
Small cell carcinoma	16.5
Large cell carcinoma	7.5

Data from Percy and Sobin (Ref. 17).

population from 1954 through 1979 revealed 292 cases of lung cancer, predominantly epidermoid tumors or adenocarcinomas (19). The proportion of small cell carcinomas fell progressively over this period to 22%, a value similar to that in the general population. If allowance is made for variation with age, it can be concluded that the incidence of tumor types in miners exposed to radon progeny is not significantly different from that in the general population (20, 21).

2.1   Cells at Risk

The tissue that lines the larynx, the trachea, and the bronchial airways is described as ciliated mucosa. This consists of a surface epithelium and underlying supporting tissue. The structure of the bronchial wall in the large airways is illustrated in Figure 7.1 (22). The epithelium is held onto a basement membrane by the triangular-shaped "basal cells." Ciliated cells extend from the basement membrane to the epithelial surface, where their cilia support and move a protective layer of mucus. Underneath the basement membrane is a layer of tissue called the lamina propria, containing blood vessels and elastic muscle fibers. The epithelium and

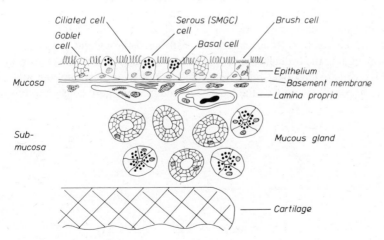

Figure 7.1. Diagrammatic section through the wall of a bronchus showing the types of cell found in the epithelium.

lamina propria together constitute the mucosa. In the bronchi, the mucosa is connected to a thick submucosa, including supporting rings of cartilage and glands that secrete most of the mucus (22, 23). The epithelium becomes progressively thinner toward the periphery of the lung. It is continuous with the epithelium of the alveolar ducts and alveoli, which is only a few microns thick (24). Airways less than about 1 mm in diameter have no cartilage rings or mucous glands and are known as bronchioles. The types of cell found in the epithelia of the bronchi and bronchioles are broadly similar, but their relative numbers differ. There are eight main types, whose characteristics and location in the epithelium are summarized in Figure 7.2.

By comparing the histological characteristics of the different types of tumor with those of normal epithelial cells, some conclusions can be drawn about the types of cell involved in the development of lung cancer. Goblet and ciliated cells are fully differentiated, do not divide, and are not involved directly in lung cancer. And, although basal cells are sometimes treated in dosimetric calculations as those whose received dose is the important one, in point of fact all the cell types other than goblet and ciliated may be involved (25). Poorly differentiated young mucous cells, characterized by small mucous granules (small mucous granule cells or SMGC in Fig. 7.1), divide in normal epithelium at a similar rate to basal cells.

There is direct histological evidence that cells containing secretory granules are implicated in epidermoid tumors (25). The development of lung cancer is usually preceded by squamous cell metaplasia (26), which is common after irritation by toxicants or after respiratory infection. Squamous metaplasia involves both hyperplasia of basal cells and incomplete differentiation of intermediate cells (Fig. 7.2). These cells have no mucous granules and no cilia, but persisting mitotic activity. Squamous metaplasia is also characterized by increased mitotic activity in small mucous granule cells (25).

In the peripheral airways (bronchioles), basal cells are rare and the mitotic activity is thought to be provided by Clara cells. These cells are probably involved in the development of adenocarcinoma (21). It can be concluded that cells at risk for the development of lung cancer are distributed throughout the bronchial airways, including the bronchioles (21). Even in the large airways, it is probable that sensitive cells extend over the whole thickness of the epithelium and are not restricted to basal locations on the basement membrane. These considerations deter-

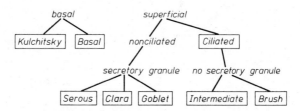

Figure 7.2. The eight epithelial cell types classified on the basis of location, presence of cilia, or type of secretory granule.

mine that the average radiation dose to epithelial cells is probably more relevant to the assessment of lung cancer risk than the dose to basal cells alone (21).

3 STRUCTURE OF THE RESPIRATORY TRACT

3.1 Functional Regions

The respiratory tract can be divided into three regions on the basis of anatomy and function (Fig. 7.3) (24). The structure and airflow in each region determine the fractional deposition of inhaled aerosol particles and of unattached radon progeny. For decay by alpha-particle emission, the radiation dose absorbed by sensitive tissue in each part of the respiratory tract is also influenced by the thickness of the epithelium.

The nasopharyngeal (N-P) region begins at the anterior nares (nostrils) and includes the respiratory airway down to the larynx. The nose functions primarily to humidify inspired air and also to protect the lower respiratory tract by filtering dust and aerosol particles. Although nasal deposition of radon progeny must be considered because of its potential to reduce the dose to the lower respiratory tract, there is no evidence from mining populations that exposure to radon progeny increases the risk of nasal cancer. The main risk is always that of bronchogenic cancer. Thus, it is less important to evaluate the dose to the nasal epithelium. In any case, the procedure for estimating the dose to cells at risk in the nose is not yet well established.

The tracheobronchial (T-B) region begins at the larynx and includes the trachea and the ciliated bronchial airways, down to and including the terminal bronchioles. The branching structure of the T-B region is illustrated in Figure 7.4 (24). There are about 10 branchings or generations of large airways (bronchi), followed by approximately five generations of bronchioles. Finally, the bronchioles branch into

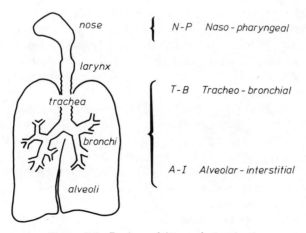

Figure 7.3. Regions of the respiratory tract.

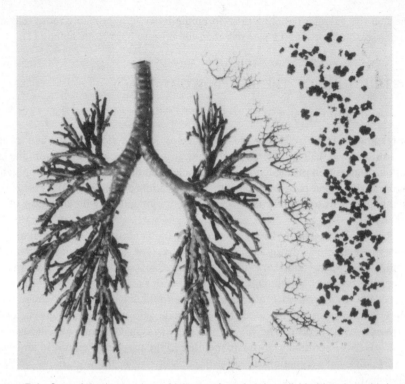

Figure 7.4. Cast of the human bronchial tree after trimming, divided into bronchi down to 3-mm diameter, small bronchi, and terminal segments of the lung, including bronchioles and alveolar ducts. (Reprinted, with permission, from O. G. Raabe, Deposition and clearance of inhaled aerosols, in *Mechanisms in Respiratory Toxicology*, Vol. I, H. Witschi and P. Nettesheim, Eds., CRC Press, Inc., Boca Raton, FL, 1982, p. 27.)

alveolated airways where gas exchange takes place in the lung. The T-B region is both ciliated and provided with mucus-secreting glands or cells, so that deposited particles can be cleared rapidly by mucociliary action to the throat for swallowing. However, soluble material may be absorbed rapidly into the blood. This pathway must also be considered when assessing the fraction of deposited radon progeny that is retained in the airway wall and thus is able to irradiate bronchial epithelium more efficiently.

The alveolar-interstitial (A-I) region of the lung consists of alveolar ducts and terminal sacs and the associated blood capillaries and lymphatic drainage ducts (23, 24). The region is characterized by the absence of cilia and a thin barrier of tissue—only a few microns thick—between the adjacent alveoli. Hence, even for alpha particles with a range of 50–80 microns in tissue, the A-I region can be considered to be homogeneous. On average, all types of cells in this region will absorb similar radiation doses.

Intact particles are cleared from the A-I region by two routes: in macrophages to the ciliated airways and via lymphatic drainage ducts to regional lymph nodes.

Neither of these pathways is important in the case of the short-lived radon progeny. Only absorption into the blood needs to be considered. It serves as a mechanism both for lung clearance and for translocation of activity to other organs.

3.2 Airway Dimensions

The first step in evaluating absorbed doses is to calculate the fraction of inhaled radon progeny deposited on airway surfaces within the lung. To do this it is necessary to adopt a simplified geometrical model of airway size and branching. A number of models available for this purpose have been summarized by Raabe (27).

Most authors have used the so-called Weibel "A" model of symmetrical branching (28). This model gives the diameter and length of bronchial and respiratory airways, assuming that airways at each level of branching are identical. Diameter and length are represented by simple formulae in terms of the generation number, z. The number of airways in each generation is given by 2^z, where $z = 0$ for the trachea and 23 for the alveolar sacs. Airway dimensions were measured from a sample of whole human lung inflated and fixed at about three-quarters of the maximum capacity. This corresponded to a lung volume of about 4800 mL.

More extensive measurements of airway size were made by Yeh and Schum (29). They prepared a replica cast by injecting silicone rubber under pressure into a lung in situ in the thorax of a human cadaver. This procedure preserved the in vivo shape of the lung. However, it gave rise to some enlargement of the airways which the authors considered equivalent to a lung inflated to total lung capacity, or about 6000 mL lung volume. Yeh and Schum recommended that their reported airway dimensions be scaled down to correspond with the volume of the lung in the normal respiratory range. To compare the aerosol deposition predicted theoretically from various lung models for a standard lung volume, Yu and Diu (30) carried out such a scaling procedure. They scaled the airway dimensions of the Weibel A and Yeh-Schum lung models to a total volume of 3000 mL, corresponding to the normal functional residual capacity (FRC) of an adult man (31). Their assumption that the caliber of bronchial airways increases in proportion to the cube root of lung expansion is supported by observations on ventilated lungs (32).

More recently, Phalen et al. (33) have reported measurements of airway sizes from replica casts of 20 lungs. These were taken from subjects aged between 11 days and 21 years. The casts were made by filling the lungs with saline in situ in the thorax and replacing the saline with silicone rubber. Airway sizes in the adult lungs were smaller than those given by the Weibel A and Yeh-Schum models before scaling, and it can be assumed that the dimensions reported by Phalen et al. approximate more closely those in lungs at normal FRC. These authors also derived regression formulae giving the variation in airway diameter and length as a function of body height. The expressions apply over the whole age range from newborn to adult. They can be used to estimate airway dimensions in children on a standard basis for the purpose of calculating lung deposition. For convenience below, the airway sizes reported by Phalen et al. for a 70-kg adult of height 175 cm are referred to as the University of California at Irvine (UCI) lung model.

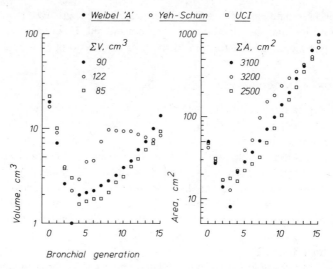

Figure 7.5. Volumes and surface areas of airways in each bronchial generation of the Weibel A, Yeh-Schum, and UCI lung models. The total volumes and areas are denoted by ΣV and ΣA, respectively.

The residual differences in airway sizes between the Weibel A and Yeh-Schum lung models scaled to the standard FRC (31) and the UCI model are shown in Figure 7.5. The volumes and surface areas of some airway generations differ by quite large factors. It is not known which model is the most realistic overall. The range of values given by these models can be regarded as an indication of uncertainty. Thus, it is useful to examine their effect on calculated lung deposition and on the estimation of dose from inhaled radon progeny. This is done later for each model. Meanwhile, Table 7.3 shows the mean airway dimensions and the relative standard deviations among models.

According to the average dimensions at normal FRC given in Table 7.3, the adult trachea has a surface area of about 50 cm²; the bronchi (generations 1–10) a total surface area of about 560 cm²; and the bronchioles (generations 11–15) an area of about 2300 cm². The total volume of these airways constitutes the anatomical dead space and is about 100 mL. During normal breathing, the bronchi would expand to give a mean surface area of about 600 cm², and the bronchioles about 2500 cm².

3.3 Epithelial Thickness

In the T-B region, radon progeny are deposited on the layer of mucus lining the airway surface, whereas the sensitive cells are within the epithelium. Because of the short range of alpha particles in tissue, the dose absorbed by sensitive epithelial cells depends rather critically on the thickness of the epithelium and on the loca-

TABLE 7.3   Average Airway Dimensions from Three Lung Models

Airway generations	Diameter		Length	
	Mean (cm)	Rel. SD (%)	Mean (cm)	Rel. SD (%)
Trachea				
0	1.65	7	9.1	12
Bronchi				
1	1.20	10	3.8	7
2	0.85	14	1.5	6
3	0.61	18	0.83	25
4	0.44	18	0.90	18
5	0.36	26	0.81	13
6	0.29	21	0.66	23
7	0.24	23	0.60	36
8	0.20	27	0.53	36
9	0.16	25	0.44	28
10	0.13	20	0.37	25
Bronchioles				
11	0.11	17	0.32	19
12	0.086	10	0.27	15
13	0.071	5	0.22	7
14	0.059	7	0.18	7
15	0.050	10	0.16	12

tions of the targets within it. Tissue thickness must be considered in relation to the alpha-particle ranges, which are given in Table 7.4.

Few measurements have been made of the thickness of bronchial epithelium. The most extensive were reported by Gastineau et al. (34), who studied clinically normal biopsy specimens. Epithelial thickness was found to be variable in airways of a given caliber, leading Gastineau et al. to report frequency distributions. Their data are summarized in Table 7.5 (35).

TABLE 7.4   Ranges in Tissue of Alpha Particles Emitted by Radon and Thoron Progeny

Nuclide	Energy (MeV)	Range (μm)
Rn-222 (radon)	5.49	41
Po-218 (RaA)	6.00	48
Po-214 (RaC')	7.69	71
Rn-220 (thoron)	6.29	52
Po-216 (ThA)	6.78	58
Bi-212 (ThC)	6.06 (36%)	49
Po-212 (ThC')	8.78 (64%)	89

TABLE 7.5   Normal Distribution of Epithelial Thickness (μm)

Airway classification (approx. generations)	Mean	SD
Main bronchi (1)	80	6
Lobar bronchi (2)	50	12
Segmental bronchi (3–5)	50	18
Transitional bronchi (9, 10)	20	5
Bronchioles (11–15)	15	5

Data from Gastineau et al. (Ref. 34); Wise (Ref. 35).

3.4   Dose from Decay of Radon Progeny

Calculation of the dose to cells in the alveolar-interstitial region is straightforward. The average dose is given by

$$D_{\text{A-I}} = \frac{nE_\alpha}{m_{\text{A-I}}} \tag{1}$$

where n is the number of decays, E_α is the alpha-particle energy, and $m_{\text{A-I}}$ is the mass of the A-I region. To obtain $D_{\text{A-I}}$ in the SI unit Gy, E_α in MeV must be multiplied by the conversion factor 1.6×10^{-13} J/MeV, and $m_{\text{A-I}}$ must be in kg.

The number of decays is calculated from the number of radon progeny atoms inhaled, the fractional deposition in the A-I region, and the proportion of progeny atoms not cleared to the bloodstream to decay elsewhere.

Calculation of absorbed dose for airways in the T-B region is more complicated. Various levels of sophistication can be employed, ranging from grossly simplified estimates of energy absorbed in some fairly arbitrary mass of tissue to detailed calculations of the number of decays and dose to specified targets in each airway, taking into account movement from the site of deposition by ciliary action. The results of these extreme approaches are compared later.

The energy absorbed by target cells is calculated by employing an idealized model of the airway geometry (36, 37), including the airway radius, the thickness and location of the radioactive source (usually mucus), and the depth of the target cells below the source. The energy-loss characteristics of alpha particles in tissue can be represented adequately (38) for this purpose by analytical approximations to range-energy tables (39). Figure 7.6 shows the variation of dose to target cells at given depths in the epithelium, calculated in this way for one decay of each of the radon and thoron progeny per unit area of airway surface. The figure shows that slightly different values are obtained for bronchi and bronchioles, where the latter have an epithelium less than 30 μm thick. The slightly higher doses in bronchioles arise because the mucous source is thinner and also the path length in air for alpha particles emitted from the far wall is shorter. Otherwise, curvature of the airway wall has little influence on dose. The main factors are the alpha-particle energy and the depth of target cells; dose decreases rapidly from the epithelial surface to zero at the end of the alpha-particle range.

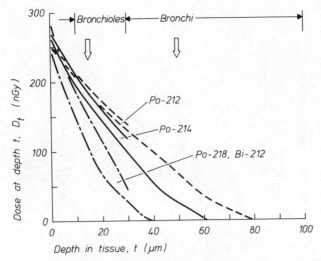

Figure 7.6. Doses to target cells at depth t in bronchial and bronchiolar epithelium from radon and thoron progeny decay in mucus, assuming 1 decay / cm² surface area. The curves extending only up to 30 μm are those for bronchioles, whereas the curves for bronchi extend up to the full range of the alpha particles considered.

Figure 7.7 shows the result of averaging doses to cells at all depths in the epithelium, again for radon and thoron progeny decaying in mucus. In this case, doses depend much less on the thickness of the epithelium. The mean dose remains finite even for a very thick epithelium. As discussed in Section 2, it is probably more relevant for risk assessment to evaluate doses to epithelial cells in this way, rather than focus only on the dose to basally located cells.

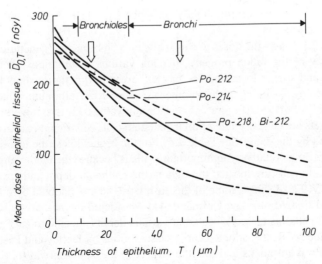

Figure 7.7. Doses averaged over all epithelial cells from radon and thoron progeny decay in mucus, assuming 1 decay / cm² surface area.

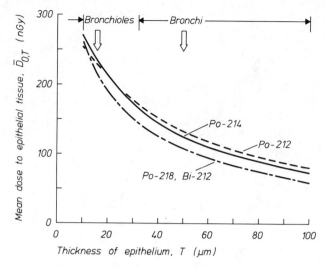

Figure 7.8. Doses averaged over all epithelial cells from radon and thoron progeny decay in mucosal tissue, assuming 1 decay / cm² surface area.

Transfer of radon and thoron progeny to mucosal tissue modifies the dose received by epithelial cells. Figure 7.8 shows the mean doses to all epithelial cells resulting from one decay per unit surface area, for activity distributed throughout the mucosa. It is assumed that the mucosal thickness is twice that of the epithelium and that a concentration gradient is present, falling to zero concentration at the base of the mucosa where blood capillaries are found (see Figure 7.1). However, this assumption is not critical, as similar results are obtained when the concentration of activity in the mucosa is assumed to be uniform. It is found that doses to epithelial cells depend only slightly on alpha-particle energy when the progeny decay in the mucosa.

Figure 7.9 shows the doses to stem cells in each bronchial generation that result from decay of the radon progeny, making various assumptions about epithelial thickness and source location. The hatched areas in this figure show the range of doses given by assuming decay in mucus (Figure 7.6—minimum values) or decay entirely in the mucosa (Figure 7.7—maximum values). It is assumed that the sensitive targets are cells capable of division (stem cells) distributed at various depths, determined by the data from Table 7.5. For the bronchioles, the location of radon progeny decay is relatively unimportant. This is because the epithelium is thin and also the stem cells are located throughout the epithelial depth and are not basal.

Figure 7.9 also shows some of the dosimetric factors adopted by other authors. Jacobi and Eisfeld (40) and Hofmann (41) considered the activity to be in mucus, with basal cells, as targets, located at various depths specific to each airway generation. The NCRP (6) adopted earlier assumptions by Harley and Pasternack (42) that activity is in mucus and that the targets in the upper airways are ''shallow'' basal cells at a depth of 22 μm. Targets in airways below the ninth generation were assumed to lie at a depth of 10 μm. Clearly, these different assumptions about

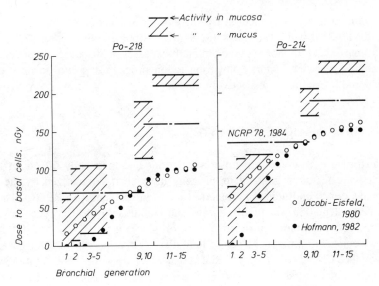

Figure 7.9. Doses to stem cells (mainly basal) in each bronchial generation from 1 decay of the radon progeny per cm^2 airway surface.

source-target geometry will influence the evaluation of doses and must be borne in mind when comparing published dosimetric studies, as is done in the next section.

Finally, the range of dosimetric factors that results when all epithelial cells are considered sensitive, and doses are averaged, is shown in Figure 7.10. In this case

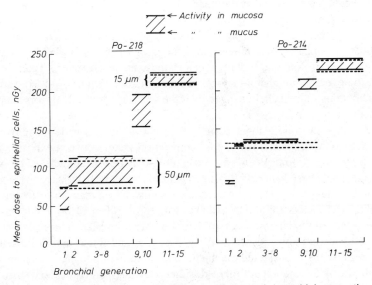

Figure 7.10. Doses averaged over all epithelial cells in each bronchial generation from 1 decay of the radon progeny per cm^2 airway surface.

there is much less dependence on the thickness and location of the source, especially for Po-214, which is always the main contributor to lung dose. In Section 7 the dosimetric factors shown for epithelial thicknesses of 50 and 15 μm are adopted to evaluate reference factors converting radon progeny exposure to dose in the bronchi and bronchioles, respectively.

4 REVIEW OF DOSE ESTIMATES

The historical development of dose calculations and their early use to set limits for exposure to radon gas and its progeny have been summarized by the U.S. National Council on Radiation Protection and Measurements (NCRP) (6). The first published calculation was that by Evans and Goodman (43). They recommended limiting the concentration of radon gas in workplace air to 10 pCi/L (370 Bq/m^3) (44), by considering the incidence of lung disease in miners from Schneeberg and Jacimov (see Chapter 8). They calculated that exposure to this concentration would give a dose of 10 mrad (0.1 mGy) per year to alveolar tissue. The ICRP first set an exposure standard for radon based mainly on a dosimetric evaluation in 1959 (45). This focused on irradiation of bronchial tissue following deposition of the radon progeny and adopted the experimental work of Chamberlain and Dyson (46). The results of Chamberlain and Dyson's study and of subsequent attempts to model lung dose from exposure to radon progeny are summarized in Table 7.6.

Chamberlain and Dyson based their calculation on measurements of deposition by diffusion of the unattached and aerosol fractions of radon progeny in a hollow cast of the trachea and main bronchi. They observed that the deposition efficiency for unattached progeny was much higher than that for condensation nuclei. Accordingly, they estimated that the dose to the bronchial epithelium was due principally to deposition of unattached Po-218 (RaA), or Pb-212 (ThB) in the case of the thoron progeny. For exposure to radon progeny, they estimated a dose, averaged over the alpha-particle ranges, corresponding to 360 mGy/WLM. When the small fraction of potential alpha energy in the unattached state is taken into account, the overall conversion factor is reduced to about 8 mGy/WLM. Table 7.6 shows how this estimate has changed over the years as additional factors have been modeled.

The first point to note about Table 7.6 is that it shows a wide range of values in the last column, that is, the overall conversion factor between exposure to potential alpha energy (unit WLM) and dose (unit mGy or 0.1 rad) derived by various authors. The lowest value of 0.8 mGy/WLM was given by Jacobi (51), who applied the standard ICRP lung clearance model to estimate dose to bronchial epithelium which was assumed to have a mass of 100 g. This is equivalent to assuming an epithelial thickness of 250 μm. The highest values, 110 and 96 mGy/WLM, were given respectively by Wise (35) and Haque and Collinson (49), partly because they considered the unattached fraction of potential alpha energy to be high. In order to compare these dosimetric studies on equivalent terms, it is necessary to extract the different dose conversion factors for the unattached and

TABLE 7.6 Summary of Published Dose Calculations for ^{222}Rn Progeny

Author (ref.)	Notes/ model	Exposure condns.	Target tissue	Unattached fraction f_p	Unattached fraction Diam. (μm)	Attached fraction AMD (μm)	Eq. factor (F)	Dose conversion factor (mGy/WLM) Fraction Unatt.	Fraction Attached	Overall
Chamberlain & Dyson, 1956 (46)	a	Mine: nose	Trachea & main bronchi (av. 45 μm depth)	2%	0.001	Not eval.	—	360	—	8
Altshuler et al., 1964 (47)	—	Mine: nose mouth	Segmental bronchi (at 35 μm depth)	2%	0.001	0.1–6.0	0.6	200 400	11 18	15 27
Jacobi, 1964 (48)	b	Home: mouth	Lobar to subsegmental bronchi (at 20 μm depth)	5%	0.001	0.09	0.5	70	29	31
Haque & Collinson, 1967 (49)	c	Home: nose	Segmental bronchi (at 30 μm depth)	12%	0.001	0.1	0.5	Not available		96
Walsh, 1970 (50)	b	Mine: nose	Bronchial region (av. 36 μm depth) (i.e., mass ca. 20 g)	2%	0.001	c.0.1	0.6	Not available		16
Jacobi, 1972 (51)	b	Mine: nose: dusty clean	Bronchial region (i.e., mass ca. 100 g)	0.7% 45%	0.001	0.05–0.2	0.3 0.04	8	0.7	0.8 4
Harley & Pasternack, 1972 (52)	c	Mine: nose	Segmental bronchi (at 22-μm depth)	0.9%	0.001	0.3	0.3	240	1.4	3.6

TABLE 7.6 *(Continued)*

Author (ref.)	Notes/model	Exposure condns.	Target tissue	Unattached fraction f_p	Diam. (μm)	Attached fraction AMD (μm)	Eq. factor (F)	Dose conversion factor (mGy/WLM) Fraction Unatt.	Attached	Overall
Jacobi & Eisfeld, 1980 (40)	—	Mine: nose	Bronchial region (basal cells)	1–5%	0.001	0.25	0.5	36	3.8	5
McPherson, 1980 (53)	b	Home: nose	Bronchial region (av. over α range) (i.e., mass ca. 3 g)	1%	0.001	0.1	1.0	500	4	c.10
Hofmann, 1982 (41, 54)	—	Home: nose	Bronchial region (basal cells)	4.5%	0.001	0.08	0.5	Not available		6
		Mine: nose		0.9%	0.001	0.17	0.6	140	c.7	c.8
James et al., 1982 (55)	J-B	Mine: nose	Bronchial region (stem cells)	1–5%	0.0008	0.1–0.5 (0.2)	0.15	100	c.5	5–8
	J-E				0.003		0.6	35	c.4	(c.6)
Wise, 1982 (35)	—	Mine: nose: Underground	Segmental bronchi (basal cells)	0.9%	0.001	0.17	0.3	200	13	15
		Open cut		50%		0.23	0.1		10	110

Study		Exposure	Target region							
Harley & Pasternack, 1982 (42)	[c]	Home: nose	Segmental bronchi (at 22-μm depth)	1%	0.003	0.12	0.7	Not available		5.2
					0.001					5.7
NEA Experts Report, 1983 (38)			Bronchial region (stem cells)							
	J-B	Mine: nose		1–5% (2.5%)	0.0008	0.1–0.5 (0.2)	0.4	100	c.5	5–8 (c.6)
	J-E							35	c.4	
	J-B	Home: nose		1.5–6% (2.5%)	0.003	0.1–0.2 (0.17)	0.4	67	3.5	4–5 (c.4)
	J-E							20	3.6	
NCRP Report No. 78, 1984 (6)	H-P [c]	Mine: nose,	Segmental bronchi (at 22-μm depth)	0.9%	0.001	0.3	0.3	200	2.4	4 (c.5)
		mouth						500		7
		Home: nose		1%	0.001	0.125	0.7	140	6	7

[a] Equilibrium factor F not specified. Value of 0.5 assumed here to derive f_p.
[b] Deposition not calculated. Authors assumed values from elsewhere.
[c] Single particle size assumed for aerosol fraction, not size distribution.

275

aerosol fractions of potential alpha energy. When possible, this is done in the penultimate columns of Table 7.6.

Considering first the dose conversion for the attached fraction of potential alpha energy, Table 7.6 shows a range of values from 0.7 to 29 mGy/WLM, both from Jacobi (48, 51). The low value again arises because the bronchial thickness is drastically overestimated. The high value arises from a combination of shallow target cells (20 μm) and small particle size (0.09 μm). Clearly, a large number of permutations of assumptions are involved in these studies, each more or less realistic. However, it is notable that since 1980 studies have converged somewhat to give estimates of dose per unit exposure to attached radon progeny in the range from about 2 to 13 mGy/WLM. Variation within this range is determined by the assumed aerosol size and depth of target cells.

Estimates of dose per unit exposure to unattached progeny also vary over a substantial range. Excluding the study that assumes a 250-μm-thick epithelium (51), the values range from about 35 mGy/WLM according to Jacobi and Eisfeld (40) to about 500 mGy/WLM according to McPherson (53) and NCRP (6). It is shown in Sections 5 and 6 that Jacobi's low value arises from a combination of special treatments of deposition and clearance. The high values arise because of the deposition estimates used (53) or the special assumptions of mouth breathing and shallow basal cells in segmental bronchi as targets (6). Despite these extremes, most estimates of the dose conversion factor for unattached radon progeny are in the range 100–200 mGy/WLM exposure.

Table 7.6 shows that authors have adopted quite different values for the unattached fraction of potential alpha energy, the size of unattached progeny, and the size distribution of the aerosol fraction. Both home and mine environments have been considered, but with little consensus on the atmospheric characteristics of each. However, some of these studies have included analyses of the sensitivity of dose estimates to aerosol and other factors (6, 35, 38, 51, 54, 55). A further potential source of variation between estimates of dose is the choice of target tissue (bronchial region or segmental bronchi) and depth of target cells.

4.1 Radon Progeny Equilibrium

There has been much confusion about the importance of the degree of radioactive equilibrium among the radon progeny in determining the dose conversion factor. The quantity potential alpha energy was devised to avoid the problem that a given activity of each of the progeny implies a different number of decays and amount of energy absorbed in the lung (56). A further source of confusion is the quantity used to specify unattached progeny. Jacobi and Eisfeld (40) showed that the dose to the bronchial region increases strictly in proportion to f_p, the unattached fraction of the total potential alpha energy, and independently of the equilibrium factor, F. Figure 7.11 shows that this simple relationship also applies to the dose in segmental bronchi, as calculated by various different models (labeled H-P, J-E, and J-B) (5). In this figure the different shaped symbols refer to three values of F, 0.15, 0.37, and 0.72. Four values of the unattached fraction of Po-218 activity, f_A, are considered, 0.05, 0.1, 0.15, and 0.2, leading to 12 different values of the unat-

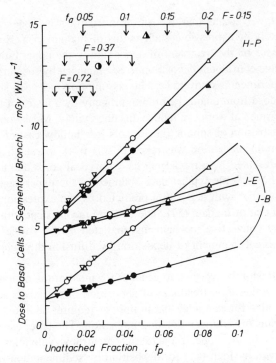

Figure 7.11. Dose to basal cells in segmental bronchi calculated as a function of f_p and equilibrium factor, F, using different dosimetric models [Harley-Pasternack (H-P), Jacobi-Eisfeld (J-E), and James-Birchall (J-B)]. The open symbols represent unattached Po-218 particles of 1-nm diameter and the solid symbols represent particles of 3-nm diameter.

tached fraction of potential alpha energy, f_p. It is seen that for each model and assumed particle size, the unattached fraction of potential alpha energy uniquely defines the dose conversion factor. However, when f_A is used to specify the unattached fraction, the dose also depends substantially on the equilibrium factor, F.

5 LUNG DEPOSITION

The studies summarized in Table 7.6 included diverse methods of estimating deposition efficiency for inhaled radon progeny. In this section recent developments in the calculation and experimental verification of aerosol deposition in lung are noted and their application to calculate deposition of radon progeny is examined.

5.1 Aerosol Deposition: Comparison of Predictions with Measurements

Diffusion is the dominant mechanism of lung deposition for radon progeny aerosols. It is generally assumed that airflow in the smaller airways is laminar at the low velocities involved and that deposition in each airway generation can be calculated adequately by expressions such as that of Ingham (57). However, there is no such consensus on the treatment of deposition in the upper bronchi. Some authors (6, 40) have considered deposition to be enhanced by secondary flow, on the basis of an experimental study (58). This assumption has been shown to reduce the calculated dose from unattached radon progeny by a factor of two (59).

Recent experimental work can reduce this uncertainty. Measurements have been made of the deposition of submicron aerosols in a hollow cast of human bronchi (60). An important precaution was taken in this work to establish realistic flow conditions, represented by a model larynx with vocal cords and a cyclical simulation of tidal flow. Some typical data obtained in the experiment are shown in Figure 7.12, together with deposition predicted by the expression of Martin and Jacobi (58) and that of Ingham (57). The data are inconsistent with the substantial enhancement by convective mechanisms predicted by the former, whereas they support the classical treatment of deposition by diffusion throughout the airways (57).

Although diffusion is expected to account for most of the overall deposition of radon progeny in the lung, treatment of deposition of the larger aerosol particles present in dirty air—for example, that in mines—requires additional consideration of the mechanisms of sedimentation and impaction. The latter especially may enhance deposition in the upper bronchi, where airflow velocities are high. The expression derived by Pich (61) for deposition by sedimentation in tubes is considered adequate (62). However, it is not possible to treat deposition by inertial impaction analytically without knowing the complex flow patterns present in the upper airways. Egan and Nixon (63) have avoided this problem by fitting an em-

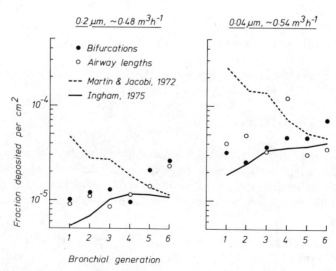

Figure 7.12. Deposition of submicron aerosols measured by Cohen et al. (60) for cyclical flow through a hollow cast of the human bronchial tree, compared with calculated values.

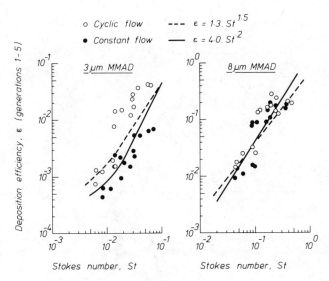

Figure 7.13. Deposition of aerosol particles measured by Schlesinger et al. (64) for both constant and cyclical flow through a hollow cast of the human bronchial tree, compared with values calculated from empirical expressions of the efficiency of deposition by impaction.

pirical expression to deposition measured in hollow casts of the upper bronchi (64). The techniques employed in these experiments were similar to those of Cohen et al. (60). Typical data obtained are shown in Figure 7.13. Deposition was found to differ between conditions of cyclical inspiration and those when air was drawn at constant velocity through the cast. Egan and Nixon fitted a simple expression in terms of the Stokes number [defined by Raabe (27)] to deposition under constant flow. A modified expression is needed to describe deposition in cyclical flow. These two expressions are seen in Figure 7.13 to represent measured values reasonably well.

Precise measurements of the total deposition of aerosols in many human subjects are now available and can be used to verify deposition calculations (30). Figure 7.14 shows data from five subjects exposed by mouth to monodisperse aerosols under carefully controlled breathing conditions (65), at a constant airflow velocity of 250 mL/s or at a constant tidal volume of 1000 mL. In these respective experiments, the tidal volume was varied over the wide range from 250 mL to 2000 mL or the breath frequency varied over the range from 3.75 to 30/min. The curves shown for comparison with these data are calculated by applying the deposition functions just described to the dimensional models of the human bronchial tree reviewed in Section 3. Dimensions of the alveolated airways are based on the model of Yeh and Schum (29). In this calculation, the airways are expanded in proportion to the mean tidal volume, and penetration of tidal air to various airway generations is represented (66, 67). The small contribution to deposition made by the oral cavity and larynx over this aerosol size range is included by applying the empirical expressions given by Rudolf et al. (68). Figure 7.14 shows that such

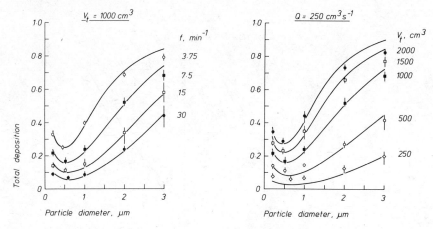

Figure 7.14. Comparison of calculated deposition in the respiratory tract with experimental data of Heyder et al. (65) for subjects breathing through the mouth under controlled conditions.

calculations can reproduce the total deposition of aerosols measured in human subjects remarkably closely, over a wide range of breathing conditions.

More recently, data have been published on respiratory tract deposition of submicron particles, covering the size range of the attached radon progeny (69) and extending almost down to the size of unattached progeny (70, 71). Figure 7.15 compares these data with the results of modeling deposition. Egan and Nixon (72) have used a sophisticated treatment of the penetration and mixing of tidal air within the lung, based on the work of Taulbee and Yu (73). However, the results obtained

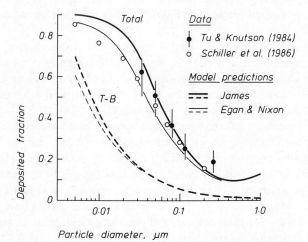

Figure 7.15. Comparison of calculated deposition in the respiratory tract with experimental data for submicron aerosols from Tu and Knutson (69) and Schiller et al. (70).

by the calculations adopted here are similar. Both are consistent with the data. Figure 7.15 also shows the proportion of deposition calculated to occur in the T-B region. It is notable that almost all particles of 0.005-μm diameter are deposited in the bronchi. The proportion increases to total bronchial deposition at 0.001 μm, the size of unattached progeny.

5.2 Deposition of Radon Progeny

For radon progeny attached to aerosol particles, loss by filtration in the nose or mouth can safely be neglected. However, a few direct measurements on human subjects indicate that about half of the unattached progeny inhaled through the nose are deposited there (74). This is consistent with the recent experimental data of Schiller (71), who estimated nasal deposition of about 15% at a particle size of 0.005 μm. Schiller's data indicate that nasal deposition increases with the square root of the diffusion coefficient, under constant breathing conditions, as expected when deposition depends on diffusion (75).

The influence of breathing rate and airway dimensions on nasal deposition of unattached progeny is uncertain. For given nasal dimensions, deposition will probably increase with the square root of the transit time through the nasal passages (75). Thus, the fraction of inhaled progeny deposited in the nose should decrease at higher breathing rates. It must presently be assumed that nasal deposition in children is similar to that in adults at a comparable level of physical exertion.

Figure 7.16 shows the results of applying the model described earlier, and estimates of nasal deposition, to calculate the fraction of inhaled radon progeny de-

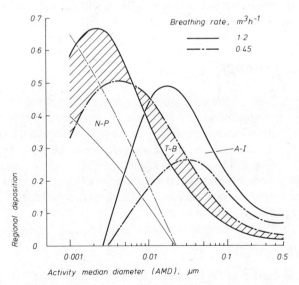

Figure 7.16. Fractional deposition of radon progeny in regions of the adult respiratory tract, calculated as a function of aerosol size and for two breathing rates.

posited in the three regions of the adult respiratory tract. The breathing rates and tidal volumes considered correspond to those of a man at work (3) and resting (31).

For aerosol sizes larger than about 0.01 μm activity median diameter (AMD), it is seen that fractional deposition in the T-B region decreases with breathing rate. The converse applies to alveolar deposition. The AMD of attached radon progeny in ordinary room air is approximately 0.1 μm (see Chapter 5). At this size, about 8% of the inhaled activity is deposited in the T-B region and almost 20% in alveoli. These values are to be contrasted with deposition of approximately 50% of unattached progeny in the T-B region, with none in the alveoli.

These regional deposition values can be used to make rough estimates of doses. Exposure to 1 WLM of potential alpha energy at an intermediate breathing rate (1, 38) of 0.75 m^3/h is equivalent to inhaling 1.65×10^{10} MeV of potential alpha energy. If all this were attached to aerosol particles, approximately 3×10^9 MeV of potential alpha energy would be deposited in the alveolar region. Most of this would be absorbed as dose by the 1 kg of tissue, giving approximately 0.5 mGy per WLM exposure. Approximately 10^9 MeV of potential alpha energy would be deposited in the T-B region. Roughly half of this would be absorbed in the epithelium, which is about 50 μm thick. The mass of tissue involved is roughly 15 g, resulting in a dose of approximately 5 mGy/WLM exposure. If all the potential alpha energy were carried by unattached progeny, about 8×10^9 MeV would be deposited in the T-B region. This would result in a dose of approximately 40 mGy/WLM, or 10 times higher than that from attached progeny.

These very approximate estimates are refined in Section 7 by calculating the deposition of radon progeny in individual airway generations, their subsequent clearance, and doses absorbed by target cells. It will be seen, however, that such detailed considerations do not give substantially different values.

6 LUNG CLEARANCE

In the bronchial tree, radon and thoron progeny are deposited on the surface of mucus. They can be moved toward the throat by the normal process of mucociliary clearance—with the additional possibility of absorption through the epithelium and elimination by the bloodstream. In the alveolar-interstitial (A-I) region, progeny are deposited onto a thin layer of surfactant fluid (24) in close contact with blood capillaries. Direct measurements of the elimination of thoron (^{220}Rn) progeny from human and animal lungs have been made. These enable the relative importance of the clearance pathways to be assessed.

6.1 Experimental Data

The rate of elimination of Pb-212 from the lungs of human subjects was measured by Jacobi et al. (76). They found a biological half-time of about 8 h, due principally to absorption from the alveolar region into the blood. Similar half-times (about

10 h) were found by Booker et al. (77) and Hursh and Mercer (78) in humans, and by Bianco et al. (79) in the dog. The latter study was concerned specifically with absorption from the bronchial region—bronchial deposition was achieved by exposing dogs to freshly formed unattached progeny. In contrast, elimination of the ^{222}Rn progeny cannot be measured directly as it is difficult to assess their initial deposition and rapid radioactive transformations. Attempts have been made by measuring the state of radioactive equilibrium in rodent (80) and dog (81) lung at sacrifice. These are not reliable, but suggest a shorter biological half-time, on the order of 10 min.

Greenhalgh et al. (82) investigated the clearance processes acting on Pb-212 ions and on insoluble particles in nasal mucosa of the rat. Ions and particles were instilled together using a very small amount of water, and their respective rates of clearance by mucociliary action were measured, together with the rate of absorption of Pb-212 into the blood. Typical observations are shown in Figure 7.17. A small proportion (about 10%) of the Pb-212 ions was absorbed rapidly into the blood—with a half-time of approximately 15 min. This rapidly absorbed fraction can be neglected in calculating lung dose. Most of the particles were cleared by mucus, but a smaller proportion of the ions followed this pathway. The authors concluded that some ions are retained in the epithelium with a relatively long half-time.

6.2 Models

Most of the dose calculations summarized in Table 7.6 assume that radon and thoron progeny are insoluble and are cleared with mucus. However, Jacobi and

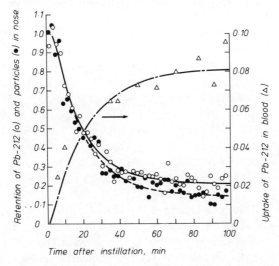

Figure 7.17. Retention of Pb-212 ions and insoluble particles (labeled with Y-88) in the nose of a rat and uptake of Pb-212 into the blood, expressed as fractions of the activities instilled at time zero.

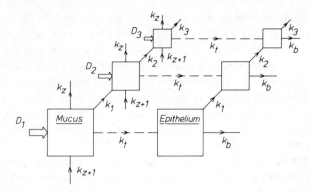

Figure 7.18. General compartment model of deposition D_z, clearance, and radioactive decay through a series of progeny (denoted by k_1, k_2, and k_3) in a bronchial generation, z. Additional symbols are defined in the text.

Eisfeld (40) have modeled the effect on lung dose of absorption into the blood, and James and Birchall (38) the effect of transfer to the epithelium. Clearance and decay of radon and thoron progeny in each generation of the bronchial tree can be represented generally by a series of compartments with associated rates of elimination, as shown in Figure 7.18. The amount of each of the progeny, D_z, deposited in generation, z, can be calculated as a function of the aerosol size distribution, as discussed in the previous section. Mucous clearance can be represented by a series of rate constants, k_z, or mathematically equivalent transit times through each generation. Absorption into the blood can be represented by a transfer rate, k_t, competing with mucous clearance (40). The number of decays of each radon or thoron progeny is evaluated using the respective radioactive decay constants, k_1, k_2, and k_3.

Jacobi and Eisfeld (40) assumed that unattached ions are absorbed much faster than progeny attached to aerosol particles. Thus, unattached Po-218, Pb-212, and their respective progeny are absorbed rapidly into the blood—with a 15-min half-time determined by the biological rate constant, k_b. This has the effect of reducing doses calculated for unattached progeny by about half (38, 59). However, special treatment of absorption for unattached ions is not supported by the experimental clearance studies (79, 82). For the attached progeny, Jacobi and Eisfeld assumed that the rate of absorption is limited by "desorption" from the carrier particles with a half-time of about 10 h. Absorption at this rate has no effect on doses from attached radon progeny, but it reduces lung doses calculated for thoron progeny by about half.

The dose calculations summarized in Table 7.6 also incorporate different assumptions about mucous clearance velocity and its variation throughout the bronchial tree. The range of values adopted is illustrated in Figure 7.19. Yeates et al. (83) based their values on observations of bronchial retention in human subjects coupled with a theoretical model of aerosol deposition. Mucous velocities vary between individuals and also decrease markedly from the trachea to the terminal bronchioles.

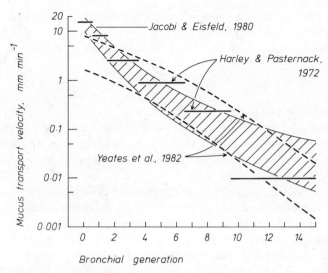

Figure 7.19. Ranges of mucous velocities taken by various authors to represent clearance from each bronchial generation. Yeates et al. (83) derived the range shown from different clearance times observed between human subjects.

The absorption characteristics of radon and thoron progeny remain uncertain, as do the rates of mucous transport at various levels in the bronchial tree. To examine the effect of these uncertainties, the range of doses given by the following rather extreme models is evaluated in Sections 7 and 8: (i) insoluble progeny transported in mucus, with the mean velocities reported by Yeates et al. (83); (ii) insoluble progeny, with no clearance; and (iii) partially soluble progeny, with 30% transferred to mucosal tissue (38, 59).

7 DOSE TO LUNG TISSUES PER UNIT EXPOSURE TO RADON PROGENY

7.1 Unattached and Aerosol Fractions

The unattached and aerosol fractions of radon progeny are characterized by two bands of particle size. Unattached progeny generally vary in size from about 1 nm for free atoms to about 3 nm for small ion clusters (84), although they may occasionally form clusters as large as 10 nm (see Chapter 5). The larger aerosol fraction will always be distributed in particle size. The parameter determining lung deposition, and thus dose, is then the activity median diameter (AMD) of the particle size distribution. The aerosol AMD will depend on the source and subsequent aging characteristics in room air (85). To assess doses under all conditions it is necessary to consider a wide range of AMD. Doses are calculated below for aerosols with AMD between 0.01 μm and 0.5 μm. For this purpose it is assumed that the geometric standard deviation of the aerosol size distribution increases progressively from 1.5 for the smallest aerosol to a maximum value of 2.0 for AMD of 0.05 μm and larger (86).

The intake of potential alpha energy for an exposure E_p is given by

$$I_p = E_p B \qquad (2)$$

where B is the breathing rate.

It is assumed here that an average breathing rate of 0.75 m^3/h characterizes domestic exposure of adult males (1, 38). This is higher than the reference value for resting man (31) of 0.45 m^3/h, but lower than 0.9 m^3/h, the value adopted by NCRP (6).

Calculated doses, averaged over all epithelial cells in the bronchial and A-I regions of the lung, are shown in Figure 7.20 on logarithmic scales as a function of particle size and for exposure to 1 WLM potential alpha energy. Bronchial dose from unattached progeny changes relatively little with particle size. However, for the aerosol fraction, it decreases markedly as the aerosol size becomes larger. Doses to the A-I region are always less than 10% of those to bronchi and can safely be neglected.

Figure 7.20 shows bands of doses that reflect the impact of assumed clearance behavior and different models of airway size. For radon progeny attached to aer-

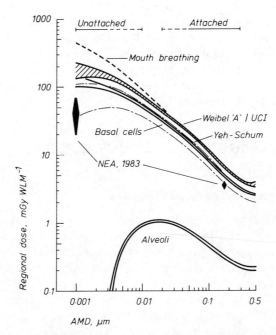

Figure 7.20. Doses averaged over all epithelial cells in the bronchial and alveolar regions of the lung per unit exposure to potential alpha energy as a function of aerosol size. Doses to basal cells and the values derived by the NEA (38) are shown for comparison.

osols, the uncertainty in calculated doses due to clearance is entirely negligible. The corresponding uncertainty in bronchial doses from unattached progeny is higher, but still only about ±30%. Doses calculated using the Weibel A or UCI airway dimensions are uniformly about 30% higher than values obtained with the Yeh-Schum model.

Figure 7.20 also shows the effect on dose of habitual mouth breathing. The maximum calculated dose, which occurs for "unattached" sizes, is twice the value for nasal breathing. This is because about half the progeny inhaled at a particle size of 1 nm (0.001 μm) are filtered by the nose, but only a small fraction would be removed by the mouth and larynx. Nasal filtration is negligible for progeny attached to aerosol particles.

The range of doses calculated when only basal cells are assumed at risk is also shown in Figure 7.20. For unattached progeny, doses are approximately one-half, and for attached progeny three-quarters, of values derived by averaging over all cells. These doses are to be compared with the range derived by the NEA (38). Reference values recommended by the NEA and adopted by UNSCEAR (1) lie at the bottom of the range of doses to basal cells derived here.

These calculations assume that the size distribution of radon progeny aerosols measured in ambient air does not change in the humid conditions of the respiratory tract. There is some evidence that such particles may grow rapidly in the nose or upper bronchi to about double their ambient size (74, 87). Table 7.7 lists values of mean dose to bronchial epithelium, obtained by weighting equally the results from all three lung models and clearance assumptions, for the two cases, where the ambient aerosol size is either maintained or doubled. These are proposed as representative values.

For aerosols in the size range 0.05–0.2 μm—the range reported for room air under normal conditions (85)—it can be concluded that mean bronchial dose is inversely proportional to the AMD. However, in absolute terms, bronchial dose from radon progeny attached to aerosols could be as low as half that indicated by the ambient aerosol size. It would be useful to resolve experimentally the degree of particle growth within the respiratory tract.

TABLE 7.7 Representative Values of Mean Bronchial Epithelial Dose from Exposure to ^{222}Rn Progeny Potential Alpha Energy in Homes

Ambient aerosol size (AMD, μm)	Dose per Unit Exposure (mGy/WLM)	
	Size maintained	Size doubled
Unattached	ca. 150	ca. 100
0.05	20	10
0.1	10	5
0.15	7	4
0.2	5	ca. 3
0.3	4	ca. 4
0.4–0.5	ca. 3	ca. 5

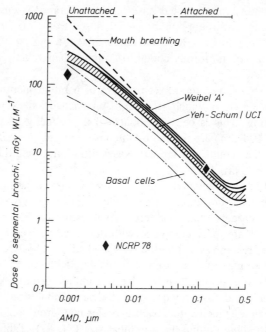

Figure 7.21. Doses averaged over epithelial cells in segmental bronchi per unit exposure to potential alpha energy. Doses derived by the NCRP (6) are shown for comparison.

The range of doses calculated for segmental bronchi (generations 3–5), rather than the average over the whole bronchial region, is shown in Figure 7.21. Doses are again averaged over all epithelial cells. In this case, the Yeh-Schum and UCI lung dimensions give similar results, whereas the Weibel A model alone gives values about 30% higher. The dose to shallow basal cells assumed by the NCRP (6) to represent exposure to the domestic aerosol (0.125 μm diameter) lies within the range of values calculated here. Figure 7.21 also shows that doses averaged over all epithelial cells in segmental bronchi are uniformly double those to basal cells only. In the case of unattached progeny, basal cell doses calculated here are similar to the value of 130 mGy/WLM assumed by the NCRP. Table 7.8 lists representative values of dose averaged over all epithelial cells in segmental bronchi, derived in the same way as those in Table 7.7 for mean bronchial epithelial dose.

It can be seen by comparing Figures 7.20 and 7.21 that doses averaged over all cells or to basal cells alone are within a factor two of each other. Table 7.7 and 7.8 show that, irrespective of aerosol size, doses in segmental bronchi are similar to the average value for the whole bronchial region. Within certain bounds, the effect of increasing the size of carrier aerosol particles (the attached radon progeny) is to reduce lung dose proportionally. The position is more complex for unattached progeny. Increasing particle size in this range serves to reduce proportionally dose

TABLE 7.8   Representative Values of Dose to Epithelium of Segmental Bronchi from Exposure to ^{222}Rn Progeny Potential Alpha Energy in Homes

Ambient aerosol size (AMD, μm)	Dose per Unit Exposure (mGy/WLM)	
	Size maintained	Size doubled
Unattached	ca. 200	ca. 100
0.05	14	7
0.1	7	4
0.15	5	3
0.2	4	ca. 3
0.3	3	ca. 4
0.4–0.5	ca. 3	—

to the segmental bronchi (Table 7.8). However, this has the effect of increasing deposition and dose in smaller airways, resulting in a relatively small overall decrease in mean dose for larger particles (Table 7.7).

7.2   Influence of Breathing Rate

Figure 7.22 relates average doses to epithelial cells at various breathing rates. Doses are normalized to values calculated at each aerosol size for the case of occupational exposure of a miner, assumed to breath at a reference (2) rate of 1.2

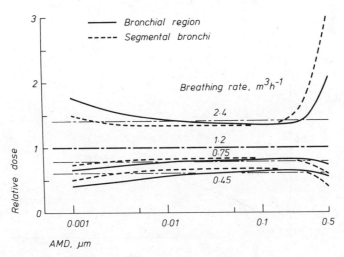

Figure 7.22. Epithelial doses in the bronchial region and segmental bronchi calculated as a function of breathing rate, relative to values for occupational exposure (e.g., uranium miners) at a breathing rate of 1.2 m^3/h.

m^3/h. Apart from the values at unusually large aerosol sizes, results for both the bronchial region as a whole and for segmental bronchi are remarkably constant at each breathing rate. They are represented well by the fine broken lines, which show values proportional to the square root of breathing rate. This relationship results from the combination of intake rate (simply proportional to breathing rate) and deposition probability—which has been shown in human subjects to be proportional to the square root of residence time in the airways when deposition occurs predominantly by diffusion (75).

It can be concluded that uncertainties or variations in breathing rate are relatively unimportant in determining lung dose and that dose varies with particle size in much the same manner over the whole physiological range of breathing rates.

7.3 Age Dependence

The main parameters influencing lung dose as a function of age are the breathing rate and lung dimensions. Adams (88) estimated breathing rates from dietary intake as a function of age. He assumed that oxygen consumption is proportional to energy expenditure, and thus dietary intake, and derived the following expression to relate the energy expenditure rate in a child of age t (years) and mass M_t (kg) to that of an adult.

$$R = (M_t/70) \exp\left[0.047(21 - t)\right] \qquad t \leq 21 \qquad (3)$$

Using this expression, with data on body weight as a function of age (89), gives the breathing rates relative to adult values shown in Figure 7.23. These correspond

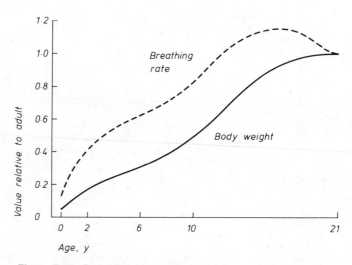

Figure 7.23. Breathing rate and body weight as a function of age.

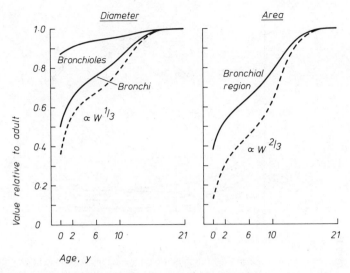

Figure 7.24. Diameters and surface areas of bronchial airways as a function of age, according to the UCI lung model.

to rates of 0.095, 0.34, 0.48, and 0.61 m³/h at birth, 2, 6, and 10 years, respectively—relative to an adult value of 0.75 m³/h. The NEA and NCRP have assumed generally lower rates of intake by children (6, 38).

The UCI lung model includes measurements of airway diameter and length throughout the bronchial tree in lungs taken from children or young adults at various ages, including neonatal specimens (33). Scaling factors for diameter and area derived from these measurements as a function of age are shown in Figure 7.24.

It is seen that the diameters of bronchioles (averaged over generations 11–15) change little with age. The increase in bronchial size is greater, but still less than might be expected if airways are simply scaled for overall body dimensions (illustrated by the dashed curves in Figure 7.24). Since bronchiolar diameter does not change much with age, it is also likely that the thickness of bronchiolar epithelium is relatively constant. However, for the bronchi it is reasonable to assume that epithelial thickness is proportional to bronchial diameter, and it is necessary to use age-dependent conversion factors between the surface density of alpha decays and dose to cells. Likewise, some assumption must be made about clearance rates as a function of age, but this is not critical. It is most reasonable to assume a constant mucous velocity, implying faster rates of clearance from shorter airways.

The effect of these considerations on mean dose to epithelial cells at various ages, relative to adult values, is shown in Figure 7.25. It is seen that the mean bronchial dose is only marginally increased in young children. This effect is smaller than the age dependence considered earlier (6, 38) and can surely be regarded as insignificant. A greater age dependence of dose to segmental bronchi emerges (Fig. 7.25), but this is still not large.

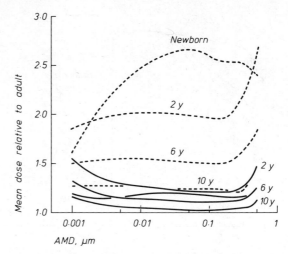

Figure 7.25. Epithelial doses in the bronchial region (solid curves) and in segmental bronchi in newborn infants and children of various ages relative to values for adults.

8   DOSES IN LUNGS AND DOSE EQUIVALENTS FOR RADON PROGENY IN HOMES AND MINES

Dose absorbed by bronchial tissue, D_B, is determined principally by the exposure to potential alpha energy, E_p, and the fraction of this energy in the unattached form, f_p. These quantities are related by the following expression.

$$D_B = E_p \left[f_p D_u + (1 - f_p) D_a \right] \tag{4}$$

where D_u and D_a are the values of dose per unit exposure to unattached and attached potential alpha energy, respectively.

Both D_u and D_a increase with breathing rate (Fig. 7.22), but relatively slightly. It is seen from Tables 7.7 and 7.8 that D_a also varies somewhat with the size of ambient aerosol and thus with environmental conditions. However, the dose per unit exposure to unattached progeny, D_u, is more than an order of magnitude greater than D_a. Just a few percent of potential alpha energy in the unattached form will therefore significantly increase the bronchial dose per unit exposure.

8.1   Reference Factors for Exposure in Homes or in Mines

The range over which the important environmental parameters may vary in homes and in mines is summarized in Table 7.9. The resulting estimates of dose conversion factors are also given, with suggested "Reference" values to characterize exposure under these different conditions.

Reineking et al. (85) studied the variation in unattached fraction of potential alpha energy, f_p, and size distribution of the aerosol fraction in a number of homes

TABLE 7.9   Ranges of Environmental Parameters in Homes and Underground Mines; Resulting Estimates of Bronchial Epithelial Dose and Proposed Reference Values for Exposure to ^{222}Rn Progeny Potential Alpha Energy

| | f_p (%) | AMD (μm) | Dose per Unit Exposure (mGy/WLM) | |
			Bronchial region	Segmental bronchi
		Home		
Range	2–15	0.02–0.2	6–26	6–27
Reference	5	0.1	ca. 13	ca. 13
		Mine		
Range	1–7	0.15–0.3	7–18	6–18
Reference	3	0.2	ca. 10	ca. 10

under different conditions. They found that the values of both parameters change substantially when strong aerosol sources are present. Smoking, cooking, or the operation of an electric motor all produce a high concentration of particles, leading to a low value of f_p of approximately 2%. Smoking and cooking also give rise to large aerosols with AMD of approximately 0.2 μm. This combination of values can be taken to define the lower bound of the dose conversion factor for room air. If intermediate values of the conversion factors D_u and D_a given in Tables 7.7 and 7.8 are assumed, this results in a lower bound estimate of 6 mGy/WLM exposure—both for epithelial dose averaged over the whole bronchial region and for dose to segmental bronchi (Table 7.9). When no strong sources of aerosol were present in room air, Reineking et al. found that f_p varied in the range 5–15%. The AMD of the aerosol fraction was then found to be about 0.1 μm. This combination of values can be taken to define an upper bound of the dose conversion factor under ordinary conditions. According to the conversion factors from Tables 7.7 and 7.8, similar values are again obtained for average bronchial dose and for dose to segmental bronchi. The ordinary upper bound is about 26 mGy/WLM when f_p is high at 15%. However, the value of f_p and thus the dose conversion factor can be even higher under "special" conditions when efficient air-cleaning devices are used (see Chapter 11).

It is difficult to specify values of f_p and aerosol AMD to "typify" indoor exposure, but values of 5% and 0.1 μm, respectively, are probably the best current estimates. These would give a conversion factor of about 13 mGy/WLM exposure for bronchial dose, with approximately half of this dose arising from unattached progeny. The values derived earlier by the NEA (38) and the NCRP (6) were shown in Table 7.6 to be lower—at about 4 and 7 mGy/WLM, respectively. In both cases, this is due mainly to the smaller dose attributed to unattached progeny. For example, the NCRP derived dose conversion factors for the unattached and aerosol fractions similar to those given in Table 7.8, but assumed an extremely low value of 1% for f_p.

The range of values for f_p and aerosol AMD shown for underground mines in Table 7.9 was estimated by the NEA (38). According to the conversion factors from Table 7.7 and 7.8, increased by 25% to allow for the higher occupational breathing rate (Section 7), this gives a band of bronchial epithelial doses from about 6 to 18 mGy/WLM exposure. Typical values of 3% for f_p (90) and 0.2 μm for the aerosol AMD (38) give an overall conversion factor to bronchial dose of about 10 mGy/WLM exposure. The value derived by NEA (38) was 6 mGy/WLM and that by NCRP was 5 mGy/WLM (Table 7.6). Again, the latter relatively low values arose from the assumption of an extreme value of 0.7% for f_p. Increasing this to 3% gives a dose conversion factor of 8 mGy/WLM, which is similar to the value given in Table 7.9.

The dosimetric analysis developed here indicates that the dose per unit exposure in homes is typically higher than that in mines, but probably only marginally so. This supports the estimate of relative doses made by the NCRP (6), but absolute values are probably about a factor two higher.

8.2 Dose Related to Radon Gas Concentration

In practice, it is often neither possible nor convenient to monitor exposure to potential alpha energy, E_p, the quantity related above to dose. However, monitoring of exposure to radon gas from the time integral of the radon concentration in air is relatively straightforward (91). Thus, the additional parameter F, known as the equilibrium factor, has been devised for practical application (1). This expresses the airborne concentration of potential alpha energy as a fraction of the highest possible value—achieved when the progeny have the same activity concentration as the measured radon gas. Thus, the potential alpha-energy concentration is 1 WL when the radon concentration is 3700 Bq/m^3, $F = 1$, and the progeny are in radioactive equilibrium with the gas. The annual exposure to potential alpha energy, E_p, is then related to the average radon concentration, C_{Rn}, by the following expression.

$$E_p[\text{WLM/y}] = \frac{8760 n F C_{Rn}}{(170)(3700)} \tag{5}$$

where C_{Rn} is in Bq/m^3; n = fraction of time spent indoors (occupancy); 8760 = number of hours per year; and 170 = number of hours per working month.

Taking n to be 0.8 (1, 38), the annual exposure to potential alpha energy is given by $0.011 \times F C_{Rn}$ in the conversion unit WLM/y per Bq/m^3.

This conversion procedure can be used with dosimetric factors chosen from Tables 7.7 and 7.8 or from elsewhere to estimate dose rates as a function of the average radon gas concentration. For that part of the exposure associated with unattached progeny, a conversion factor to average bronchial epithelial dose of 130 mGy/WLM can be assumed—with 150 mGy/WLM for segmental bronchi. For the attached fraction, a value of 0.1 μm for aerosol AMD would give respective conversion factors of about 7 and 5 mGy/WLM. The range of values of F and f_p likely to occur in room air has been modeled by Porstendörfer (9) and

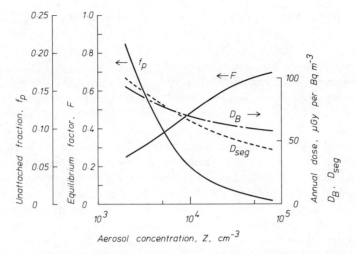

Figure 7.26. Variation of unattached fraction of potential alpha energy and equilibrium factor according to Porstendörfer's (9) model of room aerosol behavior and the effect on bronchial dose rates per unit radon gas concentration.

confirmed by other experimental studies (92). Figure 7.26 shows the variation of F and f_p found in room air, the probable relationship between these parameters, and its effect on dose per unit exposure to radon gas.

The equilibrium factor, F, generally increases with aerosol concentration (Fig. 7.26). This will lead to a proportionally higher total exposure to potential alpha energy for a given concentration of radon gas. However, the fraction of the exposure associated with unattached progeny, f_p, decreases dramatically for high F. The overall effect of these changes is that the dose rate for a given radon concentration is relatively independent of room conditions—it is not correlated with the equilibrium factor F. On this basis, a single conversion factor between radon gas concentration and bronchial dose rate can be recommended. A value of approximately 50 μGy/y per Bq/m^3 radon concentration appears to be appropriate.

8.3 Doses to Other Organs of the Body

Transfer of radon (^{222}Rn) gas and progeny from the lung gives rise to some irradiation of tissues outside the respiratory tract. However, the doses calculated for these tissues are about 2 orders of magnitude lower than that to bronchial epithelium (38, 40); they can safely be neglected for the purpose of estimating risk. Somewhat higher doses to other tissues arise from exposure to thoron (^{220}Rn) progeny, and are considered in Section 10 of this chapter.

8.4 Effective Dose Equivalent

The doses evaluated above are simply measures of the amount of energy absorbed by tissue per unit mass. However, the biological effectiveness of absorbed dose varies with the type of radiation. To represent biological effectiveness, the modified quantity "dose equivalent," is used (4). In the case of energy absorbed from alpha particles, a multiplying "quality factor" of 20 is recommended (4). Thus, an absorbed dose of 1 gray (Gy) from alpha particles is equivalent to a dose of 20 Gy from gamma rays, X rays, or beta particles. Dose modified by the quality factor is expressed in the unit sievert (Sv); thus, 1 Gy of alpha dose is represented by 20 Sv tissue dose equivalent. The quantity "tissue dose equivalent" is symbolized by H_T.

When the whole body is uniformly irradiated, for example by an external source of gamma rays, the total risk of premature death among the irradiated population and their immediate descendants is assumed by ICRP to be proportional to the dose equivalent (4). However, different organs of the body are known to vary in sensitivity. The main components of overall risk contributed by individual organs have been estimated by ICRP from various sources of human epidemiology (Chapter 8). In the case of uniform external irradiation, the ICRP considers that a fraction 0.12 of the total risk will arise from lung cancer. If the various organs of the body absorb different dose equivalents, the overall risk to the individual must be determined by weighting each component by the relative tissue sensitivity. The special concept of an "effective dose equivalent," given the symbol H_E, was developed by ICRP to place limits on the total exposure by adding all its components, from radionuclides in discrete tissues and from external exposure. Thus, the effective dose equivalent is given by the following expression:

$$H_E = \sum_T w_T H_T + H_d \qquad (6)$$

where w_T is the tissue weighting factor for tissue T; H_T is the mean tissue dose equivalent; and H_d is the dose equivalent from penetrating external radiation.

The weighting factor of 0.12 for dose equivalent to lung tissue is derived from estimates of the lifetime risk of lung cancers among atomic bomb survivors (1, 4). In this case, the alveolar and bronchial regions of the lung were each exposed to the same dose, and their relative contributions to overall risk are unimportant. However, for exposure to radon progeny bronchial tissue absorbs a high dose and alveolar tissue almost none. To assess risk for this nonuniform irradiation, the ICRP has assumed that the sensitivities of bronchial and alveolar tissue are the same—implying that half the overall weighting factor of 0.12 is contributed by each tissue (2, 93). Adopting this convention, dose absorbed from radon or thoron progeny decay in bronchial or alveolar tissue (in Gy) must be multiplied by 20 × 0.06 (by 1.2) to evaluate the contributions to effective dose equivalent (in Sv).

In terms of effective dose equivalent, the reference conversion factors between dose absorbed in the bronchial region and exposure to radon progeny, proposed in Table 7.9, become approximately 15 mSv/WLM for domestic exposure and 12 mSv/WLM for exposure in mines. The value for mines is not significantly different from that of 10 mSv/WLM adopted by ICRP (2). However, the value of 15 mSv/WLM for domestic exposure is substantially higher than that of 5 mSv/WLM adopted by UNSCEAR (1) and commonly used. In view of the uncertainties involved, it is reasonable to apply a single rounded conversion factor of 10 mSv/WLM to evaluate the effective dose equivalent for exposures in either environment.

Using Equation 5 and a typical value of the equilibrium factor, F, in the range 0.4–0.5 (1), the conversion factor between radon gas concentration in a home, averaged over a year, and the annual effective dose equivalent to the occupants is given the value 50 μSv/y per Bq/m^3. It was shown in Figure 7.26 that this value can be applied to relate radon gas concentration to dose, irrespective of the actual value of F under different conditions. For example, an average radon concentration of 20 Bq/m^3 can be converted generally to an annual effective dose equivalent of 1 mSv/y.

9 RISK ESTIMATES

9.1 Effective Dose Equivalent

The ICRP (4) evaluates risk from 1 Sv effective dose equivalent as a total likelihood of 1.65×10^{-2} of inducing a fatal malignant disease in the exposed individual or a serious hereditary defect in the individual's descendants. In the case of exposure to radon progeny, only the lung receives a significant dose—giving a likelihood of 1.65×10^{-2} per Sv of inducing lung cancer. The total risk over an individual's lifetime of premature death from lung cancer is built up from the effective dose equivalents received each year. A person exposed to radon progeny from birth at the rate of 1 mSv/y will accumulate an additional lifetime risk of approximately 60 (1.65×10^{-5}), or 0.1%, of dying from lung cancer. This value takes into account reduced effectiveness of exposure in the age range 50–70 years because of latency and competing causes of death. The overall risk from exposure to radon progeny is assumed to increase proportionally with dose and to add to other sources of risk such as smoking.

In most European and North American countries, the mean radon concentration in homes is in the range from about 20 to 60 Bq/m^3, with higher mean values of about 100 Bq/m^3 in Finland, Norway, and Sweden (1, 94). The corresponding range of lifetime risks attributed to radon progeny exposure is approximately 0.1–0.5%. These estimated risks account very approximately for between 2% and 10% of the lung cancer incidence in the respective countries.

9.2 Extrapolation from Lung Cancer Rates in Miners

Two methods can be used to estimate the risk from exposure to radon progeny in homes on the basis of the epidemiological data from mining, the so-called absolute and relative models of risk (Chapter 8). In an absolute model, it is assumed that there is no correlation between the excess rate of lung cancer induced by radiation and the normal rate of appearance of lung cancer, which is strongly related to age and smoking habit. Lung dose from radon progeny at a given age is assumed to cause, after some time lag, an excess rate of lung cancer, which remains constant in each year of remaining life. In a relative model, the assumption is made that the normal rate of appearance of lung cancer is simply increased in proportion to radiation dose. The application of this model is straightforward once the constant of proportionality has been established, but uncertainty exists whether the risk persists until the end of life. Both methods of extrapolating the lung cancer rates seen in miners to the general population have been reviewed by a Task Group of the ICRP (94).

9.2.1 *Absolute Risk.*

The ICRP Task Group considered the best current estimate of the absolute rate of lung cancer incidence in miners, related to radon progeny exposure, to be 10^{-5}/y per WLM. They reduced this value slightly to allow for the small additional doses contributed by external gamma rays and inhalation of ore dusts in mine environments, yielding an estimate of 8×10^{-6}/y per WLM attributable to radon progeny (94). Two further factors must be considered to derive a risk estimate for domestic exposure: the different age distributions of miners and the general population and any difference in doses per unit exposure. The effect of population age distribution is to increase marginally the estimate of risk—the longer time available to express lung cancers caused by irradiation in childhood is largely offset by incomplete expression of risk from irradiation in middle and old age. The ICRP considered the dose per unit exposure in homes to be 80% of that in mines. This gives a projected lifetime risk of 1.1% for an exposure to radon progeny of 1 WLM each year in the home.

The revised dosimetry given in Section 8 (Table 7.9) indicates that dose per unit exposure is similar or even slightly higher in homes than in mines, leading to a somewhat higher risk estimate of 1.5% from domestic exposure at the rate of 1 WLM/y. Using Equation 5, this can be converted to an estimate of 1.5% risk from lifetime exposure in a home to a radon gas concentration of 200 Bq/m^3. The value so obtained reinforces the estimate of 1% derived above purely on the bases of lung dosimetry and the standard ICRP risk factors (4).

9.2.2 *Relative Risk*

The ICRP Task Group (94) estimated the proportional increase in the normal rate of appearance of lung cancer among miners to be 0.8%/WLM exposure to radon progeny. For domestic exposure of adults they reduced this estimate to 0.64%/WLM on dosimetric grounds and assumed a factor 3 higher risk from exposure in childhood. On the basis of the revised dosimetry given here, such a reduction for adults is not justified. The adult value would be increased marginally, to give an estimated 1% increase in lung cancer rate per WLM exposure. For domestic exposure at the rate of 1 WLM/y integrated over a lifetime (or for chronic exposure to a radon concentration of 200 Bq/m^3), this would approximately double the normal rate of lung cancer (94). However, this estimated risk factor attributable to radon may well be too high—the incremental value of 1% each year per WLM exposure assumes that the effect of exposure early in life is maintained through to old age, when most lung cancers occur. It is probably more realistic to consider the effect of radon exposure to be limited to a shorter period of, say, 40 years. The ICRP Task Group's model then gives an estimated risk from exposure over a whole lifetime about a factor 3 lower (C. R. Muirhead, National Radiological Protection Board, personal communication). The chronic radon progeny exposure needed to double the normal rate of lung cancer may therefore be estimated to lie in the range 1–3 WLM/y (corresponding to 200–600 Bq/m^3 chronic radon concentration). The ICRP considers the approach of modeling relative risk to be the most appropriate for estimating lung cancer rates in sections of the population with different normal incidences of lung cancer: that is, in men compared with women and in smokers compared with nonsmokers (94).

9.3 Interaction with Smoking

Smoking may affect bronchial clearance, but this was shown in Section 7 to have a very small effect on lung dose. Smoking may also cause changes in the thickness of mucus and of bronchial epithelium. Since the relevant dose is now considered to be the average over all epithelial cells, including superficial and not just basal cells, changes in the tissue induced by smoking are not likely to affect the dose per unit exposure markedly. The overriding interaction with smoking is therefore the multiplicative effect of dose from radon progeny on the much higher incidence of lung cancer experienced by smokers (7). This is quantified by the relative-risk approach to modeling (94).

The ICRP Task Group considered the baseline frequency of lung cancer in nonsmokers to be 80 cases/10^6 persons per year, averaged over both sexes. This gives a lifetime expectation of lung cancer among nonsmokers of about 0.6%, which may vary between countries by about a factor 2 either way. Chronic exposure in the home to a radon concentration of 200 Bq/m^3 (equivalent to 1 WLM/y or 10 mSv/y) is estimated above to increase the normal risk of lung cancer by at least one-third and possibly to double it. On the basis of the epidemiological data from mining, therefore, the risk for nonsmokers attributable to radon progeny exposure at this rate is estimated to lie in the range 0.2–0.6%. This range corresponds to between one-fifth and about one-half the value derived purely from dosimetric analysis and the standard ICRP risk factors (4).

The normal incidence of lung cancer in smokers may be 10–20 times higher than that in nonsmokers. The multiplicative concept of relative risk implies an additional incidence of lung cancer in smokers due to radon exposure that is higher in the same proportion. The lifetime risk for smokers attributable to chronic exposure of 1 WLM/y may therefore have a lower bound in the range 2–4%, which is between about two times and four times higher than that derived purely from dosimetry. If the effect of radon exposure early in life were maintained through to old age, these estimated risk values for smokers would be increased.

10 THORON PROGENY

There is relatively little information on the characteristics of the thoron progeny aerosol in room air and the degree of radioactive equilibrium. The first progeny,

Po-216, will always be close to equilibrium with thoron gas, because of its very short half-life (0.16 s). The second progeny, Pb-212, will not approach equilibrium with thoron, because its half-life of 10.6 h is much longer than the effective rate of removal from room air by ventilation or loss to surfaces. Estimates of the activity of Pb-212 in indoor air relative to that of thoron gas have ranged from approximately 2% (38, 95) to about 10% (96). The activity of the third progeny, Bi-212 (half-life 61 min), again will be only a fraction of that of its parent. In general, therefore, more than 90% of the potential alpha energy associated with thoron progeny in indoor air is carried by Pb-212. Although the activity concentration of Po-216 may be 50 times higher, the associated fraction of potential alpha energy is minute and the dosimetric consequence of inhaling this activity (even as unattached particles) is negligible. The quantity related primarily to dose is the intake of potential alpha energy in air (38). The annual exposure to potential alpha energy can be related adequately to the mean activity concentration of Pb-212 in the air by the following expression:

$$E_p[\text{WLM/y}] = \frac{8760 n C_{\text{Pb-212}}}{(170)(300)} \tag{7}$$

where $C_{\text{Pb-212}}$ is in Bq/m^3; n = fraction of time spent indoors (occupancy); 8760 = number of hours per year; 170 = number of hours per working month; and 300 = number of Bq/m^3 Pb-212 per WL.

Taking n to be 0.8, the annual exposure to potential alpha energy is given as 0.14 WLM/y per Bq/m^3 Pb-212 concentration. The average concentration of Pb-212 in indoor air may be typically about one-fortieth that of radon gas (1). In this case, comparison of Equations 5 and 7 indicates that, on average, exposures to potential alpha energy from thoron progeny are roughly half those to the radon progeny. A mean ratio of about 0.6 has been reported from measurements in homes (96). See Chapter 1, Section 8.4 for further discussion.

10.1 Dose Conversion Factors

10.1.1 Lung Doses. Doses to lung tissue calculated for 1 WLM exposure to thoron progeny, according to the models applied above (Section 7), are shown in Table 7.10. The range of aerosol size considered is that of the thoron progeny likely to be found in indoor air (38). The size of unattached Pb-212 particles is expected to be similar to that of the radon progeny, Po-218 (Chapter 6). However, the thoron progeny are generally expected to be attached to a larger aerosol than radon progeny (Table 7.9), because of the longer time available for particle coagulation. It is likely that the ambient Pb-212 aerosol has an activity median diameter (AMD) in the range 0.2–0.3 μm (38, 40).

Table 7.10 gives conversion factors between exposure in the home (at an adult breathing rate of 0.75 m^3/h) and (i) the mean dose to epithelial cells throughout the bronchial region; (ii) the mean dose to A-I tissue; and (iii) the mean dose to epithelial cells in the segmental bronchi. The range of values given for a particular

TABLE 7.10 Representative Values of Bronchial Epithelial and Alveolar Doses from Exposure to Thoron (^{220}Rn) Progeny Potential Alpha Energy in Homes

Ambient aerosol size (AMD, μm)	Dose per Unit Exposure (mGy/WLM)		
	Bronchial region	Alveolar-interstitial region	Segmental bronchi
Unattached (Pb-212)	ca. 25	0	ca. 40
0.2	3–1.5	ca. 0.1	2–1.5
0.3	2–1.5	ca. 0.1	ca. 1.5

aerosol size takes into account the possibility that the ambient aerosol may double in size within the respiratory tract (74, 87). The variation in estimates based on different anatomical lung models (28, 29, 33) is not shown, but amounts to about $\pm 20\%$. The possible variation in bronchial doses due to clearance behavior is somewhat larger. In the extreme case of no clearance (mucous stasis) the bronchial doses would be about 50% higher than those shown in Table 7.10 for exposure to the aerosol fraction and substantially higher for the unattached fraction of exposure.

It is seen from Table 7.10 that dose to the A-I region from thoron progeny can be neglected in comparison with that to bronchial tissue. These bronchial doses are less than one-third of the doses given in Tables 7.7 and 7.8 for 1 WLM exposure to radon progeny. The conversion factors to dose averaged over the bronchial region for thoron progeny are approximately 25 mGy/WLM for the unattached fraction of potential alpha energy and 2 mGy/WLM for the aerosol fraction. Assuming an unattached fraction of 2%, the overall conversion factor is approximately 2.5 mGy/WLM. It can be shown that this value increases approximately in proportion to the square root of the breathing rate, as discussed for radon progeny in Section 7.

The corresponding contribution to effective dose equivalent from 1 WLM exposure to thoron progeny is approximately 3 mSv/WLM. In terms of the average concentration of Pb-212 in indoor air, the effective dose equivalent contributed each year by lung irradiation is approximately 0.4 mSv/y per Bq m^{-3} (see Equation 7).

10.1.2 Doses to Other Tissues.
Because of its long radioactive half-life, a substantial proportion of the Pb-212 activity deposited in the alveolar-interstitium can be absorbed into the blood and carried to other organs of the body. This can be taken up and retained by various organs, where decay of the subsequent progeny, Bi-212, will irradiate tissue with alpha particles. It is therefore more important with thoron progeny to assess doses absorbed by tissues outside the lung to evaluate all components of the effective dose equivalent than was the case for radon progeny.

The rate at which Pb ions are absorbed from human lung into the blood has been determined. It corresponds to a biological half-time of about 10 h (76–78).

This is similar to the radioactive half-life of Pb-212 and will result in absorption into the blood of approximately half the activity deposited in the alveolar-interstitium. From Figure 7.16, the fraction of inhaled Pb-212 activity deposited in the alveolar-interstitium is approximately 10% (for an aerosol AMD in the range 0.2–0.5 μm). Thus, it can be assumed that about 5% of inhaled Pb-212 is absorbed into the blood. The ICRP has estimated that Pb is transferred relatively rapidly by the blood to other tissues (with a half-time of 6 h) (97), so that approximately two-thirds of the Pb-212 activity entering the blood (or 3% of the inhaled activity) is taken up by these tissues. Of this, fractions 0.55, 0.25, and 0.02 are considered to concentrate in the skeleton, liver, and kidneys, respectively (38, 97), where complete decay will occur through the progeny Bi-212.

Doses to these tissues can be calculated using the standard ICRP models (3). Thus, in the skeleton, Pb-212 is assumed to deposit uniformly over all bone surfaces. Half of the alpha particles from decay of the progeny Bi-212 are assumed to irradiate sensitive cells in the marrow cavities of bone; the other half harmlessly irradiate bone mineral. Half the energy of alpha particles emitted into the marrow cavities is assumed to be absorbed in the thin layer of tissue lining the bone surface; for adult man, the mass of bone surface tissue is taken to be 0.12 kg. The remaining energy (one-quarter of that from all alpha decays in bone) is absorbed in red bone marrow, where dose is averaged over a total mass of 1.5 kg. The mass of the liver is taken to be 1.8 kg and that of the kidneys 0.31 kg. The calculated values of absorbed doses per unit exposure, expressed in mGy/WLM, the tissue weighting factors recommended by ICRP (4), and the resulting contributions from each tissue to effective dose equivalent (see Equation 6) are given in Table 7.11.

The values of dose for individual tissues, given in Table 7.11, are all small compared with that of about 2.5 mGy/WLM for bronchial epithelium. Furthermore, the contribution to effective dose equivalent from all tissues outside the lung is negligible compared with that from bronchial irradiation. The dose conversion factors given in Table 7.11 correspond to about one-quarter of those derived elsewhere for occupational exposure at a breathing rate of 1.2 m^3/h (40, 98). This difference arises simply from the combination of higher intake per unit exposure, which is proportional to breathing rate (factor 1.6×), and a higher fractional deposition assumed for the alveolar-interstitium (factor 2.5×).

TABLE 7.11 Values of Doses and Effective Dose Equivalents for Tissues Outside the Lung from Exposure to Thoron (^{220}Rn) Progeny Potential Alpha Energy in Homes

Tissue	Absorbed dose (mGy/ WLM)	w_T	Effective dose equivalent (mSv/WLM)
Bone surface	0.09	0.03	0.05
Red bone marrow	0.007	0.12	0.02
Liver	0.01	0.06	0.01
Kidney	0.005	0.06	0.006
Total	—	—	ca. 0.1

10.2 Risk Estimates

The risk of lung cancer from domestic exposure to thoron progeny can be estimated directly from the effective dose equivalent, which is approximately 3 mSv/WLM (0.4 mSv/y per Bq/m^3 Pb-212). Alternatively, risk can be assessed relative to that from exposure to radon progeny, on the basis of the relative doses to bronchial epithelium. The value of 2.5 mGy/WLM estimated for thoron progeny is approximately one-fifth of that estimated for radon progeny (Table 7.9). The risk that lung cancer will be induced by thoron progeny is therefore projected to be about one-fifth that from the same exposure to radon progeny.

11 SUMMARY

1. Consideration of the variety of lung cancer types in miners exposed to radon progeny and their similarity to lung cancers in the general population indicates that various types of cell in the bronchial epithelium are at risk. This implies that dose averaged over the whole epithelial thickness is relevant to the induction of lung cancer and not just that to deep-lying basal cells, as generally assumed historically.

2. Sufficient data are available on deposition of aerosol particles in human lung to improve procedures for modeling; lung deposition of radon and thoron progeny can now be modeled realistically for a range of breathing conditions, subject age, and aerosol characteristics.

3. Application of improved dosimetric models to recent data on the range of aerosol characteristics in homes, which indicate for radon progeny a significant fraction of potential alpha energy in the unattached state, points to an increased estimate of the conversion factor between exposure and bronchial dose.

4. It is likely that the dose from a given exposure to radon progeny in homes is similar to or marginally higher than that in mine atmospheres. The corresponding lifetime risks from exposure are probably similar for the two environments. These can be evaluated by converting an exposure of 1 WLM potential alpha energy to an effective dose equivalent of 10 mSv. Dose for a given exposure is not significantly higher in children than in adults.

5. Consideration of the inverse relationship between the unattached fraction of potential alpha energy in room air and the degree of radioactive equilibrium between radon gas and its progeny indicates that dose is closely related to the concentration of radon gas averaged over a period of exposure. This has beneficial implications for domestic and occupational monitoring schemes. The annual effective dose equivalent can be assessed from the average concentration of radon gas in a home, using the conversion factor 20 Bq/m^3 is equivalent to 1 mSv/y.

6. It is likely that the risk from exposure to thoron progeny is about one-fifth of that from radon progeny, per unit potential alpha energy. Only bronchial epithelium is irradiated significantly in both cases, leading to an increased risk of lung cancer.

REFERENCES

1. United Nations Scientific Committee on the Effects of Atomic Radiation (1982). *Ionizing Radiation: Sources and Biological Effects*, Annex D, Report to the General Assembly, UN, New York, p. 141.

2. International Commission on Radiological Protection (1981). *Limits for Inhalation of Radon Daughters by Workers*, ICRP publication 32, *Ann. of ICRP*, **6**(1).

3. International Commission on Radiological Protection (1979). *Limits on Intakes of Radionuclides by Workers*, ICRP publication 30, Part 1, *Ann. of ICRP*, **2**(3/4).

4. International Commission on Radiological Protection (1977). *Recommendations of the International Commission on Radiological Protection*, ICRP Publication 26, *Ann. of ICRP*, **1**(3).

5. James, A. C. (1984). Dosimetric approaches to risk assessment for indoor exposure to radon daughters, *Radiat. Prot. Dosim.*, **7**, 353.

6. National Council on Radiation Protection and Measurements (1984). *Evaluation of Occupational and Environmental Exposures to Radon and Radon Daughters in the United States*, NCRP report no. 78, Bethesda, MD.

7. Jacobi, W., and Paretzke, H. G. (1985). Risk assessment for indoor exposure to radon daughters, *Sci. Total Environ.*, **45**, 551.

8. Ellett, W. H., and Nelson, N. S. (1985). Epidemiology and risk assessment. In R. B. Gammage and S. V. Kaye (eds.), *Indoor Air and Human Health*, Lewis, Chelsea, p. 79.

9. Porstendörfer, J. (1984). Behaviour of radon daughter products in indoor air, *Radiat. Prot. Dosim.*, **7**, 107.

10. Royal College of Physicians (1983). *Health or Smoking?* Pitman, London.

11. Doll, R., and Peto, R. (1981). The causes of cancer: Quantitative estimates of avoidable risks of cancer in the United States today, *J. Natl. Cancer Inst.*, **66**, 1191.

12. Schneiderman, M. A., Découfle, P., and Brown, C. C. (1979). Thresholds for environmental cancer, biologic and statistical considerations. *Ann. NY Acad. Sci.*, **329**, 92.

13. Peto R., and Doll, R. (1985). The control of lung cancer, *New Scientist*, no. 1440, 26.

14. Spencer, H. (1977). *Pathology of the Lung*, Pergamon, Oxford.

15. Kreyberg, L. (1967). Histological typing of lung tumours. In *International Histological Classification of Tumours*, no. 1, World Health Organisation, Geneva, p. 1.

16. World Health Organisation (1981). Histological typing of lung tumours. In *International Histological Classification of Tumours*, no. 1, 2nd ed., Geneva.

17. Percy, C., and Sobin, L. (1983). Surveillance, epidemiology and end result lung cancer data applied to the World Health Organisation's classifications of lung tumors, *J. Natl. Cancer Inst.*, **70**, 663.

18. Saccomanno, G., Archer, V. E., Saunders, R. P., James, L. A., and Beckler, P. A. (1964). Lung cancer of uranium miners on the Colorado Plateau, *Health Phys.*, **10**, 1195.

19. Saccomanno, G., Archer, V. E., Auerbach, O., Kuschner, M., Egger, M., Wood, S., and Mick, R. (1982). Age factor in histological type of lung cancer among uranium miners, a preliminary report. In M. Gomez (ed.), *Radiation Hazards in Mining: Control, Measurement and Medical Aspects*, Soc. Mining Engrs., New York, p. 675.

20. Greenberg, E. R., Korson, R., Baker, J. Barrett, J., Baron, J.A., and Yates, J. (1984). Incidence of lung cancer by cell type: A population-based study in New Hampshire and Vermont, *J. Natl. Cancer Inst.*, **72**, 599.

21. Masse, R. (1984). Cells at risk. In H. Smith and G. Gerber (eds.), *Lung Modelling for Inhalation of Radioactive Materials*, Commission of the European Communities, EUR-9384, Brussels, p. 227.

22. Jeffery, P. K. and Reid, L. M. (1977). The respiratory mucous membrane. In J. D. Brain, D. F. Proctor, and L. M. Reid (eds.), *Respiratory Defence Mechanisms*, Part I, Dekker, New York, p. 193.

23. Gil, J. (1982). Comparative morphology and ultrastructure of the airways. In H. Witschi and P. Nettesheim (eds.), *Mechanisms in Respiratory Toxicology*, Vol. I, CRC Press, Boca Raton, FL, p. 3.

24. Phalen, R. F. (1984). *Inhalation Studies: Foundations and Techniques*, CRC Press, Boca Raton, FL, Chapter 2.

25. Trump, B. F., McDowell, E. M., Glavin, F., Barrett, L. A., Becci, P., Schurch, W., Kaiser, H. C., and Harris, C. C. (1978). The respiratory epithelium IV. Histogenesis of epidermoid metaplasia and carcinoma in situ in the human, *J. Natl. Cancer Inst.*, **61**, 563.

26. Saccomanno, G. (1982). Cancer of the lung in uranium miners. In M. Gomez (ed.), *Radiation Hazards in Mining: Control, Measurement and Medical Aspects*, Soc. Mining Engrs., New York, p. 203.

27. Raabe, O. G. (1982). Deposition and clearance of inhaled aerosols. In H. Witschi and P. Nettesheim (eds.), *Mechanisms in Respiratory Toxicology*, Vol. I, CRC Press, Boca Raton, FL, p. 27.

28. Weibel, E. R. (1963). *Morphometry of the Human Lung*, Academic Press, New York.

29. Yeh, H. C., and Schum, G. M. (1980). Models of human lung airways and their application to inhaled particle deposition, *Bull. Math. Biol.*, **42**, 461.

30. Yu, C. P., and Diu, C. K. (1982). A comparative study of aerosol deposition in different lung models, *Am. Ind. Hyg. Assoc. J.*, **43**, 54.

31. International Commission on Radiological Protection (1975). *Reference Man*, ICRP publication 23, Pergamon, Oxford.

32. Hughes, J. M. B., Hoppin, F. G., and Mead, J. (1972). Effect of lung inflation on bronchial length and diameter in excised lungs, *J. Appl. Physiol.*, **32**, 25.

33. Phalen, R. F., Oldham, M. J., Beaucage, C. B., Crocker, T. T., and Mortensen, J. D. (1985). Postnatal enlargement of human tracheobronchial airways and implications for particle deposition, *Anat. Rec.*, **212**, 368.

34. Gastineau, R. M., Walsh, P. J., and Underwood, N. (1972). Thickness of bronchial epithelium with relation to exposure to radon, *Health Phys.*, **23**, 857.

35. Wise, K. (1982). Dose conversion factors for radon daughters in underground and open-cut mine atmospheres, *Health Phys.*, **43**, 53.

36. Haque, A. K. M. M. (1967). Energy expended by alpha particles in lung tissue II. A computer method of calculation, *Br. J. Appl. Phys.*, **18**, 657.

37. Harley, N. H. (1971). Spatial distribution of radon daughter and plutonium-239 alpha lung dose based on experimental energy absorption measurements, Ph.D. thesis, New York University, New York.

38. Nuclear Energy Agency Group of Experts (1983). *Dosimetry Aspects of Exposure to Radon and Thoron Daughter Products*, OECD, Paris.

39. Armstrong, T. W., and Chandler, K. C. (1973). SPAR, a FORTRAN program for computing stopping powers and ranges for muons, charged pions and heavy ions, report ORNL-4869, Oak Ridge National Laboratory, Oak Ridge, TN.

40. Jacobi, W., and Eisfeld, K. (1980). Dose to tissues and effective dose equivalent by inhalation of radon-222, radon-220 and their short-lived daughters, GSF report S-626, Gesellschaft für Strahlen-und Umweltforschung, Munich-Neuherberg, West Germany.

41. Hofmann, W. (1982). Cellular lung dose for inhaled radon decay products as a base for radiation-induced lung cancer risk assessment: I: Calculation of mean cellular doses, *Radiat. Environ. Biophys.*, **20**, 95.

42. Harley, N. H., and Pasternack, B. S. (1982). Environmental radon daughter alpha dose factors in a five-lobed human lung, *Health Phys.*, **42**, 789.

43. Evans, R. D., and Goodman, C. (1940). Determination of the thoron content of air and its bearing on lung cancer hazards in industry, *J. Ind. Hyg. Toxicol.*, **22**, 89.

44. Evans, R. D. (1981). Inception of standards for internal emitters, radon and radium, *Health Phys.*, **41**, 437.

45. International Commission on Radiological Protection (1959). *Permissible Dose for Internal Irradiation*, ICRP publication 2, Pergamon, Oxford.

46. Chamberlain, A. C., and Dyson, E. D. (1956). The dose to the trachea and bronchi from the decay products of radon and thoron, *Br. J. Radiol.*, **29**, 317.

47. Altshuler, B., Nelson, N., and Kuschner, M. (1964). Estimation of lung tissue dose from the inhalation of radon and daughters, *Health Phys.*, **10**, 1137.

48. Jacobi, W. (1964). The dose to the human respiratory tract by inhalation of short-lived Rn-222 and Rn-220 decay products, *Health Phys.*, **10**, 1163.

49. Haque, A. K. M. M., and Collinson, A. J. L. (1967). Radiation dose to the respiratory system due to radon and its daughter products, *Health Phys.*, **13**, 431.

50. Walsh, P. J. (1970). Radiation dose to the respiratory tract of uranium miners—A review of the literature, *Environ. Res.*, **3**, 14.

51. Jacobi, W. (1972). Relations between the inhaled potential alpha-energy of Rn-222 and Rn-220 daughters and the absorbed alpha-energy in the bronchial and pulmonary lung, *Health Phys.*, **23**, 3.

52. Harley, N. H., and Pasternack, B. S. (1972). Alpha absorption measurements applied to lung dose from radon daughters, *Health Phys.*, **23**, 771.

53. McPherson, R. B. (1980). Environmental radon and radon daughter dosimetry in the respiratory tract, *Health Phys.*, **39**, 929.

54. Hofmann, W. (1982). Personal characteristics and environmental factors influencing lung dosimetry of inhaled radon decay products. In M. Gomez (ed.), *Radiation Hazards in Mining: Control, Measurement and Medical Aspects*, Soc. Mining Engrs., New York, p. 669.

55. James, A. C., Jacobi, W., and Steinhäusler, F. (1982). Respiratory tract dosimetry of radon and thoron daughters: The state-of-the-art and implications for epidemiology and radiobiology. In. M. Gomez (ed.), *Radiation Hazards in Mining: Control, Measurement and Medical Aspects*, Soc. Mining Engrs., New York, p. 42.

56. Bale, W. F. (1980). Memorandum to the files, March 14, 1951: Hazards associated with radon and thoron, *Health Phys.*, **38**, 1061.

57. Ingham, D. B. (1975). Diffusion of aerosols from a stream flowing through a cylindrical tube, *Aerosol Sci.*, **6**, 125.

58. Martin, D., and Jacobi, W. (1972). Diffusion of small-sized particles in the bronchial tree, *Health Phys.*, **23**, 23.

59. James, A. C. (1985). Dosimetric assessment of risk from exposure to radioactivity in mine air. In H. Stocker (ed.), *Occupational Radiation Safety in Mining*, Vol. 2, Canadian Nuclear Assoc., Toronto, p. 415.

60. Cohen, B. S., Harley, N. H., Schlesinger, R. B., and Lippmann, M. (in press). Non-uniform particle deposition on tracheobronchial airways: Implications for lung dosimetry, *Ann. Occup. Hyg.*

61. Pich, J. (1972). Theory of gravitational deposition of particles from laminar flow in channels, *Aerosol Sci.*, **3**, 351.

62. Heyder, J., and Gebhart, J. (1977). Gravitational deposition of particles from laminar aerosol flows through inclined circular tubes, *J. Aerosol Sci.*, **8**, 289.

63. Egan, M. J., and Nixon, W. (1985). A model of aerosol deposition in the lung for use in inhalation dose assessments, *Radiat. Prot. Dosim.*, **11**, 5.

64. Schlesinger, R. B., Gurman, J. L., and Lippman, M. (1982). Particle deposition within the bronchial airways: Comparisons using constant and cyclic inspiratory flows, *Ann. Occup. Hyg.*, **26**, 47.

65. Heyder, J., Armbruster, L., Gebhart, J., Grein, E., and Stahlhofen, W. (1975). Total deposition of aerosol particles in the human respiratory tract for nose and mouth breathing, *J. Aerosol Sci.*, **6**, 311.

66. Altshuler, B. (1959). Calculation of regional deposition of aerosol in the respiratory tract, *Bull. Math. Biophys.*, **21**, 257.

67. Altshuler, B. (1969). Behaviour of airborne particles in the respiratory tract. In G. E. W. Wolstenholme and J. Knight (eds.), *Circulatory and Respiratory Mass Transport*, Churchill, London, p. 215.

68. Rudolf, G., Gebhart, J., Heyder, J., Schiller, C., and Stahlhofen, W. (1986). An empirical formula describing aerosol deposition in man for any particle size, *J. Aerosol Sci.*, **17**, 350.

69. Tu, K. W., and Knutson, E. O. (1985). Total deposition of ultrafine hydrophobic and hygroscopic aerosols in the human respiratory tract, *Aerosol Sci. Technol.*, **3**, 453.

70. Schiller, C., Gebhart, J., Heyder, J., Rudolf, G., and Stahlhofen, W. (in press). Deposition of monodisperse insoluble aerosol particles in the 0.005 to 0.2 μm size range within the human respiratory tract, *Ann. Occup. Hyg.*

71. Schiller, C. (1985). Diffusionsabscheidung von Aerosolteilchen im Atemtrakt des Menshen, Ph.D. thesis, J.W. Goethe-Universität, Frankfurt/Main, West Germany.

72. Egan, M. J., and Nixon, W. (in press). Mathematical modelling of fine particle deposition in the respiratory system. In W. Hofmann (ed.), *Proc. 2nd Int. Symp. on Deposition and Clearance of Aerosols in the Human Respiratory Tract*, Int. Gesellschaft für Aerosole in der Medizin, Salzburg, Austria.

73. Taulbee, D. B., and Yu, C. P. (1975). A theory of aerosol deposition in the human respiratory tract, *J. Appl. Physiol.*, **38**, 77.

74. George, A. C., and Breslin, A. J. (1969). Deposition of radon daughters in humans exposed to uranium mine atmospheres, *Health Phys.*, **17**, 115.

75. Gebhart, J., and Heyder, J. (1985). Removal of aerosol particles from stationary air within porous media, *J. Aerosol Sci.*, **16**, 175.

76. Jacobi, W., Aurand, K., and Schraub, A. (1957). The radiation exposure of the or-

ganism by inhalation of naturally occurring radioactive aerosols. In G. C. de Hevesy, A. G. Forssberg, and J. D. Abbott (eds.), *Advances in Radiobiology*, Oliver and Boyd, Edinburgh, p. 310.

77. Booker, D. V., Chamberlain, A. C., Newton, D., and Stott, A. N. B. (1969). Uptake of radioactive lead following inhalation and injection. *Br. J. Radiol.*, **42**, 457.

78. Hursh, J. B., and Mercer, T. T. (1970). Measurement of the Pb-212 loss rate from human lungs, *J. Appl. Physiol.*, **28**, 268.

79. Bianco, A., Gibb, F.R., and Morrow, P. E. (1974). Inhalation study of a submicron size lead-212 aerosol. In *Proc. 3rd Int. Congress of the International Radiological Protection Association*, CONF-730907, United States Atomic Energy Commission, Washington, DC, p. 1214.

80. Pohl, E. (1965). Biophysikalische untersuchungen uber die inkorporation der naturlich radioaktiven emanation und desen zerfallsprodukte, *Sitzungsber Osterr. akad. Wiss. Wien IIA*, **174**, 309.

81. Morken, D. A., and Scott, J. K. (1966). The effects on mice of continual exposure to radon and its decay products on dust, report UR-669, University of Rochester, Rochester, NY.

82. Greenhalgh, J. R., Birchall, A., James, A. C., Smith, H., and Hodgson, A. (1982). Differential retention of Pb-212 ions and insoluble particles in nasal mucosa in the rat, *Phys. Med. Biol.*, **27**, 837.

83. Yeates, D. B., Gerrity, T. R., and Garrard, C. S. (1982). Characteristics of tracheobronchial deposition and clearance in man, *Ann. Occup. Hyg.*, **26**, 245.

84. Raes, F. (1985). Description of the properties of unattached Po-218 and Pb-212 particles by means of the classical theory of cluster formation, *Health Phys.*, **49**, 1177.

85. Reineking, A., Becker, K. H., and Porstendörfer, J. (1985). Measurements of the unattached fractions of radon daughters in houses, *Sci. Total Environ.*, **45**, 261.

86. Davies, C. N. (1974). The size distribution of atmospheric particles, *Aerosol Sci.*, **5**, 293.

87. Martonen, T. B., and Patel, M. (1981). Modelling the dose distribution of H_2SO_4 aerosols in the human tracheobronchial tree, *Am. Ind. Hyg. Assoc. J.*, **42**, 453.

88. Adams, N. (1981). Dependence on age at intake of committed dose equivalents from radionuclides, *Phys. Med. Biol.*, **26**, 1019.

89. Altman, P. L., and Dittmer, D. S. (1972). *Biology Data Book*, Vol. 1, Federation of American Societies for Experimental Biology, Bethesda, MD, p. 195.

90. Stranden, E., and Berteig, L. (1982). Radon daughter equilibrium and unattached fraction in mine atmospheres, *Health Phys.*, **42**,, 479.

91. Nuclear Energy Agency Group of Experts (1985). *Metrology and Monitoring of Radon, Thoron and Their Daughter Products*, OECD, Paris.

92. Vanmarcke, H., Janssens, A., and Raes, F. (1985). The equilibrium of attached and unattached radon daughters in the domestic environment, *Sci. Total Environ.*, **45**, 251.

93. Cross, F. T., and Bair, W. (1984). Mean dose versus local dose to the respiratory tract: Implications for radiological protection. In H. Smith and G. Gerber (eds.), *Lung Modelling for Inhalation of Radioactive Materials*, EUR-9384, Commission of the European Communities, Brussels, p. 303.

94. International Commission on Radiological Protection (1987). *Lung Cancer Risk from*

Environmental Exposures to Radon Daughters, Report of a Task Group, ICRP publication 50, *Ann. of ICRP*, **17**(1).

95. Steinhäusler, F. (1975). Long term measurements of ^{222}Rn, ^{220}Rn, ^{214}Pb and ^{212}Pb concentrations in the air of private and public buildings and their dependence on meteorological conditions, *Health Phys.*, **29**, 705.

96. Schery, S. D. (1985). Measurements of airborne ^{212}Pb and ^{220}Rn at varied indoor locations within the United States, *Health Phys.*, **49**, 1061.

97. International Commission on Radiological Protection (1980). *Limits for Intakes of Radionuclides by Workers*, ICRP publication 30, suppl. to Part 2, *Ann. of ICRP*, **5**(1-6).

98. Jacobi, W., and Eisfeld, K. (1982). Internal dosimetry of radon-222, radon-220 and their short-lived daughters. In K. G. Vohra, U. C. Mishra, K. C. Pillai, and S. Sadasivan (eds.), *Natural Radiation Environment*, Wiley Eastern, New Delhi, p. 131.

▬ 8

Epidemiological Evidence of Radon-Induced Health Risks

F. STEINHÄUSLER

Institut für Allgemeine Biologie, Biochemie und Biophysik, Universität Salzburg, Salzburg, Austria

Whoever wishes to investigate medicine properly should proceed thus: in the first place to consider the seasons of the year, and what effects each of them produces. Then the winds, the hot and the cold, especially such as are common to all countries, and then such as are peculiar to each locality. In the same manner, when one comes into a city to which he is a stranger, he should consider its situation, how it lies as to the winds and the rising of the sun; for its influence is not the same whether it lies to the north or the south, to the rising or to the setting sun. One should consider most attentively the waters which the inhabitants use, whether they be marshy and soft, or hard and running from elevated and rocky situations, and then if saltish and unfit for cooking; and the ground, whether it be naked and deficient in water, or wooded and well watered, and whether it lies in a hollow, confined situation, or is elevated and cold; and the mode in which the inhabitants live, and what are their pursuits, whether they are fond of drinking and eating to excess, and given to indolence, or are fond of exercise and labor.

HIPPOCRATES, On Air, Waters and Places

1 INPUT DATA REQUIRED FOR EPIDEMIOLOGICAL STUDIES RELATED TO RADON EXPOSURE

1.1 Introduction

Epidemiology can be defined as the investigation of those parameters which determine the distribution and the frequency of occurrence of a given disease in defined human population subgroups (1). It uses input data from a wide range of subjects, including the following (2–4):

1. Medical characteristics of the disease
2. Frequency of occurrence of the disease as a function of observation time

311

3. Distribution of the disease in the population investigated
4. Cofactors influencing the distribution pattern
5. Mathematical methods for data analysis
6. Demographical data on the population under investigation as well as on the matching exposed control group

A primary task in epidemiological research is to determine the validity of the data used, including the sources and the methods employed to obtain and analyze the data.

The collection of epidemiological data from defined population groups exposed to radon can be carried out in the following ways:

1. As a cohort study where data on a (rare) exposure to a hazardous agent from individual subjects and from nonexposed controls are used. In a retrospective cohort study (case history study) the groups are defined after the disease has already occurred, thereby providing results from presently available data. A prospective cohort study (forward study) uses data from groups that are identified before the occurrence of the disease. The group members are followed until they die, thereby necessitating observations into the future.

2. As a case control study for which individual subjects are selected for the study on the basis of nondisease and disease, thereby evaluating a number of exposures in relation to one (mostly rare) disease; this approach is mainly used with hospital data.

At this point the importance of the choice of a comparable nonexposed control group is emphasized. This group should represent all the characteristics that can be identified in the exposed group—ranging from age and sex distribution to socioeconomic factors—with the exception of the exposure itself.

The overall objective of an epidemiological study is to obtain information about the disease under investigation based on biological inferences derived from quantitative assessment of the disease phenomena in selected population groups. Ideally the results should be independent of the method employed; i.e. those obtained from a retrospective study should be the same as the results from a forward study.

By comparing the incidence rate among the members of the exposed group with the rate of incidence in the nonexposed control group, it may be possible to identify factors associated with the cause(s) of the disease. Within the constraints mentioned above, this permits quantitative assessment of levels of risk due to exposure to the identified hazardous agent. However, it must be cautioned that epidemiology is not able to provide indisputable proof that there is a causal relationship between the effect observed in the exposed group and the factor investigated.

In view of the increasing number of politicosocioeconomic decisions concerning public health that are based on epidemiological investigations, it is stressed that the accuracy of the results obtained with this methodology depends on the quality of the input data used. Owing to the many uncertainties involved in obtaining some of the demographical data and health statistics, epidemiological data are to be considered as "soft" data; i.e., they belong to the lowest class of data with regard to reproducibility and overall accuracy (5).

1.2 Epidemiology of Radon-Induced Lung Cancer

Unlike the incidence of cancer at any other site of the human body, lung cancer is generally increasing in the industrialized countries among both males and females. Without reference to the potentially causal relationship with smoking habits and deterioration of environmental conditions, it is important to realize that any additional lung cancer cases due to elevated radon decay product (Rn-d) exposure have to be detected against this high background of "spontaneous" lung cancer cases in the general population, itself exposed to varying levels of Rn-d due to the natural radiation environment. Therefore, strict quality control of the input data used for such a study is essential in order to avoid erroneous conclusions about the potential hazard due to Rn-d exposure.

This is particularly true for the problem of low-level Rn-d exposure. To carry out an epidemiological study on the lung cancer risk associated with Rn-d exposure at environmental levels, the following conditions should ideally be met:

1. Determination of the individual doses due to Rn-d inhalation in the exposed group with a high degree of reliability
2. Identification of a specific type of lung cancer induced by Rn-d only
3. Definition of a control group matching the exposed group in all aspects, but itself not exposed to Rn-d

In reality none of these conditions can be met completely. Even in cases where actual exposure measurements have been carried out, reliable individual dose assessment is still a complex task owing to the number of physical and biological variables involved and their large variability with time and/or space (6). Therefore, epidemiologists often have to rely on mean group values rather than individual values; in some cases measurements are missing altogether and exposure estimates are used as input data.

There have been repeated attempts to correlate the distribution of lung cancer types with past Rn-d exposure, suggesting increased occurrence of oat cell type with increasing exposure (7). However, these associations are both questionable due to potential bias and subject to time-dependent changes. Lung cancer induced by low-level Rn-d exposure cannot be distinguished with histological-cytological methods from lung cancer initiated by other carcinogens, such as tobacco smoke (cf. Chapter 7, Section 2).

Also, the third condition mentioned above cannot be fulfilled as there is no "zero Rn-d exposure" group to serve as a control. Everyone is subject to exposure from the natural radiation environment. Furthermore, individual susceptibility to radiation exposure can vary considerably with age, sex, and hormonal-enzymatic status. Therefore, it is impossible to ensure that the exposed and nonexposed study groups comply with the requirement for homogeneity.

For a detailed discussion of the implicit limitations of epidemiological studies in general, and of those relevant to Rn-d exposure carried out hitherto, see Section 3 of this chapter.

In general, one must compromise the ideal situation by accepting unavoidable deficiencies. Figure 8.1 shows schematically the radiological, demographical, and

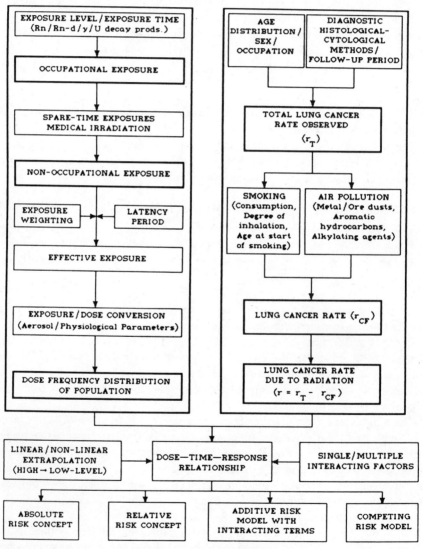

Figure 8.1. Scheme of radiological, demographical, and medical data needed for control and test populations for risk assessment of lung cancer induction due to Rn-d exposure. (Reprinted with permission from Ref. 8.)

medical data needed for lung cancer epidemiology with an Rn-d-exposed group and a nonexposed control population (8).

The radiological data group provides information on the total radiation dose from all internal and external sources during occupational and nonoccupational exposure. A complication arises from the fact that the latent period between the initial Rn-d exposure that induces lung cancer and the macroscopic expression of the pulmonary malignancy ranges from less than 10 years (for smokers) to over 50 years (for nonsmokers), with a mean value of about 20 years (9, 14). The length of the latent period has significant influence on the lifetime risk. Depending on the assumed risk model, increasing the latent period by a factor of 4 causes a reduction of the estimate of lifetime risk by about 50% (15). This is also of particular importance for continuous low-level Rn-d exposure: in the case of nonoccupational exposure of the public, a lengthy latent period may extend beyond an individual's life expectancy.

Depending on the atmospheric characteristics (e.g., aerosol particle size) during exposure and physiological parameters (e.g., respiratory minute volume), exposure is converted to dose by applying the appropriate conversion factor. With individual dose data the dose-frequency distribution can be calculated for a given population. Two examples for presentation of data on Rn-d concentration and respectively resulting dose are shown in Figures 8.2 and 8.3 (16, 17).

The second group of input data for such an epidemiological study is composed of medical data on lung cancer diagnosis, demographical information (e.g., age and sex distribution), as well as quantitative characteristics of smoking habits and

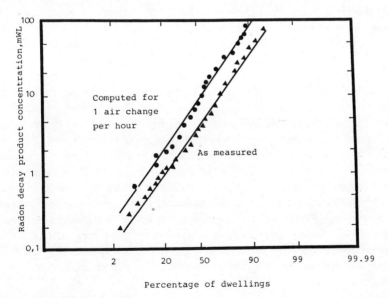

Figure 8.2. Cumulative frequency distribution of Rn-d concentration in air in the living areas of some dwellings in Cornwall (1 mWL = 10^{-3} working level = 2.08×10^{-8} J m^{-3}.) (Reprinted with permission from Ref. 17.)

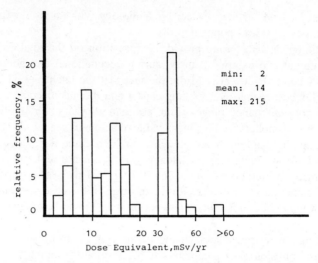

Figure 8.3. Frequency distribution of the mean annual dose equivalents to the bronchial epithelium basal cells of segmental and subsegmental bronchioles for 729 test persons in Salzburg. (Reproduced from *Health Physics*, Vol. 45, p. 331, by permission of the Health Physics Society.)

the presence of potential or known carcinogenic atmospheric pollutants other than Rn-d. The total observed lung cancer rate is corrected for the contributions of other carcinogens to determine the number of lung cancers induced by Rn-d only.

As the biological effect of low-level Rn-d exposure cannot be detected directly against the high background of "spontaneous" or "natural" lung cancer in the general population, it is necessary to extrapolate down to low dose levels from human data obtained at high dose levels, or to use information derived from animal inhalation studies, the latter being the subject of Chapter 9. A conservative approach, applied, for example, by the International Commission on Radiological Protection (ICRP), assumes a linear no-threshold dependence between dose and effect; i.e., only zero dose will guarantee no Rn-d-induced lung cancer. Based on information from radiobiological and epidemiological investigations (e.g., cellular repair effects or cell killing), there is also the possibility of assuming a nonlinear correlation between dose and effect, even with the potential existence of an apparent threshold value (18); the latter possibility, however, is rejected for reasons of microsimetry (45). The establishment of a dose-response-time relationship can be further complicated if additional factors acting as cocarcinogens—e.g., tobacco smoke, diesel exhaust, ore dust—are known to be present. In this case the observed lung cancer rate is the result of the interaction of mutually superimposed agents, which may lead to a synergistic effect with, for example, a multiplicative interaction.

Assessment of the lung cancer risk to the Rn-d-exposed group requires knowledge of the lung cancer incidence rate as a function of age of the exposed persons. Figure 8.4 shows the time distribution of excess lung cancer for two different concepts (15).

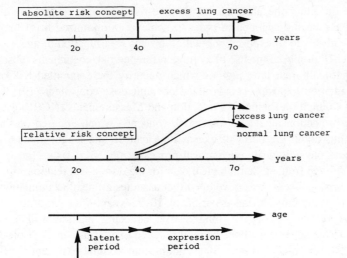

Figure 8.4. Comparison of lung cancer incidence based on absolute- versus relative-risk concepts as a function of age assuming a single exposure at the age of 20 years. (From Ref. 15. Reproduced with permission.)

The absolute-risk concept is based on the assumption that the excess risk is dose-dependent and additive to the "normal" lung cancer risk (R_0), the latter being independent of dose D. The total observed risk, R_{obs}, can be determined from the equation

$$R_{obs} = R_0 + aD \tag{1}$$

where a = absolute-risk factor, i.e., the number of additional lung cancer cases in relation to the number of exposed persons normalized by the dose. With this concept it is not possible to differentiate lung cancer incidence among members of the exposed group from lung cancer incidence due to Rn-d exposure; i.e., in a subgroup lung cancer may be induced from Rn-d exposure or from other carcinogens present as well.

In the relative-risk concept the integral observed risk, R'_{obs}, is calculated based on the assumption of a no-threshold linear increase of risk with dose D:

$$R'_{obs} = R_0 (1 + bD) \tag{2}$$

where b = relative-risk factor, relating the ratio of lung cancer rate among the Rn-d-exposed group and the lung cancer rate among the nonexposed group. Relative risks (bD) $\ll$ 1 indicate a weak association with Rn-d exposure, and vice versa.

Based on either the absolute- or relative-risk concept, several modified risk models have been developed in order to achieve an optimized fit of lung cancer incidence observed in exposed population groups as a function of age.

The ICRP proposed the use of average reference risk coefficients (absolute-risk concept) for different lung regions which quantify the committed risk of cancer due to radiation exposure standardized per unit dose equivalent (19). The U.S. National Council on Radiation Protection and Measurements (NCRP) used an excess-risk projection model (absolute-risk concept), which is based on theoretical assumptions about the onset of excess lung cancer, the length of its expression period, and physiological cell removal processes (20, 21). Using linear approximations derived from epidemiological data for the dose-effect relationship, a model (absolute-risk concept) was developed that assumes a linear accumulation of lung tumors to occur only during a period of 10–25 years after exposure (22). In a further development of the relative-risk concept, maximum-likelihood and weighted-least-squares methods were introduced to establish an exposure-response dependence for epidemiological data, taking into account exponential cell killing (23). Another model based on the relative-risk concept, the proportional-hazard model, uses the similarity between the observed age distribution of the radiation-induced lung cancer rate and the expected rate ''without radiation'' (24); to correct for the promoting influence of smoking, this model applies the results of correlations between smokers and nonsmokers in the general population.

Each of the above models neglects the influence of nonradiological lethal risks competing with mortality from Rn-d-induced lung cancer, such as, for example, accidents, nonmalignant diseases, and suicide, all contributing to the normal mortality rate. Furthermore, the use of ''unexposed'' controls always includes an unjustified assumption about a negligible, but in reality unknown, component of risk due to Rn-d exposure received predominantly indoors (see also Section 1.1).

2   HUMAN EXPOSURES TO RADON AND ITS PROGENY

2.1   Introduction

The history of epidemiological studies on Rn-d-exposed population groups is a tragic example of the slow process of understanding a causal relationship between exposure to an unknown hazard and its detrimental health effect, as well as a lack of communication between members of the international scientific community.

Historically, the first evidence of health risks associated with Rn-d exposure dates back to medical observations by Paracelsus and Agricola in the sixteenth century, when it was noted that the mining population in parts of Germany (Schneeberg) and Bohemia (St. Joachimsthal), C.S.S.R., were suffering from a widespread fatal lung disease known as ''mala metallorum'' or ''Schneeberger *Krankheit*'' (25). It was not until the nineteenth century that lung cancer was identified as the primary cause of death for about 75% of all miners in the Schneeberg region (9, 26, 82); it took about another 50 years until a similar medical diagnosis was published for the miners in St. Joachimsthal (27, 57). With the increasing use of uranium for military purposes (nuclear weapons production) and later also for peaceful uses (electricity production), the lung cancer incidence rate of uranium mining populations received worldwide attention. Unfortunately, the association between radon emanating from the radium (^{226}Ra)-bearing rocks in the C.S.S.R. mines and the observed endemic lung cancer incidence hypothesized as early as 1921 was not accepted for another 30 years (27, 28). Finally in the 1950s the significance of exposure to Rn-d rather than inhalation of radon gas itself was established on theoretical grounds and from experimental investigation as the causative agent for the observed excess lung cancer in Europe and the United States (29, 30).

Owing to this historical development, most of the relevant epidemiological studies are based on occupationally exposed populations with high Rn-d exposures obtained under mining conditions. Equivalent studies on nonmining populations are rare and were not begun until the late 1970s, although as early as 1956 the importance of Rn-d indoor exposure for the general public was pointed out (31). This delay was partially due to the fact that the dose contribution by Rn-d to the total dose from the natural radiation environment had been generally underestimated despite the timely availability of relevant information indicating high local doses in part of the respiratory tract due to inhomogeneous nuclide deposition (32).

Another reason that epidemiological studies of nonmining populations are rare is the difficulty of conducting such studies owing to the inherent statistical problems associated with low-level exposure. A feasibility analysis was conducted to investigate the minimum detectable risk for 10,000 nonoccupationally exposed individuals with an unrealistically high lifetime exposure rate of 1 WLM y^{-1} (1 WLM (working-level month) = 12.95 J m^{-3} s; see Chapter 1, Section 8.1) in comparison to an identical nonexposed cohort of 10,000 individuals (33, 34). The results showed that even for a follow-up period of 40 years the smallest detectable risk at the 95% significance level is still 4×10^{-6} y^{-1} WLM^{-1}. Thus, even with satisfactory individual dose records, the apparent epidemiological threshold below which excess lung cancer cannot be detected is too high to provide adequate results.

Therefore, only limited attempts have been made thus far to investigate the low-level dose-effect relation for the general public. In the rest of this section, epidemiological surveys on human Rn-d exposure are described for mining and nonmining population groups, considering exposure conditions, population characteristics, and data collection, with emphasis on low-level exposure data.

Results for mining populations at low exposures, i.e., below about 200 WLM, are given in Table 8.1. For results at higher exposures, cf. reports of individual studies given below. (A summary of recent studies and analyses is given as an Editors' Note at the end of this chapter.)

2.2 Mining Populations

2.2.1 U.S. Uranium Miners

2.2.1.1 Exposure conditions. U.S. uranium miners represent one of the best-studied population groups with past occupational Rn-d exposure. The quality of

Table 8.1   **Comparison of Observed Versus Expected Number of Lung Cancer Cases for Uranium Miners and Nonuranium Miners Receiving Rn-d Exposures Below 239 WLM**

Population/cumulative exposure (WLM)	Number of lung cancer cases		Remarks
	Observed	Expected	
Uranium Miners			
1. United States 0–119	3	3.96	
120–239	7	2.24[a]	
2. CSSR < 50	33.2	16.6	All values are "frequency/10^3
50–99	21.2	13.2	miners"
100–149	34.0	13.8	
3. Canada 0.1–10	14	9.5	No prior gold mining
10.1–40	15	17.4	experience; zero years lag
40.1–100	12	13.2	assumed
Nonuranium Miners			
1. Newfoundland 0	7	7	Fluorspar miners; comparison
1–9	3	2.02	with surface miners
10–239	13	0.5	
2. Norway 1–19	3	0.50	Niobium miners; all smokers (up
20–79	4	0.58	to 150 g tobacco/week)
80–119	2	0.07	

[a]Not statistically significant at 1% level, marginally at 5% (15).

the Rn-d exposure data is characterized by a significant improvement over the past 30 years, ranging from estimated values supposedly representative for a whole mine in the 1950s to individual miner exposure data derived from statistically designed sampling plans used in the 1980s (35–38).

In the pre-World War II period, uranium was mined in the United States as a by-product of mining for vanadium. During the 1940s this was followed by intensified mining of uranium as the mineral of primary interest for military purposes. In 1950 a level of employment of about 500 miners was reached with a daily production rate of 600 tons of ore. In this early phase only sporadic radon measurements were carried out. These measurements indicated a wide range of possible exposure conditions, with median radon values from 13 kBq/m^3 to 185 kBq/m^3 and maximum values at the work sites of 1900 kBq/m^3.

Most mines were ventilated only by natural ventilation, causing wide spatial and temporal variations of Rn-d values and equilibrium factors within a given mine. All individual exposures of miners for that period were derived from educated guesses based on radon concentration values interpolated from regional averages or estimated from measurements in mines of similar location, ore grade/type, depth, and ventilation. By 1952 a survey of several mines showed that about 44% of the miners were exposed to Rn-d in excess of 10 WL (37 kBq/m^3 equilibrium-equivalent concentration). Average Rn-d exposure in 10% of the mines would be above 50 WL.

In the following years Rn-d measurements were performed at irregular intervals (long-term average: one measurement per mine per year) (39). The analytical method applied was based on the Kusnetz method, with a total uncertainty of at least 30% due to the method itself. Frequently the site selected for measurement was chosen because concentration values were expected to be high and the objective was to identify the problem. Although after 1960 Rn-d measurements were carried out more frequently, by 1967 50% of all exposure data were still only estimates, partially based on the individual recall of employment period and mine location. The work force was characterized by a high degree of mobility, which at one stage caused a discrepancy between the actual total number of uranium miners reported by the Colorado Bureau of Mines and the number employed. The job classification "uranium miner" is associated with some uncertainties because some miners categorized as "uranium miner" had previous hard-rock experience or changed to non-uranium mining after their employment in a uranium mine, in both cases leading to unknown Rn-d exposures during the pre- or posturanium mining period.

Because of these uncertainties with regard to the estimated mean Rn-d exposure and the length of active employment at a given time (i.e., the length of Rn-d exposure), the assignment of exposure rates in different studies on U.S. uranium miners can differ by as much as a factor of 24 for the same miner (40).

Figure 8.5 shows the long-term trend of average exposure of U.S. uranium miners, using mainly estimated data for the period before the mid-1960s (41). At present, average Rn-d exposure is significantly below the exposure estimated as typical for the period 1950–1960.

The occupational exposure of U.S. uranium miners to external gamma radiation has generally been assumed to result in a dose equivalent of 10 mSv/y (13, 37). This component of radiation exposure cannot be neglected because individual mean values up to 30 mSv/yr can be attained for miners working in uranium mines having ore grades between 0.06 and 0.35% (49). In addition, even when individual gamma-exposure data are available, there can be a discrepancy by more than a factor of 4 between the average exposure rate derived from individual badge dosimeters as compared to data derived from site monitoring. The reasons may be self-shielding of the miners, self-shielding of the badges, as well as different residence times of the miners at various locations.

Another source of radiation exposure hitherto considered only of secondary importance is inhaled uranium and its long-lived daughters; these can deliver up to 10% of the dose allowed for short-lived decay products (50).

Apart from Rn-d exposure, several nonradioactive air pollutants are known to occur in mines, such as aromatic hydrocarbons, alkylating agents, metal dusts, deposits of soot from diesel engines, Zn and Pb from blasting primers, S from black powder fuse, and welding fumes (37, 42). The significance of exposure to these potentially or known harmful agents for the induction of lung cancer is controversial and has not yet been quantified.

So far none of the epidemiological studies carried out on U.S. uranium miners has taken into consideration all the above components in addition to Rn-d exposure itself.

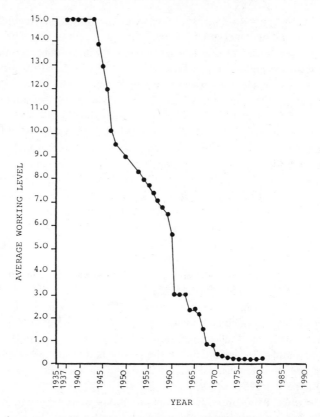

Figure 8.5. Average potential alpha-energy concentration (in units of working level) to which U.S. underground uranium miners were exposed (41). (Reproduced by permission of American Institute of Mining, Metallurgical and Petroleum Engineers.)

The most important nonradioactive carcinogen to which U.S. uranium miners were exposed is tobacco smoke. Since smoking is thought to be the single most significant cause of lung cancer induction, any lung cancer epidemiology has to pay particular attention to the contribution of this factor to the overall observed lung cancer rate.

About 70% of the U.S. uranium miners were smokers, twice the value for the general public (37). In order to take the contribution from smoking into consideration, it is essential to quantify the use and consumption of tobacco, the degree of inhalation, and the age when smoking began. Also the temporal changes of the tobacco blends used over the past 30 years have to be accounted for.

For further discussion on possible synergistic effects between various hazardous agents and Rn-d, see Section 3.

The size of the U.S. uranium miner population reached a maximum of about 4000 persons by 1964, taking into account only those with an underground employment period of at least 1 month. From this population a study group was formed consisting of 3336 white and 780 mostly Indian underground uranium miners, of whom more than half were hired between 1952 and 1957 (12, 13, 46, 47). The median age of the white miners at first uranium mining was 30 years.

These miners showed a high degree of job-related mobility as well as independent work habits. The majority of the miners worked less than 10 years in uranium mines. Periods of working overtime were followed by vacations. Mine operation was variable and workdays irregular. Therefore, it is unclear to what extent the individual exposure was fractionated as intermittent, rather than continous, dose rates.

2.2.1.2 Data on Lung Cancer. The first information on increased lung cancer among U.S. uranium miners was obtained in the early 1960s, when the rate among these miners was found to be a factor of 10 higher than that in the general public (35, 43). Although an unsuitable control population had been chosen in this study, epidemiological methods were improved in the following years. A case-comparison study revealed 116 "definite" and five unidentified "possible" lung cancer cases among uranium miners during 1949–1969. These cases were compared to lung cancer cases in nonuranium miners serving as controls and considered to be matching in age and smoking status (44). That matching was not achieved completely may explain the inconclusive result: a 67% excess of small cell carcinoma among uranium miners is in contradiction to the 50% excess of squamous cell carcinoma observed among the control group. In the following years reports have been published repeatedly on the lung cancer incidence rate among the miners and histological information on this study group. However, there is a discrepancy, perhaps caused by including living cases, with regard to the number of lung cancer cases observed by the cutoff date September 30, 1977 (15). The numbers quoted range from 119 to 159 cases following an assumed 10-year latency (47, 48, 51). The latest mortality data on these miners refer to 185 cases among the 950 persons deceased by December 31, 1977 (12); this is consistent with the higher number quoted above only if it also includes miners who were exposed for less than 10 years. This discrepancy has a significant impact on the risk factors derived from these data (see Section 4). In 33 cases the death certificate is still outstanding. By this time the cohort, with a median cumulative exposure of 430 WLM (mean = 821 WLM), had been followed on average for 19 years.

It has been argued for the past 20 years that Rn-d-induced lung cancer is associated with an unusual cell type frequency distribution; in particular, small cell carcinoma is supposed to be typical for past Rn-d exposure. As this issue is one of the main arguments used in questioning the value of presently used risk assessment, the significance of quality control of medical data used for quantification of the observed "effect" is discussed in the following paragraphs. As discussed in Chapter 7, there is evidence, in any case, that the overall cell-type distribution for the miner lung cancers may be similar to that for the general public, but with different histological types appearing at different times.

Lung carcinomas are not specific for a particular region of the lung, but may arise in any part of the respiratory tract. Lung tumors themselves are heterogeneous, with frequent mixing of all four categories of lung cancer. Therefore, all types are actually present in some cases. Histopathological investigations are subject to many errors during the initial phase of obtaining the tissue sample, as well as during histological typing of the lung tumors.

In view of the above, it is understandable that lung cancer diagnosis generally has a low degree of reliability, taking into account additional uncertainties due to inter- and intraobserver variability. For further details, see Section 3.

For the U.S. uranium miners, associations of a certain lung cancer cell type distribution with Rn-d exposure are questionable for the following additional reasons (7, 151):

1. Observer variability in tissue classification: a panel of pathologists identified twice as many small cell carcinomas, as compared to a single pathologist.
2. Source term influence: almost 60% more small cell carcinomas were found in tissue slides from an autopsy series in comparison to slides from a biopsy series.

Furthermore, 4% ''possible'' lung cancers were included, but not identified as such.

When death certificates were used as the source of data, changes in cause of death from that on the death certificate to something else occured in both directions in 15% of all cases; only 82% of the original pathological findings were confirmed as lung cancer (37). Many of these miners had ''chronic cough.'' It is possible that some deaths were actually due to lung cancer but erroneously attributed to tuberculosis or silicosis. The latest results indicate that the lung cancer cell type frequency distribution changes with follow-up time, possibly reflecting changing external exposure cofactors, such as aerosol characteristics or smoking habits (7).

2.2.2 C.S.S.R. Uranium Miners

2.2.2.1 Exposure Conditions. The Bohemian study group consists of miners from the Jachymov (formerly St. Joachimsthal) area, covering the period 1948–1975 (52). Radon measurements started as early as 1924 with concentration values in the mines ranging from 12 kBq/m^3 to 331 kBq/m^3 (53).

During the 1930–1940 period, most mines had Rn values below 13 kBq/m^3. Data on the conditions in the following years have not been published. From 1948 until 1975, an average of 100 radon measurements were made annually for every uranium mine (10, 54).

Little information is available about the sources of the altogether ''120,000 reliable Rn measurements.'' No data exist on the equilibrium factor and its uncertainty, required for the assessment of Rn-d exposure based only on Rn measurements.

In view of the large spatial and temporal variability of the exposure caused by the simultaneous influence of several parameters (e.g., ventilation conditions, ore content, groundwater seepage, and so forth), there are two suspicious aspects of these data (55, 56). First, the variation of the mine-year specific measurements is surprisingly small: the coefficient of variation is less than or equal to 20%. Additional Rn-d measurements have been performed since 1960. The mean exposure is 310 WLM, covering a wide range from about 20 WLM to 1000 WLM. This leads to the second interesting aspect: in contrast to probabilistic expectations, the rates/WLM in all groups are in exceptional agreement, despite the large standard deviations of the single values; for further details, see Section 3.

Exposure of the C.S.S.R. uranium miners to nonradioactive hazardous agents is well documented (57). Miners inhaled various toxic metal ore dusts (cobalt, nickel, manganese) differing in their quartz content, as well as fungi growing in the damp, cold mines. Furthermore, the ore dust contained elevated levels of arsenic, known to induce lung cancer and skin cancer. There is also an indirect indication that toxic levels of arsenic were present in these mines: a highly significant increase of skin cancer has been observed among the C.S.S.R. uranium miners (58). This is in contrast to comparable, but arsenic-free Rn-d exposures in U.S. uranium mines, where skin cancer was not observed to occur at a higher rate than among controls.

The number of miners in the C.S.S.R. study group was originally 4364, each of whom started uranium mining in the period from 1948 to 1957; a selected study subgroup A comprises 2433 miners (52, 59).

2.2.2.2 Data on lung cancer.

During the period 1928–1938, 63 autopsy and histological samples were available from diseased miners of St. Joachimsthal. Lung cancer was diagnosed in about 45% of these cases (53). An additional 16 cases of lung cancer in this population group were registered during World War II (60), and in the years 1945–1966 another 73 lung cancer cases were diagnosed. It should be noted, however, that the actual number of cases is likely to be higher because during the Communist takeover after World War II in the C.S.S.R. many inhabitants of German origin were forced to leave the country, making the lung cancer cases observed until 1958 representative for the remaining Czech part of the population only. Also, it is known that political prisoners were used occasionally as miners in particularly high Rn-d exposure conditions and it is uncertain to what extent they were included in the study population.

In 1971 the first report on increased lung cancer incidence among C.S.S.R. uranium miners was published, with updates issued in 1976 and 1979 (11, 54, 59). Using the standardized information on lung cancer incidence as published, together with the data on the population size, it can be concluded that, during the average follow-up period of about 26 years, about 280 lung cancer cases have occurred in the total study group.

Histopathological information on the C.S.S.R. uranium miner data is scarce and inconclusive. There is no description of the source of the tissue samples (e.g., age of patient), the method of preparation of the tissue slides, or the quality control employed in applying histopathological classification methods.

With regard to the question of the potential existence of a distribution of cancer cell type related to Rn-d exposure, the following inconclusive observations have been reported (61): In comparison to controls, C.S.S.R. uranium miners show a deficit of epidermoid tumors, no difference for adenocarcinomas, and an excess of small cell anaplastic tumors. Although one expects to see an increase of each lung cancer cell type with an increased level of cumulative Rn-d exposure, the fact that a deficit of a certain cancer cell type was observed with increased radiation exposure may be an indication of the need for histopathological reclassification. In view of the fact that a certain number of tissue samples were reported as "unclassifiable," together with the above-noted lack of important histopathological data, it appears questionable whether any statistically valid conclusion concerning a change of cell type distribution due to elevated Rn-d exposure can be drawn from these data.

2.2.3 Canadian Uranium Miners

2.2.3.1 Exposure Conditions. In 1955, mining of uranium ore was started in the province of Ontario, Canada. At this time no Rn-d measurements were carried out, and only occasionally, in some of the mines, was Rn measured (62). The uranium mining industry reached its peak productivity within a few years, and by the beginning of the 1960s a maximum number of about 11,000 miners was employed, declining equally rapidly to about 2000 thereafter (63). Rn-d exposures within mines and among mines are known to have varied considerably. In view of these large variations and the lack of appropriate data, it was attempted to calculate a range of "best estimates" rather than a single value for each miner, assuming that for the period until 1967 the true value for each worker lies within this range (64). Mean cumulative Rn-d exposure was estimated to be about 60 WLM, i.e., only 7% and 20%, respectively, of the corresponding values for the U.S. and C.S.S.R. uranium miners. After 1967, individual exposure assessments were carried out, and Rn-d exposures were found to average below 1 WLM/year. Figure 8.6 shows the temporal change of the Rn-d exposure for a given mine for the period 1955–1977, indicating the peak exposure time to be around 1965 (65). The Ca-

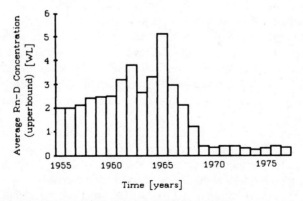

Figure 8.6. Example of temporal change: Annual radon progeny concentrations in Canadian uranium mines (Elliot Lake Area, Ontario). (Adapted, with permission, from Ref. 65.)

nadian uranium miners differ in another important job-related aspect from the U.S. and C.S.S.R. uranium miners. The average employment period of a Canadian uranium miner (median of 1.5 years) is only about 15% of the average time U.S. and C.S.S.R. miners worked in uranium mines, indicating a high degree of job mobility. Therefore, miners were exposed at an elevated rate in the pre-1967 period.

Retrospective Rn-d exposure is further complicated by the fact that some of the Canadian uranium miners had gold mining experience prior to their employment in the uranium industry. Ontario gold miners, and other miners who worked in various types of ore, show a significantly increased lung cancer risk (64).

Data on exposure to contaminants other than Rn-d (e.g., arsenic, asbestos, blasting fumes, radioactive ore dust, diesel exhausts) are not available yet. No data exist on past thoron decay product exposure or on exposure to long-lived alpha emitters. Doses due to external irradiation have not been taken into consideration.

The severe limitations associated with the retrospective assessment of individual Rn-d exposures based on educated guesses rather than Rn-d measurements are comparable to those indicated in Sections 2.2.1 and 2.2.2; for further discussion see also Section 3.

2.2.3.2 Data on Lung Cancer.

In the Canadian uranium miner studies no data on the histopathology of lung cancer tissue samples are yet available (64–66). Instead, death information is derived from the Canadian Mortality Data Base plus additional manual resolution, relying on death certificates only. For the period January 1955–December 1981 different International Classification of Diseases (ICDA) codes were used: the seventh revision from 1955 to 1968; the eighth revision from 1969 to 1978 and the ninth revision from 1979 to 1981. Altogether, death information on the uranium miners is categorized into 45 groups of death causes. With regard to malignant neoplasms of the respiratory system, this classification system differentiates between neoplasms of "trachea, bronchus, lung," "larynx," "nose, nasal cavities, etc.," and "other." Despite the differences between the three revised codes, death information was not recoded to avoid any bias in comparing the results with the mortality data of the control population.

By 1981, after an average follow-up period of 15 years, a total of 121 malignant neoplasms were registered as the cause of death in the study group of 15,984 uranium miners; in 119 of these the neoplasm was cancer of the ICDA category "trachea, bronchus, lung." In this context it is interesting to note that in 11 additional cases "silicosis, chronic interstitial pneumonia" was declared as cause of death. In a subgroup of uranium miners (about 13,400) who had not previously been working in gold mines, 82 lung cancer cases were observed during the same period of observation. Data on smoking characteristics are not yet available.

2.2.4 Others

2.2.4.1 French Uranium Miners.

Although uranium mining in France started as early as 1947, it was only in 1985 that preliminary results of an epidemiological study of uranium miners were published (67). This study suffers from an unknown uncertainty with regard to individual exposures to Rn-d for two reasons. First, from 1947 to 1955 no individual survey of the exposure to Rn and Rn-d was carried out. Estimates, taking into account ore characteristics, ventilation, and working methods, as well as a few radon measurements, range from 1 to 10 WLM for the average monthly exposure for this period in the 11 different mines. The uniformity of the estimated values for a period of up to 8 years is somewhat unusual (e.g., the monthly average exposure for mine Henriette was 10 ± 0 WLM, and for mine Lachaux it was 1 ± 0 WLM), when one takes into consideration the frequent change of ventilation conditions and long-term changes in mining methods.

The second reason for an unquantifiable uncertainty is due to the methodology used in the subsequent years. After 1956, area monitoring of Rn and radioactive ore dust concentration was introduced, resulting in about 20–30 measurements per miner per year for the period 1957–1970 and finally reaching 57–70 Rn measurements per miner per year for the period 1971–1985. Despite these favorable conditions, individual Rn-d exposure assessment is uncertain because Rn-d exposure is estimated from a "global value" for the equilibrium factor of 0.22, assumed to be valid for the total period 1956–1980 as well as for all French uranium mines. This value of the equilibrium factor represents an increase of the previously assumed value by 30% in order to account for the general underestimation of the individual exposure if derived from area monitoring only. At present, the mean or median cumulative exposure cannot be calculated.

Because of national regulations, the use of national cancer statistics is limited. Only lung cancer cases identified as occupational disease can be verified by histopathological methods. In all other cases only the life status (dead or alive) can be used as a source of information.

The study group consists of 1957 miners with a mean employment period of 11.4 years, covering the period 1947–1983. Average annual Rn-d exposure ranged from 2.5 WLM to 4.3 WLM for the years 1956–1970, and from 1.6 WLM to 3.2 WLM for the period 1971–1980. Annual average exposure to radioactive ore dust was higher by a factor of 2 during the 1960s as compared to the corresponding value of 82 Bq h m^{-3} in 1980. Except for the period 1960–1963, when mean values reached up to 17 mSv/y, the average gamma exposure decreased continuously over the years from about 10 mSv/y to less than 5 mSv/y in 1980.

With an average follow-up period of 25.9 years, a total of 36 lung cancer cases had been identified as cause of death by December 1983.

No information is available about smoking characteristics or exposure to nonradioactive carcinogens in mine atmospheres.

2.2.4.2 Swedish Hard-Rock Miners. In the iron ore mining community of Grängesberg, Sweden, lung cancer case-reference studies were carried out, examining the incidence in the periods 1957–1977 and 1966–1977 (68, 69). The reason for repeating these studies was to account for the increasing lung cancer rate through the early 1960s, which leveled off thereafter. The source of information on lung cancer was the parish death and burial register. No histopathological data are available. Smoking information is not quantitative with regard to tobacco consumption, number of years of smoking, age when smoking was started, and so forth, but is limited to the indication that the ratio of smoking miners to nonsmoking miners ranges from 1.5 to 2.0 for the different studies. Miners were known to have received exposure to silica; however, data were not available to account for this quantitatively.

Rn-d exposure data have large associated uncertainties. Together with the relatively small number of observations, this raises questions about the feasibility of carrying out a study for quantitative risk assessment. Using mining company records Rn-d exposure data were estimated retrospectively. For instance, it was assumed that all workers aged 50 years and above had been exposed to an average level of 0.5 WL, based on a few area measurements.

Other studies among Swedish metal miners all suffer from the same severe uncertainties with regard to the Rn-d exposure assessment as outlined above for the iron ore study group, as they rely on "qualified guesses" and "estimates" rather than actual exposure measurements (70–72). (Cf. Editors' Note at the end of this chapter for discussion of a more recent Swedish study.)

2.2.4.3 Newfoundland Fluorspar Miners.

Since 1933, calcium fluoride has been mined in St. Lawrence, Newfoundland, in over a dozen different mines. Mining operations frequently involved the use of natural ventilation only, with large variations over the years for a given mine as well as between different mines. The two main mines were extremely wet, with groundwater being the principal source of radon in the mine atmosphere. The first Rn/Rn-d measurements, taken in 1959/60, indicated a large range of values for a given mine, from below the limit of detection to almost 200 WL. Subsequently, mechanical ventilation was introduced. Rn-d exposure estimates are available for each miner for the post-1960 period with Rn-d levels generally well below 1 WL. Pre-1960 Rn-d exposure measurements are not available; recently reestimates have been carried out, indicating a range of average values from 2.5 to 10 WL (73). The study group consists of 2120 miners, millers, and surface workers. Average exposure was estimated to be about 204 WLM for the underground miner subgroup (47).

Since the first discovery in the early 1950s of an unusually large number of lung cancer cases among members of this mining community, the results of epidemiological studies on this group have been updated twice (74–76). Incidence data on the lung cancer mortality are derived from death certificates. All miners not found through the National Death Index were considered to be alive. By 1978 a total of 104 lung cancer cases had been observed in the study group, with more than two-thirds of the cases occurring among the underground miners. An additional investigation using sputum cytology revealed that of 29 miners with lung cancer, 90% had squamous cell carcinoma; small cell carcinoma occurred in only 7% of the cases (77). Information on individual smoking characteristics of the members of the study group was collected in four surveys between 1960 and 1978, categorizing members into "nonsmokers," "ex-smokers," "light smokers," and "heavy smokers"; pipe and cigar smokers were grouped with nonsmokers. The results of these studies showed that about 80% of the miners belonged to the group of heavy smokers.

Because of the many uncertainties noted with regard to the retrospective exposure assessment, this study cannot be used for a quantitative exposure-effect assessment.

2.2.4.4 South African Gold/Uranium Miners. In South Africa, uranium has been produced as a by-product of gold mining since 1952, reaching a production peak in 1960 (78). By 1971 about 20,000 white miners and 250,000 nonwhite miners had received Rn-d exposure; external irradiation is generally low because of low average ore grade (about 0.05% uranium). Owing to extreme environmental conditions underground, ventilation is high in these mines, thereby causing Rn-d levels to be mostly below 0.3 WL. Measurements were carried out on 12 mines, providing the database for "guesstimates" of the Rn-exposure levels in 119 mines. It was concluded that in 96% of these mines, exposure levels ranged from 0.1 to 0.7 WL. In 1967 a study group of 575 white underground miners was formed to investigate the lung cancer incidence. These miners are subject to a high degree of job mobility not only between different mines, but also between different work activities within the same mine. For organizational reasons, a period of observation from 1960 to 1967—during which the average cumulative exposure was about 36 WLM—was chosen.

From the Medical Research Council, data on work history were obtained for 352 miners with lung cancer who had been employed in underground gold mines. Together with estimated data on the populations at risk, an average annual rate of lung cancer deaths of 2.96 per 10,000 miners was calculated. Additional histopathological investigations indicate an increase of small cell carcinoma in selected miners as compared to nonminers. No quantitative information on quality control of the histopathology used or on the exposure to nonradioactive hazardous agents (tobacco smoke, diesel fumes), radioactive ore dust, and thoron decay products is available.

The usefulness of this study for quantitative exposure-effect appraisal is limited for the same reasons indicated above.

2.2.4.5 Norwegian Niobium Miners. At Ulefoss, Norway, niobium was produced from an underground mine for a limited period, from 1957 to 1965. In addition to niobium oxide, the ore contained uranium and thorium. A study group of 318 workers was formed, of which 77 men were underground miners; about 27 men of the latter group had previous hard-rock experience (79). About 15% of the workers could not be identified. Based on a series of Rn-d and thoron (^{220}Rn) decay product (Tn-d) measurements, taken over a 2-day period at a few sites during the winter in 1959 under exceptionally good ventilation conditions, individual exposures were estimated to range from about 1 to 4 WL for Rn-d and about 0.2 to 0.4 WL for Tn-d. Questions remain about the reliability of the exposure data: the measurement techniques; the unknown contribution of the nonoccupational exposure in the homes (possibly of similar magnitude as the occupational exposure), which is of particular importance in such low-level exposure studies; and pre-niobium-mining exposure, which can reach up to 50 WLM for some miners.

Data on lung cancer incidence were obtained from the Norwegian Cancer

Registry, based on reports from medical institutions. During the period from the beginning of 1953 to the end of 1981 (equivalent follow-up periods ranged from 16 to 28 years), a total of 12 cases of lung cancer were observed in the study group; 75% of them occurred in the subgroup of underground miners. From pathology reports it can be concluded that only 25% of the lung cancers were probably small cell carcinoma, whereas almost 75% were squamous cell carcinomas.

Smoking characteristics were determined quantitatively for the study group, characterizing members as nonsmokers, medium smokers (lifetime tobacco consumption from 20 to 200 kg), and heavy smokers (more than 200 kg lifetime consumption); it is important to note that lifetime tobacco consumption up to 20 kg was considered as "nonsmoking." Among the underground miners, 85% were smokers. As indicated above for other similar epidemiological studies, the many uncertainties associated with the exposure data prohibit the use of these results for quantitative assessment of any exposure-effect relationship.

2.2.4.6 British Nonuranium Miners. Mining in Britain dates back to pre-Christian times, resulting in numerous mines of varying size with large areas of old workings and open stopes. Some mines have historic tunnel systems, partially still in connection with currently operated sections, with a total length of up to 140 km (80, 81, 185). It is common to use either natural ventilation only or low-volume mechanical ventilation. The results of a nationwide survey showed that of all underground miners (population size: about 190,000 employees) about 1300 noncoal miners are exposed on average to between 1 and 4 WLM/y (total mean exposure of noncoal miners: 2.6 WLM/y). The rest of the miner population, predominantly coal miners, receive a significantly lower annual mean exposure, ranging from 0.12 to 0.24 WLM.

Epidemiological studies have been carried out on hematite miners in Cumberland and tin miners in Cornwall (186, 187). In both cases increased lung cancer incidence could be correlated with elevated Rn-d levels, using death certificates and comparing lung cancer rates of the underground miners with those of the general public or surface miners. However, it is not possible to establish a dose-effect relationship for Rn-d exposure from these data for the following reasons:

1. Rn-d exposures are only estimated owing to the lack of sufficient measurements;
2. iron ore dust itself is a suspected carcinogen, i.e., contributing an unknown amount to the observed excess cancer in hematite miners;
3. tin miners are exposed to high levels of ore dust, resulting in a high mortality rate due to silicosis;
4. no quantitative data on individual smoking characteristics are available.

2.3 Nonmining Populations

2.3.1 General. In contrast to the multiple epidemiological surveys that have been carried out among miners, equivalent data for the general public are scarce.

As early as the 1950s interests centered on the investigation of potential biological effects among residents of areas with elevated natural radioactivity, such as monazite sand areas in coastal regions of India and Brazil (83).

About 20 years later, in Europe, such research was carried out among workers and inhabitants of radon spas, where patients are irradiated deliberately with radon-containing water and air as therapeutic agents in the course of treatment of various diseases (84).

At the end of the 1970s, the first radon surveys were completed for indoor Rn-d exposure of the general public either on a detailed local scale or as large national studies (85). These studies result mainly in data on the frequency distribution of radon or Rn-d indoor concentrations for different population groups. Only a few investigations have included individual dose assessments (86). Inherent methodological problems and high cost generally limit the number of epidemiological studies on lung cancer induced by low-level Rn-d exposure (see also Sections 2.1 and 3). Therefore, it is unlikely that in the near future more such studies on nonmining populations will be carried out. (Cf. Editors' Note at the end of this chapter.)

2.3.2   Radon Spa Workers and Inhabitants.

Worldwide, water or air containing elevated levels of radon is used by parts of the medical profession as a therapeutic agent for bathing and inhalation; this has occurred, for example, in Austria, Bulgaria, the C.S.S.R., France, Germany (East and West), Italy, Japan, the United States, and the U.S.S.R. (84, 87). In many cases this treatment is even paid for by national public health insurance. In the U.S.S.R., for instance, if patients are unable to go to so-called "radon spas," automatically produced radon sources are made available to them. The treatment is not limited to adults only: e.g., in Bulgaria even children are deliberately exposed to elevated levels of radon as a form of medical treatment.

In these radon spas it is usually not the patients, but rather the employees and people who live nearby, who can receive a significantly increased dose due to Rn-d inhalation. Exposures occur in association with the collection and supply of water as well as during treatment in bathrooms, pools, inhalation rooms, and so forth. Radon either emanates directly from the water, or it is transported from inhalation therapy facilities into the atmosphere. Although tourists and even patients generally receive only a small additional radiation burden owing to the short exposure times, occupational exposure for spa workers and nonoccupational exposure for some residents can be significantly elevated, thereby resulting in an increased risk for lung cancer induction (88).

Despite the increased dose from Rn-d exposure for these population groups, the small numbers of persons exposed at the higher levels limit the statistical significance of such epidemiological studies. In addition, spa employees generally show a high degree of job mobility, leading to relatively high annual dose rates but low accumulated dose levels over a lifetime. Furthermore, their Rn-d exposure is heterogeneous in accordance with their different life-styles and residence time in various spa areas, where Rn-d levels show pronounced spatial and temporal fluctuations. None of the studies carried out so far used integrating methods or personal dosimeters for determination of individual Rn-d dose values in order to account for this variability.

In Austria the natural radiation environment of the Gastein Valley with the radon spas Badgastein and Bad Hofgastein has been the subject of several studies in the past 25 years (89–91). Based on several-thousand area grab sample measurements of Rn and Rn-d, the mean annual Rn-d exposure was calculated for different population groups. For instance, the population of Badgastein (approximately 6300 inhabitants) receives a mean exposure ranging from about 0.2 to 2.7 WLM/y. Prior to the 1970s, occupational exposure of spa workers (about 150 persons) was typically between 1 and 5 WLM/y, but in some cases (about 10 persons) exposure could exceed 10 WLM/y. However, in recent years ventilation techniques have been modified to reduce occupational exposure levels.

For inhabitants whose residence time in the area exceeded 10 years, lung cancer incidence was studied. During the observation period 1949–1978, lung cancer frequency doubled, correlating with the increased use of radon-containing thermal water due to increased tourism. However, no causal relationship can be inferred from this result because over the same period air pollution in the valley due to traffic increased by more than a factor of 10. Of the 176 lung cancer cases observed in this study period, only three patients were occupationally exposed to high Rn-d levels; two of these were heavy smokers.

Employees in Bulgarian radon spas underwent sputum tests (92). The results indicated that there is a statistically significant increase in the frequency of atypical cells in sputum samples of spa workers as compared to controls. However, no data are available on the individual Rn-d exposure.

In other studies of Austrian, Italian, and Japanese employees, as well as residents of radon spas, Rn-d-related biomedical chromosome aberrations or levels of $^{210}Po/^{210}Pb$ in teeth and urine were increased in comparison to control populations (93, 94).

2.3.3 General Public.

Members of the general public can be exposed to elevated Rn-d levels mainly owing to radon entry from the ground into houses, by radon exhalation from building materials into the room air, and by the use of radon-containing water for cooking, consumption, or sanitary purposes.

So far the only epidemiological evidence for a potentially increased risk is indirect, based on correlation studies of the domestic use of drinking water and the incidence of cancer in Iowa (95, 96). Both studies use the radium (^{226}Ra) content of drinking water and the lung cancer incidence rate from death certificates as input parameters to investigate the existence of a causal relationship between these two variables. It could be shown that the lung cancer rates for consumers of water with elevated radium content are higher than those for users of water with low radium content (Fig. 8.7) (96). No data are available on actual individual doses due to Rn-d exposures; it is assumed that the amount of radon deemanated from the drinking water into the room air is correlated directly with the radium content of the water supply. Differences in water consumption and ventilation rate, as well as the

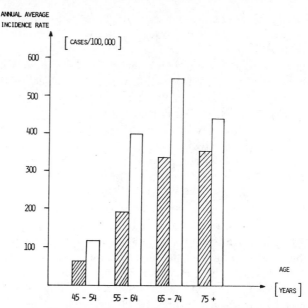

Figure 8.7. Age-specific male lung cancer incidence rates (Iowa), classified according to the mean radium (^{226}Ra) levels in drinking water. ▨ = radium concentration < 111 Bq/m³; ☐ = radium concentration > 111 Bq/m³. (Reproduced with permission from Bean, J. A., Isacson, P., Hahne, R. M. A., and Kohler, I., Drinking water and cancer in Iowa: II. Radioactivity in drinking water, *American Journal of Epidemiology*, **116**, 924, 1982.)

degree of deemanation in the course of varying activities, are not taken into consideration. The widespread use of water softeners in these areas (e.g., such units are installed in 42% of all Iowa homes) represents another unknown variable, since water softening is known to result in a significant reduction of the radium level in drinking water (97, 98). An additional water treatment-related effect can arise from the chlorination of water because the resulting formation of trihalomethane has also been associated with lung cancer (99).

No quantitative data are available on individual smoking habits and tobacco consumption. However, it was noted in the Iowa study that no local geographical difference in smoking characteristics paralleled the geographical difference in radioactivity of water supplies.

Similar exposure conditions can be found in Finland, where drinking-water supplies with radon values up to 44 MBq/m³ have been found (100). Therefore, drinking water can represent a major source of indoor radon pollution, causing chromosomal aberrations in some of the consumers. However, the fundamental methodological problems indicated earlier (small number of exposed persons, problems of individual dose assessment resulting from past and present indoor exposure, and high cost due to long follow-up periods) have made an epidemiological study among the Finnish users of water from drilled wells unfeasible so far (101).

A nationwide indoor survey was carried out in 13 cities in Canada (102). Altogether 9999 homes—chosen on a statistically valid grab-sample basis—were investigated for Rn- and Rn-d levels in buildings. The geometric mean Rn values for the 13 cities ranged from 5.2 Bq/m^3 to 32.6 Bq/m^3; the corresponding Rn-d values were 0.9 to 3.6 mWL. As the study was performed during June–August 1977 and 1978 the results obtained are typical for the summer season only. The Rn-concentration data were correlated with the lung cancer incidence in the various regions, using data from death certificates. No statistically significant correlation could be established, although over 5% of all buildings had Rn-d values exceeding 20 mWL. It was not within the scope of this study to aim for individual dosimetry, or for the quantitative assessment of other confounding factors, such as smoking habits or air pollution. (Recent studies among the general public are summarized briefly in the Editor's Note at the end of this chapter.)

2.3.4 High Background Radiation Areas.

High background radiation areas are defined as such if at least one of the following conditions is met (103):

1. the annual exposure rate from external terrestrial sources (over extended areas) is greater than 52×10^{-6} C/kg;
2. the long-lived alpha activity ingested with the local diet and water is greater than 1.8 Bq/d;
3. the radon concentration of potable water is greater than 185 kBq/m^3;
4. the radon (^{222}Rn and ^{220}Rn) concentration in the atmosphere is greater than 30 Bq/m^3.

Until now all attempts to correlate external exposure rate with regional cancer mortality have failed to demonstrate any conclusive and statistically significant results; some data contradict previous results, even though they are obtained from the same population (104–107). Taking into account additional subcompartments of these special ecological systems (e.g., geology, hydrology, biology), more defined epidemiological studies have been carried out mainly in Pocos de Caldas (Brazil), and Kerala (India). However, these studies generally lacked the holistic approach needed for such a task, i.e., taking into consideration additional cofactors other than radiation exposure (e.g., socioeconomic situation, life-style, and so forth) which potentially contributed to the observed health effects. In addition, the use of cancer mortality proved to be unsuitable to identify subtle dose-related differences in the radiation-induced biological effects between selected population subgroups, indicating the need for more sensitive histocytological methods (108–114). Furthermore, these studies generally lacked the application of recent advances in dosimetry, relying on whole-body concepts rather than cellular or even microdosimetric approaches, thereby disregarding age- and sex-dependent differences in dose distribution. Although it was possible to determine the dose-dependent effect of exposure resulting in chromosomal aberrations, a causal relationship between cancer incidence and radiation exposure, particularly with regard to radon, has not been established.

3   LIMITATIONS OF EPIDEMIOLOGICAL STUDIES

3.1   Introduction

At present it is assumed—relying mainly on epidemiological research—that between 60% and nearly all of the cancer incidence observed in humans is due to the influence of environmental factors and chemical carcinogens (115, 116). Genetic factors and oncogenic viruses are generally considered to be of considerably lesser significance. The methodology used in epidemiological studies to infer a causal relationship between one or more environmental agents and a specific malignant disease is based on observations rather than controlled experiments, thereby missing the important elements of randomization and controls. In addition, the frequent failure to apply rigorous methods of statistical inference has led to criticism of some major epidemiological surveys (117, 118).

A cautious approach is also necessary in the interpretation of epidemiological studies dealing with the problem of lung cancer induction due to long-term low-level Rn-d exposure for the following reasons:

1. association can be identified erroneously with cause, i.e., emphasizing the role of radon exposure only but underestimating simultaneous exposure to other carcinogens present in the atmosphere;
2. accurate and reliable quantification of the biological end point under investigation over observation periods of several decades is difficult to achieve; i.e., comparability of lung cancer diagnosis and classification over the past 50 years and/or between different societies (e.g., United States versus C.S.S.R.) is unlikely.

In the following subsections the significance of the input parameters "exposure" and "effect" and the uncertainties associated with them are discussed for studies of Rn-d-induced lung cancer incidence.

3.2   Uncertainties of Past Radon Progeny Exposure Assessment

Knowledge of individual exposure to the carcinogen Rn-d, prior to the detection of lung cancer, is of utmost importance if a statistically significant dose-effect relationship is to be obtained in an epidemiological study. At present none of the available retrospective studies on Rn-d-exposed population groups is able to provide this vital information with a compelling degree of accuracy and reliability. Most of these surveys are based on indirect estimates of past Rn-d exposure levels; in many cases they are even unable to give more than a "guesstimate" of annual average exposure for a given time. Instead of actual measurements, similarities between retired and presently accessible mines in ore content or mining techniques have to be used to infer past Rn-d levels. The shortcomings of such methods, even under controlled situations, are well documented. The unique role of Rn-d control in mine engineering and ventilation problems is readily acknowledged (119).

In the few studies where measurements have been carried out, area grab samples have been employed. Using these data to assign the necessary individual dose values is associated with many uncertainties, as is discussed below.

3.2.1 Comparability of Measurement Techniques. Different techniques for Rn-d measurements have a large range of intrinsic uncertainties due to the analytical procedures and instrumentation employed (120). For instance, data from the widely used Kusnetz method are very erratic in comparison to continuous Rn-d monitoring owing to pronounced variations of the Rn-d levels in mines (130). Attempts to achieve intercalibration of various types of Rn and Rn-d measuring equipment under ideal laboratory conditions revealed significant discrepancies between participants (121, 122). In routine surveillance programs, however, exposure measurements based on area grab sampling are carried out frequently by different personnel using different instruments. Another factor causing significant variability in Rn-d readings is the sensitivity of some instrumentation to changing environmental conditions (130, 131).

3.2.2 Validity of Potential Alpha-Energy Concentration (PAEC) Measurements. Often PAEC measurements are used, together with the occupancy time as reported, e.g., by the miner himself or his foreman, to evaluate individual exposure. This procedure is valid only if the nuclide concentration is constant in time and space during the stated period. Knowledge of the precision and accuracy of the measurement method itself, as well as that of the recorded time, is also required. Owing to the variety of different activities during a work shift, there is no mean exposure value that can be assigned to a typical uranium miner. Exposure for a miner in production is up to 30 times the exposure value for a miner with shop duties (123). Owing to varying ventilation rates and effectiveness, physical actions (blasting, hauling, drilling), and pressurization of the mine, Rn-d exposure levels can vary within the same mine by an order of magnitude even in modern mines with largely controlled working conditions (128, 130).

With regard to compensation for spatial and temporal variability, it is necessary to take 10–30 grab sample measurements at a given site in order to assess the mean site-specific value with 50% accuracy at the 95% confidence level (40). Temporal changes of Rn-d levels alone account for a range of the coefficient of variation from typically 5% to 95% under mining conditions (124).

Owing to an unpredictable variation of mixtures of ^{218}Po, ^{214}Pb, and ^{214}Bi, simple correlations between equilibrium factors, Rn-d product mixtures, and age of air are impossible to find, adding a significant element of uncertainty for retrospective exposure assessments (125). Knowledge of the equilibrium factor for assessment of individual Rn-d exposure values is most important in cases where only Rn data are available. In a comprehensive mine survey over 1 year it was found that values of the equilibrium factor ranged from 0.08 to 0.93, indicating that it is inaccurate to assume a single value (134).

3.2.3 Area Versus Personal Monitoring. Until recently no country employed personal Rn-d monitors in order to assess the individual Rn-d exposure, but instead used area monitoring. A large-scale survey in France indicates, however, that area monitoring generally overestimates low-level Rn-d exposures and underestimates high individual exposures (126, 152). Comparing the annual means of Rn-d exposure as assessed by individual dosimetry versus area monitoring, a difference of 45% between the two methods was revealed: area monitoring generally underestimated the collective dose. In the case of individual doses, the factor of underestimation ranged from 5 to 20 (126, 127).

Taking into account the pronounced short- and long-term variations of Rn-d values in mines (128, 129), together with all the mentioned uncertainties, it appears rather optimistic to calculate an individual Rn-d exposure value in retrospect for each subject of an epidemiological survey based, for example, on personal recall of the miner of place and period of occupation or Rn-d values measured in other mines having similar uranium ore grade. This is particularly true for low-level exposures where past-estimated occupational exposure levels are of a similar magnitude as nonoccupational Rn-d exposures occurring during spare-time activities indoors. It is a common characteristic of all attempts carried out hitherto to reconstruct past Rn-d exposure levels in mines that insufficient attention has been paid to the dynamic nature of such working environments. The frequent change of working conditions and work activities causes Rn-d levels to change markedly. As examples, the rate of increase in Rn-d levels might be 1 WL/h when air is turned off for scaling, and Rn-d levels typically drop by a factor of 50 from the scaling phase to the drilling phase (132).

Recently, in a study aiming to improve retrospective exposure estimates in mining environments, the key factors affecting Rn-d variability were analyzed, together with a critical analysis of the reliability of the various sources of information for reconstructing such data (133). It was concluded that historical records from mining companies, as well as government records, are difficult to obtain and are often subject to destruction or neglect. Data derived from worker interviews require a cautious approach and are generally the least reliable part of the information collected. With regard to estimating Rn-d levels, it was revealed that calculated Rn emanation rates based on laboratory measurements are usually significantly lower than those actually measured in mines. This means that Rn-d values derived from laboratory Rn emanation data underestimate the actual Rn-d exposure. Of particular importance in this study was the observation, derived from experiments as well as theoretical modeling, that the relatively small amount of compressed air introduced to the heading caused a considerable reduction of the Rn-d levels around the workmen. Together with the other uncertainties mentioned above, one must seriously question the validity of early exposure estimates for occupational exposure to Rn-d.

3.3 Uncertainties of Lung Cancer Incidence Data

The most common database for quantification of the parameter ''effect'' in mortality studies is derived from death certificates. In the case of lung cancer, with its high probability of fatality, mortality statistics can be used as a reliable indicator for lung cancer incidence. In order to assess the accuracy of the observed effect, it is important to know the accuracy of death certification. A comparison of lung cancer incidence and mortality shows fluctuations in the observed mortality from primary lung cancer due to inconsistencies in classification and application of WHO-coding practices (135). Comparing mortality with morbidity, it can be demonstrated, for example, that the number of unspecified lung cancer cases represents 26% of the mortality series, but only 5% of the morbidity series, indicating frequent insufficient information in death certificates. Sometimes malignant cases, as inferred from autopsied cases, are overlooked clinically, leading to the conclusion that statistics on cancer morbidity should never be based on data derived from death certificates only (136).

Using National Cancer Registry facilities as the primary data source for lung cancer incidence data leads to errors due to overregistration (about 2% of the cases), errors as to site classification (about 4%), and incorrect recording in the benign list (about 2%; all figures referring to Sweden) (137). In this Swedish study it was found that the recorded histological diagnosis "epidermoid carcinoma" was incorrect in 21–54% of all cases, depending on the type of lung cancer.

Lack of standardized methods in tissue typing generally causes low reliability in histological type registration. Intercomparability tests of histological classification results of lung cancer confirm that bronchial carcinoma is one of the most difficult lesions with respect to histological typing. In a survey, a panel of 15 pathologists, experienced in bronchial carcinoma typing, agreed in only 38% of all samples; the rest of the results showed unacceptable differences in individual classifications, differing up to a factor of 38 between the minimum and maximum number classified as a particular cancer type (138). Especially in cases where small cell carcinoma of the lung is combined with other types of lung carcinoma, histological typing is in disagreement with cytological subtyping (139). Tests on the reliability of diagnosing various morphological subtypes of small cell carcinoma of the lung showed that unanimity of three participating histopathologists varied between 38% and 54% of the classified cases (140). As shown in several independent studies, these inconsistencies are not attributable to one pathologist, but rather are common to all of them and reflect the wide range of possibilities for error in lung cancer diagnosis (144–146).

Furthermore, many lung cancer cases are not diagnosed before autopsy (141). Based on postmortem examinations compared to antemortem diagnosis, 40% of primary lung cancer cases are missed altogether by diagnosis of clinicians and about 30% are false positives (142, 143).

There are several reasons for these rather disturbing findings:

1. *Tissue sample preparation:* Tissue preparation for histopathological classification is a source of considerable uncertainty in itself: crush artifacts occur in about 25% of all biopsies, causing misclassifications as "small cell carcinomas" (147); the time between sampling and fixation is decisive for the outcome; the type of histochemical staining used influences the number of carcinomas diagnosed as adenocarcinomas by a factor of 3 (148).

2. *Histological typing:* The World Health Organization has defined four categories with 24 types of malignant lung cancer (149). Examples of misclassification include the following: spindle cell type of squamous cell carcinoma is frequently

confused with carcinosarcoma; in the case of small cell carcinoma it is difficult to distinguish subtypes even with cytological methods; special care is needed to exclude metastases from primary adenocarcinoma in other sites; poorly differentiated adenocarcinoma cannot be readily distinguished from large cell carcinoma; it is often difficult to differentiate between epithelial mesotheliomas and adenocarcinomas; several lesions (mycoses, parasitic infections, vascular malformations) resemble lung tumors.

3. *Ultrastructure:* Lung tumors are generally heterogeneous. Intermixing of the four major categories of lung carcinomas is frequent: squamous cell carcinomas, adenocarcinomas, small cell carcinomas, and large cell carcinomas are actually all present, if the correct microscopic investigation method is used (150).

3.4 Smoking

Among the various causes of lung cancer, smoking is generally considered dominant among nonradiation factors, supposedly causing about 83% of all lung cancer among men and about 43% among women (116, 163). Although it is not within the scope of this chapter to review the validity of this hypothesis, we consider it necessary to point out that the same weaknesses found in epidemiological studies discussed earlier also apply here. Some of these studies, for example the Doll-Hill survey (153, 154), are typical examples of ill-conducted epidemiological research. The authors of this postal survey considered it sufficient to collect data on name, age, address, and smoking history to infer causality from association. Questions of comparability of the different groups with regard to physiological or socioeconomic factors remained unanswered; the survey thereby disregarded an elementary rule of statistical inference, comparing the mortality trends in a group of self-selected British doctors and all men in England and Wales (118).

Often the argument is used that results of randomized animal experiments confirm the carcinogenic effect of tobacco condensate as well as a dose-effect relationship (157, 158). However, this disregards the known difficulties in extrapolation from animal to humans, the general problem with extrapolation from the high doses used in animal experiments to low-dose values occurring in human exposure conditions, and the fact that these substances were usually applied in a strictly nonphysiological way. Our present understanding of smoking-induced lung cancer still leaves some issues unresolved, such as:

- how cigarette smoking causes lung cancer;
- why it is so difficult to induce lung cancer in rodents by smoke inhalation;
- what is the reason for contradicting incidence rates of lung cancer in different countries with regard to differences in tobacco consumption, i.e., low consumption per capita but high lung cancer rate and vice versa;
- what causes lung cancer in nonsmokers, with an annual incidence rate ranging from 40 to $100/10^6$ persons (160, 161).

However, despite these unanswered questions, it is assumed in the following that smoking results in an increased prevalence of respiratory tract lesions, therefore representing a higher risk of lung cancer induction (163–165).

Irrespective of the strength of the association between smoking and lung cancer, it is essential for an epidemiological survey that any assessment of the lung cancer resulting from the carcinogen "tobacco smoke" in the presence of the other suspected carcinogen Rn-d is based on data of the following variables:

- consumption of tobacco (rate and total amount);
- degree of inhalation;
- age when smoking began and stopped.

This assumes that the carcinogenic characteristics of tobacco remain constant with time. However, in reality the tobacco blends of cigarettes have changed significantly in the past. The ratio of tar to nicotine has been lowered—thereby reducing the risk for lung cancer induction from tobacco smoke (163). However, this has not been taken into account in studies on Rn-d-exposed smokers.

Also, the merely qualitative categorization used in some Rn-d epidemiological studies, such as, for example, "heavy smokers," is insufficient, since the lung cancer mortality rate can vary up to a factor of 4 with any of the above smoking related variables (159). Definitions used for "nonsmokers," including never-smokers, pipe or cigar smokers, or "occasional" smokers (consumers of up to 20 kg of tobacco in a lifetime), also are unsuitable in quantifying the respective specific contributions by smoking and Rn-d inhalation to the overall observed lung cancer incidence.

Apart from lacking complete data on smoking habits, results from such epidemiological studies are difficult to compare because they are not standardized with regard to how the information was obtained (by mail survey or personal interview), how questions were worded, and when the information was obtained (at the time of medical examination or in retrospect from the recall of relatives).

Furthermore, the topic of sex- and age-dependent individual "dose assessment" in relation to tobacco smoke inhalation has been neglected (155, 156). Although extensive dosimetric modeling has been carried out with the one carcinogen, Rn-d, accounting for physical and biological parameters (162), the results of such a sensitivity analysis have not been applied to the other carcinogen, tobacco smoke, in Rn-d epidemiologies.

The generally low quality of the input data used for quantifying the effect of smoking is reflected, for example, in the results of a study relating the frequency of bronchogenic carcinomas to cumulative cigarette consumption (7): the number of epidermoid cancers observed in "nonsmokers" is about 50% too high, compared to the corresponding number derived from extrapolation of the "smoker" curve down to zero cigarette consumption; in the case of small-cell undifferentiated cancers, the corresponding number is about 40% too low.

3.5 Synergism

In order to differentiate between the carcinogenic effect of Rn-d exposure and exposure to cigarette smoking, it is necessary to investigate the possibility of interaction between both carcinogens. This is particularly important in the case of epidemiological research carried out on a population group, such as miners, that has a higher percentage of smokers than the general public. In cases of low-level Rn-d exposure it may be impossible to quantify even a presumed interaction, if superimposed on a known strong carcinogen, such as cigarette smoke. In reality, the interaction of the two carcinogens may be very complex.

Special attention has focused on the possibility of synergistic interaction between Rn-d and smoking, defined as the cooperative action of both carcinogens such that the total combined effect exceeds the sum of the two effects taken independently (166).

In order to address this question, a working hypothesis for lung cancer induction is adopted in the following discussion, based on a stochastic multistep theory of carcinogenesis (Fig. 8.8) (167, 168). The process of cell transformation is assumed to include one or more intermediate reversible steps during cell development from an initially normal lung cell into the final, irreversible stage of a malignant lung cell. The potential existence of reversibility in carcinogenesis after exposure to the two carcinogens of interest here is indicated by the capability of cells to stimulate repair activities after alpha-particle exposure, as well as by the decreased lung cancer incidence rate among ex-smokers (169–171). Characteristic of this model is the assumed interaction between an initiator and a promoting agent. In the case of Rn-d exposure, alpha radiation causes the initial cellular damage, which is then promoted by the influence of other carcinogenic substances, e.g., those contained in cigarette smoke (88, 172, 178). This may explain the reduction of the latent period, as observed among smoking miners (173, 174).

Epidemiological evidence exists for and against synergism, ranging from data suggesting additivity to those indicating a multiplicative type of interaction. Dosimetric considerations are equally contradictory. On the one hand, it is suggested that the increased thickness of the epithelial mucous layer found in smokers causes an overall reduction of dose to epithelial cells from penetrating alpha particles, i.e., an antagonism between Rn-d and smoking; on the other hand, the delayed lung clearance rate of carcinogens contained in the inhaled smoke leads to a dose increase, i.e., synergism (39, 173, 175–177). Furthermore, smoke inhalation can cause a large and variable reduction of mucociliary clearance, even down to zero (182); often this reduction is accompanied by a regionally pronounced loss of homogeneity of the viscous film.

The issue is further complicated by inconsistent results from animal inhalation experiments. Simultaneous exposure of dogs to Rn-d and tobacco smoke confirmed results from human epidemiological studies indicating antagonistic interaction (179). However, exposure of rats to cigarette smoke following their exposure to Rn-d resulted in synergism between the two carcinogens, particularly at low levels of Rn-d exposure (180); this effect could not be demonstrated when the order of exposure to Rn-d and smoke was reversed. Direct application of these results to humans is difficult for the following reasons:

1. in the study using dogs, Rn-d exposure levels exceeded human occupational exposure levels by orders of magnitude;

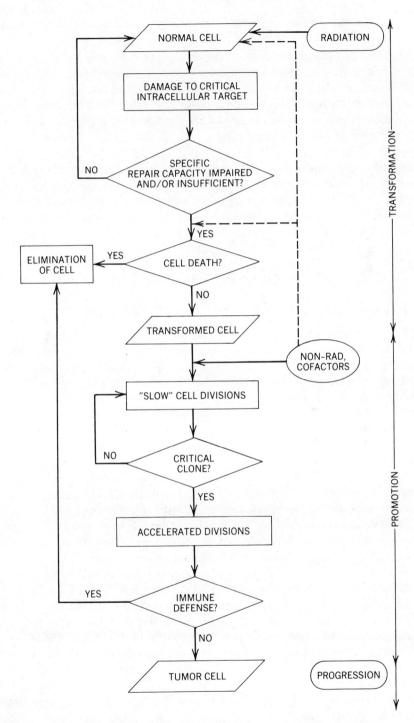

Figure 8.8. Scheme for cancer induction due to radiation exposure.

343

2. exposure to smoke was not standardized between the two studies; e.g., the exposure to tar particles was relatively low in the study with rats;

3. large interspecies differences exist between humans, dogs, and rats with regard to the dose resulting from inhalation of alpha particles as well as smoke particles, e.g., with respect to particle deposition and clearance in the lung, and physiology of the biological target cells (183, 184). For instance, particle deposition in humans due to smoking one pack per day for 20 years is equivalent to rats smoking seven cigarettes per day for 2.5 years (181).

Summarizing, it can be concluded that, in view of the many uncertainties, the question of synergism remains unresolved. From the available data one cannot justify a quantitative assessment of the potential synergistic effect. This is also shown in the large range of estimated correction factors—which differ by 300%— used to account for reduced lung cancer risk for nonsmoking miners (47).

4 ASSESSMENT OF RISK FROM INDOOR RADON EXPOSURE

4.1 Introduction

"Hazard" can be defined as a situation or activity that involves events with undesirable consequences of partially or completely unknown degree and uncertain occurrence in the future (188). The probability of accidents occurring as a result of an existing hazardous situation, termed "risk," can lead to property damage, bodily harm, or even death.

The evolution of humans is significantly influenced by their capability of identifying individual sources of risk and developing means of reducing or even avoiding them altogether. These countermeasures to increase safety concern natural hazards in the environment (e.g., floods, avalanches, fires) as well as man-made hazards (e.g., arms, machinery). However, it was only in this century that mathematical methods were developed for practical application to quantifying risk-benefit-cost assessments. This enabled society to make objective comparisons between the magnitude of risks associated with different hazards (e.g., different sources of energy production) and alternative countermeasures concerning the same risk (e.g., different vaccines against a certain infectious disease).

In order to assess the lifetime risk of a member of the general public resulting from exposure to a carcinogenic agent in the environment, such as Rn-d, the length of the latent period, which is followed by a period of lung tumor expression, has to be quantified (see also Fig. 8.4). This requires that the follow-up period of the study group be sufficiently long to include all Rn-d-induced lung cancer cases, particularly those occurring in the low-level exposure group. As several members of the epidemiological study groups described in Sections 2.2 and 2.3 are still alive, all studies carried out until now represent essentially truncated studies with incomplete follow-up, with the C.S.S.R. and U.S. uranium miners representing the most complete data.

Data from the C.S.S.R. uranium miners indicate a finite period of excess lung cancer, starting about 10 years after initial Rn-d exposure. After about 20 years a maximum value is reached, whereas excess lung cancer diminishes to control values by about 25–30 years after Rn-d exposure has started (10). Data on U.S. miners show a peak in excess deaths due to lung cancer 15–20 years after initial Rn-d exposure, dropping to about 70% of this value over the following 10 years (12). However, it is questionable whether this type of time-dependent response can also be applied for low-level chronic exposure, since it is likely that both groups of uranium miners received their Rn-d exposures at high exposure rates over a period of a few years during the early phase of uranium mining (13, 41). Nonoccupational Rn-d exposure, by contrast, occurs typically at considerably lower exposure rates but throughout a lifetime, resulting in a possibly increased latent period and thereby reduced lifetime risk (see also Section 1.2). Application of the proportional hazard model to the miners' data, however, shows that for a given cumulative dose, lower dose rates appear to be more harmful than higher dose rates (192). International review committees differ significantly in their respective results with regard to the problem of latency, i.e., assuming either a mean manifestation period of about 30 years (ICRP), a 40-year period for the full expression of pulmonary malignancy after an initial exposure to Rn-d (UNSCEAR), or even the possibility of a continued risk of lung cancer induction throughout life (BEIR) (13, 19, 47). This spread of values may be caused by combining information from heterogeneous data, i.e., individuals with different rates of accumulated exposure as well as different biological responses. The resulting statistical association between exposure and latent period has been criticized as potentially meaningless in biological terms (191). In view of the uncertainties associated with the database of these estimates, a conservative approach is often taken in accordance with standard radiation protection practices. In the following discussion, this approach is followed, and a period of 40 years is assumed for the combined latency and expression period associated with nonoccupational Rn-d exposure.

With regard to the choice of the model for assessment of the lifetime risk, the decision is not essential at present and is often overrated in importance, given the large and often unquantifiable uncertainties associated with the input data. Provided that complete follow-up data are available, absolute and relative risk models will give the same result for lifetime risk assessments (47). Figure 8.9 shows the increase of cumulative lung cancer risk due to continuous Rn-d exposure for members of the general public at a constant exposure rate, assuming a latent period, l, and a constant incremental risk, a, per year of exposure (15). Assessment of the lifetime risk requires the deduction of the last l years of "wasted" Rn-d exposure prior to death. The total cumulative risk is represented by the area under curve A. For comparison, the cumulative risk is also indicated for the case of a finite expression period of Rn-d-induced lung cancer (curve B).

In the following subsections, lung cancer risk assessments as derived from epidemiological studies of miners, and their applicability to nonoccupationally exposed members of the general public, are discussed.

4.2   Lung Cancer Risk Assessment for Miners

In order to judge the validity of the results from the reanalysis of epidemiological data using mathematical models of varying complexity, it is important to review

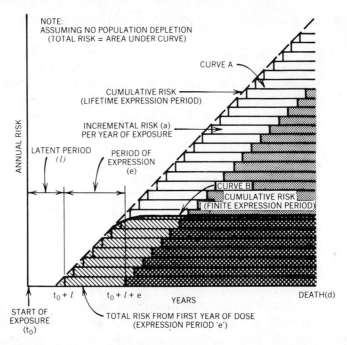

Figure 8.9. Schematic illustration of cumulative absolute risk from continuous exposure. (From Ref. 15. Reproduced with permission.)

the conclusions of some of the major studies. Authors of epidemiological studies have repeatedly stated caveats, indicating that their data are neither intended, nor suited for, a deduction of a quantitative dose-effect relationship in terms of risk assessment, without exercising extreme caution; for example:

> . . . This analysis is most emphatically not offered as a basis for any estimate of risk per unit dose . . . . (62)

> . . . The study was not designed . . . to demonstrate that low levels of exposure cause any detectable increase in the lung cancer incidence rate . . . . (37)

> . . . should be looked upon as a first and very crude approximation . . . neglect confounding factors . . . and effects of environmental factors other than radioactivity . . . assume that all 'excess' lung cancer deaths observed in this population are solely the result of exposure to the short-lived daughters of radon-222 . . . . (190)

> It is therefore not considered appropriate to extrapolate at present from the truncated period of observation to lifetime risk . . . '' (64)

> . . . it is not possible to draw any conclusions about dose and effect below about 100 WLM due to the considerable uncertainty in exposure and statistical error . . . . (70)

In Figure 8.10 data from lung cancer epidemiologies are compiled for several groups of miners. Individual, largely estimated, cumulative exposures cover more

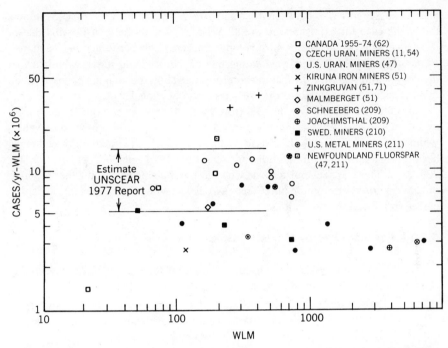

Figure 8.10. Number of excess lung cancer cases for mining populations (standardized per unit of Rn-d exposure) as a function of cumulative exposure. (Reproduced, with permission, from Ref. 55.)

than two orders of magnitude; owing to the large uncertainties and potential bias discussed earlier, it is not possible to give meaningful error bars for these values. Despite these severe limitations, it will be attempted to make use of these data to draw some conclusions on the carcinogenic risk resulting from chronic low-level Rn-d exposure. The data in Figure 8.10 can be interpreted as a three-stage dose-effect relationship:

1. up to about 100 WLM: linear dependence, typical for many radiation dose-effect functions;
2. between 100 and about 500 WLM: plateau region;
3. above 500 WLM: curvilinear downward trend, possibly due to reduced life expectancy (24).

For the purpose of estimating the risk for low-level Rn-d exposure, lung cancer cases observed in this exposure group have been summarized for uranium and nonuranium miners in Table 8.1, which shows that miners in general are at an elevated risk for lung cancer induction above an estimated Rn-d exposure value of about 100 WLM.

The large uncertainties associated with such risk estimates are shown, for example, in the fact that Canadian miners do not express a statistically significant higher lung cancer risk between 40.1 and 100 WLM; in the case of U.S. miners this is the case for exposures up to 239 WLM. It should be kept in mind that in these epidemiological studies most comparisons are made between miners and men of the general public, thereby violating one of the principal requirements in epidemiological research, i.e., that the control group should match the exposed group in all aspects except for Rn-d exposure (see also Section 1.2).

Absolute risk factors (a) derived from these studies range from about 2 to 30 excess lung cancer cases annually per WLM per 10^6 persons, with most values within the range $5 \leq a \leq 15$; based on these data, lifetime risks for miners have been estimated to range from 200 to 600 cases per WLM per 10^6 persons (13, 47, 209–211). There are several reasons why these risk values may be either too high or too low to describe the "pure" risk associated with Rn-d exposure, as is discussed in the following sections.

4.2.1 The Risk Factor May Be Overestimated

a. The individual radiation exposure of some of the miners may have actually been higher than the value assigned in the epidemiological studies:

  i. Early information on exposure of U.S. miners was derived from mine operators, representing Rn-d levels in known problem areas; occasionally higher exposures were underreported.

  ii. Miners were exposed—simultaneously with the short-lived Rn-d—to external gamma radiation, thoron (^{220}Rn) decay products, and long-lived Rn-d products.

  iii. Many miners had previous hard-rock mining experience where they were also exposed to the above components, contributing to their cumulative dose. This factor can be decisive to the outcome of an epidemiological survey of a mining population, as can be seen by comparing the lung cancer incidence rate in Canadian uranium miners with and without prior gold mining experience.

b. Miners were also exposed to potential or known carcinogenic cofactors.

c. Taking into account only lung cancer incidence data in the groups exposed to 100 WLM or less, the difference between the observed and expected number of cases is not statistically significant, even when comparing miners with men of the general public.

4.2.2 The Risk Factor May Be Underestimated

a. The final number of lung cancer cases may continue to grow further:

  i. Epidemiological and radiobiological studies show that the Rn-d exposed cohort has to be followed until extinction, particularly in the case of low-level exposure with extended latency periods; all miner studies represent truncated cohorts.

  ii. Supralinearity has been suggested for the Rn-d-induced lung cancer relationship (212).

b. The actual number of Rn-d-induced lung cancer cases may be higher than the number observed hitherto:

    i. Whenever results are derived from autopsy material (e.g., as is the case for 80% of the U.S. results), it is possible that lung tumors can be missed, since the bronchial sections are very small.

    ii. Many miners had a "chronic cough"; this makes it possible that some deaths attributed to tuberculosis, silicosis, or unspecified cancer were actually due to lung cancer.

In view of the multiple sources of bias and uncertainty in the risk values, and also considering the possibility of mutual, partially compensatory effects between some of the above factors, it seems appropriate to err on the safe side for the particular risk, ensuring the protection of the exposed individual, rather than minimizing economic losses; this, of course, has to be in balance with regard to expenditures concerning the protection against other risks; i.e., one should aim for an optimization in minimizing health detriments from many sources of risk. Therefore, in the following discussion it is assumed that the most probable value of a is 10 excess lung cancer cases per WLM per 10^6 person-years ($\pm 100\%$ uncertainty) used for men occupationally exposed in mining environments.

Detailed sensitivity analysis of the influence of the various factors contributing to the overall uncertainty of the risk assessment is not yet available. However, a first approximation indicates that—independent of the underlying risk concept— the range of uncertainties in the number of Rn-d-related lung cancer cases (i.e., mean $\pm$ one standard deviation) is at least of the same order of magnitude as the total number of lung cancer cases to be expected (196). Using a mean exposure-dose conversion factor of 6 mGy/WLM for mining environments, the average bronchial dose due to alpha-particle irradiation of the basal cells in the bronchial epithelium can be assessed (162). Together with the above exposure-related absolute risk coefficient, a, this results in a dose-related average value of 1.7 excess lung cancer cases per million person-years per mGy (with an uncertainty of about $\pm 100\%$) for miners.

In Figure 8.11 the data on the relative risk (b, in units 10^{-2} per WLM) are summarized for the three most comprehensive studies on uranium miners (51, 64). In the lower exposure group (< 200 WLM), which is of particular interest to lifetime exposure conditions of members of the general public, values cover the approximate range $0.5 \leq b \leq 2$; the average value is about $b = 1$. Applying the same exposure-dose conversion factor as above, the relative increase in risk of lung cancer in uranium miners is 0.17%/mGy (with a range of uncertainty of about $\pm 50\%$).

4.3 Lung Cancer Risk Assessment for the General Public

In recent years several attempts have been made to estimate the lung cancer risk due to Rn-d exposure for nonoccupational exposure situations, using data from miner epidemiological studies or nonsmoker lung cancer incidence. Estimates for

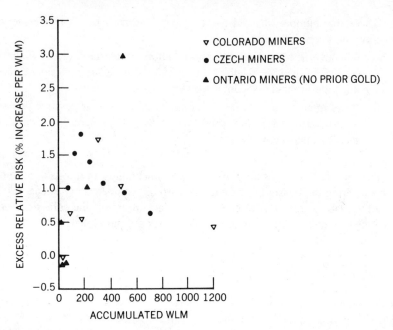

Figure 8.11. Relative risk of Rn-d-induced lung cancer for uranium miners as a function of cumulative exposure. (Adapted, with permission of the Canadian Nuclear Association, from Refs. 51 and 64.)

the annual lung cancer incidence due to Rn-d exposures for members of the public range from about 20 to $230/10^6$ persons, with nonsmokers at values below 100 (20, 21, 195, 207).

However, it is not justified to propose a numerical basis for the "pure" Rn-d-induced lung cancer risk for the general public for the following reasons:

1. All available risk data have large associated uncertainties with regard to dose as well as effect. In addition, they were derived from population groups with high past Rn-d exposure levels. No data are available from nonoccupationally Rn-d-exposed members of the public. To assess the low-level exposure risk of this latter group by extrapolating from uncertain high-level exposure data would only introduce even larger uncertainties due to the lack of information on the shape of the dose-effect relationship, the influence of time-dependent dose distribution, and the latency period (193, 194).

2. No information exists on the individual response of children, chronically ill persons, old people, or women in general with regard to Rn-d exposure and lung cancer. Risk data derived from miners represent risk for a male population subgroup only, for which the "healthy worker effect" has been observed (64, 204). The use of values averaged over age- and sex-dependent differences introduces yet another element of uncertainty in the already uncertain risk assessment.

3. The problem of synergism between Rn-d and the most common lung carcin-

ogen, cigarette smoke, is unresolved. However, even less information is available on several other important cofactors: the nature and actual ''dose'' levels resulting from other organic and inorganic air pollutants found indoors (205); the interaction between Rn-d and these lung irritants; the influence of other factors associated with lung cancer occurrence (e.g., ethnicity, socioeconomic class, population density, life-style) (206). Therefore, it is concluded that the present lack of knowledge prohibits isolating Rn-d as *one* component among several suspected or identified lung carcinogens in the environment of humans, by proposing a risk factor for Rn-d without any degree of acceptable accuracy.

However, it is possible to estimate a value for the upper bound of Rn-d-associated risk in line with the well-established principle of health physics practices mentioned earlier, i.e., accepting the possibility of potentially overestimating the actual risk by adopting a value for the upper limit of risk.

A first approximation of such an upper limit for nonoccupational Rn-d exposure is represented by the risk factor derived from the miner studies discussed earlier.

This value includes not only the risk from the ''pure'' Rn-d alpha-radiation dose, but also an element of risk resulting from simultaneous exposure to other radiation sources (external gamma radiation, internal exposure to long-lived alpha emitters). In view of the higher-than-average percentage of smokers among miners as compared to the general public, these values also include an additional safety margin, particularly for nonsmokers.

Of course, the risk factors derived from epidemiological studies of miners describe the risk resulting from Rn-d exposure conditions that normally do not exist for members of the general public, neither in absolute exposure levels, nor in terms of exposure rate. It has been indicated that they may be even further restricted, i.e., they could apply only to miners who smoke (13). The following arguments, concerning demographical and physiological differences as well as differences in exposure conditions between mining and indoor environments, can be used against the application of these risk factors for estimating the risk for members of the public:

1. respiratory minute volume is higher for hard manual labor in mines than for inhabitants of dwellings;
2. miners investigated were adult men only, whereas indoor exposure includes children and women as well;
3. past Rn-d levels in mines are 1–2 orders of magnitude higher than ''normal'' indoor levels;
4. mine atmospheres contain other suspected or known carcinogens besides Rn-d (e.g., ore dust, diesel and acid fumes, etc.) which may act synergistically with Rn-d; also, physical characteristics of aerosols and Rn-d in mine atmospheres differ from those in homes (e.g., aerodynamic median diameter, unattached fraction, equilibrium factor);
5. occupational Rn-d exposure of miners is short-term (typically 10 years) and

intermittent (40 h/week), but nonoccupational indoor exposure is long-term (i.e., over lifetime) and chronic.

Arguments no. 1–3 are essentially taken into account when individual Rn-d exposure is converted into mean bronchial alpha dose. This step considers physiological differences (age, sex, physical activity) and atmospheric exposure conditions (aerosol characteristics) (162). With regard to argument no. 4, it is emphasized that the most important cofactor for carcinogenesis, i.e. smoking, is likely to affect miners in the same manner as it affects members of the general public. Furthermore, additional carcinogens due to traffic- and industry-related air pollution can also be found in urban environments. The possibility of a significant influence of dose rate (argument no. 5) cannot be ruled out at this time, since analysis of epidemiological data from U.S. and C.S.S.R. miners shows that for equivalent cumulative doses, lower dose rates can be more strongly related to lung cancer induction than higher dose rates (11, 192).

Another possibility to assess an upper limit for the Rn-d-induced lung cancer risk for the general public is the use of lung cancer incidence data for nonsmoking members of the public. In this manner the risk resulting from exposure to all lung carcinogens occurring in a nonmining environment, including Rn-d exposure, is taken into account. Studies of this kind are scarce and difficult because lung cancer among nonsmokers occurs very infrequently. The probability of obtaining a statistically significant result with such a study is a function of the ratio between the true excessive risk and the standard deviation of the observed lung cancer incidence (189). Difficulties in dealing with such a rare event are reflected in the large discrepancies between age-specific lung cancer rates among nonsmokers derived from various studies: values differ by up to 100%, particularly for the age group 55–75 years (197–202). It is a common characteristic, however, that lung cancer death rates among nonsmokers increase with age, ranging from about 20 cases per 10^6 men per year at age 40 years up to about 300 cases per 10^6 men per year at age 75 years. Female rates are about half these values, possibly owing to lower susceptibility (197). As Rn-d-related risk data for occupational Rn-d exposure of females are not available, male data are considered to be applicable to female members of the general public, allowing an additional safety margin.

A third possibility consists of determining the Rn-d dose frequency distribution for a given urban population, applying the risk value derived for miners, and comparing the theoretically derived result with actually observed incidence data. The above-mentioned differences between Rn-d exposure conditions for miners and the general public are taken into account by using the appropriate exposure-dose conversion factor. The number of lung cancer cases to be expected from Rn-d risk assessment was calculated using the lower value of the most probable theoretical range of values for miners (200×10^{-6}/WLM). It could be shown that this theoretically calculated number represents about 15% of the actually observed total number of cases (16). This is in good agreement with the current assumption that about 75% of the total number of observed lung cancer cases can be attributed to smoking only (116). These results were corroborated by a case-referent study, comparing the expected lung cancer rate (based on national incidence data) with the incidence rate of inhabitants of dwellings with Rn-d levels >50 Bq/m^3 and ≤ 50 Bq/m^3 respectively (203). Only persons having lived at the same address for 30 years or more were considered. The results demonstrated that about 30% of the lung cancer cases could be attributed to elevated Rn-d exposure.

In order to facilitate the understanding of the magnitude (rather than the precise value, which is impossible to give at present) of the risk of Rn-d-induced lung cancer, a general comparison with other risks is shown in Table 8.2 (208). It can be seen that risk from exposure at the "normal" value found in European houses is comparable to the mean risk resulting from occupational radiation exposure; the latter itself is as low as the risk resulting from occupational activities as a civil servant. However, at the other end of the scale, Rn values that have been found in problem buildings, i.e., 100 times higher than average, present a risk considered unacceptably high, such as the lung cancer risk resulting from daily consumption of one packet of cigarettes. Development of such a risk perspective is one element in devising strategies for coping with the wide range of radon concentrations to which the public is exposed (cf. Chapter 12).

Editors' Note

In recent times, stimulated by national needs to formulate action programs, new analyses have been performed on the entire range of epidemiological data and these results projected onto the exposures received by the general population. This chapter cites two examples of the former, performed by international (13) and national (47) committees. It also indicates the wide range of estimated risk for the general population, as well as the large uncertainties for these, in Section 4. Considerable efforts are now being devoted to reconciling differences among the primary epidemiological studies and to understanding better how to apply the results to the general population. The dosimetric analysis set forth in Chapter 7 is a primary example of the latter effort, since it provides a basis for examining specifically the difference in doses to miners and members of the general public for the Rn-d exposures they receive. As an example of the former, the U.S. National Academy of Sciences' Committee on the Biological Effects of Ionizing Radiation (BEIR) has attempted to gather together the raw data on exposures and lung cancer incidence from the main miner epidemiological studies, with the objective of reanalyzing the entire body of information in a consistent framework (213).

During the period over which these efforts have been undertaken, other analyses, or "appreciations," have appeared. The most public has been that set forth in the guidance provided to U.S. residents by the Environmental Protection Agency (EPA) (214). This pamphlet provides the estimate that people who spend 75% of their time, over a 70-year lifetime, in a home with 4 pCi/L (150 Bq/m^3) of radon suffer, on the average, an associated risk of dying from lung cancer of 1.3–5.0%. This risk range extends to values that appear consistent with the raw data but that considerably exceed risk estimates of the radiological community, as may be seen by attempting to reduce them to a common mode of expression (which must be

Table 8.2 Magnitude of Risk of Rn-d Lung Cancer, Compared with Other Risks[a]

Mortality risk per year per million affected persons	Radon daughter content in housing (Bq/m³)	Risks from radon	Risks from other radiation	Other risks	Action by society
100,000	40,000	Maximum from ground in housing			
10,000	4,000	Action level, existing housing in Sweden	Limit value for radiation work; limit value in Swedish mines	Smoking one pack/day, all health risks; Smoking one pack/day, lung cancer risk	Society intervenes
1,000	400	Limit value, new housing in Sweden	Mean value in Swedish mines; one intestinal X-ray per year, max. gamma radiation in housing	Work in ore mines; Motor traffic accidents	Society takes certain actions

354

Scale	Radon	Other risks	Society response
100	Limit value for general public from artificial radiation; Mean value for advanced radiation work; Mean value for light radiation work	Building work; Work in public service	Society provides information; private individuals attempt to take preventive action
40	"Normal" for European housing		
10		Train accidents	Private individuals are not worried to any noteworthy extent
4	Outdoors		
1	Expected upper limit for population close to nuclear power stations (normal operation)	Wasps, snakes, lightning	
0.4	Fallout from nuclear weapons testing		
0.1			

[a]Risks from radon according to the Swedish Radon Commission, compared with other risks. Left-hand scale reflects risk of premature death. Note that the risk is influenced both by the radon decay product content and by the occupancy time. (Assumption: Risk factor = $2.5/10^3$ persons exposed to 1 kBq/m^3 during 1 year.) (Reproduced with permission from Ref. 208.)

recognized as a potential pitfall, as noted below). Like most analyses, the EPA estimate assumes a 50% Rn-d equilibrium factor, from which the risk figure can be transformed to 2.4–9.4 deaths per 10^4 WLM.

As noted in Section 4.2, lifetime risks for miners were earlier summarized as 200 to 600 cases per WLM per 10^6 persons (13, 47), which we may transform directly to 2–6 cases per 10^4 WLM, covering the lower half of the EPA range, since lung cancer cases are almost always fatal. In contrast, a somewhat more recent review of the National Council on Radiation Protection and Measurements cites a risk of 1–2 cases per 10^4 WLM in general and, for exposures that occur throughout a lifetime, as for the general public, the risk is expressed in their report as 9.1×10^{-3} cases per WLM/y exposure over a lifetime (215). For a lifetime of 70 years, this may be converted to approximately 1.3 cases per 10^4 WLM, below the range cited by the EPA. It must be emphasized, however, that conversions to a common expression for risk, as is done in this note, entail the possibility of misinterpretation by projecting risk factors onto a general population without recognizing (implicitly) different assumptions about population mix and age distribution.

Chapter 7 provides the basis for another such comparison. There, in Section 9.2, is provided an estimate of 1.5% lifetime risk of lung cancer for domestic exposures of 1 WLM/y, based on estimates of the International Council on Radiological Protection, as adjusted upwards based on the dosimetric calculations of Chapter 7. This may be converted to our common units as 2.1 cases per 10^4 WLM. Chapter 7 also estimates a relative risk factor, based on the same premises, of 1% increase in lung cancer rate per WLM exposure, consistent with the approximate risk cited in this chapter and with the central region of the data in Figure 8.11.

This relative risk factor is significantly different from that obtained by a recent common analysis of data from several of the primary epidemiological studies, which yielded a relative risk factor from the miners of 2.3% per WLM (216). Furthermore, when the resulting model was applied to the case of homes with an Rn-d concentration of 0.02 WL (74 Bq/m^3), equivalent to the radon concentration of 4 pCi/L (150 Bq/m^3) used for the EPA risk estimate cited above, the authors obtained a lung-cancer risk of 2%, assuming an occupancy factor of 17 hours per day. However, in obtaining this estimate, the authors had presumed that the dose per WLM for the general public was half that for the miners, based on differences in breathing rate. If this modifying factor is removed, consistent with recent dosimetry (Ref. 215 and Chapter 7), the risk estimate presumably doubles to 4%. This may be converted to an absolute risk factor of 8.0 per 10^4 WLM, which is comparable to the high end of the EPA range of risks.

Thus even systematic examinations of the full range of epidemiological data and associated evidence can yield substantially different risk factors, either for miners or the general public. These differences appear to arise more from the manner in which the data are utilized than in the inherent uncertainties in the data discussed in detail in this chapter. The factors contributing to the range of estimates include, at this point, only modest differences in the dosimetry and appear to arise more from differences in the underlying risk model employed, i.e., absolute versus relative (or intermediate forms), and—perhaps most importantly—in treatment of the dependence of added lung-cancer risk on age and smoking habits. For example, both Chapter 7 and another recent analysis point out that the importance of smoking in connection with radon risks depends very substantially on whether an absolute or relative risk model is used (217) and differences in treatment can greatly affect resulting estimates; thus treatment of the U.S. miner data, taking smoking explicitly into consideration, yielded a relative risk factor of 0.3% per WLM (218), far less than the estimate of Ref. 216. (One may note from Figure 8.10 that the U.S. miner data has raw risk factors that are somewhat lower than for some other studies, but this does not appear to be the main reason for the contrast between these estimates.) Such difficulties can be compounded when trying to apply risk factors from the miners to the general public, because proper description of each of these populations is necessary—particularly in respect to age and smoking habits—if one is to avoid a blanket presumption that they are similar.

These difficulties cause many scientists to greet risk estimates, particularly for the general public, with a good deal of skepticism, reasons for which are clear from this chapter. Many scientists have particular difficulty with the higher range of risk estimates sometimes used for the general public, since they imply that radon can markedly increase the total risk of lung cancer. An estimate of 4 or 5% risk (e.g., for homes with 150 Bq/m^3 of radon) is a substantial fraction of the risk attributed even to smoking. Considering that regions are being discovered where this is the *average* concentration, some expect that a substantial indication of such risks would be apparent, even from cursory examinations of lung cancer rates by locale. Furthermore, some are skeptical because, even for more typical indoor levels, the corresponding risk is comparable to the total risk of lung cancer of nonsmokers. This does not mean, however, that all of the nonsmoker risk would be accounted for by radon exposures, since—at least in a relative risk model—most of the incidence associated with radon would appear among those who smoke (and who therefore have a much higher "baseline" risk of lung cancer).

One may hope that improved information from epidemiological studies (as well as from basic biological investigations of mechanisms of carcinogenesis) will improve this picture. From individual studies of miners, however, there appears to be little convergence. For example, one of the more recent studies, focusing on Swedish iron miners, extracts distinct risk factors for smokers and nonsmokers (219). The attributable risk appears to be comparable for the two groups, in contrast to the expectation of a relative risk model, which would predict much higher added risk for the smokers. The BEIR committee's analysis of data from four important studies produced a dose-response model couched in terms of relative risk, with a multiplicative interaction between smoking and Rn-d exposure (213). For the U.S. population, this representation yields approximately 3.5 deaths per 10^4 WLM, higher than the NCRP or ICRP estimates, but in the lower half of the EPA range.

The alternative method for understanding the extent to which radon affects lung cancer risk is, of course, to conduct epidemological studies examining the correlation between radon exposures and lung cancer incidence among the general public. This approach has the difficulties of any epidemiological study, plus that associated with the low exposures of the general public as compared with those of uranium miners. The roughly order-of-magnitude difference in exposures poses what might be an insurmountable difficulty, unless the risk factors are at the high end of the range cited above.

As discussed in Section 2.3.3, studies among the general public have provided little information. Nonetheless, such studies are being undertaken, sometimes at a level of sophistication and effort that is considerably greater than for earlier studies. Thus the studies summarized in this chapter (as well as those in Refs. 220–223) provide a preliminary look at the approaches that might be taken in large-scale case-control studies among the general public in areas that have higher-than-average indoor radon concentrations. Such studies have been undertaken in the United States among the heavily exposed populations of Pennsylvania and New Jersey. Whether they and other studies provide information beyond that from the miner studies depends critically, not on the design and conduct of the studies, but on the actual amount of risk induced by environmental radon exposures. If this is at the lower end of the range summarized above, the studies are unlikely to reduce the uncertainty in present risk estimates, even if they do indicate that some radon-related incidence occurs.

REFERENCES

1. *Epidemiology—A Guide to Teaching Methods* (1973). Churchill Livingstone, New York.

2. Roht, L. H., Selwyn, B. J., Holguin, A. H., and Christensen, B. L. (1982). *Principles of Epidemiology*, Academic Press, New York.

3. Monson, R. R. (1980). *Occupational Epidemiology*, CRC Press, Boca Raton, FL.

4. Lilienfeld, D. E. (1978). Definitions of epidemiology, *Am. J. Epidemiol.*, **107**, 87.

5. Committee on Data for Science and Technology (CODATA) (1975). International Council of Scientific Unions, CODATA bull. no. 16.

6. Hofmann, W. (1981). Personal characteristics and environmental factors influencing radiation carcinogenesis due to inhaled radon decay products. In M. Gomez (ed.), *Proc. Int. Conf. on Radiat. Hazards in Mining: Control, Measurement and Medical Aspects*, Soc. of Mining Engineers, New York, p. 669.

7. Saccomanno, G., Archer, V. E., Auerbach, O., Kuschner, M., Egger, M., Wood, S., and Mick, R. (1981). Age factor in histological type of lung cancer among uranium miners, a preliminary report. In M. Gomez (ed.), *Proc. Inter. Conf. on Radiat. Hazards in Mining: Control, Measurement and Medical Aspects*, Soc. of Mining Engineers, New York, p. 675.

8. Steinhäusler, F., and Pohl, E. (1984). Lung cancer risk for miners and atomic bomb survivors and its relevance to indoor radon exposure, *Radiat. Prot. Dosim.*, **7**, 389.

9. Härting, F. H., and Hesse, W. (1879). Der Lungenkrebs, die Bergkrankheit in den Schneeberger Gruben, Teil I, *Eulenbergs Vierteljahrschr. Gerichtl. Med. öffentl. Gesundheit.*, Neue Folge, **30**, 296.

10. Sevc, B., and Placek, V. (1973). Lung cancer risk in relation to long-term exposure

to radon daughters. In E. Bujdoso (ed.), *Proc. IRPA Second Europ. Congr. Radiat. Prot.*, Akademiai Kiado, Budapest, Hungary, p. 129.

11. Kunz, E., Sevc, J., Placek, V., and Horacek, J. (1979). Lung cancer in man in relation to different time distribution of radiation exposure, *Health Phys.*, **36,** 699.

12. Waxweiler, R. J., Roscoe, R. J., Archer, V. E., Thun, M. J., Wagoner, J. K., and Lundin, F. E. (1981). Mortality follow-up through 1977 of the white underground miners cohort examined by the US-Public Health Service. In M. Gomez (ed.), *Proc. Int. Conf. Radiat. Hazards in Mining: Control, Measurement and Medical Aspects,* Soc. of Mining Engineers, New York, p. 823.

13. United Nations Scientific Committee on the Effects of Atomic Radiation (UNSCEAR) (1977). Sources and effects of ionizing radiation, report to the General Assembly with Annexes, United Nations, New York.

14. Radford, E. P., and St. Clair Renard, K. G. (1984). Lung cancer in Swedish iron miners exposed to low doses of radon daughters, *N. Engl. J. Med.*, **310,** 1485.

15. Senes Consultants Ltd. (1984). Assessment of the scientific basis for existing federal limitations on radiation exposure to underground uranium miners, report for the American Mining Congress, Toronto, Ontario, Canada.

16. Steinhäusler, F., Hofmann, W., Pohl, E., and Pohl-Rüling, J. (1983). Radiation exposure of the respiratory tract and associated carcinogenic risk due to inhaled radon daughters, *Health Phys.*, **45,** 331.

17. Wrixon, A. D., Brown, L., Cliff, K.D., Driscoll, M. H., Green, B. M. R., and Miles, J. C. H. (1984). Indoor radiation surveys in the UK, *Radiat. Prot. Dosim.*, **7,** 321.

18. Luckey, T. D. (1980). *Hormesis with Ionizing Radiation*, CRC Press, Boca Raton, FL.

19. International Commission on Radiological Protection (ICRP) (1981). *Limits on Inhalation of Radon Daughters by Workers*, Annals of the ICRP, publication 32, vol. 6, no. 1, Pergamon Press, Oxford, England.

20. National Council on Radiation Protection and Measurements (NCRP) (1984). Exposures from the uranium series with emphasis on radon and its daughters, NCRP rep. no. 77, Bethesda, MD.

21. National Council on Radiation Protection and Measurements (NCRP) (1984). Evaluation of occupational and environmental exposures to radon and radon daughters in the United States, NCRP rep. no. 78, Bethesda, MD.

22. Stewart, C. G. (1983). A model for the accumulation of cases of pulmonary malignancy in time when dose is accumulated in time, Atomic Energy of Canada Ltd., rep AECL-7155, Chalk River Nuclear Laboratories, Chalk River, Ontario, Canada.

23. Thomas, D. C., and McNeill, K. G. (1982). Risk estimates for the health effects of alpha radiation, report INFO-0081, Atomic Energy Control Board, Ottawa, Ontario, Canada.

24. Jacobi, W., Paretzke, H. G., and Schindel, F. (1985). Lung cancer risk assessment of radon-exposed miners on the basis of a proportional hazard model. In H. Stocker (ed.), *Proc. Internat. Conf. Occup. Radiat. Safety in Mining*, Canadian Nuclear Assoc., Toronto, Ontario, Canada, p. 17.

25. Agricola, G., *De Re Metallica*, Dover Publications, New York. Translated by Hoover, H. C., and Hoover, L. H. (1950) (in English).

26. Härting, F. H. and Hesse, W. (1879). Der Lungenkrebs, die Bergkrankheit in den Schneeberger Gruben, Teil II, *Eulenbergs Vierteljahresschr. Gerichtl. Med. öffentl. Gesundheit.*, *Neue Folge*, **31**, 102, 313.

27. Uhlig, M. (1921). Über den Schneeberger Lungenkrebs, *Virchows Arch.*, **230**, 76.

28. Bale, W. F. (1980). Hazards associated with radon and thoron. Memorandum to the files, March 14, 1951, *Health Phys.*, **38**, 1062.

29. Aurand, K., Jacobi, W., and Schraub, A. (1955). Zur biologischen Strahlenwirkung des Radon und seiner Folgeprodukte, *Sonderbände Strahlenther.*, **35**, 237.

30. Bale, W. F., and Shapiro, J. V. (1956). Radiation dosage to lungs from radon and its daughter products. In *Proc. Internat. Conf. on Peaceful Uses of Atomic Energy*, *Geneva*, United Nations, New York.

31. Hultquist, B. (1956). Studies on naturally occurring ionizing radiations with special reference to radiation doses in Swedish houses of various types, *Kungl. Svenska vetenskapsakademius handligar*, **Bd 6/3.**

32. Pohl, E. (1965). Biophysikalische Untersuchungen über die Inkorporation der natürlich Radioaktiven Emanationen und deren Zerfallsprodukte, *Sitzungsber. Österr. Akad. Wiss.*, *Math.-nat. Klasse*, **Abt. II**, 174, Heft 8-10.

33. James, A.C. (1984). Personal communication.

34. Webb, G. A. M., O'Riordan, M. C., Reissland, J. A., and Hill, M. D. (1983). Natural radiation and waste disposal, report NRPB-R 156, National Radiological Protection Board, Chilton, England.

35. Wagoner, J. K., Archer, V. E., and Carroll, B. E. (1964). Cancer mortality patterns among US uranium miners and millers, 1950 through 1962, *J. Natl. Cancer Inst.*, **32**, 787.

36. Holaday, D. A. (1969). History of the exposure of miners to radon, *Health Phys.*, **16**, 547.

37. Congress of the United States (1967). *Joint Committee on Atomic Energy*, Part 1 and 2.

38. Stocker, H. (1985). *Proc. Int. Conf. Occup. Radiat. Safety in Mining*, Canadian Nucl. Assoc., Toronto, Ontario, Canada.

39. Lundin, F. E., Wagoner, J. K., and Archer, V. E. (1971). *Radon Daughter Exposure and Respiratory Cancer, Quantitative and Temporal Aspects*, Nat. Inst. Occup. Safety and Health/Nat. Inst. Env. Sciences, joint monograph no. 1, US Dept. Health, Education and Welfare, Public Health Service (NTIS, no. PB 204871), Washington, DC.

40. Dory, A. B. (1979). *Practical Difficulties Related to Implementation of ICRP-Recommended Dose Limitation in Uranium Mines*, IAEA conf. no. IAEA-SR-36/7, International Atomic Energy Agency, Vienna, Austria, p. 287.

41. Swent, L. W. (1981). Statement of principles. In M. Gomez (ed.), *Proc. Int. Conf. Radiat. Hazards in Mining: Control, Measurement and Medical Aspects*, Soc. of Mining Engineers, New York, p. 823.

42. Jackson, P. O. (1981). Statement of principles. In M. Gomez (ed.), *Proc. Int. Conf. Radiat. Hazards in Mining: Control, Measurement and Medical Aspects*, Soc. of Mining Engineers, New York, p. 1031.

43. Archer, V. E., Magnusson, H. J., and Holaday, D. A. (1962). Hazards to health in uranium mining and milling, *J. Occup. Med.* **4**, 55.

44. Saccomanno, G., Archer, V. E., Auerbach, O., Kuschner, M., Saunders, R. P., and Klein, M. B. (1972). Histologic types of lung cancer among uranium miners, *Cancer*, **27**, 515.

45. Katz, R., and Hofmann, W. (1982). Thresholds in radiobiology, *Phys. Med. Biol.*, **27**, 1187.

46. Archer, V. E., Wagoner, J. K., and Lundin, F. E. (1973). Lung cancer among uranium miners in the United States, *Health Phys.*, **25**, 351.

47. U.S. National Academy of Sciences, National Research Council BEIR III (1980). *The Effects on Populations of Exposure to Low Levels of Ionizing Radiation*, Washington, DC.

48. Archer, V. E., Gilliam, J. D., and Wagoner, J. D. (1976). Respiratory disease mortality among uranium miners, *Ann. NY Acad. Sci.*, **217**, 280.

49. Utting, R. E. (1981). Assessment of gamma doses absorbed by underground miners in Canadian uranium mines. In M. Gomez (ed.), *Proc. Int. Conf. Radiat. Hazards in Mining: Control, Measurement and Medical Aspects*, Soc. of Mining Engineers, New York, p. 533.

50. Harley, N. H., Bohning, D. E., and Fisenne, I. M. (1981). The dose to basal cells in bronchial epithelium from long-lived alpha emitters in uranium mines. In M. Gomez (ed.), *Int. Conf. Radiat. Hazards in Mining: Control, Measurement and Medical Aspects*, Soc. of Mining Engineers, New York, p. 36.

51. Archer, V. E., Radford, E. P., and Axelson, O. (1978). Factors in exposure-response relationship of radon daughter injury. In *Proc. Conf./Workshop on Lung Cancer Epid. in Industr. Appl. of Sputum Cytology*, Colorado School of Mines, Golden, CO, p. 324.

52. Schüttmann, W. (1982). Ionisierende Strahlung und Bronchialkarzinom, *Z. Erkrank. Atm. Org.*, **159**, 3.

53. Behounek, F. (1970). History of the exposure of miners to radon, *Health Phys.*, **19**, 56.

54. Sevc, J., Kunz, E., and Placek, V. (1976). Lung cancer in uranium miners and long-term exposure to radon daughter products, *Health Phys.*, **30**, 433.

55. Cohen, B. L. (1981). Failures and critique of the BEIR-III lung cancer risk estimate. In M. Gomez (ed.), *Proc. Int. Conf. Radiat. Hazards in Mining: Control, Measurement and Medical Aspects*, Soc. of Mining Engineers, New York, p. 114.

56. Petersen, G. R., and Sever, L. E. (1982). An appraisal of selected epidemiologic issues from studies of lung cancer among uranium and hard rock miners, U.S. Uranium Registry, rep. no. USUR-02 HEHF-35.

57. Lorenz, E. (1944). Radioactivity and lung cancer: A critical review of lung cancer in the miners of Schneeberg and Joachimsthal, *J. Natl. Cancer Inst.*, **5**, 1.

58. Sevcova, M., Sevc, J., and Thomas, J. (1978). Alpha irradiation of the skin and the possibility of late effects, *Health Phys.*, **35**, 803.

59. Sevc, J., Placek, V., and Jerabvek, J. (1971). Lung cancer risk in relation to long-term radiation exposure in uranium mines. In *Proc. 4th Conf. on Radiat. Hyg.*, Jasna Pod Chopkom, C.S.S.R, Part II, p. 315.

60. Horacek, J. (1969). Der Joachimsthaler Lungenkrebs nach dem zweiten Weltkrieg (Bericht über 55 Fälle), *Z. Krebsforsch.*, **72**, 52.

61. Horacek, J., Placek, V., and Sevc, J. (1977). Histologic types of bronchogenic cancer in relation to different conditions of radiation exposure, *Cancer*, **40**, 832.

62. Ham, J. M., Hume, F. R., Gray, C.C., Gladstone, A. L., Beaudry, J., Perry, E. A., and Riggin, R. P. (eds.) (1976). Report of the Royal Commission on the health and safety of workers in mines, Ministry of the Attorney General, Ontario, Canada.

63. Myers, D., and Stewart, C. G., (1978). Some health aspects of Canadian uranium mining. In *Proc. Conf./Workshop on Lung Cancer Epid. in Industr. Appl. of Sputum Cytology*, Colorado School of Mines, Golden, CO.

64. Muller, J., Wheeler, W. C., Gentleman, J. F., Suranyi, G., and Kusiak, R. (1985). Study of mortality of Ontario miners. In H. Stocker (ed.), *Proc. Internat. Conf. Occup. Radiat. Safety in Mining*, Canadian Nuclear Assoc., Toronto, Ontario, Canada, p. 335.

65. Muller, J., Wheeler, W. C., Gentleman, J. F., Suranyi, G., and Kusiak, R. (1983). *Study of Mortality of Ontario Miners*, Part 1, Rep. Ontario Ministry of Labour, Ontario Workers' Compensation Board, Atomic Energy Control Board of Canada.

66. Smith, M. E. (1981). Health hazards in mining: The files and facilities. In M. Gomez (ed.), *Proc. Int. Conf. on Radiat. Hazards in Mining: Control, Measurement and Medical Aspects*, Soc. of Mining Engineers, New York, p. 836.

67. Tirmarche, M., Brenot, J., Piechowski, J., Chameaud, J., and Pradel, J. (1985). The present state of an epidemiological study of uranium miners in France. In H. Stocker (ed.), *Proc. Internat. Conf. Occup. Radiat. Safety in Mining*, Canadian Nuclear Assoc., Toronto, Ontario, Canada, p. 344.

68. Edling, C. (1982). Lung cancer and smoking in a group of iron ore miners, *Am. J. Ind. Med.*, **3**, 191.

69. Edling, C., and Axelson, O. (1983). Quantitative aspects of radon daughter exposure and lung cancer in underground miners, *Br. J. Ind. Med.*, **40**, 182.

70. Snihs, J. O. (1973). The approach to radon problems in non-uranium mines in Sweden. In *Proc. Third Internat. Congr. Internat. Radiat. Prot. Assoc. (IRPA)*, USAEC conf. 73097-P.2, Washington, DC, p. 909.

71. Axelson, O., and Sundell, L. (1978). Mining, lung cancer and smoking, *Scand J. Work Environ. Health*, **4**, 46.

72. Axelson, O. (1982). *Epidemiology of Occupational Cancer: Mining and Ore Processing*, Occupat. Safety & Health Series, no. 46, Internat. Labour Organ., Geneva, Switzerland, p. 135.

73. Corkill, D. A., and Dory, A. B. (1984). *A Retrospective Study of Radon Daughter Concentrations in the Workplace in the Fluorspar Miners of St. Lawrence, Nfld.*, Atomic Energy Control Board of Canada, Ottawa.

74. De Villiers, A. J., and Windish, J. P. (1964). Lung cancer in a fluorspar mine community; I. Radiation, dust and mortality, *Br. J. Ind. Med.*, **21**, 94.

75. Morrison, H. I., Wigle, D. T., Stocker, H., and De Villiers, A. J. (1981). Lung cancer mortality and radiation exposure among the Newfoundland fluorspar miners. In M. Gomez (ed.), *Proc. Int. Conf. on Radiat. Hazards in Mining: Control, Measurement and Medical Aspects*, Soc. of Mining Engineers, New York, p. 322.

76. Morrison, H. I., Semenciw, R. M., Mao, Y., Corkill, D. A., Dory, A. B., De Villiers, A. J., Stocker, H., and Wigle, D. T., Lung cancer mortality and radiation exposure among the Newfoundland fluorspar miners. In H. Stocker (ed.), *Proc. In-*

ternat. Conf. Occup. Radiat. Safety in Mining, Canadian Nuclear Assoc., Toronto, Ontario, Canada, p. 365.

77. Wright, E. S., and Couves, C. M. (1977). Radiation-induced carcinoma of the lung. The St. Lawrence tragedy, *J. Thorac. Cardiovasc. Surg.*, **74**, 495.

78. Basson, J. K., Wynham, C. H., Heyns, A. J. A., Keely, W. H., Barnard, C. P. S., Munro, A. A., and Webster, I. (1971). Lung cancer and exposure to radon daughters in South African gold/uranium mines, rep. no. PEL 209, Atomic Energy Board, Pretoria, South Africa.

79. Solli, H. M., Andersen, A., Stranden, E., and Langard, S. (1985). Cancer incidence among workers exposed to radon and thoron daughters at a niobium mine, *Scand. J. Work. Environ. Health*, **11**, 7.

80. Boyd, J. T., Doll, R., Foulds, J. S., and Leiper, T. (1970). Cancer of the lung in iron ore (haematite) miners, *Br. J. Ind. Med.*, **27**, 97.

81. O'Riordan, M. C., Rae, S., and Thomas, G. H. (1981). Radon in British mines—A review. In M. Gomez (ed.), *Proc. Int. Conf. on Radiat. Hazards in Mining: Control, Measurement and Medical Aspects*, Soc. of Mining Engineers, New York, p. 74.

82. Luedwig, P., and Lorenser, E. (1924). Untersuchung der Grubenluft in den Schneeberger Gruben auf den Gehalt an Radiumemanation, *Strahlentherapie*, **17**, 428.

83. Vohra, K. G., Pillai, K. C., Mishra, U. C., and Sadasivan, S. (eds.) (1982). *Natural Radiation Environment*, Wiley Eastern, Dehli.

84. Proc. Internat. Symposium (1979). Grundlagen der Radontherapie, Bad Münster, FRG. In I. K. Dirnagl (ed.), *Z. angew. Bäder- Klimaheilkunde*, 26/4.

85. Steinhäusler, F. (1985). European radon surveys and risk assessment. In R. B. Gammage and S. V. Kaye (eds.), *Indoor Air and Human Health*, Lewis, Chelsea, MA, p. 109.

86. Steinhäusler, F., Hofmann, W., Pohl, E., and Pohl-Rüling, J. (1980). Local and temporal distribution pattern of radon and daughters in an urban environment and determination of organ dose frequency distributions with demoscopical methods. In *Proc. Symp. Natur. Radiat. Environment III*, conf-780422, vol. 2, DOE Symp. Ser. 51, NTIS, Springfield, VA, p. 1145.

87. Steinhäusler, F. (1985). The radon dilemma. In H. Stocker (ed.), *Proc. Int. Congr. on Occup. Radiat. Safety in Mining*, Can. Nucl. Assoc., Toronto, Ontario, Canada, p. 637.

88. Uzunov, I., Steinhäusler, F., and Pohl, E. (1981). Carcinogenic risk of exposure to radon daughters associated with radon spas, *Health Phys.*, **41**, 807.

89. Pohl-Rüling, J., and Scheminzky, F. (1972). The natural radiation environment of Badgastein, Austria and its biological effects. In J. A. S. Adams, W. M. Lowder, and T. F. Gesell (eds.), *Proc. Int. Symp. The Natural Radiation Environment II*, Vol. I, conf-720805-P1, NTIS, Springfield, VA, p. 393.

90. Pohl, E., Pohl-Rüling, J., and Steinhäusler, F. (1977). The natural radioactivity of the air in the region of Badgastein/Austria, the measurement of its local and temporal fluctuations and the resulting dose to various population groups. In *Int. Symp. on Areas of High Natural Radioactivity, Pocos de Caldas, Brazil, 1975*, Acad. Brasil. Cienc., Rio de Janeiro, p. 182.

91. Pohl-Rüling, J., Steinhäusler, F., and Pohl, E. (1982). Radiation exposure and resulting risk due to residence and employment in a radon spa. In K. G. Vohra, K. C.

Pillai, U. C. Mishra, and S. Sadasivan (eds.), *Natural Radiation Environment*, Wiley Eastern, Delhi, p. 107.

92. Vaskov, L. S. (1973). Comparative clinical studies on the occupational hazards from inhaled radon daughters in workers in nonuranium mines and mineral baths. In E. Bujdoso (ed.), *Proc. IRPA 2nd Europ. Congr. Radiat. Prot.*, Akademiai Kiado, Budapest, p. 645.

93. Pohl-Rüling, J., and Fischer, P. (1983). Chromosome aberrations in inhabitants of areas with elevated radioactivity. In *Radiation-Induced Chromosome Damage in Man*, Alan R. Liss, New York, p. 527.

94. Clemente, G. F., Renzetti, A., Santori, G., Steinhäusler, F., and Pohl-Rüling, J. (1984). Relationship between the ^{210}Pb content of teeth and exposure to radon and radon daughters, *Health Phys.*, **47**, 253.

95. Bean, J. A., Isacson, P., Hausler, W., and Kohler, I. (1982). Drinking water and cancer incidence by source of drinking water and size of municipality, *Am. J. Epidemiol.*, **116**, 912.

96. Bean, J. A., Isacson, P., Hahne, R. M. A., and Kohler, I. (1982). Drinking water and cancer in Iowa: II. Radioactivity in drinking water, *Am. J. Epidemiol.*, **116**, 924.

97. Environmental Protection Agency (1977). Cost of radium removal from potable water supplies, USEPA rep. no. EPA-600/2-77-073, Washington, DC.

98. Environmental Protection Agency (1978). Manual of treatment techniques for meeting the interim primary drinking water regulations, USEPA rep. no. EPA-600/8-77-005, Washington, DC.

99. Cantor, K. P., and McCabe, L. J. (1978). The epidemiologic approach to the evaluation of organics in drinking water. In R. L. Jolley, H. Grochev, and D. H. Hamilton, (eds.), *Water Chlorination: Environmental Impact and Health Effects*, Vol. 2, Ann Arbor Science Publ., Ann Arbor, MI, p. 379.

100. Kahlos, H., and Asikainen, M. (1980). Internal radiation doses from radioactivity of drinking water in Finland, *Health Phys.*, **39**, 108.

101. Castrén, O. (1982). Radon in Finnish dwellings—Aspects of epidemiological studies and radiation protection. In G. Clemente, A. V. Nero, F. Steinhäusler, and M. E. Wrenn (eds.), *Proc. Specialist Meet. on the Assessment of Radon and Radon Daughter Exposure and Related Biological Effects*, RD Press, University of Utah, Salt Lake City.

102. Letourneau, E. G., and Wigle, D. T. (1982). Mortality and indoor daughter concentrations in 13 Canadian Cities. In G. Clemente, A. V. Nero, F. Steinhäusler, and M. E. Wrenn (eds.), *Proc. Spec. Meet. on the Assessment of Radon and Radon Daughter Exposure and Related Biological Effects*, RD Press, University of Utah, Salt Lake City, p. 239.

103. *Proc. Symp. on Areas of High Nat. Radiat.* (1977). Academia Brasileira de Ciencias, Rio de Janeiro.

104. Calapaj, G. G. (1975). Mortalita per leucemia e dose assorbita per il fondo naturale di radiazioni nella popolazione Italiana, *Statistica*, **35**, 275.

105. High Background Radiation Research Group (1980). Health survey in high background radiation areas in China, *Science*, **209**, 877.

106. Eckhoff, N. D., Shultis, S. K., Clack, R. W., and Ramer, E. R. (1974). Correlation of leukemia mortality rates with altitude in the United States, *Health Phys.*, **27**, 377.

107. Mason, T. J., and Miller, R. W. (1974). Cosmic radiation at high altitudes and U.S. cancer mortality 1950–1969, *Radiat. Res.*, **60**, 302.

108. Penna Franca, E., Costa Ribeiro, C., Cullen, T. L., Barcinski, M., and Gonzales, E. (1973). Natural radioactivity in Brazil: A comprehensive review with a model for dose-effect studies. In J. A. S. Adams, W. M. Lowder, and T. F. Gesell (eds.), *Proc. 2nd Int. Symp. on Nat. Radiat. Envir.*, conf-720805-P2, NTIS, Springfield, VA, p. 929.

109. Barcinski, M. A., do Ceu, M., Abreu, A., de Almeida, J. C. L., Naya, J. M., Fonsela, L. C., and Castro, L. E. (1975). Cytogenetic investigation in a Brasilian population living in an area of high natural radioactivity, *Am. J. Hum. Genet.*, **27**, 802.

110. Cullen, T. L., Paschoa, A. S., Penna Franca, E., Costa Ribeiro, C., Barcinski, M., and Eisenbud, M. (1980). Two decades of research in the Brazilian areas of high natural radioactivity. In *Proc. 5th Int. IRPA Congress*, Jerusalem, Israel, p. 361.

111. Gopal-Ayengar, A. R., Sundaram, K., Mistry, K. B., and George, K. P. (1977). Current status of investigations on biological effects of high background radioactivity in the monazite bearing areas of Kerala coast in south-west India. In *Proc. Int. Symp. on Areas of High Natural Radioactivity*, Academia Braziliera de Ciencias, Rio de Janeiro, Brazil, p. 19.

112. Leonard, A., Delpoux, M., and Dalebroux, M. (1980). Recherches sur les effets genetiques de la radioactivité naturelle anormale observée localement dans le sud-ouest de la France. In *Proc. Sem. on the Radiolog. Burden of Man from Natural Radioactivity in the Countries of the European Communities*, Commission of the European Communities, Brussels, p. 469.

113. Verma, I. C., Kochupillai, N., Grewal, M. S., Mallick, G. R., and Ramalingswami, V. (1977). Genetic effects of high background radiation in coastal Kerala—Chemical and cytogenetics studies. In *Proc. Int. Symp. on Areas of High Nat. Radioactivity*, Academia Braziliera de Ciencias, Rio de Janeiro, Brazil, p. 185.

114. Pohl-Rüling, J., and Fischer, P. (1979). The dose effect relationship of chromosome aberrations to alpha and gamma irradiation in a population subjected to an increased burden of natural radioactivity, *Radiat. Res.*, **80**, 81.

115. Preussmann, R. (1976). Chemical carcinogens in the human environment. Problems and quantitative aspects, *Oncology*, **33**, 51.

116. American Cancer Society (1980). Cancer facts and figures, New York.

117. Horwitz, R. I., and Feinstein, A. R. (1979). Methodological standards and contradictory results in case-control research, *Am. J. Med.*, **66**, 556.

118. Burch, P. R. J. (1978). Smoking and lung cancer: The problem of inferring cause, *J. Roy. Stat. Soc. Ser. A (General)*, **141**, 437.

119. Rock, R. L. (1974). Mine engineering and ventilation problems unique to the control of radon daughters, U.S. Dept. of the Interior, MESA-info-rep. 1001.

120. OECD-NEA Group of Experts (1985). *Metrology and Monitoring of Radon, Thoron and Their Daughters*, NEA/OECD Publication, Paris.

121. Miles, J. C., Stores, E. J., Cliff, K. D., and Sinnaeve, J. (1984). Results from an international intercomparison of techniques for measuring radon and radon decay products, *Radiat. Prot. Dosim.*, **7**, 169.

122. OECD-NEA (1986). *Proc. Intern. Workshop on Intern. Intercalibration and Inter-*

comparison for Radon, Thoron and Their Daughters Monitoring Equipment, Paris, May 1985, NEA/OECD Publication, Paris.

123. Cooper, W. E. (1981). A comparison of radon-daughter exposures calculated for U.S. underground uranium miners based on MSHA and company records. In M. Gomez (ed.), *Proc. Int. Conf. on Radiat. Hazards in Mining: Control, Measurement and Medical Aspects*, Soc. of Mining Engineers, New York, p. 292.

124. Borak, T. B., Franco, E., Schiager, K. J., Johnson, J. A., and Holub, R. F. (1981). Evaluation of recent developments in radon progeny measurements. In M. Gomez (ed.), *Proc. Inter. Conf. on Radiat. Hazards in Mining: Control, Measurement and Medical Aspects*, Soc. of Mining Engineers, New York, p. 419.

125. Holub, R. F., and Droullard, R. F. (1980). Rate of plateout in radon daughter mixture distributions in uranium mine atmospheres, *Health Phys.*, **39,** 761.

126. Zettwoog, P. (1981). State-of-the-art of the alpha individual dosimetry in France. In M. Gomez (ed.), *Proc. Int. Conf. on Radiat. Hazards in Mining: Control, Measurement and Medical Aspects*, Soc. of Mining Engineers, New York, p. 321.

127. Viljoen, J., and Balint, A. B. (1985). Comparing personal alpha dosimetry with the conventional area monitoring-time weighting methods of exposure estimations: A Canadian assessment. In H. Stocker (ed.), *Proc. Int. Conf. Occup. Radiat. Safety in Mining*, Canadian Nucl. Assoc., Toronto, Ontario, Canada, p. 285.

128. Berteig, L., and Stranden, E. (1981). Radon and radon daughters in mine atmospheres and influencing factors. In M. Gomez (ed.), *Proc. Int. Conf. on Radiat. Hazards in Mining: Control, Measurement and Medical Aspects*, Soc. of Mining Engineers, New York, p. 89.

129. Roze, V., and Raz, R. (1985). Measurement of temporal variations in radon progeny working levels in mine atmospheres. In H. Stocker (ed.), *Proc. Int. Conf. Occup. Radiat. Safety in Mining*, Canadian Nucl. Assoc., Toronto, Ontario, Canada, p. 107.

130. Briggs, M. R., King, R. H., and Franklin, J. C. (1985). In-mine evaluation of continuous radon and working-level detectors. In H. Stocker (ed.), *Proc. Int. Conf. Occup. Radiat. Safety in Mining*, Canadian Nucl. Assoc., Toronto, Ontario, Canada, p. 212.

131. Steinhäusler, F., Daschil, F., and Pfligersdorffer, P. (1985). Comparative tests of radon and radon daughter detection systems under simulated environmental conditions. In H. Stocker (ed.), *Proc. Int. Conf. on Occup. Radiat. Safety in Mining*, Canadian Nucl. Assoc., Toronto, Ontario, Canada, p. 116.

132. Scott, A. G. (1985). Recreating the uranium mining environment of the 1950's. In H. Stocker (ed.), *Proc. Int. Conf. Occup. Radiat. Safety in Mining*, Canadian Nucl. Assoc., Toronto, Ontario, Canada, p. 196.

133. Dory, A. B., and Corkill, D. A. (1985). Practical approach to retrospective estimation of radon daughter concentration in the underground mining environment. In H. Stocker (ed.), *Proc. Int. Conf. Occup. Radiat. Safety in Mining*, Canadian Nucl. Assoc., Toronto, Ontario, Canada.

134. Stranden, E., and Berteig, L. (1982). Radon daughter equilibrium and unattached fraction in mine atmospheres, *Health Phys.*, **42,** 479.

135. Larsson, S. (1971). Comparison of lung cancer morbidity and mortality in Sweden 1959–66, *Acta Pathol. Microbiol. Scand.* Sect. A, **79,** 524.

136. de Faire, U., Friberg, L., Lorich, U., and Lundman, T. (1976). A validation of cause-of-death certification in 1156 deaths, *Acta Med. Scand.*, **200,** 223.

137. Larsson, S. (1971). Completeness and reliability of lung cancer registration in the Swedish Cancer Registry, *Acta Pathol. Microbiol. Scand.* Sect. A, **79**, 389.

138. Kutschera, W., and Salzer, G. (1969). Klinische Kritik an der histologischen Klassifizierung des Bronchuskarzinoms, *Z. Erkrankungen Atmungsorgane*, **130**, 17.

139. Zaharopoulos, P., Wong, J. Y., and Stewart, G. D. (1982). Cytomorphology of the variants of small-cell carcinoma of the lung, *Acta Cytol.*, **26**, 800.

140. Hirsch, F. R., Matthews, M. J., and Yesner, R. (1982). Histopathologic classification of small cell carcinoma of the lung, *Cancer*, **50**, 1360.

141. Berge, T., and Lundberg, S. (1970). Cancer i Malmö 1958–1966, *Sv. Läk. Tidn.*, **67**, 5531.

142. Heasman, M. A., and Lipworth, L. (1966). *Accuracy of Certification of Cause of Death*, Her Majesty's Stationary Office, General Register Office: Studies on Medical and Population Subjects, no. 20.

143. Waldron, H. A., and Vickerstaff, L. (1977). *Limitations of Quality. Ante-mortem and Post-mortem diagnoses*, Nuffield Provincial Hospital Trust, London.

144. Jimenez, F., Teng, P., and Rosenblatt, M. B. (1975). Cancer of the lung in males, *Bull. NY Acad. Med.*, **51**, 432.

145. Bauer, F. W., and Robbins, S. L. (1972). An autopsy study of cancer patients. I. Accuracy of the clinical diagnosis (1955 to 1965), Boston City Hospital, *JAMA*, **221**, 1471.

146. Herrold, K. Mc. D. (1972). Survey of histologic types of primary lung cancer in U.S. veterans, *Pathol. Annu.*, **7**, 45.

147. Carr, D. T., and Lukeman, J. M. (1980). Classification of lung cancer, *Cancer Bull.*, **32**, 77.

148. Herman, D. L., and Crittenden, M. (1961). Distribution of primary lung cancer carcinomas in relation to time as determined by histochemical techniques, *J. Natl. Cancer Inst.*, **27**, 1227.

149. World Health Organization (1982). Histological typing of lung tumors, *Neoplasma*, **29**, 111.

150. Saba, S. R., Espinoza, C. G., Richman, A. V., and Azar, H. A. (1983). Carcinomas of the lung: An ultrastructural and immunocytochemical study, *Am. J. Clin. Pathol.*, **80**, 6.

151. Ives, J. C., Buffler, P. A., and Greenberg, S. D. (1983). Environmental associations and histopathologic patterns of carcinoma of the lung: The challenge and dilemma in epidemiologic studies, *Am. Rev. Respir. Dis.*, **128**, 195.

152. Piechowski, J. W., LeGac, J., Brenot, J., Nenot, J. C., and Zettwoog, P. (1982). Miner's exposures to radon daughters: Individual or ambient monitoring? In *Proc. 3rd SRP Int. Symp. Radiat. Prot. Advances in Theory and Practice*, Inverness, Great Britain, p. 488.

153. Doll, R., and Hill, A. B. (1950). Smoking and carcinoma of the lung. Preliminary report, *Br. Med. J.*, **2**, 739.

154. Doll, R., and Peto, R. (1976). Mortality in relation to smoking: 20 year's observations on male British doctors, *Br. Med. J.*, **2**, 1525.

155. Tokuhata, G. K., and Lilienfeld, A. M. (1963). Familial aggregation of lung cancer in humans, *J. Natl. Cancer Inst.*, **30**, 289.

156. Tokuhata, G. K. (1976). Cancer of the lung: Host and environmental interaction. In H. T. Lynch (ed.), *Cancer Genetics*, Thomas, Springfield, IL.

157. Davies, R. F., Lee, P. N., and Rothwell, K. (1974). A study of the dose response of mouse skin to cigarette smoke condensate, *Br. J. Cancer*, **30**, 146.

158. Peto, R., Roe, F. J. C., Lee, P. N., Levy, L., and Clack, J. (1975). Cancer and aging in mice and men, *Br. J. Cancer*, **32**, 411.

159. Fraumeni, J. F. (1975). *Persons at High Risk of Cancer*, Academic Press, New York, p. 131.

160. Doll, R. (1953). Mortality from lung cancer among nonsmokers, *Br. J. Cancer*, **7**, 303.

161. Stranden, E. (1980). Radon in dwellings and lung cancer—A review, *Health Phys.*, **38**, 301.

162. OECD-Nuclear Energy Agency (1983). Dosimetry aspects of exposure to radon and thoron daughter products, NEA Experts Report, OECD, Paris.

163. U.S. Surgeon General (1981). *The Health Consequences of Smoking, the Changing Cigarette*, US Government Printing Office, Washington, DC.

164. World Health Organization (WHO) (1975). *Smoking and Its Effects on Health*, WHO Techn. Rep. ser. no. 568, Geneva.

165. World Health Organization (1979). *Controlling the Smoking Epidemic*, WHO Techn. Rep. ser. no. 636, Geneva.

166. Taylor, C. E., and Gordon, J. E. (1953). Synergism and antagonism in mass diseases of man, *Am. J. Med. Sci.*, **255**, 320.

167. Süss, R., Kinzel, V., and Scribner, J. D. (1973). *Cancer—Experiments and Concepts*, Springer Verlag, New York.

168. Moolgavkar, S. H., and Knudson, A. G. Jr. (1981). Mutation and cancer: A model for human carcinogenesis, *J. Natl. Cancer Inst.*, **66**, 1037.

169. Dirnagl, K. (ed.) (1984). Proc. II Int. Symp., Physikal., biolog. u. med. Wirkungen niedrig dosierter ionisierender Strahlen, in *Z. Physik. Med. Baln. Med. Klimatol.*, 13/1.

170. Wynder, E. L., and Goodman, M. T. (1977). Smoking and lung cancer: Some unresolved issues, *Cancer Res.*, **37**, 4608.

171. Doll, R., and Hill, A. B. (1964). Mortality in relation to smoking: Ten years observations of British doctors, *Br. Med. J.*, **1**, 1399.

172. Uzunov, I. (1973). Some problems of maximum permissible doses by inhalation of short-lived Rn 222 daughters in mines and radon spas. In E. Bujdoso (ed.), *Proc. 2nd Europ. IRPA-Congr. on Radiat. Prot.*, Akademiai Kiado, Budapest, Hungary, p. 121.

173. Axelson, O., and Sundell, L. (1978). Mining, lung cancer and smoking, *Scand. J. Work. Environ. Health*, **4**, 46.

174. Axelson, O. (1980). Interaction between smoking and exposure to radon daughters. In W. Rom and V. Archer (eds.), *Health Implications of New Energy Technologies*, Soc. for Occup. and Environ. Health, Washington, DC, p. 23.

175. Whittemore, A., and Altshuler, B. (1976). Lung cancer incidence in cigarette smokers: Further analysis of Doll and Hill's data for British physicians, *Biometrics*, **32**, 850.

176. Axelson, O. (1980). Arsenic compounds and cancer. In V. Vainio, M. Sorsa, and K.

Hemminki (eds.), *Occupational Cancer and Carcinogens*, Hemisphere, New York, p. 309.

177. Chovil, A. C. (1979). Occupational lung cancer and smoking: Review in the light of current theories of carcinogenesis, *Can. Med. Assoc. J.*, **121**, 548.

178. Cross, F. T. (1984). Radioactivity in cigarette smoke issue, *Health Phys.*, **46**, 205.

179. Cross, F. T. (1982). Influence of radon daughter exposure rate and uranium ore dust concentration on occurrence of lung tumors. In G. Clemente, A. V. Nero, F. Stein-häusler, and M. E. Wrenn (eds.), *Proc. Specialist Meet. on the Assessment of Radon and Radon Daughter Exposure and Related Biological Effects*, RD Press, University of Utah, Salt Lake City, p. 189.

180. Chameaud, J., Perraud, R., Masse, R., and Lafuma, I. (1981). Contribution of animal experimentation to the interpretation of human epidemiological data. In M. Gomez (ed.), *Proc. Intern. Conf. on Radiat. Hazards in Mining: Control, Measurements and Medical Aspects*, Soc. of Mining Engineers, New York, p. 222.

181. Masse, R., Chameaud, J., and Lafuma, I. (1985). Cocarcinogenic effect of tobacco smoke in rats. In G. Cumming and G. Bonsignore (eds.), *Smoking and the Lung*, Plenum Press, New York and London.

182. Lippman, M. (1981). Influence of air pollutants on lung clearance. In H. Hauck (ed.), *International Symposium on Deposition and Clearance of Aerosols in the Human Respiratory Tract*, Arbeitsgemeinschaft f. Aerosole in der Medizin, Bad Gleichenberg.

183. Daschil, F., and Hofmann, W. (1984). Extrapolation model for aerosol deposition in mammalian lungs and comparison with experimental results. In B. Y. H. Liu, D. Y. H. Pui, and H. J. Fissan (eds.), *Aerosols: Science, Technology and Industrial Applications of Airborne Particles*, Elsevier, New York, p. 1042.

184. Daschil, F., and Hofmann, W. (1983). The relevance of animal models for radionuclide inhalation in man. In *Proc. Spec. Workshop "Current Concepts in Lung Dosimetry,"* report PNL-SA-11049, Battelle Pacific Northwest Laboratory, Richland, WA, p. 95.

185. Dungey, C. J. (1981). The radon problem of two Cornish mines. In M. Gomez (ed.), *Proc. Intern. Conf. on Radiat. Hazards in Mining: Control, Measurements and Medical Aspects*, Soc. of Mining Engineers, New York, p. 65.

186. Fox, A. J., Goldblatt, P., and Kinlen, L. J. (1981). A study of the mortality of Cornish tin miners, *Br. J. Ind. Med.*, **38**, 378.

187. Garrard, J. (1949). Vital capacity measurements in Cornish tin miners, *Br. J. Ind. Med.*, **6**, 221.

188. Lee, T. R. (1981). The public's perception of risk and the question of irrationality. In The Royal Society (ed.), *The Assessment and Perception of Risk*, London, p. 164.

189. Land, C. E. (1980). Estimating cancer risks from low doses of ionising radiation, *Science*, **209**, 1197.

190. Muller, J., Wheeler, W. C., Gentleman, J. F., Suranyi, G., and Kusiak, R. A. (1983). *Study of Mortality of Ontario Miners 1955–1977*, Ontario Ministry of Labour, Ontario Workers Compensation Board, Atomic Energy Control Board of Canada.

191. Hewitt, D. (1978). Biostatistical studies on Canadian uranium miners. In *Proc. Conf./Workshop on Lung Cancer Epidemiology and Industrial Applications of Sputum Cytology*, Colorado School of Mines, Golden, CO, p. 264.

192. Hornung, R. W., and Samuels, S. (1981). Survivorship models for lung cancer mortality in uranium miners—Is cumulative dose an appropriate measure of exposure? In M. Gomez (ed.), *Proc. Inter. Conf. on Radiat. Hazards in Mining: Control, Measurement and Medical Aspects*, Soc. of Mining Engineers, New York, p. 363.

193. Rossi, H. H. (1980). Comments on the somatic effects of the BEIR III report, *Radiat. Res.*, **84**, 395.

194. Pohl-Rüling, J., Fischer, P., and Haas, O. (1983). Effect of low dose acute X-irradiation on the frequencies of chromosomal aberrations in human peripheral lymphocytes in vitro, *Mutation Res.*, **110**, 71.

195. Evans, R. D., Harley, J. H., Jacobi, W., McLean, A. S., Miles, W. A., and Stewart, L. G. (1981). Estimate of risk from environmental exposure to radon 222 and its decay products, *Nature*, **290**, 98.

196. Steinhäusler, F., and Hofmann, W. (1985). Inherent dosimetric and epidemiological uncertainties associated with lung cancer risk assessment for mining populations. In H. Stocker (ed.), *Proc. Int. Conf. on Occupational Radiation Safety in Mining*, Can. Nucl. Assoc., Toronto, Ontario, Canada, p. 327.

197. Garfinkel, L. (1980). Cancer mortality in non-smokers: Prospective study by the American Cancer Society, *J. Natl. Cancer Inst.*, **65**, 1169.

198. Hammond, E. C., and Hord, D. (1958). Smoking and death rates—Report on 44 months of follow-up of 187 783 men, *JAMA*, **166**, 1294.

199. Kahn, H. A. (1966). *The Dorn Study of Smoking and Mortality Among U.S. Veterans*, Natl. Cancer Inst. Monograph 19, U.S. Dept. HEW, p. 1.

200. Hammond, E. C. (1966). *Smoking in Relation to the Death Rates of One Million Men and Women*, Natl. Cancer Inst. Monograph 19, U.S. Dept. HEW, p. 127.

201. Enstrom, J. E., and Godley, F. H. (1981). Cancer mortality among a representative sample of nonsmokers in the United States during 1966–68, *J. Natl. Cancer Inst.*, **65**, 1175.

202. Townsend, J. (1978). Smoking and lung cancer: A cohort data study of men and women in England and Wales 1935–1970, *J. Roy. Statist. Soc., Ser. A (General)*, **141**, 95.

203. Edling, C. (1983). Lung cancer and radon daughter exposure in mines and dwellings: Study no. V, Linköping University, Medical Dissertation No. 157, Dept. of Occup. Med., Linköping, Sweden.

204. Nair, R. C., Abbatt, J. D., Howe, G. R., Newcombe, H. B., and Frost, S. E. (1985). Mortality experience among workers in the uranium industry. In H. Stocker (ed.), *Proc. Int. Conf. Occup. Radiat. Safety in Mining*, Canadian Nucl. Assoc., Toronto, Ontario, Canada, p. 354.

205. Gammage, R. B., and Kaye, S. V. (eds.) (1985). *Indoor Air and Human Health*, Lewis, Chelsea, MA.

206. Eisenbud, M. (1978). *Environment, Technology and Health*, New York University Press, New York.

207. Jacobi, W. (1984). Possible lung cancer risk from indoor exposure to radon daughters, *Radiat. Prot. Dosim.*, **7**, 395.

208. Statens Stralskyddsinstitut (1984). Radon in housing, National Institute of Radiat. Prot. rep. no. A84-10, Stockholm, Sweden.

209. Archer, V. E., and Lundin, F. E. (1967). Radiogenic lung cancer in man: Exposure-effect relationship, *Environ. Res.*, **1**, 370.

210. Snihs, O. (1973). In R. E. Stanley and A. A. Moghissi (eds.), *Noble Gases*, CONF-730915, U.S. Atomic Energy Commission.

211. US National Academy of Sciences, National Research Council BEIR I (1972). *Effects on Populations of Exposure to Low Levels of Ionizing Radiation*, Washington, DC.

212. Archer, V. (1981). Perspective on cancer and radon daughters. In M. Gomez (ed.), *Proc. Int. Conf. on Radiat. Hazards in Mining: Control, Measurement and Medical Aspects*, Soc. of Mining Engineers, New York, p. 811.

213. U.S. National Academy of Sciences, Committee on the Biological Effects of Ionizing Radiation (in press). *Health Risks of Radon and Other Internally Deposited Alpha Emitters*.

214. U.S. Environmental Protection Agency (and Department of Health and Human Services) (1986). *A Citizen's Guide to Radon*, report OPA-86-004.

215. National Council on Radiation Protection and Measurements (NCRP) (1984). Evaluation of occupational and environmental exposures to radon and radon daughters in the United States, NCRP report no. 78, Bethesda, MD.

216. Thomas, D. C., McNeill, K. G., and Dougherty, C. (1985). Estimates of lifetime lung cancer risks resulting from Rn progeny exposure, *Health Phys.*, **49**, 825.

217. Ginevan, M. E., and Mills, W. A. (1986). Assessing the risks of Rn exposure: The influence of cigarette smoking, *Health Phys.*, **51**, 163.

218. Whittemore, A. S., and McMillan, A. (1983). Lung cancer among U.S. uranium miners: A reappraisal, *J. Nat. Cancer Inst.*, **71**, 489.

219. Radford, E. P., and Renard, K. G. (1984). Lung cancer in Swedish iron miners exposed to low doses of radon daughters, *New Engl. J. Med.*, **23**, 1485.

220. Hess, C. T., Weiffenbach, C. V., and Norton, S. A. (1983). Environmental radon and cancer correlations in Maine, *Health Phys.*, **45**, 339.

221. Edling, C., Kling, H., and Axelson, O. (1984). Radon in homes—A possible cause of lung cancer, *Scand. J. Work Environ. Health*, **10**, 25.

222. Pershagen, G., Damber, L., and Falk, R. (1984). Exposure to radon in dwellings and lung cancer: A pilot study. In B. Berglund, T. Lindvall, and J. Sundell (eds.), *Indoor Air* (Proc. 3rd Int. Conf. on Indoor Air Quality and Climate, Stockholm, Aug. 20–24, 1984), Swedish Council for Building Research, Stockholm, Vol. 2, p. 73.

223. Svensson, C., Eklund, G., and Pershagen, G. (1987). Indoor exposure to radon from the ground and bronchial cancer in women, *Int. Arch. Occup. Environ. Health*, **59**, 123.

▬ 9

Evidence of Lung Cancer from Animal Studies

F. T. Cross

Biology and Chemistry Department, Pacific Northwest Laboratory, Richland, Washington

1 INTRODUCTION

Animal studies have been conducted for several decades to identify the nature and levels of uranium mine air contaminants that were responsible for producing the lung cancers observed among uranium miners. Many of the initial studies were concerned with early effects or short-term pathological changes (1–3). Exposures were based primarily on radon gas concentrations, giving little or no information on the radon decay product concentrations, which have subsequently been shown to contribute the greatest radiation dose to the lung. The early studies (4–7), in which lung tumors were produced, were methodologically or statistically inadequate to show an unequivocal association of lung tumors with exposure to radon and/or radon decay products.

Beginning in the 1950s, a growing concern emerged that the increased incidence of respiratory cancer observed in the European uranium mining population would also be found in U.S. miners (8, 9). Systematic studies were subsequently begun in the United States to identify the agents responsible for the increased incidence of lung cancer in miners and to develop exposure-response relationships in animals. Investigators at the University of Rochester (UR) began to focus attention on the biological and physical behavior of radon decay products as well as on their contribution to the radiation dose to the respiratory tract (10–12). Shapiro (13) exposed rats and dogs to several levels of radon alone and in the presence of radon progeny attached to room-dust aerosols. He showed that the degree of attachment of radon decay products to carrier dust particles was a primary factor in influencing the alpha-radiation dose to the airway epithelium. He demonstrated that this dose was due primarily (>95%) to the short-lived radon progeny ^{218}Po (RaA) and ^{214}Po (RaC′), rather than to the parent ^{222}Rn.

Work supported by the U.S. Department of Energy under Contract DC-AC06-76RLO 1830.

In 1953, Cohn et al. (14) reported the relative levels of radioactivity found in the nasal passages, in the trachea and major bronchi, and in the other portions of rat lungs after exposure to radon and/or radon progeny. The respiratory tracts of animals that inhaled radon plus its decay products contained 125 times more activity than those of animals that inhaled radon alone.

Beginning in the mid-1950s, Morken, at UR, initiated a pioneering series of experiments (15–17) to evaluate the biological effects of inhaled radon and radon progeny in mice; later experiments also used rats and beagle dogs. The essentially negative biological results of these studies suggested that alpha irradiation is inefficient in producing tumors in the respiratory system.

In the late 1960s and early 1970s, other studies in France (Compagnie Générale des Matières Nucléaires, COGEMA) and the United States (Pacific Northwest Laboratory, PNL) were initiated and later proved successful in producing lung tumors from inhaled radon decay products. The French investigators exposed rats to radon decay products alone or in combination with stable cerium, with uranium ore dust, or with cigarette smoke to produce tumors in the lung (18–20). The later U.S. studies were designed to systematically determine the pathogenic role of radon decay products, alone or in various combinations with uranium ore dust, diesel engine exhaust, and cigarette smoke. These studies involved lifespan exposures of beagle dogs and Syrian golden hamsters and chronic exposures of rats (21, 22).

This report highlights the two U.S. studies (UR and PNL) and the French study (COGEMA). A review of the animal studies through 1970 appeared in the final report of Subgroup I.B, Interagency Uranium Mining Radiation Review Group (23). That report, which particularly addressed the early, acute, radon toxicity studies, concluded (as did an earlier Federal Radiation Council report) (24) that experimental work prior to the 1970s had not shown that it was possible to produce pulmonary carcinomas in animals, in a systematic way, from controlled exposures to radon and its progeny. Since that review, a discussion of the biological effects in animals of inhaled radon and radon decay products has appeared in an International Commission on Radiological Protection (ICRP) report, ICRP publication 31 (25). Even more detailed presentations of the animal studies are presented in a National Council on Radiation Protection and Measurements publication (NCRP report no. 78), *Evaluation of Occupational and Environmental Exposures to Radon and Radon Daughters in the United States* (26), and in the Senes Consultants, Ltd. report prepared for the American Mining Congress, *Assessment of the Scientific Basis for Existing Federal Limitations on Radiation Exposure to Underground Uranium Miners* (27).

We present here updated biological-effects data resulting from chronic radon inhalation exposures of mice, hamsters, rats, and beagle dogs. Emphasis is placed on the carcinogenic effects of radon and radon decay products, including the influences of radon progeny exposure rate, unattached fraction and disequilibrium, and coexposure to other pollutants. These data are correlated with estimated human epidemiological data. Plausible values for the radon (radon progeny) lifetime lung cancer risk coefficients are also provided.

2   RADON INHALATION STUDIES AT THE UNIVERSITY OF ROCHESTER (UR)

2.1   Introduction

These studies, which attempted to develop exposure-response relationships in mice, rats, and dogs from inhalation exposures to radon and radon decay products, were conducted by Morken and co-workers (12, 15–17). The exposures involved approximately 2000 mice, 100 rats, and 80 dogs, as well as control animals.

Exposures were to unfiltered laboratory room air (25°C, 50% relative humidity) which, along with radon, was circulated through an approximately 2-m³ exposure chamber. The dust concentration was on the order of 0.1 mg/m^3 (which, by inference from the PNL exposures, ought to have resulted in high unattached fractions for the radon decay products). Subsequent data from Mercer and Stowe (28) have placed the activity median aerodynamic diameter (AMAD) at $0.2 \ \mu\text{m}$ and the fraction of unattached ^{218}Po (*fa*)* at 20%. The aerosols consisted of dusts, oil, and water droplets. Radon concentrations were about $0.5 \ \mu\text{Ci/L}$ (1.8×10^7 Bq m^{-3}) in the mouse and dog experiments and about $1 \ \mu\text{Ci/L}$ (3.7×10^7 Bq m^{-3}) in the rat experiments.

2.2   Experiments with Mice

Mice of the CAF$_1$ strain, 20 weeks old at the start of exposures, were given chronic inhalation exposures for 150 h/week (for 8 weeks to life) to 2000-working-level (WL) potential alpha-energy concentration [~ 1800 working level month (WLM)/week].† Average alpha dose rates in sacrificed animals were estimated to be 5, 18, 2, 60, and 280 rad/week‡ in whole body, kidney, liver, gastrointestinal (GI) tract/stomach and contents, and lungs/trachea/bronchi, respectively. Dose to bronchial tissue was 5–10 times that to the whole lung, or as much as 2800 rad/week. The range of exposures in the dosimetry determinations was 14,000–72,000 WLM. Lung deposition of inhaled radioactivity was nearly 100%. Clearance to blood was rapid (about 10 min), suggesting that the attached radioactivity was rapidly dissolved from the carrier aerosol.

In the first experiment, lifespan exposures of male and female mice shortened lifespans by 50% as a result of the intense radiation exposures (54-week median lifespan, compared with 109 weeks for control animals). Estimated cumulative potential alpha-energy exposures were 72,000 WLM; estimated mean doses to

---

*fa refers to the fraction, or percentage, of the first decay product of ^{222}Rn (^{218}Po, historically referred to as RaA) that is unattached to a carrier aerosol.

†Working level month is an exposure equivalent to 170 h at a 1-WL concentration. Working level is defined as any combination of the short-lived radon decay products in 1 L of air that will result in the ultimate emission of 1.3×10^5 MeV of alpha energy upon decay to ^{210}Pb. Thus, working level is a unit of measure of potential alpha-energy concentration associated with short-lived radon-decay products. See Section 8.1, Chapter 1 for more on units.

‡1 rad = 100 erg/g; the SI unit for absorbed dose is the gray (Gy), where 1 Gy = 100 rad.

lung were 11,000 rad. Destructive hyperplastic and metaplastic lesions were observed in the tracheobronchial tree, but no carcinomas were noted.

Other groups of mice were similarly exposed, in a second experiment, for 15, 25, or 35 weeks. The 35-week exposures confirmed the results of the previous experiment. No lifespan shortening was noted in the 15- and 25-week exposures, which ranged from 27,000 to 45,000 WLM, producing average lung doses from 4200 to 7000 rad. In a third experiment, animals were exposed for 10, 15, 20, or 25 weeks; some were killed following completion of exposures and others, thereafter, at 10-week intervals from 60 until 110 weeks of age. Exposures ranged from 18,000 to 45,000 WLM; estimated mean doses to lung ranged from 2800 to 7000 rad.

Pathological changes observed in the second and third experiments were similar to those observed in the first experiment, but they were not as extensive. Changes were more marked in the trachea than in the large bronchi. Repair of these lesions was rapid and, by 8 weeks after exposure, tissues appeared to be normal. However, the epithelial lining of terminal bronchioles became flattened or disappeared with increased time after exposure. Lesions were variants of those that occurred spontaneously in older control animals (e.g., adenomas and foci of adenomatosis); the adenomas showed qualitative changes suggestive of malignancy.

2.3 Experiments with Rats

Four groups of 48 male, standard (STD) and specific-pathogen-free (SPF) Sprague-Dawley rats were exposed, 25 h/week for 24 weeks, to 7300 WL potential alpha-energy concentration (~ 1100 WLM/week). Cumulative exposures were approximately 26,000 WLM; estimated mean lung doses were 4400 rad.

Histopathological changes observed in irradiated STD rats were not marked nor were they greatly different from the changes observed in control animals, though some increase was noted in metaplasia, denudation of the respiratory tract, and fibrosis. One rat had an adenoma, another a squamous "tumorlet." None of the lesions appeared to be related to dose.

Histopathological changes observed in SPF rats were similar to those in STD rats, except for the absence of squamous metaplasia. Tumorlets, similar to those seen in the earlier mouse experiments, were also noted in the SPF rats. None of the histopathological changes, however, appeared to be dose-related or to progress with time. Subsequent effects included one undifferentiated carcinoma, one adenoma, and one well-differentiated, keratinizing, squamous carcinoma, which occupied nearly all of one lung lobe. The paucity of findings precludes the development of exposure-response relationships.

2.4 Experiments with Dogs

Fifty-one beagle dogs (40 exposed, four chamber-control, and seven age-control) were exposed for 1, 2, 4, 8, 15, or 50 days, at 200 WLM/day, to provide cumulative potential alpha-energy exposures ranging from 200 to 10,000 WLM. They were sacrificed at 0, 1, 2, and 3 years after exposure; none remained alive after 3 years. Other animals were used in dosimetry experiments and, in small numbers, in earlier pilot experiments.

The results of the dosimetry and pilot experiments are discussed first:

1. Average doses/unit exposure to whole lung were 0.17 rad/WLM, with a range (among nine animals) of 0.08–0.79 rad/WLM. Doses/unit exposure to tracheal epithelium, as well as to bifurcations, averaged about 5 rad/WLM, with a range from 0.3 to 21 rad/WLM. The dose to tracheobronchial epithelium from ^{218}Po was considered three to four times higher than that from ^{214}Po.

2. Exposure of one dog to 1200 WLM (estimated mean lung dose, 200 rad) produced minimal epithelial thickening in some areas of the lung; the trachea showed squamous metaplasia of epithelium without keratinization.

3. Exposures of five dogs to ~2000 WLM (four at ~1000 WLM/week, one at ~200 WLM/week) and one dog to ~3900 WLM (~400 WLM/week), with no control animals, produced subtle, diffuse histopathological changes in microscopic foci. Foci of slight hyperplasia were noted in tracheobronchial and bronchiolar epithelium, along with foci of inflammation in small bronchioles and in alveolar walls. These foci were more diffuse and less severe in animals exposed at the two lower rates of exposure, although occasionally foci were more prominent at the lower exposure rates. The somewhat similar histopathological findings in these six animals, along with the small number of animals exposed and the lack of control animals, make exposure-response relationships questionable.

The results of the large exposure-response relationship study were as follows:

1. Lesions observed for 200- to 10,000-WLM exposures were subtle, variable, diffuse, and very small, involving only a very small fraction of the lung.

2. No significant differences in neoplastic lesions were observed between age- and chamber-control dogs.

3. No significant differences from control groups were noted immediately following exposures for animals exposed to a range from 200 to 10,000 WLM radon decay products. The number of small inflammatory foci increased with exposure level in animals sacrificed at 1 and 2 years; however, by the third year of sacrifice, the relationship disappeared at the lower exposure levels and was equivocal at the higher exposure levels.

4. Small patches of thickened alveolar walls, with some metaplasia of alveolar cells and hyperplasia of bronchial epithelium, were noted. No lesions were noted in the upper bronchial region, indicating that they either rarely occurred or were rapidly repaired.

2.5 Discussion and Conclusions

These experiments were most noteworthy in establishing the exposure-to-dose relationships in whole lung or sections of lung as well as in other organs. The few early and late pathological effects did not allow establishment of carcinogenic exposure-response relationships, which subsequent experiments at COGEMA and PNL have established. In the early experiments, the only late, permanent changes apparent occurred in the alveolar and, possibly, in the bronchiolar region of the lung. They were observed for a wide range of doses, for a period of up to 3 years in the dog and 1 and 2 years in the rat and mouse, respectively. Some of these changes may have been preneoplastic, but the high-level exposures, with consequent lifespan shortening, and the early termination of experiments precluded further development. The influence of the radon decay product carrier aerosol (laboratory room air) on the results of these experiments is uncertain.

3 RADON INHALATION STUDIES AT COMPAGNIE GÉNÉRALE DES MATIÈRES NUCLÉAIRES (COGEMA)

3.1 Introduction

The studies by Chameaud and colleagues (19, 20, 29–34) were begun in the late 1960s and early 1970s to determine whether radon and its decay products induced tumors in rats, and to provide experimental data supporting the epidemiological data on radon progeny carcinogenesis.

Prior to 1972, male, SPF, Sprague-Dawley rats were exposed to ambient air, passed by a closed circuit through trays of finely ground ore containing 25% uranium. Resulting radon concentrations were 0.75 μCi/L (2.8×10^7 Bq m^{-3}); decay-product equilibrium factors were about 30%. With filters and electrostatic purifiers, the equilibrium factor was reduced to about 1%. By calculation, potential alpha-energy concentrations were on the order of 2300 and 75 WL, respectively, for the two disequilibrium conditions.

After 1972, animals were exposed to radon derived from underground barrels of radium-rich lead sulfate. Radon was pumped, by a closed circuit, into a 1-m^3 equilibration container, then to two 10-m^3 metal inhalation chambers. Up to 600 rats could be exposed for as long as 16 h when oxygen was added to the inhalation chambers. Maximum radon concentrations were 1.25 μCi/L (4.6×10^7 Bq m^{-3}), generally with decay products at 100% equilibrium. By calculation, the maximum potential alpha-energy concentration was 12,500 WL. Because of plateout on the cages and the hairs of rats, the disequilibrium of the decay products increased when the number of animals in the inhalation chambers increased. Exposure periods ranged from about 1 to 10 months; exposure rates ranged from less than ten to hundreds of WLM/week, the majority averaging approximately 200–400 WLM/week.

3.2 Results*

In two major experiments (19), rats were given inhalation exposures to stable cerium hydroxide or to 130 mg/m^3 uranium ore dust concentrations, with and with-

---

*Exposure levels in this section have been supplied by COGEMA and may be different from previously published values (35).

out radon progeny, to determine whether the presence of dust altered the carcinogenic effect of radon decay products. Exposure to stable cerium hydroxide prior to radon decay product exposures shortened the induction-latency period of tumors by 2–3 months. Uranium ore dust (given on alternate days to radon progeny exposures) appeared to have little influence on the tumorigenic process, although the number of animals used was too small to permit a firm conclusion (31). Potential alpha-energy exposures varied from 500 to 8500 WLM. The various equilibrium ratios of the decay products appeared to have no effect. These experiments confirmed that radon decay products alone induced tumors in rats.

Other changes observed in these experiments were:

1. At high potential alpha-energy exposures, large areas of diffuse interstitial pneumonia with hyaline membrane formation were noted, along with severe fibrosis of interalveolar septa surrounding capillaries. Death generally occurred between a few weeks and a few months following exposures that exceeded 6000 WLM. No lung cancers were produced.

2. Animals lived longer at lower potential alpha-energy exposures, with carcinomas appearing between the 12th and 24th month after the beginning of exposures. The time to appearance of tumors increased with decrease in cumulative potential alpha-energy exposure. Exposures of 2000–5000 WLM, delivered over 300–500 h (during 3–4 months), produced the highest incidence of tumors (50%).

3. Bronchiolar metaplasia was found at the bronchioloalveolar junction and in neighboring alveoli. It consisted of large columnar cells, with basal nuclei and light-colored protoplasms that were often ciliated. Alveolar metaplasia of cuboidal cells, with darker protoplasms, appeared in peripheral regions of the lungs.

4. Adenomatous lesions of variable sizes and cell layers covered areas of the alveolar septa.

5. Adenomas, consisting of round tumors with cells often clustered together, were observed.

6. Malignant tumors of several different types were found, often in the same animal. These included epidermoid carcinomas, not always clearly differentiated, often keratinized or necrosed, and occasionally extending into the mediastinum; bronchiolar adenocarcinomas, sometimes mucus-producing, containing numerous cellular anomalies, characterized by a high number of mitoses and invasion of other lung lobes, though they were seldom metastatic; and bronchioloalveolar adenocarcinomas, exhibiting few mitoses but frequently invading the mediastinum, diaphragm, and thoracic wall.

7. A range of intermediary lesions was noted. For example, some adenomatous lesions were clearly different from carcinomas; however, some adenomas showed malignant characteristics.

8. The exposure/tumor-incidence relationship, uncorrected for lifespan shortening, was not linear over the wide range of exposures; the incidence per unit exposure increased with decreasing high cumulative exposure.

Subsequent experiments, which confirmed the pathology observed in the two major experiments described above, also extended the potential alpha-energy ex-

TABLE 9.1. Summary of Tumors Primary to the Lungs of Rats, Median Survival Times, and Lung Tumor Risk Coefficients for Compagnie Générale Des Matières Nucléaires (COGEMA) Radon-Progeny Exposures[a]

Group mean exposure (WLM)	Nominal exposure rate (WLM/wk)	Number of animals examined	Number of animals with tumors	Tumors (%)	Group median survival time (days)	Mean lifetime risk coefficient $(10^{-4}/WLM)$[b]
20–25	2–4	~1000	25	1.7	684	7.5[c]
50	2–8	~800	30	2.9	687	5.8[c]
290	9	21	2	10	610	3.3
860	370	20	4	20	672	2.8[d]
1470	370	20	5	25	606	1.7
1800	200	50	17	34	600	1.8
1900	310	20	7	35	548	1.8
2100	220	54	23	43	593	2.0
2800	310	180	74	41	560	1.5
3000	370	40	17	43	670	1.4
4500	370	40	29	73	644	1.6

[a]Data from Chameaud et al. (31–34).
[b]Values uncorrected for lifespan differences from control animals. Lifetime risk coefficients based on raw incidence at very low exposures are considered to accurately define the initial slope of the risk coefficient curve.
[c]Value corrected for lung tumor incidence in control rats of low exposure group (0.83%); normal incidence in the absence of appreciable background radon exposure is about 0.1–0.2% (68). Median survival time of control rats of the two lowest exposure groups was 752 days.
[d]Calculated value at this exposure level is 2.3.

posures down to approximately 20–50 WLM (31, 33, 34). Tumor-incidence and survival-time data are shown in Table 9.1; the data are not sufficiently detailed to estimate uncertainties. Lifetime lung-tumor risk coefficient data are also shown in Table 9.1. Although the risk data are uncorrected for lifespan shortening, a recent hazard-function analysis demonstrates that when the data are adjusted for competing causes of death, the excess risk of developing pulmonary tumors is approximately linearly related to exposure throughout the range of exposures studied (36). Further findings are given below:

1. Tumor-latency period (defined as the time interval between start of radon decay product exposures and death, or sacrifice, of the animal) increased with decrease in cumulative potential alpha-energy exposures. Mean latency times of tumor-bearing animals were on the order of 750 days for exposures <300 WLM and 650 days for exposures exceeding 1000 WLM.

2. As with human cancers, lung cancers in rats invaded pulmonary lymph nodes, but metastases to other tissues were, again, rare. Tumor size increased with increase in cumulative WLM exposures.

3. No radioinduced oat cell carcinomas were observed in rats; however, other histological types of lung carcinomas were similar to those observed in humans.

4. Besides lung carcinomas, only two types were noted in radon-progeny-exposed rats: cutaneous epitheliomas of the upper lip and cancers of the urinary

system. The SPF Sprague-Dawley rat is known to be very sensitive to the latter type of tumor.

5. The incidence of lung cancer increased with decreasing high radon progeny exposure rate. The greatest effect was noted in exposure-fractionation experiments. Rats exposed to approximately 3000 WLM potential alpha energy, at 3000-WL concentrations, for 7 h/day, 1 or 5 days/week (average, rounded, exposure rates are calculated to be 100 and 600 WLM/week), showed a nearly fourfold increase in cancer incidence with exposure protraction.*

6. No change in tumor incidence was noted with age of adult animals at first exposure to radon decay products; however, the latency period continually shortened as the age at first exposure increased. At 3000-WLM exposures, the latency period was 640, 510, 450, and 305 days, respectively, for 150, 280, 400, and 520 days of age at first exposure.

7. Synergism was observed between inhaled radon progeny and whole-body, cigarette smoke exposures when the latter followed the total exposures to radon decay products. However, when the cumulative cigarette smoke exposures preceded the radon decay product exposures, no increase in tumor incidence was noted over that produced by radon decay products alone. The effect of cigarette smoke, therefore, depended on the time sequence of exposures and was attributed to its promoting action (30, 31). Histological types of cancers observed in the smoking experiments were not altered by cigarette smoke exposures. No data are given on whether the latency period of tumors was influenced by smoke exposures; the observation that tumors in the radon-progeny- and smoke-exposed animals were larger and more invasive than those observed in radon-progeny-only exposures may be indicative of a shorter latency period for smoking-related tumors.

3.3 Discussion and Conclusions

To date, the COGEMA studies have produced more than 800 lung cancers in about 10,000 rats exposed to ambient aerosols or to various concentrations of radon progeny alone and in mixtures with other pollutants. The exposure-response relationship data shown in Table 9.1, therefore, represent only a portion of the total data from these experiments. The derived range in mean lifetime risk coefficient, uncorrected for lifespan differences from control animals, is about $1.5-7.5 \times 10^{-4}$/WLM exposure between approximately 20- to 25- and 5000-WLM exposures. The risk decreases at higher WLM exposures owing to lifespan shortening and gradually appears to plateau at about $6-8 \times 10^{-4}$/WLM at the 20- to 50-WLM exposures. No evidence of a threshold below 20-WLM exposures was apparent (34).

These experiments have been useful in clarifying the epidemiological data. Although tumor types differ somewhat, the overall lung-tumor-incidence data in rats are similar to (and perhaps quantitatively higher than) present estimated lung-tu-

---

*Potential alpha-energy concentration and exposure rates were subsequently changed to 1500 WL and 50 and 300 WLM/week, respectively (35).

mor-incidence data in humans. (See Section 7, Comparison of Human and Animal Radon Exposure Data.)

4 RADON INHALATION STUDIES AT PACIFIC NORTHWEST LABORATORY (PNL)

4.1 Introduction

Exposures of dogs and rodents to uranium mine air contaminants were begun in the late 1960s and early 1970s at PNL to identify agents, and their levels, responsible for producing lesions of the respiratory tract similar to those observed in uranium miners. The early experiments concentrated on lifespan inhalation exposures of Syrian golden hamsters and beagle dogs to mixed aerosols of radon, radon progeny, carnotite uranium ore dust, diesel engine exhaust, and cigarette smoke. Most of the final data from these early experiments have been published (21, 37, 38). To provide data missing from the earlier dog study, follow-up studies include exposures of beagle dogs to uranium ore dust alone (but not to radon decay products alone) and exposures of male, SPF, Wistar rats to mixtures of radon, radon progeny, and uranium ore dust (22, 39–44). Because the studies in rats are designed to develop exposure-response relationships, the exposures are truncated. They are also designed to study the roles of carnotite uranium ore dust concentration and radon progeny exposure rate, unattached fraction, and disequilibrium in the production of lung lesions. Histopathology, clinical pathology, and pulmonary physiology tests were the primary means of measuring biological response in these experiments. Urinalyses have recently supplemented serum tests as more sensitive evaluations for kidney damage. Radiometric analyses of tissues have been employed to determine mean radon decay product tissue doses and the body distribution of long-lived radioactivity from the ore dust.

4.2 Experimental Methods

Male hamsters and rats were first exposed when they were approximately 12–14 weeks of age; beagle dogs (both male and female) were 2–2.5 years of age. The experimental methodology is described in previous reports (21, 37, 38, 45). Radon concentrations ranged from 0.1 to 0.3 μCi/L (3.7×10^6 to 11×10^6 Bq m^{-3}) in these experiments. The milled carnotite ore dust aerosols had mass median aerodynamic diameters (MMAD) on the order of 1.0 μm, with a geometric standard deviation (GSD) of about 2.0; the overall average AMAD of the radon decay products was about 0.5 μm, with an overall average GSD of about 2.0. The ore dust used in PNL experiments prior to late 1982 contained about 4% U_3O_8 by weight (46). Thereafter, replacement ore dust contained about 2% U_3O_8. Free silica content of both ore dust aerosols was on the order of 80%.

The exposure chambers were flow-through devices; therefore, the fractional equilibrium of the radon decay products was less than 1 and ranged from 0.1 to 0.6, depending on experimental conditions. In the hamster experiments, a diesel engine was operated to simulate patterns of engine use in mines; CO levels were held to 50 ppm, NO_2 levels to about 5 ppm, and SO_2 and aliphatic aldehyde levels remained below the 1-ppm detection limit. Cigarette smoke exposures of dogs were by mouth and nose only and varied, among animals, between 10 and 20 cigarettes/day.

When animals were found dead or were sacrificed, the lungs and selected other organs were removed and fixed in 10% neutral buffered formalin or glutaraldehyde for subsequent histopathological examination. Appropriate test statistics were used to compare survival curves and other biological data. The exposure protocols for the completed hamster and dog experiments are shown in Table 9.2. Exposure protocols for the ongoing rat experiments are too numerous to show. Essentially, they involve mixtures of radon decay products with uranium ore dust to study the roles of cumulative potential alpha energy, carnotite uranium ore dust concentration, and radon progeny exposure rate, unattached fraction, and disequilibrium in the production of lung lesions.

4.3 Lifespan Shortening and Weight Loss

Lifespan exposures of Syrian golden hamsters to radon progeny alone or in combination with uranium ore dust and diesel engine exhaust caused no significant ($p > 0.05$) changes in mortality patterns compared with those of controls. Amyloidosis, centrilobular hepatocyte degenerative changes, and renal tubular nephrosis were common in all hamsters, which may account for their median lifespan being only a little greater than 1 year. The mean potential alpha-energy exposure in the hamster experiments was on the order of 10,000 WLM. In contrast, lifespan

TABLE 9.2 Exposures in Pacific Northwest Laboratory (PNL) Hamster and Dog Lifespan Studies

Number of animals	Exposure
	Hamsters[a]
102	Controls (room air)
102	700 WL
102	800 WL, ore dust (22 mg/m³ particle concentration)
102	Ore dust (19 mg/m³ particle concentration)
102	Diesel exhaust (7 mg/m³ particle concentration)
102	800 WL, ore dust and diesel exhaust (23 mg/m³ particle concentration)
	Dogs[b]
9	Controls (room air)
20	600 WL, 13 mg/m³ ore dust
20	600 WL, 13 mg/m³ ore dust, 10 cigarettes/day (7 days/week)
20	10 cigarettes/day (7 days/week)[c]

[a]Exposed 6 h/day, 5 days/week.
[b]Radon progeny and ore dust exposures of 4 h/day, 5 days/week.
[c]Three additional dogs were given 20 cigarettes/day, 7 days/week.

exposures of beagle dogs to mixtures of radon progeny, uranium ore dust, and cigarette smoke caused significant lifespan shortening when compared with the approximately 15-year mean lifespan of controls (Table 9.3). Mean survival times of the dogs exposed to radon decay products and ore dust mixtures, with or without added cigarette smoke, was 4–5 years. Mean survival times of controls and smoke-only-exposed dogs were equivalent to one another during the same period. The mean potential alpha-energy exposure of the dogs was about 13,000 WLM.

Chronic exposure of male Wistar rats to mixtures of radon decay products and uranium ore dust also shortened lifespan (Table 9.3). Because the exposures are still in progress, the lifespan shortening and weight loss versus cumulative-exposure relationships have not yet been fully developed. The data that have been analyzed, however, generally show no significant differences in mortality patterns compared with those of controls for exposures up to about 2500 WLM. Exposures exceeding 5000 WLM have caused significant lifespan shortening, the effect increasing with exposure. In general, rats that showed lifespan shortening also showed weight loss.

Thus far, two life-shortening anomalies have been noted in the rat experiments. First, in an interim study to determine any influence of radon progeny exposure rate, rats exposed to about 640 WLM at the lowest rate (about 44 WLM/week) died earlier than other animals given comparable cumulative exposures. Second, in a study to determine the influence of unattached versus attached radon decay products, rats exposed to about 5100 WLM at the highest unattached fraction level ($fa = 24\%$) died earlier than other animals given comparable cumulative exposures. (Life table analyses of the survival time data in the unattached fraction study (43) showed that the estimated probabilities of a rat dying with a lung tumor before 600 days were 0.42, 0.65, and 0.75, respectively, for 1.6, 10, and 24% unattached ^{218}Po concentrations. When expressed as percentages of the radon concentration rather than the ^{218}Po concentration, the fraction unattached was 1.3, 5.2, and 9.5%.) Neither of these experiments has been repeated to determine whether the data are artifactual. Later experiments at 640-WLM exposures and 53-WLM/week exposure rates showed no appreciable lifespan shortening (Table 9.3).

In addition, the mean survival time of tumor-bearing rats (as in the COGEMA data) was always significantly longer than that of non-tumor-bearing rats. This is not surprising, since the induction latency period of lung tumors is a large fraction of the rat lifespan, and tumors must grow to a size sufficient for detection; the shorter-lived animals may have died too soon for tumors (if any) to be detected. In species with lifespans much longer than the tumor induction latency period (e.g., dogs and humans), lethality from neoplasms is marked.

4.4 Pathological and Clinical Responses

It is difficult to pinpoint the cause(s) of lifespan shortening in the animal experiments discussed above. Various pathological changes and clinical responses were also noted, including neoplasia. All are considered to have played some role in causing the death of the animals.

TABLE 9.3 Current Summary of Tumors Primary to the Respiratory Tracts of Rats and Dogs, Mean Survival Times, and Lung Tumor Risk Coefficients for Pacific Northwest Laboratory (PNL) Radon Decay Product Exposures

Group mean exposure (WLM)	Nominal potential alpha-energy concentration (WL)	Nominal exposure rate (WLM/wk)	Number of animals examined	Number of animals with lung tumors	Lung tumors (%)[a]	Extrathoracic tumors (%)[b]	Group mean survival time (days)[c]	Mean lifetime risk coefficient (10^-4/WLM)[d]
			Male Specific-Pathogen-Free Wistar Rats					
322[e]	1000	530	131	19	15	1	625	4.5
320[e]	1000	180	93	14	15	0	626	4.7
640[e]	1000	530	70	7	10	1	596	1.6
642[e]	1000	180	95	12	13	0	605	2.0
642[e]	500	88	32	9	28	0	652	4.4
641[e]	100	53	64	18	28	2	696	4.4
644[e]	250	44	32	5	16	0	535[f]	2.4
1,280[e]	1000	530	38	11	29	5	655	2.3
1,280[e]	100	53	32	21	66	0	730	5.1
2,630[e]	1000	530	38	13	34	0	651	1.3
2,560[e]	1000	180	62	20	32	0	603	1.3
2,580[e]	500	88	32	16	50	0	613	1.9
2,560[e]	100	53	32	22	69	0	634	2.7
3,800[g]	400	190	27	5	19	7	409	0.49
5,120[e]	1000	530	41	20	49	3	592	0.95
5,150[e]	500	260	32	17	53	3	451	1.0
5,100[h]	500	260	32	25	78	14	525	1.5
5,140[i]	500	260	32	8	25	6	335[f]	0.49
5,090[j]	500	260	32	22	69	0	526	1.4
5,120[e]	100	53	32	25	78	3	607	1.5
9,200[e]	900	440	31	22	71	3	465	0.77
10,250[e]	1000	530	52	33	63	6	466	0.62

TABLE 9.3 *(Continued)*

Group mean exposure (WLM)	Nominal potential alpha-energy concentration (WL)	Nominal exposure rate (WLM/wk)	Number of animals examined	Number of animals with lung tumors	Lung tumors (%)[a]	Extrathoracic tumors (%)[b]	Group mean survival time (days)[c]	Mean lifetime risk coefficient $(10^{-4}/\mathrm{WLM})$[d]
Male and Female Beagle Dogs								
12,700[k]	600	71	19	1	5	5	1490	0.041
13,500[l]	600	71	19	7	37	11	1520	0.27

[a]Normal lung tumor incidence in control rats is about 0.1–0.2%.

[b]Includes tumors of the nose, mouth, pharynx, and larynx.

[c]Values are underlined when survival curves of exposed animals are significantly different from those of controls.

[d]Values uncorrected for lifespan shortening. Uncertainties in lifetime risk coefficients are approximately equal to uncertainties in exposure data (standard deviations on exposure were generally less than ±20% of the means).

[e]Unattached percentage of ^{218}Po (fa) generally <3%.

[f]Survival curve was significantly different from all other groups at this exposure level.

[g]High fa [not measured; radon (radon-progeny)-only exposures].

[h]fa = 10%.

[i]fa = 24%.

[j]High radon decay product disequilibrium; equilibrium factor F = 0.1.

[k]fa < 3%, 10 cigarettes (7 days/week).

[l]fa < 3%, sham smoking.

4.4.1 Hematological Effects. The hematological effects observed were infrequent and species-dependent and differed from the lymphocytopenia that usually results from inhalation exposure to transuranics.

Hamsters exposed to high levels of radon decay products with uranium ore dust and diesel engine exhaust showed no significant changes in hematocrit, erythrocyte, leukocyte, or differential leukocyte levels when compared with levels measured in controls. In contrast, dogs exposed to high levels of radon progeny, uranium ore dust, and cigarette smoke manifested mean leukocyte values significantly higher than those of controls. The leukocytosis was exclusively the result of an absolute neutrophilia, which, in turn, probably resulted from chronic irritation and pulmonary cell death. Neutrophilia was also observed in dogs exposed to radon progeny and uranium ore dust, as well as in dogs exposed to cigarette smoke alone. Mean lymphocyte, monocyte, and eosinophil levels, as well as blood serum constituents, were not significantly different among the various exposed and control dogs. Leukocytosis has not yet been observed in the follow-up study on dogs exposed for 6 years to uranium ore dust alone.

In plutonium experiments, lymphocytopenia is considered to be primarily a result of irradiation of cells or tissues within the lungs (25). However, dogs receiving mean lung doses from radon progeny exposures comparable to mean lung doses from plutonium exposures do not manifest lymphocytopenia.

Rats exposed to approximately 300- to 10,000-WLM potential alpha energy (estimated 50- to 2000-rad mean lung dose) and uranium ore dust showed no significant changes in hematocrit, erythrocyte, leukocyte, or differential leukocyte levels when compared with levels in controls. In this respect, rats were similar to the hamsters; the beagle dog is, therefore, the most sensitive of the three animals with regard to hematological effects.

4.4.2 Renal Evaluations. Renal function was evaluated in six uranium-ore-dust-exposed and six sham-exposed dogs following 6 years of exposure for 20 h/week to 15 mg/m^3 uranium ore dust concentrations. Integrated urine samples were collected in ice-cooled containers prior to and following a 20-h period of water deprivation. Tests were conducted on urine osmolality, specific gravity, glucose, creatinine, protein, sodium, potassium, chloride, alkaline and acid phosphatases, glutamic oxaloacetic transaminase, and glutamic pyruvic transaminase; a microscopic examination was also performed.

Results of the battery of tests were equivalent for the exposed and sham-exposed dogs, with the exception of glucose. The mean for glucose excreted in 24 h by the exposed dogs was 27.3 mg versus 10.1 mg by the sham-exposed dogs ($p < 0.05$). This difference was equally apparent when glucose excretion was expressed as mg/kg of body weight or as mg/mL of urine. However, the ability of the kidneys to concentrate urine following deprivation of water for an extended period was not different between the two treatment groups. Thus, based on this series of renal tests, it appears that kidney function has not been appreciably compromised by prolonged exposure to high concentrations of uranium ore dust.

Average uranium (^{234}U and ^{238}U) concentration measured in the lungs of two sacrificed animals following 1-, 2-, 3-, 4-, and 6-year ore dust exposures was 7 nCi/kg (260 Bq kg^{-1}). ^{230}Th concentrations were higher, starting at about 35 nCi/kg (1300 Bq kg^{-1}) at 1 year and gradually increasing to about 140 nCi/kg (5200 Bq kg^{-1}) at 4–6 years of exposure (41, 42). Radionuclide concentrations in the kidneys of these animals were not measured, but limited data on kidney-to-lung radioactivity ratios in rats and dogs followed inhalation of pitchblende uranium ores can be obtained from Stuart et al. (46, 47). These investigators exposed rats to approximately 1000 mg/m^3 (25% U$_3$O$_8$) pitchblende uranium ore concentration for 2 h, twice weekly for 8 weeks. Groups of animals were sacrificed in the first, second, and eighth weeks of exposures, and in the first, ninth, and seventeenth weeks after cessation of exposures. Their data show that, at the end of the first week, ^{238}U levels in the kidneys of rats were about one-twentieth of those in the lung, with ^{230}Th levels only one-tenth those for ^{238}U. The initial preponderance of uranium in the kidneys reflected the preferential solubilization of uranium from the lungs. Urine samples during the same period contained two to five times more uranium than thorium. Thorium levels in the kidneys, however, continued to build during exposures, and the rapid removal of uranium from the tissue after cessation of exposure brought its level to nearly equal that of thorium 2 and 4 months later.

Subsequent data in dogs, following exposures to this same ore at 100 mg/m^3 concentrations, for 1 h, five times weekly for 5 months, showed the radioactive concentrations of thorium in the kidneys to be twice those of uranium. Ratios of kidney-to-lung concentrations were about 0.37 and 0.14 for ^{238}U and ^{230}Th, respectively.

4.5 Respiratory Tract Lesions

In the radon-progeny-exposed animals, the lesions observed in organs other than the lung were considered spontaneous, or only indirectly exposure-related, in contrast to the case for most alpha emitters, which translocate from the lung to irradiate other organs. (A possible exception is the appearance of two osteosarcomas in a group of approximately 100 hamsters exposed to radon decay products and uranium ore dust.)

4.5.1 Nonneoplastic Lesions.

Pulmonary fibrosis and, to a lesser extent, emphysema are common findings in hamsters, rats, and dogs exposed to radon decay products and uranium ore dust. Alveolar septal fibrosis was noted in hamsters exposed to radon progeny, uranium ore dust, and diesel exhaust (this was also true of ore-dust-only exposures, giving the impression that ore dust alone was responsible for this finding). However, another group of hamsters exposed to comparable levels of ore dust and radon decay products did not show alveolar septal fibrosis. There was no explanation for this finding.

Pulmonary fibrosis was prevalent in all dogs exposed to radon progeny and uranium ore dust. Alveolar septal fibrosis was apparent to a slight degree in dogs exposed to 1800-WLM potential alpha energy plus 13 mg/m^3 uranium ore dust concentrations, becoming progressively worse after longer exposures. The condition was characterized by large fibrotic areas in the parenchyma, occasionally involving the major portion of some lung lobes. While the cause of this fibrosis was being investigated, radon-progeny-exposed dogs were compared, on a radiation dose basis, with plutonium-exposed dogs. The prevalence and severity of both emphysema and fibrosis were comparable when dogs were matched as to similar estimated peripheral lung doses. Because the ore dust was absent from the plutonium experiments, the tentative conclusion is that the radiation doses were responsible for the production of these lesions. This conclusion is supported by a current experiment with dogs exposed to uranium ore dust alone. For comparable cumulative exposures to uranium ore dust without the radon progeny exposures, the most notable pulmonary lesions observed were vesicular emphysema (but of less severity than when radon decay products were present), peribronchiolitis, and pneumoconiosis. The degree of pulmonary interstitial fibrosis was slight. Thus, a more rapid development of fibrotic lesions occurred when radon decay products were combined with uranium ore dust.

The only significant pulmonary function change observed in these ore-dust-exposed dogs was an increased slope of the single-breath N_2 washout curve, suggesting an uneven distribution of ventilation. This change was observed in dogs exposed for less than 1 year and continued without increase through 5 years of exposure. Measurements of pulmonary resistance, made through 5 years of exposure, showed slight age-related changes and increasing differences between control and exposed animals with duration of exposure. These two changes are suggestive of bronchitis, similar to the "industrial" bronchitis of mine workers.

The degree and severity of pulmonary fibrosis in rats as a function of radon progeny exposure level are currently under study. Exposures to about 5000-WLM potential alpha energy plus uranium ore dust produced about a 40% incidence of diffuse fibrosis. Only trace to small amounts were noted in animals exposed to less than 1200-WLM potential alpha energy. Thus, the incidence, if not the severity, of this lesion appears comparable to that observed in dogs.

In addition, animals exposed to radon decay products alone or in mixtures with other uranium mine air pollutants commonly had adenomatous lesions that progressed to squamous metaplasia of alveolar epithelium. Bronchioloalveolar and bronchogenic carcinomas followed this and other preneoplastic changes in the lung. Hyperplasia and squamous metaplasia of nasal epithelium, with eventual development of squamous cell carcinoma, were also noted in experiments (generally in rodents) when the unattached fraction of radon progeny was high (39, 43). Low or intermediate unattached fractions produced nasal carcinoma in dogs; either their nasal tissue is more sensitive to carcinogens, or nasal deposition was higher in dogs, compared with rodents (38).

4.5.2 Neoplastic Lesions. In the lifespan studies with dogs, animals with tumors of the respiratory tract generally had cumulative potential alpha-energy exposures exceeding 13,000 WLM; the exposure rate was 71 WLM/week. Under the conditions of the experiment, concomitant exposure to cigarette smoke had a mitigating effect on radon-progeny-induced tumors. This was possibly due to a thickening of the mucous layer as a result of smoking and a stimulatory effect of cigarette smoke on mucociliary clearance, although no empirical evidence was collected during the experiments to substantiate these possibilities. The overall incidence of tumors primary to the lung was 21% for a mean potential alpha-energy exposure of 13,100 WLM; the incidence was 37% in the group exposed to radon progeny and uranium ore dust, but only 5% in the comparably exposed group that also received cigarette smoke exposures. The overall incidence of nasal carcinoma was 8%. The lung cancers were about 70% bronchogenic carcinoma and 30% bronchioloalveolar carcinoma (22). The simplified convention used was that epidermoid tumors and mucus-staining adenocarcinomas were considered bronchogenic carcinomas, whereas tumors of Clara cell or type II alveolar cell origin, as well as non-mucus-staining adenocarcinomas, were considered bronchioloalveolar carcinomas.

Lifespan inhalation exposures of male hamsters produced severe radiation pneumonitis but only four squamous carcinomas (three in the radon-progeny-only group, one in the group exposed to radon progeny and uranium ore dust) in 306 radon-progeny-exposed animals (1.3% incidence). Squamous carcinoma occurred only in association with squamous metaplasia of alveolar epithelium, which, in turn, occurred only in hamsters receiving exposure to radon decay products. Thus, it appears that exposure to radon progeny, development of squamous metaplasia, and development of carcinoma were related. Because so few lung cancers were produced in these high-exposure experiments, perhaps, in part, due to the animals' short median lifespan, it was concluded that the Syrian golden hamster was an inappropriate model for further study of the carcinogenic potential of inhaled (in contradistinction to instilled) mine air pollutants.

Over 4000 male, SPF, Wistar rats have received chronic exposures to ambient air or to mixtures of radon progeny and uranium ore dust since 1978. Many of these animals are still alive. The histopathology data are still accumulating, but some general trends can be observed.

An increasing trend (sometimes significant) was observed in lung cancer risk per cumulative potential alpha-energy exposure with: (i) a decrease in potential alpha-energy exposure rate, (ii) an increase in unattached fraction of radon progeny, and (iii) an increase in radon progeny disequilibrium. The lung cancers observed between exposures of approximately 300 and 5000 WLM were about 70% bronchogenic carcinoma and 30% bronchioloalveolar carcinoma, using the simplified convention of classification (22). The locations of the tumors were most often estimated (by sizing associated bronchi and bronchioles) to be about 50% proximal (bronchus-associated) and 50% distal (bronchiole- and alveolus-associated), in contrast to the nearly 100% proximal location of human lung cancers (48, 49). The prevalence of nasopharyngeal squamous metaplasia and, generally, carcinoma increased with increased levels of unattached radon decay products.

Incidence data on tumors primary to the respiratory tracts of rats and dogs from various potential alpha-energy exposures are also shown in Table. 9.3. Data on approximately 2800 rats currently on experiment are omitted from this table. The data are, as yet, inadequate to draw definitive conclusions regarding the effect of exposure rate and the magnitude of the lifetime risk coefficient below 100-WLM exposure. Some of the rats currently under study have been exposed at about 5 WLM/week, approximately the average exposure rates of former miners.

The data in Table 9.3 also indicate an increasing lifetime lung tumor risk coefficient with decreasing cumulative potential alpha-energy exposure. Like the CO-GEMA data, the PNL risk coefficient data have not been corrected for lifespan shortening due to competing causes of death, such as radiation pneumonitis (see footnote *b*, Table 9.1). Nor can it be concluded, at present, that the increase in the risk coefficient continues with further decrease in cumulative exposure and exposure rate. The PNL experiments contain exposures as low as 20 WLM, a value comparable to estimated mean lifetime indoor exposures of humans.

The multispecies PNL experiments have also been very useful in clarifying the epidemiological data. (See Section 7, Comparison of Human and Animal Radon Exposure Data.) The tumor incidence data, especially those derived from high-exposure-rate experiments, are similar not only to those from COGEMA but also to present, estimated, lung-tumor-incidence data in humans.

There are no firm explanations, at present, for the relative insensitivity of hamsters, compared with rats and dogs, to the induction of lung cancers following radon progeny inhalation exposures. It could be that their generally shorter lifespan, compared with that of rats, decreases their chance of developing lung cancer. However, rats receiving exposures comparable to those of hamsters develop far more lung cancers, even within a period comparable to the lifespan of hamsters. It is also uncertain whether the radiation sensitivity of nonsmoking dogs differs from that of rats, since we can plot only one datum at high radon progeny exposure.

5   SUMMARY AND DISCUSSION OF RADON INHALATION STUDIES IN ANIMALS

5.1   Summary

The studies of the three laboratories, described above, were undertaken to determine exposure-response relationships under controlled exposure conditions and, where possible, to define the correlation between exposure and absorbed dose in respiratory tissue.

At UR, mice received cumulative inhalation exposures to 14,000–72,000 WLM of potential alpha energy from radon decay products in laboratory room air at approximately 1800 WLM/week, over 10 to 35 weeks; dogs received 200–10,000 WLM, at 200 WLM/day, or average exposure rates of 1000 WLM/week, over 1 to 50 days; rats received about 26,000 WLM over 24 weeks, at approximately 1100 WLM/week. Destructive, hyperplastic, and metaplastic lesions appeared in the lungs of all three species. Adenomas and tumorlets (presumably adenomatoses or preneoplastic, bronchiolized alveolar lesions) appeared in mouse lungs, and chronic inflammation appeared in dog lungs, but in neither were there frank carcinomas. Late effects in rat lungs included tumorlets, two adenomas, and two carcinomas.

At COGEMA, rats developed lung cancer between 12 and 24 months after the start of 3- to 4-month exposures (with environmental dust and uranium ore dust) totaling 500–8500 WLM of potential alpha energy. Later experiments included cigarette smoke exposures and radon progeny exposures as low as approximately 20–25 WLM potential alpha energy. Exposure rates varied from less than 10 to several hundred WLM/week, the majority centering around 200–400 WLM/week. Observed pulmonary cancers included epidermoid (squamous) carcinoma, bronchiolar adenocarcinoma, bronchioalveolar adenocarcinoma, and "mixed" carcinoma. Cancer incidence depended on both exposure rate and cumulative potential alpha-energy exposure.

At PNL, chronic inhalation exposures of rats, hamsters, and dogs to 10–1000 WL of potential alpha energy with no added ore dust, or with variable uranium ore dust concentrations, diesel engine exhaust, and cigarette smoke, produced pulmonary fibrosis, emphysema, and neoplastic lesions of the respiratory tract. Exposures ranged from about 20 to 16,000 WLM; exposure rates ranged from a few WLM/week to about 500 WLM/week. Respiratory tract cancers included squamous carcinoma and bronchioloalveolar carcinoma in dogs receiving $4-4\frac{1}{2}$ years of exposure to radon decay products with uranium ore dust (with or without concomitant cigarette smoke exposures) at cumulative potential alpha-energy exposures of 12,000–16,000 WLM. Very few squamous carcinomas were observed in Syrian golden hamsters exposed to 10,000 WLM of potential alpha energy from radon progeny alone and in mixtures with uranium ore dust and diesel engine exhaust. The SPF rats exposed to variable concentrations of radon progeny and uranium ore dust have developed squamous cell carcinoma, adenocarcinoma, and mixed carcinoma, the incidence depending on both the rate and cumulative potential alpha-energy exposure. As in the COGEMA data, tumor incidence at very high exposures was low as a result of lifespan shortening.

5.2 Discussion

Five variables emerge as influences on the tumorigenic efficiency of radon progeny in the animal studies: (i) cumulative potential alpha-energy exposure; (ii) radon progeny exposure rate; (iii) radon progeny unattached fraction; (iv) radon-progeny disequilibrium; and (v) concomitant exposures to other pollutants.

The COGEMA and PNL data indicate that tumor incidence increased with an increase in cumulative potential alpha-energy exposure (WLM) and a decrease in exposure rate (WLM/week). In an overview, Chameaud et al. (31) concluded that lung cancer incidence at comparable cumulative exposure increased as the potential alpha-energy concentrations decreased from 12,000 to less than 3000 WL. In a related dose fractionation study with cumulative exposures of 3000 WLM and potential alpha-energy concentrations of 1500 WL, an approximately fourfold increase in lung cancers was observed when the exposure rate decreased from about

300 to 50 WLM/week.* Whether this exposure rate dependence persists at the far lower rates formerly received by miners may be answered by the results of the current PNL exposure rate experiments. The miners' exposures were estimated to average a few WLM/week or less. However, according to the National Academy of Sciences (Committee on the Biological Effects of Ionizing Radiations; BEIR) (50), before 1960, U.S. miners were exposed to much higher levels, with potential alpha-energy concentrations ranging generally from 10 to 100 or more WL. A trend toward increasing tumor risk with decreased exposure rate was noted in the earlier PNL rat experiments (40, 43) when the rates changed from 180 to 88 WLM/week and 44 WLM/week. The fact that the increase was not significant and that results were somewhat equivocal at 44 WLM/week (as a result of life-span shortening in that group) suggested that the exposure rate dependence in rats may taper off at the lower weekly rates of exposure. However, more recent data, shown in Table 9.3, confirm the increase in lung tumor risk with decreased exposure rate down to 53 WLM/week.

Data on rats at PNL also indicate an increase in the risk of primary lung tumors with increase in the radon decay product unattached fraction and disequilibrium (43). The risk increase from 1.6% unattached ^{218}Po to 10% unattached ^{218}Po is significant ($p \leq 0.05$), but the trend reverses at 24% unattached ^{218}Po as a result of lifespan shortening in that group. In contrast to the COGEMA experiments, the increase is also significant with radon progeny disequilibrium (an equilibrium factor of 10% versus 40%) when the total numbers of neoplastic lesions of the lung are compared. However, the increasing trend is of borderline significance ($p = 0.10$) when the total numbers of rats with lung tumors are compared. The data on nasal carcinoma show an increasing (but not significant) trend with unattached ^{218}Po and, as with the neoplastic lesions of the lung, a reverse trend at 24% unattached ^{218}Po. There is no indication that high-disequilibrium (low equilibrium factor) radon progeny exposures, without concomitant high unattached ^{218}Po, produce more nasal carcinoma than low-disequilibrium radon progeny exposures.

The role of concomitant exposures to other pollutants depends not only on the nature of the pollutant, but also on the time sequence of exposures. Simultaneous or same-day exposure to radon progeny and uranium ore dust, diesel engine exhaust or cigarette smoke increased the incidence of preneoplastic lesions but, with the exception of cigarette smoke, did not seem to change the incidence of lung tumors in the PNL experiments. In the COGEMA rat experiments, cigarette smoke was cocarcinogenic with radon progeny when exposure to smoke followed completion of exposure to the decay products (20). This effect was not seen, however, when smoking preceded the decay product exposures. In the PNL dog experiments, lung tumor incidence decreased when animals were given alternate (but same-day) exposures to radon decay products and cigarette smoke.

The absorbed doses/unit exposure (rad/WLM), calculated or measured by various investigators, help to clarify the extrapolation of animal data to humans. Doses/unit exposure in hamster airway epithelium were conservatively calculated

---

*See footnote in Section 3.2 regarding these exposure rates.

by Desrosiers et al. (51) to range from 0.1 to 0.3 rad/WLM (1–3 mGy/WLM), with 0.1 rad/WLM (1 mGy/WLM) to "4th airway group basal cells." At the UR, Morken (17) measured about 0.17 rad/WLM (1.7 mGy/WLM) for the whole lungs of mice and dogs; he considered doses to the bronchial tissue of mice to be 5–10 times the mean lung dose and doses to the dog trachea to be 30 times this value. No absorbed doses were measured in the COGEMA rat studies. Preliminary measurements of absorbed dose at PNL indicated 0.2–0.4 rad/WLM (2–4 mGy/WLM) in whole lungs of dogs (52). These figures are, at first glance, fairly consistent, and the values for animals are similar to the values calculated for humans [0.3–1 rad/WLM (3–10 mGy/WLM) for bronchial epithelium, with whole-lung doses 5–10 times smaller; see also Chapter 7] (53–57). Dosimetric agreement does not necessarily suggest that cancer incidence data in animals can be directly extrapolated to humans because of possible differences in tissue sensitivities and affected sites in the lung. However, the apparently reasonable agreement of both dosimetric and carcinogenic data, at least at the higher exposure rates and for exposure levels exceeding about 100 WLM, suggests that the animal models (particularly rats) are reasonable surrogates for humans.

6 EXPOSURE-EFFECT RELATIONSHIPS FOR MAJOR BIOLOGICAL EFFECTS

6.1 Introduction

In this section we discuss the data for the major biological effects observed in the radon inhalation studies, with emphasis on the PNL data for nonneoplastic lesions. Because the radon inhalation studies are still in progress, the data are incomplete, especially in regard to low-exposure and low-exposure-rate effects. Following is a summary of species-specific effects:

- Lifespan shortening—uncommon in hamsters; common in dogs and rats
- Pulmonary emphysema—uncommon in rats; common in dogs and hamsters
- Pulmonary fibrosis—common in dogs, hamsters, and rats
- Respiratory cancer—uncommon in hamsters; common in dogs and rats.

The complete data are summarized in the following sections.

6.2 Lifespan Shortening

- Hamsters: No significant lifespan shortening for potential alpha-energy exposures to 10,000 WLM
- Dogs: 4- to 5-year mean survival time for potential alpha-energy exposures averaging 13,000 WLM (mean lifespan of control dogs is about 15 years)
- Rats: No significant lifespan-shortening for potential alpha-energy exposures

<2500 WLM; significant lifespan shortening above 5000 WLM, increasing with length of exposure.

6.3 Pulmonary Emphysema

- Hamsters: Early finding—approximately 40% incidence with exposures to ore dust alone, to diesel engine exhaust alone, to radon progeny alone, and to mixtures with radon decay products. Not found with radon-progeny-only potential alpha-energy exposures <7000 WLM
- Dogs: Smoke-only exposures—barely perceptible to moderate; ore-dust-only exposures—slight to moderate; smoke, ore dust, and radon progeny exposures—moderate to severe; 100% incidence at 13,000 WLM
- Rats: Rare in animals exposed to mixtures of ore dust and radon progeny with potential alpha-energy exposures <10,000 WLM.

6.4 Pulmonary Fibrosis

- Hamsters: Approximately 20% incidence with exposure to both ore dust alone and ore dust, diesel engine exhaust, and radon decay products. Rare with exposure to diesel engine exhaust alone, radon progeny alone, or radon progeny plus ore dust.
- Dogs: Smoke-only exposures—equivocal findings; ore-dust-only exposures—slight, increasing with duration of exposure; smoke, ore dust, and radon progeny exposures—marked with exposure to 13,000 WLM potential alpha energy, slight with exposure to 1800 WLM
- Rats: Ore dust and radon progeny exposures—trace amounts to essentially none at <600 WLM cumulative potential alpha-energy exposure; trace to small amounts at 1000 WLM; small to moderate amounts in about 40% of animals at 5000 WLM; moderate amounts in 100% of animals at 10,000 WLM. Radon-progeny-only exposures—approximately 60% incidence at 3800-WLM cumulative potential alpha-energy exposure.

6.5 Lung Cancer

The mean lifetime, lung tumor risk (uncorrected for lifespan differences from control animals) is plotted against the potential alpha-energy exposure data of Tables 9.1 and 9.3 in Figure 9.1. The PNL data do not include values for the high-unattached-fraction and high-disequilibrium data on rats, or for the data on the two groups of rats that showed life-shortening anomalies. The generally higher tumor efficiencies in the PNL studies (in contrast to the COGEMA studies) is probably due to the lower average exposure rates of the PNL experiments. Error bars are omitted because of the difficulty in estimating them for the COGEMA radon experiments.

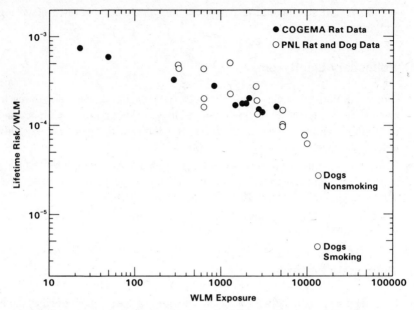

Figure 9.1. Lifetime lung tumor risk coefficients for radon progeny exposure.

The uncertainties in the PNL lung cancer incidence and risk coefficient data are considered to be close to the uncertainties in the exposure data (standard deviations were generally well within ±20% of the means). Whenever PNL exposure conditions were duplicated, reproducibility of tumor incidence data was also generally within ±20% of the mean, which included the uncertainties in the exposure data. Because the normal lung tumor incidence in the absence of appreciable background radon exposures is very low (<0.2%) in the COGEMA and PNL rats, the risk coefficient data, except for the 20- to 50-WLM COGEMA group of rats, have not been corrected for the incidence in control animals.

Current experiments at PNL, which involve mixtures of radon decay products and uranium ore dust, will further define the shape of the risk coefficient curve for very low exposures and exposure rates. For the present, COGEMA data at low exposure and low exposure rates indicate a leveling off of the risk to a value between 6 and 8×10^{-4}/WLM.

7   COMPARISON OF HUMAN AND ANIMAL RADON EXPOSURE DATA

The epidemiological data derived from many types of underground mining show a relatively consistent relationship between lung cancer incidence (nearly the same as death rate from lung cancer) and exposure to radon decay products (50, 58–63). This underlying consistency is probably related to the relatively narrow range of

bronchial dose/unit cumulative potential alpha-energy exposure under various exposure conditions in the mines. The few differences result partly because the radon
progeny exposures of miners are imperfectly known, and partly because of the
influence of both exposure rate and the presence of other mine air pollutants. The
unattached fraction and disequilibrium differences are probably second-order influences.

The comparison of animal data with human data that follows is not meant to
constitute proof, in humans, of effects (or absence of effects) that are demonstrated
in animals. We merely suggest explanations of provisional human data and potential findings in humans. The hamster data are excluded from this comparison in
view of the known low carcinogenic sensitivity of hamsters to inhaled radionuclides.

1. In rats, tumor production/unit exposure at very high exposures (uncorrected
for competing causes of death) was lower than at moderate exposures (Tables 9.1
and 9.3). However, the recent analysis of the COGEMA radon data by Gray et al.
(36) suggests that the age-specific prevalence of pulmonary tumors continues to
increase with exposure, even at very high exposures, when the data are adjusted
for life shortening. Miners exposed to the highest radon progeny levels in underground mines had the lowest attributable lung cancer rates/unit exposure (50).

2. In both the human and rat studies, tumor production appeared to increase
with decreasing exposure rate (31, 40, 43, 48, 64). However, the analysis of the
human data by Kunz et al. (64) suggests that the exposure rate dependence may
taper off at environmental and occupational rates and levels of exposure.

3. In a small group of Swedish zinc/lead miners, a lower lifetime incidence of
lung cancer was observed in those who smoked and were exposed to radon progeny
than in the nonsmokers similarly exposed (65). This is tentatively ascribed to the
protective effect of either increased mucus production from smoking or of the
thickened mucosa resulting from smoker's bronchitis. A similar result was observed in dogs (38). In rats, cigarette smoke was found to be cocarcinogenic with
radon decay products when exposure to smoke followed completion of exposure
to the decay products (20). This effect was not observed, however, when smoking
preceded the radon progeny exposure (31). Such disparities may partially explain
discrepancies in interpreting tentative epidemiological data.

4. Emphysema and fibrosis have been attributed to radon progeny exposure in
animals—hamsters, rats, and dogs (21, 39)—and in underground miners (66).
Simultaneous exposure of animals to ore dust or diesel engine exhaust generally
increased the incidence of emphysema and fibrosis but did not appear to increase
the number of tumors produced when exposure to radon progeny exceeded 300
WLM cumulative potential alpha energy (21, 31, 40, 45).

5. For equivalent cumulative potential alpha-energy exposures, the older the
animal at the start of exposure, the shorter the time-to-tumor period and, in humans
(the data suggest), the higher the associated risk (31, 50). The highest risk coefficient calculated in humans, about 50×10^{-6} lung cancers y^{-1} WLM^{-1}, is for
persons first exposed when over 40 years of age (50).

6. The predictions of the various dosimetric models appear to be borne out in the various species. The tumors induced in experiments with animals are commonly more distal than those in humans. Desrosiers' (51) modeling of Syrian golden hamster lungs showed that peripheral basal and Clara cells may receive doses approximately equal to or greater than those received by basal cells in the central airways. Human tumors have appeared almost exclusively in the upper generations of the bronchial tree. Some absorbed-dose calculations show that basal cells in human upper airways received the highest dose from radon decay products (53, 54, 67).

7. Lifetime, lung tumor risk coefficients are similar in animals (rats, primarily) and humans. Data are inadequate and insufficient to provide lifetime, lung tumor risk coefficients versus cumulative potential alpha energy exposure of mice, hamsters, and dogs. The coefficients based on rat data, uncorrected for lifespan shortening, appear to range between approximately 1 and 5×10^{-4}/WLM for all lung tumors (benign and malignant) at cumulative exposures between 100 and 5000 WLM (Tables 9.1 and 9.3). At exposures considerably less than those where mean lifespan is significantly shortened (< 500 WLM), the lifetime risk coefficient in the earlier PNL experiments was about 2×10^{-4}/WLM for malignancies and ranged between 2 and 4×10^{-4} for all lung tumors (22). Recent rat data at 20- to 50-WLM exposures, at low exposure rates, indicate that the lifetime risk coefficient ranges between 6 and 8×10^{-4}/WLM (33). A summary of estimated human lifetime lung cancer risk coefficients appears in Table 9.4.

8. Except for the greater prevalence of solid alveolar tumors and bronchioloalveolar carcinomas observed in the animals and, possibly, the oat cell (K-cell) type of tumors observed in humans, the tumor data are not dissimilar. Although K-cell carcinomas were not found in the animal experiments, Masse (68) considers that K cells are involved in pretumoral lesions, with species-dependent phenotypic expression. Chameaud et al. (32) postulated that, in rats, K cells convert to mucus-secreting cells, which may eventually become adenocarcinomas.

TABLE 9.4 Summary of Lifetime Lung Cancer Risk Coefficients per Cumulative Potential Alpha-Energy Exposure of Humans[a]

Risk coefficient (WLM^{-1})	Ref.
2–4.5×10^{-4}	61
2×10^{-4}	69
2×10^{-4}	70[b]
2–14×10^{-4c}	50
1.5–4.5×10^{-4}	63
$\leq 1 \times 10^{-4}$	71[b]
1–2×10^{-4}	26[b]

[a]Unless otherwise specified, values pertain to occupational exposures of underground miners.
[b]Environmental exposures.
[c]Values were converted from published annualized coefficients, assuming 30 years for cancer expression.

Data observed in animals that are not unequivocally demonstrated in human exposures to radon progeny are: (i) the increase in tumor production with increase in radon progeny unattached fraction and disequilibrium, and (ii) the importance of the temporal sequence of exposures to cigarette smoke and radon progeny. (The absence of these findings, however, does not constitute proof that similar data might not be in human exposures, but may rather reflect the paucity of this type of human data.)

REFERENCES

1. Jansen, H., and Schultzer, P. (1926). Experimental investigations into the internal radium emanation therapy. I. Emanatorium experiments with rats, *Acta Radiol.*, **6**, 631.

2. Read, J., and Mottram, J. C. (1939). The "tolerance concentration" of radon in the atmosphere, *Br. J. Radiol.*, **12**, 54.

3. Jackson, M. L. (1940). *The Biological Effects of Inhaled Radon*, master's thesis, Massachusetts Institute of Technology, Cambridge, MA.

4. Huech, W. (1939). Kurzer Bericht über Ergebnisse Anatomischer Untersuchungen in Schneeburg, Z. *Krebsforschung*, **49**, 312.

5. Rajewsky, B., Schraub, A., and Schraub, E. (1942). Uber die toxische Dosis bei Einatmung von Ra-Emanation, *Naturwissenschaften*, **30**, 489.

6. Rajewsky, B., Schraub, A., and Schraub, E. (1942). Zur Frage der Toleranz-Dosis bei der Einatmung von Ra-Em, *Naturwissenschaften*, **30**, 733.

7. Kushneva, V. S. (1959). *On the Problem of the Long-Term Effects of Combined Injury to Animals of Silicon Dioxide and Radon*, TR-4473, US Atomic Energy Commission, Division of Technical Information, Washington, DC, p. 21.

8. *Proc. Seven State Uranium Mining Conference on Health Hazards.* (1955). Hotel Utah, Salt Lake City, UT.

9. Wagoner, J. K., Archer, V. E., Carroll, B. E., and Holaday, D. A. (1964). Cancer mortality patterns among U.S. uranium miners and millers, 1950 through 1962, *J. Natl. Cancer Inst.*, **32**, 787.

10. Bale, W. F. (1951). Hazards associated with radon and thoron, Memo dated March 14, 1951, Division of Biology and Medicine, Atomic Energy Commission, Washington, DC. (Also found in *Health Phys.*, **38**, 1061.)

11. Harris, S. J. (1954). Radon levels in mines in New York State, *Arch. Ind. Hyg. Occup. Med.*, **10**, 54.

12. Morken, D. A. (1955). Acute toxicity of radon, *AMA Arch. Ind. Health*, **12**, 435.

13. Shapiro, J. (1954). *An Evaluation of the Pulmonary Radiation Dosage from Radon and Its Daughter Products*, project report UR-298 to the US Atomic Energy Commission, University of Rochester, Rochester, NY.

14. Cohn, S. H., Skow, R. K., and Gong, J. K. (1953). Radon inhalation studies in rats, *Arch. Ind. Hyg. Occup. Med.*, **7**, 508.

15. Morken, D. A., and Scott, J. K. (1966). *Effects on Mice of Continual Exposure to Radon and Its Decay Products on Dust*, project report UR-669 to the US Atomic En-

ergy Commission, University of Rochester, Rochester, NY, National Technical Information Service, Springfield, VA.

16. Morken, D. A. (1973). The biological effects of the radioactive noble gases. In R. E. Stanley and A. A. Moghissi (eds.), *Noble Gases*, CONF-730915, National Technical Information Service, Springfield, VA, p. 469.

17. Morken, D. A. (1973). The biological effects of radon on the lung. In R. E. Stanley and A. A. Moghissi (eds.), *Noble Gases*, CONF-730915, National Technical Information Service, Springfield, VA, p. 501.

18. Perraud, R., Chameaud, J., Masse, R., and Lafuma, J. (1970). Cancer pulmonaires expérimentaux chez le rat après inhalation de radon associé à des poussières non radioactives, *Compt. Rend. Ser. D.*, **270**, 2594.

19. Chameaud, J., Perraud, R., Lafuma, J., Masse, R., and Pradel, J. (1974). Lesions and lung cancers induced in rats by inhaled radon-222 at various equilibriums with radon daughters. In E. Karbe and J. F. Park (eds.), *Experimental Lung Cancer. Carcinogenesis and Bioassays*, Springer-Verlag, New York, p. 411.

20. Chameaud, J., Perraud, R., Chretien, J., Masse, R., and Lafuma, J. (1980). Combined effects of inhalation of radon daughter products and tobacco smoke. In C. L. Sanders, F. T. Cross, G. E. Dagle, and J. A. Mahaffey (eds.), *Pulmonary Toxicology of Respirable Particles*, CONF-791002, National Technical Information Service, Springfield, VA, p. 551.

21. Cross, F. T., Palmer, R. F., Filipy, R. E., Busch, R. H., and Stuart, B. O. (1978). *Study of the Combined Effects of Smoking and Inhalation of Uranium Ore Dust, Radon Daughters and Diesel Oil Exhaust Fumes in Hamsters and Dogs*, PNL-2744, Pacific Northwest Laboratory, Richland, WA, National Technical Information Service, Springfield, VA.

22. Cross, F. T., Palmer, R. F., Busch, R. H., Dagle, G. E., Filipy, R. E., and Ragan, H. A. (1987). An overview of the PNL radon experiments with reference to epidemiological data. In R. C. Thompson and J. A. Mahaffey (eds), *Life-Span Radiation Effects Studies in Animals: What Can They Tell Us?* 22nd Hanford Life Sciences Symposium, September 27-29, 1983, Richland, WA, National Technical Information Service, Springfield, VA, p. 608.

23. Richmond, C. R., and Boecker, B. B. (1971). *Experimental Studies*, final report of Subgroup I.B, Interagency Uranium Mining Radiation Review Group, Environmental Protection Agency, Rockville, MD.

24. Federal Radiation Council (1967). *Guidance for the Control of Radiation Hazards in Uranium Mining*, staff report no. 8 (Revised), US Government Printing Office, Washington, DC.

25. International Commission on Radiological Protection (ICRP) (1980). *Biological Effects of Inhaled Radionuclides*, ICRP publication 31, Pergamon Press, New York.

26. National Council on Radiation Protection and Measurements (NCRP) (1984). *Evaluation of Occupational and Environmental Exposures to Radon and Radon Daughters in the United States*, NCRP report no. 78, National Council on Radiation Protection and Measurements, Bethesda, MD.

27. Senes Consultants, Ltd. (1984). *Assessment of the Scientific Basis for Existing Federal Limitations on Radiation Exposure to Underground Uranium Miners*, Report prepared for the American Mining Congress, Senes Consultants Ltd., Willowdale, Ontario, Canada.

28. Mercer, T., and Stowe, W. A. (1970). Radioactive aerosols produced by radon in room air. In W. H. Walton (ed.), *Inhaled Particles III*, Vol. II, Unwin Bros. Ltd., Gresham Press, Old Woking, p. 839.

29. Chaumeaud, J., Perraud, R., Masse, R., Nenot, J. C., and Lafuma, J. (1976). Lung cancer induced in rats by radon and its daughter nuclides at different concentrations. In *Biological and Environmental Effects of Low Level Radiation*, Vol. II, IAEA STI/PUB/409, International Atomic Energy Agency, Vienna, p. 223.

30. Chaumeaud, J., Perraud, R., Chretien, J., Masse, R., and Lafuma, J. (1978). Experimental study of the combined effect of cigarette smoke and an active burden of radon-222. In *Late Biological Effects of Ionizing Radiation*, Vol. II, IAEA STI/PUB/489, International Atomic Energy Agency, Vienna, p. 429.

31. Chameaud, J., Perraud, R., Masse, R., and Lafuma, J. (1981). Contribution of animal experimentation to the interpretation of human epidemiological data. In M. Gomez (ed.), *Proceedings of the International Conference on Radiation Hazards in Mining: Control, Measurement and Medical Aspects*, Kingsport Press, Inc., Kingsport, TN.

32. Chameaud, J., Perraud, R., Lafuma, J., and Masse, R. (1982). Cancers induced by Rn-222 in the rat. In G. F. Clemente, A. V. Nero, F. Steinhäusler, and M. E. Wrenn (eds.), *Proceedings of the Specialist Meeting on Assessment of Radon and Daughter Exposure and Related Biological Effects*, RD Press, Salt Lake City, UT, p. 198.

33. Chameaud, J., Masse, R., and Lafuma, J. (1984). Influence of radon daughter exposure at low doses on occurrence of lung cancer in rats, *Radiat. Prot. Dosim.*, **7**, 385.

34. Chameaud, J., Masse, R., Morin, M., and Lafuma, J. (1984). Lung cancer induction by radon daughters in rats (present state of the data on low-dose exposures). In H. Stocker (ed.), *Proceedings of the International Conference on Occupational Radiation Safety in Mining*, Canadian Nuclear Association, Ontario, Canada, p. 350.

35. Chameaud, J. (1986). Personal communication, Compagnie Générale Des Matières Nucléaires, Razes, France.

36. Gray, R. H., Lafuma, J., Parish, S. E., and Peto, R. (1987). Radon inhalation by rats: An examination of the dose-response relationship for induced pulmonary tumors and of the exposure parameters and cofactors affecting risk. In R. C. Thompson and J. A. Mahaffey (eds.), *Life-Span Radiation Effects Studies in Animals: What Can They Tell Us?* 22nd Hanford Life Sciences Symposium, September 27-29, 1983, Richland, WA, National Technical Information Service, Springfield, VA, p. 592.

37. Cross, F. T., Palmer, R. F., Busch, R. H., Filipy, R. E., and Stuart, B. O. (1981). Development of lesions in Syrian golden hamsters following exposure to radon daughters and uranium ore dust, *Health Phys.*, **41**, 135.

38. Cross, F. T., Palmer, R. F., Filipy, R. E., Dagle, G. E., and Stuart, B. O. (1982). Carcinogenic effects of radon daughters, uranium ore dust and cigarette smoke in beagle dogs, *Health Phys.*, **42**, 33.

39. Stuart, B. O., Palmer, R. F., Filipy, R. E., and Gaven, J. (1978). Inhaled radon daughters and uranium ore dust in rodents. In D. L. Felton (ed.), *Pacific Northwest Laboratory Annual Report for 1977 to the DOE Assistant Secretary for Environment*, PNL-2500, Part 1, National Technical Information Service, Springfield, VA, pp. 3.70-3.72.

40. Cross, F. T., Palmer, R. F., Busch, R. H., and Buschbom, R. L. (1982). Influence of radon daughter exposure rate and uranium ore dust concentration on occurrence of lung tumors. In G. F. Clemente, A. V. Nero, F. Steinhäusler, and M. E. Wrenn,

(eds.), *Proceedings of the Specialist Meeting on Assessment of Radon and Daughter Exposure and Related Biological Effects*, RD Press, Salt Lake City, UT, p. 189.

41. Cross, F. T., Buschbom, R. L., Dagle, G. E., Filipy, R. E., Jackson, P. O., Loscutoff, S. M., and Palmer, R. F. (1983). Inhalation hazards to uranium miners. In D. L. Felton (ed.), *Pacific Northwest Laboratory Annual Report for 1982 to the DOE Office of Energy Research*, PNL-4600, Part 1, National Technical Information Service, Springfield, VA, p. 77.

42. Cross, F. T., Buschbom, R. L., Dagle, G. E., Jackson, P. O., Palmer, R. F., and Ragan, H. A. (1984). Inhalation hazards to uranium miners. In D. L. Felton (ed.), *Pacific Northwest Laboratory Annual Report for 1983 to the DOE Office of Energy Research*, PNL-5000, Part 1, National Technical Information Service, Springfield, VA, p. 41.

43. Cross, F. T., Palmer, R. F., Dagle, G. E., Busch, R. E., and Buschbom, R. L. (1984). Influence of radon daughter exposure rate, unattachment fraction, and disequilibrium on occurrence of lung tumors, *Radiat. Prot. Dosim.*, **7**, 381.

44. Cross, F. T. (1984). *A Review of Radon Inhalation Studies in Animals with Reference to Epidemiological Data*, Research Report for Senes Consultants, Ltd., Ontario, Canada, Battelle, Pacific Northwest Laboratories, Richland, WA.

45. Palmer, R. F., Stuart, B. O., and Filipy, R. E. (1973). Biological effects of daily inhalation of radon and its short-lived daughters in experimental animals. In R. E. Stanley and A. A. Moghissi (eds.), *Noble Gases*, CONF-730915, National Technical Information Service, Springfield, VA, p. 507.

46. Stuart, B. O., and Jackson, P. O. (1975). The inhalation of uranium ores. In *Proceedings, Conference on Occupational Health Experience with Uranium*, National Technical Information Service, Springfield, VA.

47. Stuart, B. O., and Beasley, T. M. (1967). Non-equilibrium tissue distributions of uranium and thorium following inhalation of uranium ore by rats. In C. N. Davies (ed.), *Inhaled Particles and Vapours II*, Pergamon Press, Oxford/New York, p. 291.

48. Archer, V. E. (1978). Summary of data on uranium miners. In J. E. Turner, C. F. Holoway, and A. S. Loebl (eds.), *Proceedings, Workshop on Dosimetry for Radon and Radon Daughters*, ORNL-53481, Oak Ridge National Laboratory, Oak Ridge, TN, National Technical Information Service, Springfield, VA, p. 23.

49. Schlesinger, R. B., and Lippman, M. (1978). Selective particle deposition and bronchogenic carcinoma, *Environ. Res.*, **15**, 424.

50. National Academy of Sciences (1980). *The Effects on Populations of Exposure to Low Levels of Ionizing Radiation* (BEIR-III Report), National Academy Press, Washington, DC.

51. Desrosiers, A. E., Kennedy, A., and Little, J. B. (1978). ^{222}Rn daughter dosimetry in the Syrian golden hamster lung, *Health Phys.*, **35**, 607.

52. Palmer, R. F., Jackson, P. O., Gaven, J. C., and Stuart, B. O. (1976). Dosimetric studies of inhaled radon daughters in dogs. In D. L. Felton (ed.), *Pacific Northwest Laboratory Annual Report for 1975 to the ERDA Division of Biomedical and Environmental Research*, BNWL-2000, Part 1, National Technical Information Service, Springfield, VA, p. 53.

53. Harley, N. H., and Pasternack, B. S. (1972). Alpha absorption measurements applied to lung dose from radon daughters, *Health Phys.*, **23**, 771.

54. Harley, N. H., and Pasternack, B. S. (1982). Environmental radon daughter alpha dose factors in a five-lobed human lung, *Health Phys.*, **42**, 789.

55. Hofmann, W. (1982). Cellular lung dosimetry for inhaled radon decay products as a base for radiation induced lung cancer risk assessment. I. Calculation of mean cellular doses, *Radiat. Environ. Biophys.*, **20**, 95.

56. Jacobi, W., and Eisfeld, K. (1980). *Dose to Tissues and Effective Dose Equivalent by Inhalation of Radon-222, Radon-220 and Their Short-Lived Daughters*, Gesellschaft für Strahlen-und Umweltforschung MBH, report GSF S-626, Institut für Strahlenschutz, München-Neuherberg.

57. James, A. C., Jacobi, W., and Steinhäusler, F. (1981). Respiratory tract dosimetry of radon and thoron daughters: The state-of-the-art and implications for epidemiology and radiobiology data. In M. Gomez (ed.), *Proceedings of the International Conference on Radiation Hazards in Mining: Control, Measurement and Medical Aspects*, Kingsport Press, Inc., Kingsport, TN, p. 42.

58. Archer, V. E., Radford, E. P., and Axelson, O. (1979). Radon daughter cancer in man: Factors in exposure response relationship. In *Proceedings, Workshop on Lung Cancer Epidemiology and Industrial Applications of Sputum Cytology*, Colorado School of Mines Press, Golden, CO, p. 324.

59. National Institute for Occupational Safety and Health/National Institute of Environmental Health Sciences (1971). *Radon Daughter Exposure and Respiratory Cancer—Quantitative and Temporal Aspects*, joint monograph no. 1, National Technical Information Service, Springfield, VA.

60. National Academy of Sciences (1972). *The Effects on Populations of Exposure to Low Levels of Ionizing Radiation* (BEIR Report), National Academy Press, Washington, DC.

61. United Nations Scientific Committee on the Effects of Atomic Radiation (1977). *Sources and Effects of Ionizing Radiation*, United Nations, New York.

62. Radford, E. P. (1981). Radon daughters in the induction of lung cancer in underground miners. In R. Peto and M. Schneiderman (eds.), *Quantification of Occupational Cancer*, Banbury report 9, Cold Spring Harbor Laboratory, Cold Spring Harbor, NY, p. 151.

63. International Commission on Radiological Protection (ICRP) (1981). *Limits for Inhalation of Radon Daughters by Workers*, ICRP publication 32, Pergamon Press, New York.

64. Kunz, E., Sevc, J., Placek, V., and Horacek, J. (1979). Lung cancer in man in relation to different time distribution of radiation exposure, *Health Phys.*, **36**, 699.

65. Axelson, O., and Sundell, L. (1978). Mining, lung cancer and smoking, *Scand. J. Work Environ. Health*, **4**, 46.

66. Archer, V. E., Carol, B. E., Brinton, H. P., and Saccomanno, G. (1964). Epidemiological studies of some non-fatal effects of uranium mining. In *Radiological Health and Safety in Mining and Milling of Nuclear Materials*, Vol. 1, IAEA Symposium, August 26-31, 1963, International Atomic Energy Agency, Vienna, p. 21.

67. Altshuler, B., Nelson, N., and Kuschner, M. (1964). Estimation of lung tissue dose from the inhalation of radon and daughters, *Health Phys.*, **10**, 1137.

68. Masse, R. (1980). Histiogenesis of lung tumors induced in rats by inhalation of alpha emitters: An overview. In C. L. Sanders, F. T. Cross, G. E. Dagle, and J. A. Mahaffey

(eds.), *Pulmonary Toxicology of Respirable Particles*, CONF-791002, National Technical Information Service, Springfield, VA, p. 498.

69. Jacobi, W. (1977). Interpretation of measurements in uranium mines: Dose evaluation and biomedical aspects. In *Personal Dosimetry and Area Monitoring Suitable for Radon and Daughter Products*, Proceedings of NEA Specialist Meeting, Nuclear Energy Agency, OECD, Paris, p. 33.

70. Cliff, K. D., Davis, B. L., and Riessland, J. A. (1979). Little danger from radon, *Nature*, **279**, 12.

71. Evans, R. D., Harley, J. H., Jacobi, W., McLean, A. S., Mills, W. A., and Stewart, C. G. (1981). Estimate of risk from environmental exposure to radon-222 and its decay products. *Nature*, **290**, 98.

PART FOUR

CONTROLLING INDOOR EXPOSURES

— 10

Preventing Radon Entry

ARTHUR G. SCOTT
American Atcon/Arthur Scott and Associates, Mississauga, Ontario, Canada

1 HISTORICAL REVIEW OF MITIGATION MEASURES

1.1 Introduction

The field of radon mitigation has undergone considerable changes in approach and theory over the past 15 years. Initially, it was directed entirely toward those sites where man's actions had raised local radium concentrations, e.g., by the use of uranium mill tailings as a construction material, but as the realization grew that elevated building radon concentrations could occur in areas of "normal" radioactivity, mitigation work became necessary to deal with naturally occurring radon. The approaches used for these different cases are now fairly well standardized, but it is informative to briefly review the events that led us to our present understanding of the causes of radon entry into buildings and of the best ways to prevent that entry.

The first major radon mitigation program was at Grand Junction, Colorado, where uranium mill tailings containing up to 6000 Bq/kg radium had been used as fill and as a replacement for sand. Many buildings stood on a layer of tailings used to level the site or had tailings as backfill against the basement walls, causing radon levels in excess of 200 Bq/m^3. The preferred mitigative action was to remove the radon source (1). As the radium concentration in tailings was much higher than local environmental levels, the tailings could be located by surface and bore-hole gamma-ray surveys, augmented by radon flux measurements on walls and floors to indicate the direction of the radon source (2). Removal of the tailings reduced the radon concentrations in the buildings.

In some buildings, the concrete itself had been made with tailings instead of sand, and in others, removal of the tailings was not practicable for structural reasons. Accordingly, seamless epoxy coatings were developed for use as a barrier to prevent radon diffusion through concrete surfaces (3). The success of this diffusion barrier in reducing radon levels even when the source was known to be tailings outside the building (4, 5)—was taken as confirmation of the general assumption that radon migrated into buildings by diffusion down the concentration gradient between a high-activity radon souce and the structure interior.

407

The validity of this concept appeared to be confirmed when a similar mitigative program was carried out at Port Hope, Ontario, where the source was soil contaminated with radium refinery wastes. Gamma surveys and radon flux measurements located high activity sources, which were then removed by excavation (6, 7).

When it was discovered that many houses and buildings in three major Canadian mining towns also had elevated radon levels (>200 Bq/m^3) (8, 9), mitigation programs were started in those towns. It was assumed that the cause was contamination by high activity mine or refinery wastes, and that ''standard'' investigative and mitigative methods would be useful in reducing these levels.

The first major project to get underway was at Elliot Lake, Ontario, where it was found that although many houses had driveways covered with up to 20 cm of mine waste rock giving gamma fields in excess of 1 μGy/h (100 μR/h), removal of this material did not reduce the radon levels. There was little correlation between surface gamma fields and radon, for many houses with elevated radon had background (0.1 μGy/h) fields. This indicated that the source was entirely buried, and more elaborate investigative methods would be required (10).

An extensive source location study of 15 of these houses was carried out, involving excavations to the depth of the footings, gamma logging of multiple boreholes, plus soil radium and soil gas radon measurements. At the same time an internal route-of-entry survey was carried out to measure the radon flux from walls, floors, exposed uraniferous rocks, sumps, and floor drains.

Results from the source location survey were disappointing. No high-activity source could be located. The fill around all these houses was similar in size distribution and radioactivity (40 Bq/kg Ra) to undisturbed soil exposed in local aggregate pits, with no trace of mine or mill wastes (11, 12). There was no sign of the steep radon concentration gradients in the soil that would be expected if there were deep buried radon sources (13).

The route-of-entry survey found that the radon fluxes from concrete walls, floors, and exposed rocks were all similar (10^{-3} Bq m^{-2}s^{-1}), remarkably constant, and too low by a factor of at least 10 to provide the radon supply needed to explain the observed radon levels in the houses. In addition, the exterior soil gas concentrations were too low to produce the observed concrete flux rates by diffusion. The only high fluxes found were measured over sumps, drains, and openings that connected directly to the soil.

1.2 Identification of Soil Gas as the Cause

The maximum radon concentrations of 30 kBq/m^3 found in sumps and drains were high enough that entry of 1–2 m^3/h of that air into the house would explain the observed indoor radon levels. These concentrations were comparable to the higher radon concentrations found in soil gas outside the house, which suggested that radon was present in drains and sumps because it had been carried there by soil gas.

A test with a small electric pump showed that soil gas containing 30 kBq/m^3 radon could be withdrawn from an internal peripheral drain connection at 1 m^3/h by a very small suction (< 3 Pa). This was comparable to the pressure differential between the inside and the outside of a building produced by wind and thermal forces, which are normally a few Pa (see Chapter 2), and therefore the soil gas flows produced by these pressure differentials could provide all the radon needed to give the observed levels in these houses. The implications of this were considerable.

First there was no longer any need to search for "the source." High activities to provide high radon concentration gradients were no longer needed if mass flow of soil gas containing radon, rather than diffusion, was the transport mechanism. There was sufficient radium in the soil within a few meters of the basement walls to provide all the radon that entered any house, and so the local soil could easily be the source. If this was the case, source removal was not a viable mitigative option, and other methods would have to be found.

Second, a much wider implication was that as the radium content of the local soils was "average" (40 Bq/kg), there might be many other areas with elevated radon concentrations in housing.

Third, the low radon fluxes from the walls and floors indicated that intact concrete was an effective barrier to soil gas movement and radon entry, and therefore attention could be devoted entirely to the openings in these surfaces, and not to the surfaces themselves.

Fourth, if the radon was brought in by a mass flow of soil gas, then making the openings airtight should reduce the radon supply and the radon concentrations in the house. At the time these conclusions were so surprising that an experimental program was thought needed to verify them.

1.3 Demonstration Program

1.3.1 Concrete as a Barrier.
The minimal importance of environmental radon transport through concrete was demonstrated by measuring the radon flux from the interior surface of poured concrete basement walls both below and above grade and on the above-grade exterior surface (Fig. 10.1). The fluxes were the same at all three positions, demonstrating not only that there was no significant diffusional flow of radon from the soil through the wall, but that the radon flux measured was due to the radium present in the aggregate used to build the wall. A theoretical examination of this case (14) found that very high external radon concentrations were needed before radon diffusion through concrete equaled the diffusion rate produced by concrete aggregates of average radioactivity.

1.3.2 Air Barriers as a Mitigative Measure.
The ability of air barriers to reduce radon concentrations was tested by building two small plywood enclosures over concrete joints in a basement and a third over an intact concrete floor to serve as a control. The concentrations in the first two enclosures were initially 1000–2000 Bq/m^3, compared to 200 Bq/m^3 in the control, where the supply was entirely by diffusion. Closing the joint in the concrete with tape, silicone, or butyl caulking, or expanding urethane foam, reduced the concentrations to levels com-

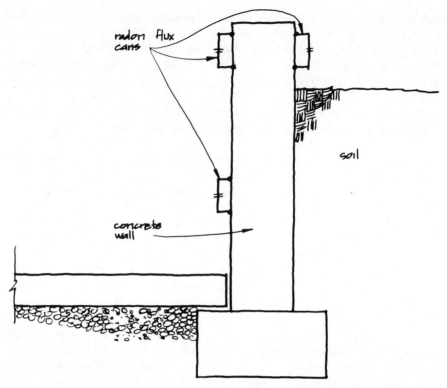

Figure 10.1. Measurement of radon flux from and through concrete walls.

parable with the control. The differences between materials could be attributed entirely to their ability to produce an airtight seal (15).

As a final demonstration, the most accessible soil connections in 25 houses were closed using expanding urethane foam. The average potential alpha-energy concentration was reduced by at least 50% in 18 of these houses, returning to its previous value when the foam plug was removed (16, 17).

1.4 Summary

These results confirmed that elevated environmental radon levels could be produced in houses by the entry of soil gas containing radon through openings in the concrete basement structures and could be reduced by reducing the soil gas flows. As the radon supply by diffusion through concrete was negligible compared to the supply via soil gas, epoxy diffusion barriers were not required, for the concrete itself was an effective barrier against soil gas. Mitigation measures against environmental radon would therefore have to be based on controlling the movement of soil gas, rather than preventing radon diffusion (18). The validity of this understanding has been demonstrated since by the success of mitigative work based on this approach carried out in Canada (18–20), Sweden (21–24), and the United States, particularly New York State (25, 26) and, more recently, Eastern Pennsylvania, New Jersey, and the Pacific Northwest (27).

The work in Canada was carried out in three uranium mining areas, with average soil radium. In all, about 850 houses were treated, and 400 new houses were modified for radon exclusion. Sealing and soil ventilation were used about equally, and 60 houses were fitted with forced ventilation systems. The Swedish work is in alum shale areas, where the soil radium is elevated, and soil ventilation, plus some sealing, has been used in more than 100 houses. In the Pennsylvania and New York projects (24 houses each), soil ventilation has been used exclusively, because the basement houses were constructed of hollow concrete block and could not be sealed. Soil radium levels were significantly elevated in Pennsylvania, but were normal in the New York project. In the Pacific Northwest, a broader range of techniques was employed—although in a smaller number of homes (14)—turning them on and off and modifying them to elucidate their effect on the indoor concentration. And although the indoor concentrations in the area of concern—the Spokane River Valley—are far higher than normal, soil radium concentrations were found to be average or below average, illustrating the importance of soil gas flow and the related parameter, permeability (cf. Chapter 2).

2 BASIC MITIGATION METHODS

The fundamental mitigation methods fall into four categories. The first is source removal, which is practicable only in cases where the source has been introduced into the local environment by man's actions. The second is to increase the resistance of the building fabric to soil gas entry, generally called "sealing." The third is to increase the rate of removal of radon from the building by increasing the structure ventilation rate, and the fourth is to reduce the soil gas flow by reducing the pressure differential between the building and the soil. The last category generally is called soil ventilation.

As will become clear below, this last approach is typically the most important one for the case of high radon concentrations occurring from ordinary soil and rock. Often it has to be supplemented by sealing, which—by itself—is typically not able to effect the radical reductions often seen with soil ventilation. Source removal is usually not practical for natural soils. And, it is also worth pointing out, soil ventilation itself has a variety of forms. These often involve depressurization of the layer of material immediately below the house, but sometimes involve just the opposite—i.e., pressurization of this layer, which might be thought of as creating a pressure barrier between the bulk of the soil and the house—and other times entail ventilation (or even pressurization) of special components of the structure, such as the drain tile system or hollow concrete block walls, if present.

The complexities and costs of mitigation are due, not only to the variety of possible methods, but also mainly to the difficulties of applying these methods to existing buildings. Tasks that could have been performed at low cost if the problem had been identified before construction, e.g., source removal, can approach a major fraction of the building cost when they have to be carried out in or around completed buildings. For the more likely case of naturally occurring radium, the soil ventilation approach is more likely, and this too is much more easily implemented when the building is being constructed, rather than as a remedial measure.

2.1 Source Removal

If the cause of elevated radon levels is highly active radium-bearing materials—such as uranium mine waste rock, uranium mine tailings, or uranium/radium refinery wastes—then experience is that the removal of this material out to 3 m from the building foundation effectively and permanently reduces the radon concentration (7). In this respect, it is the ideal mitigative measure and, therefore, has been favored by government-funded mitigation projects where high first cost was less important than obtaining a long-term solution. However, as anyone with experience in remedial programs will confirm, the simplicity of the concept is rarely equaled in the execution.

For example, in cases where the radon source is known to be radium wastes, the hygiene standards and radioactive contamination control procedures required for removal are quite outside the normal scope of the earth-moving trades. The training and supervision required is a powerful argument in favor of the use of specialist teams.

The contaminated material removed from the site has to be transferred to an acceptable storage area. In uranium mining areas where there are mill tailings areas available, this can be a minor problem. If the material is radium refinery waste, no acceptable local storage areas may be available, and opposition to creation of a site, or even to transport of the wastes to an acceptable site, may delay removal almost indefinitely. Examples of these kinds of delay have occurred in Montclair, New Jersey, and Scarborough, Ontario, Canada.

Material removal is often surprisingly expensive. Much of the excavation has to be done by hand, as limited clearances around buildings can prevent the use of machinery. Even when mechanical equipment can be used, excavation adjacent to buildings is difficult. Active material used as backfill may be mixed with local excavated material containing rubble, boulders, or broken rock. Below-ground services may require considerable protection or rerouting. Additions to buildings may not have proper foundations, and the below-ground portions of structures may become unsafe when their ground support is removed. The sides of the excavations may require considerable support for safety reasons. Contractor's personnel may accidentally damage the building structure with their equipment.

Finally, when all active material is removed and replaced, extensive landscaping is required to restore the area, particularly shrubbery and flower beds, to its original appearance. Costs are highly site-dependent, but generally lie in the range of $5000–$15,000 to remove material from round a house.

To remove material from beneath a building, the concrete floor slab must be removed. The space is rarely large enough to use mechanical equipment for this.

The concrete must be broken into pieces of less than 50 kg so that it can be man-handled. This requires air-powered jackhammers. If the slab is thick, a large dia-mond-blade saw may be needed to cut the concrete into sections. In all cases, considerable mess is generated, and major efforts are required to limit redecoration to just the work area. The radioactive material exposed often has to be removed by hand owing to insufficient space for a mechanical excavator, and extensive manual work is required to replace the fill and the concrete slabs. Again, costs are highly site-dependent, but are not likely to be less than $5000 and can be much higher if extensive restoration of finish is needed.

If the building foundation rests on source material, the building must be sup-ported during and after removal. In favorable circumstances local support can be provided and the removed material replaced with concrete. In other cases, it may be cheaper to support the entire building superstructure while the foundation struc-ture and the source material are removed and replaced. The costs of this work are highly site-dependent, but are estimated to range from at least $5000 to $20,000. As a result of these high costs, material is not always removed from beneath foot-ings, and source removal is often supplemented by soil gas exclusion methods.

2.2 Sealing

2.2.1 *Routes of Soil Gas Entry.* The discovery that solid concrete was es-sentially impermeable to soil gas containing radon led naturally to the development of methods to seal the openings through which soil gas enters a structure. It was soon found that the subgrade structure of most buildings was not airtight. Con-ventional building styles and the actions of the building trades produce many open-ings through which soil gas containing radon can flow freely from the soil into the building interior. In order of importance, examples of these are hollow concrete block basement walls, exterior perimeter drains brought into the building to sumps, untrapped interior floor drains heading to soakaways, openings left in the floor slab of single story buildings to assist in the installation of plumbing fixtures or service entries, junctions between walls and floors, and junctions between floor slab sec-tions. Other openings are produced as a side effect of architectural features in houses, such as sunken living rooms, sunken baths, or unpaved crawl spaces. In some cases there are concealed openings in floor slabs made to correct errors in plumbing installations. Cracks through the building materials themselves, caused by shrinkage or settling, can be significant.

In buildings with poured concrete basements, the major joint connecting to the soil is the wall/floor joint (Figure 10.2). The concrete floor is poured after the walls have been erected and touches the walls when the concrete is wet. As it sets, the floor shrinks away from the walls, leaving a small gap around the entire perim-eter of the basement. The fraction of this crack that connects to the soil, and hence its importance as a route of soil gas entry, depends very much on the circumstances during the pour and the curing conditions for the concrete afterward. The gap can be much less than 1 mm—or as large as 3 mm—and the total effective open area can be several hundred cm^2. Sometimes a compressed fiberboard "expansion joint"

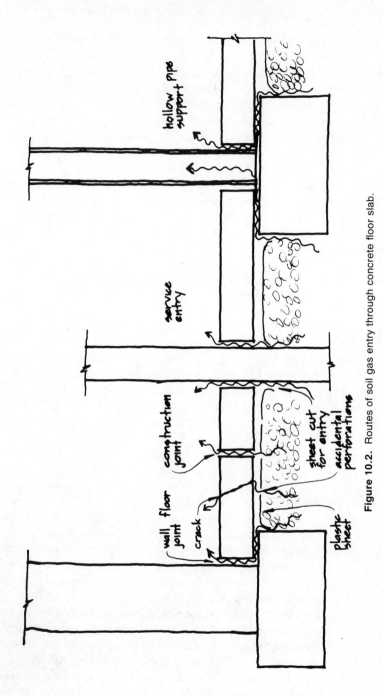

Figure 10.2. Routes of soil gas entry through concrete floor slab.

414

is placed here before pouring the floor. This creates an even larger direct connection to the soil.

The basement floor is often poured late in the construction of the building, when the building supports, furnace, oil tank, and stairs are resting on the subfloor fill. The concrete beneath or around these areas often has openings in it. If the building supports are hollow steel or concrete block columns, they can provide major soil gas entry routes via the column centers.

Poured concrete floor slabs and basement walls sometimes crack as the result of restraint during curing, or by unbalanced forces created by settlement. In general, these cracks are small, and they are minor routes of entry, particularly if the floor slab was poured over plastic sheet. Curing cracks are produced by shrinkage tension forces in the slab, and they tend to radiate from floor openings, drains, or service entries, where there are also openings in the subfloor plastic sheeting. The presence of this kind of crack makes it difficult to seal the opening, because the cracks provide a bypass round the sealant.

Concrete that covers large areas is poured in sections to minimize shrinkage stresses. New sections are butted against the old sections and can shrink away as far as 1 mm on setting. The openings pass completely thorough the slab, but may not reach the soil if a plastic sheet was laid beneath the slab for moisture control. This is an effective barrier to soil gas.

If the foundation walls are of hollow concrete block, there are a large number of potential openings (Figure 10.3). Soil gas can enter the concrete block walls through openings in the mortar joints between the blocks and footing and between the blocks, through porous mortar, and through cracks or openings in the wall created by soil movement. Once within the walls, the gas moves through the interconnecting block cavities and can pass into the building through openings in interior mortar joints, cracks, or open block cavities at the top of the walls. As concrete block walls are literally a collection of inaccessible holes held together by cement, it is futile to hope that all these openings could be sealed effectively (28). Sealing is not a valid mitigation measure for concrete block foundations.

In some areas, a gap of 4–5-cm width is left between the edge of the floor slab and the inner surface of concrete block basement walls. This "French drain" intercepts water leaking through the walls and drains it to the subfloor fill to keep the floor dry, even if the walls are wet. This is a very large opening to the house from the soil and, if present, accentuates the problems of concrete block construction.

The equivalent leakage area of all openings in standard house basements with poured concrete walls and floor areas of 120–200 m^2(1200–2000 ft^2) can be up to several hundred square centimeters. Most of the resistance to soil gas movement is in the soil itself, so a major reduction in the area of subgrade openings is needed to reduce the soil gas flow rate significantly. Experience suggests that the total effective leakage area within the building substructure must be reduced to less than 1 cm^2 to produce a major reduction in average radon concentration (29).

In modern communities with a relatively uniform style of construction it has

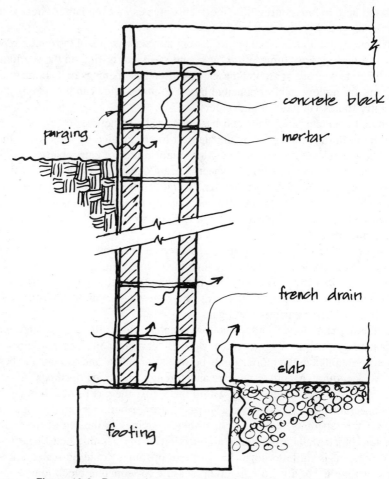

Figure 10.3. Routes of soil gas entry through concrete block walls.

been possible to identify a number of routes that are routinely produced by the building techniques used, and to develop standard methods to close the most common of these. In older communities, the variation in building styles, techniques, and materials may be too great to develop standard methods or, by producing many different routes, may make sealing too expensive or impractical as a remedial technique. Examples of these include rural communities where concrete blocks are used extensively for foundations, old houses with bare earth beneath suspended floors and no ventilation in the space, or cellars with fieldstone or random rubble walls and floors of bare earth, exposed rock, or flagstone.

2.2.2   Sealing Materials.   The ground on which a building stands is not stable. For example, in Northern areas of North America, the annual freeze/thaw cycle changes the volume of the upper soil layers over a year, and in Southern areas with clay soils a similar shrinkage/swell cycle takes place in response to seasonal rainfall variation. Although foundations are placed at a depth chosen to minimize the movements, a significant amount of relative movement can still take place in the foundations, and a few cracks are common. Water often leaks in at a crack, so the concrete there is usually damp.

Ten potential sealants were laboratory tested (30) for their ability to form an airtight seal to both dry and damp concrete, to maintain their seal in the presence of water, and to withstand movement of the substrate. Satisfactory materials included two catalyzing rubber-based sealants that use a primer coat to prepare the surface and one solvent hardening primerless rubber/asphalt sealant. One rubber sealant was intended for use in channels; the other two sealants were intended to form watertight membranes over surfaces. In areas where limited movement takes place, and where large openings such as service entries need to be filled, an asphalt/solvent mix (roofing cement) was found to seal to concrete with minimum surface preparation (31).

The other materials examined were not flexible enough. Epoxy materials are good sealants, but they are rigid and so strong that new cracks will often form adjacent to old epoxy-filled joints as a result of stresses from soil movement. Flexible sealants allow the building to cycle while maintaining their seal and do not produce new stresses that might cause new cracks.

2.2.3 Sealing Methods.

Joints can be sealed either by opening them with a power chisel wide enough to allow a channel-type sealant to be inserted, or by cleaning the concrete surface on either side of the joint for adhesion, and placing a membrane type sealant over the joint (32).

The wall/floor joint is the most difficult to seal, for the sealant must form a good seal to both the horizontal floor and the vertical wall. The optimal solution for all joints and cracks is to use a formed-in-place membrane sealant of sufficient viscosity and film strength that it can be applied to vertical wall surfaces as well as to the floor. Preparation involves removal of the surface layer of concrete on either side of the joint with a powered chipping gun, vacuum removal of dust, application of a primer, and the "painting" of a catalyzing urethane rubber layer over the joint.

This elaborate preparation is needed because the concrete surface is covered by a coating of laitance (a thin layer of cement with poor adhesion) and is often painted. It is virtually impossible to obtain a permanent bond between this surface and a sealant. All paint and loose material must be removed to expose a fresh concrete surface before a reliable bond can be obtained.

To ensure bonding, most sealants require the fresh surface to be treated with a primer, a highly solvent material that penetrates the concrete pores and forms a thin skin of material on the surface that is firmly bonded to the surface below. The sealant adheres to this primer (33).

The sewer and water connections are normally brought into a building through a formed opening in the concrete floor slab. The material (paper, fiber insulation) that was packed around the pipe to keep the concrete away is usually left in place and provides very little resistance to soil gas movement. This route can be closed by removing the packing material and pouring a sealant into the annular opening between the pipe and the concrete.

A similar opening exists beneath the toilets on concrete floor slabs, but is concealed by the foot of the bowl. The toilet can be lifted to expose the opening and a sealant poured into it.

Baths on concrete floor slabs have their drains placed in a large formed opening that is concealed by the bath. Access to the area can usually be gained by cutting through an adjacent frame wall to fill the opening to a depth of 2 cm or more with a pourable sealant. A highly solvent asphaltic material was found satisfactory, for the solvent penetrates the concrete over time and so forms a good bond despite the presence of dirt and laitance on the vertical sides of the opening.

In many areas the exterior peripheral groundwater drainage tile (weeping tile) is connected to an internal sump or a basement floor drain (Figure 10.4). This results in a direct entry route for soil gas: it can enter the perforated weeping tiles and move into the building via the drain connection. In other areas floor drains are not connected to the sanitary sewer, but to an untrapped soakaway, which collects soil gas as effectively as the drain tiles.

This entry can be closed by replacing the drain or sump with one that incorporates a water trap and connecting a priming line to a regularly used fixture (e.g., a laundry tub or toilet) to maintain the water seal. A lower-cost alternative is to close the drain or sump with a plastic water-trap adaptor, and either rely on drainage water to maintain the seal or routinely pour water into the trap. However, often the junction between the drain pipe and the edge of the sump crock or the floor is not airtight, and additional sealing is needed at these locations.

2.2.4 Epoxy Sealants. All cracks and joints in a basement can be sealed if the entire basement surface is coated with a multilayer seamless epoxy coating material. As epoxy will not adhere properly to laitance and old paint, the entire basement surface has to be ground to expose fresh concrete, and then at least two coats of epoxy must be applied to ensure a continuous film. The massive disruption, the toxic fumes released during application, and the cost make this a method of last resort. It is only useful in areas where the ground is sufficiently stable that seasonal movement will not rupture the epoxy film at cracks or joints. It is only in the unique case where the concrete contains high levels of radium, and is itself a major radon source, that these epoxy sealants are the first choice.

2.2.5 Costs. To provide an indication of the costs of these mitigation measures, the approximate cost of work in houses utilizing contractors' personnel with some experience are given on page 420.

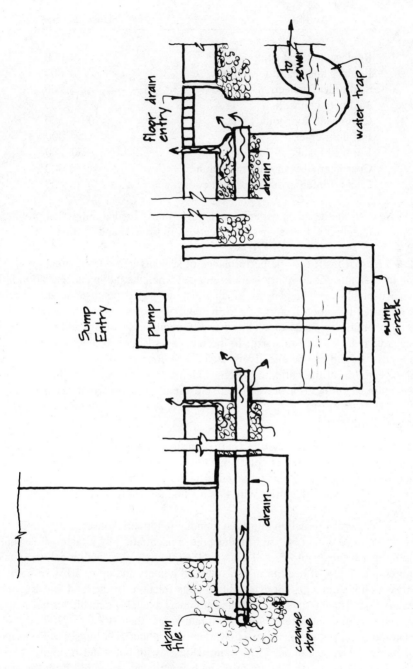

Figure 10.4. Routes of soil gas entry via drainage system.

Action	Cost ($U.S.)
Replace and seal sump	1,000
Replace and seal floor drain	800
Seal toilet connection	200
Seal bath connection	200
Close wall/floor joint	1,500–3,500
Fill floor crack	50–200
Fill wall crack	50–200
Coat internal wall with membrane	5,000
Coat all internal surfaces with epoxy	15,000

These costs are based on experience in government-funded mitigation programs in approximately 300 houses in three locations in Canada and Florida.

2.2.6 Performance. The performance of sealants in a retrofit situation is difficult to evaluate, for normally work is stopped when the radon concentration falls to an acceptable level. In general, closing just the major openings, such as drains, has produced reduction factors of 3–5 in about 50% of housing where sealing is a reasonable mitigative measure. The other 50% required sealing of additional routes to achieve reductions of this size. In the few cases where all the soil connections are accessible and can be effectively sealed, the concentration may be reduced to that expected from the building materials alone. In more usual retrofit situations, a reduction factor of 5 is achievable with closure of the larger obvious entry routes.

2.3 Ventilation

2.3.1 General. Increasing the ventilation flow rate in a building to reduce the radon concentration is the simplest method of all and has the advantage that it requires no knowledge of foundation construction, soil conditions, or identification of entry routes. The difficulties with this method are entirely practical ones.

1. The natural ventilation rate even in modern northern houses, is typically 25–50 L/s (50–100 cfm) (34), so to reduce the concentration by a factor of 3 would require an air supply of 75–150 L/s (150–300 cfm). The additional air would require up to 7 kW of heating in areas of cold winters and up to 3 kW of cooling in areas of hot summers. These constitute large fractions of the total house energy consumption. The energy cost, and the equipment available suitable for house use, limit the maximum additional ventilation rate to less than 100 L/s (200 cfm).

The practical reduction factor is no more than about 2 in houses with forced-air heating, which act as one large room. Houses with hot-water heating may act as two compartments, and the upstairs can be ventilated separately from the basement. Reduction factors of as high as 10 can be obtained in such cases by supplying fresh air to the upstairs alone.

2. In practice, the effect of adding ventilation is hard to predict. If a supply fan is used, the additional air forced in tends to lower the building neutral plane (the plane above which the air flows out of the building, and below which the air flows in) and so reduces the natural ventilation rate. As a result, the total ventilation flow does not increase by as much as the amount of air blown in by the fan (35).

3. In partial compensation for (2) the lowering of the neutral plane decreases the pressure difference between the building and the soil, and so decreases the inflow of soil gas. The effect of this reduction in radon supply rate can decrease the radon concentration in the building by much more than the increase in ventilation rate (36). Similarly, an exhaust fan raises the neutral plane, increases the building-soil pressure differential, and can increase the radon supply enough to compensate for the increased ventilation rate (37).

These pressure-induced changes in radon supply rate can lead to changes in radon concentration much larger than those expected from the changes in ventilation flows. Unfortunately, the size of the change is hard to predict, for it depends on the total building leakage area and its distribution among building surfaces, factors that vary considerably from building to building.

4. The noise resulting from the addition of fans, or changes in the speed of existing fans, can be unacceptable to the occupants.

5. In cold-weather areas, pressurization of the building will cause increased leakage of warm moist air into the building walls and roof structure. The water condensed from this air when it reaches cold portions of the structure can induce mold growth and rot in wooden parts of the structure.

6. Satisfactory and effective ventilation systems are remarkably difficult to achieve in retrofit situations, even when competent and qualified design assistance is available. Careful and informed inspection is a necessity.

Notwithstanding the difficulties listed above, in some circumstances ventilation may be the only effective mitigation measure available (38). Examples of some situations where it has been used are given below.

2.3.2 Crawl-Space Ventilation.
Structures with crawl spaces often have high radon concentrations in the crawl space owing to a combination of large areas of exposed soil and low ventilation rates. The natural circulation airflows distribute crawl-space air to the rest of the building (39, 40). Mitigative work is often difficult owing to poor access and limited space.

Where winters are not severe, the crawl space is often unheated and is essentially outside the building. In those cases, significant concentration reductions can be made by increasing the ventilation area, or installing a small fan, and closing the major openings in the floor to reduce the air exchange between the crawl space and the living area. Additional insulation to reduce heat loss through the floor may be needed because improved ventilation will lower the temperature of the crawl space.

Heated crawl spaces that are essentially part of the building interior present the greatest problems for mitigation by ventilation. Services and heating ducts are often run through these spaces, so they cannot be simply ventilated by outside air without adding insulation. If the furnace and air ducting are in the crawl space, major work may be required to isolate them from the crawl-space air. The preferred mitigative method is soil ventilation, but if this is not feasible, owing to limited access, then there are two ventilation strategies.

The first is direct introduction of fresh outside air. This not only dilutes the radon present in the crawl space, but in addition slightly pressurizes the crawl space and reduces the exhalation rate of radon from the soil. In cold climates, the air may have to be heated to avoid cold floors or even freezing water services in the crawl space. The high costs of a heater unit and of energy make this an unattractive approach for individuals, but it has been used on government-sponsored projects.

The second approach is to exhaust the crawl space, creating a small negative pressure so that the normal flow of air is from the building to the crawl space. The radon concentration in the crawl space tends to increase, so the effectiveness of this method depends entirely on the fan being large enough to ensure that leakage is from the building into the crawl space.

2.3.3 Structure Ventilation.
The ventilation in a building can be increased conveniently by a small fan blowing unconditioned outside air into the building. If an existing air system is used to distribute the air, the amount of air that can be delivered by this means is limited by the capacity of the heating/cooling system to accept this inflow without upsetting temperature control. A separate fan is not needed in houses with forced-air systems, for the circulating fan can be run at low speed continually, going to full speed only when the thermostat calls for heating or cooling. Outside air is drawn in through a pipe connected to the return air duct close to the fan. The volume of air drawn in through the pipe can be regulated by an orifice, or by a two-position electrically controlled damper.

In modern "tight" homes and buildings, quite small airflows can provide significant reductions in radon concentration owing to the pressurization effect reducing radon inflows, but in older buildings the required flows are likely to be more than the temperature control systems can tolerate. If mitigation is used for these structures, a supplementary heating or cooling system, or at least an air-to-air heat exchanger, will be needed.

If only small reduction in radon concentration is required, an air-to-air heat exchanger may be satisfactory, for it operates with nominally balanced supply and exhaust flows. The pressure in a building is unchanged by its operation, and both the natural ventilation rate and soil gas flows are unchanged. Consequently, the radon concentration in a building is reduced by the increase in the ventilation rate, a factor of no more than 2 or 3: there is no pressurization to reduce the supply rate.

In order for heat exchangers to be effective, structures must be relatively airtight. If the natural ventilation rate is high, the size of the unit required for a significant reduction may prove uneconomical or impracticable. Most older buildings are not airtight; hence heat exchangers have limited use as a mitigative measure for existing buildings. In fact, it is not certain that they are cost-effective, as compared to a simple fan.

The ventilation rate can be increased by a small fan exhausting air from the building. The discharged air must ultimately come from outside the building, so the limit on the amount of air that can be exhausted is still the capacity of the heating/cooling system to maintain temperature control. As decreased pressure tends to increase the radon supply into the space, exhaust is useful as a mitigative method only where spaces can be closed off from the occupied part of the structure, e.g., inaccessible crawl spaces.

2.4 Soil Ventilation

2.4.1 *General*. When the soil connections are so many or so inaccessible (as in the case of concrete block walls) that sealing them is impractical (28, 41, 42), the only ways to decrease the radon entry rate are (i) to decrease the flow of soil gas by reducing the pressure differential between the building and soil, or else (ii) to reduce the radon concentration in the soil gas near the building. These effects can be achieved simultaneously by the use of a soil ventilation system.

This system consists of a perforated pipe network beneath and around the building that is maintained at a pressure lower than the building pressure, either by a small fan or by a passive vented stack. The local reversal of the pressure difference causes air to flow out from the building through the soil to the collection system, thus effectively preventing the entry of soil gas through the house-to-soil connections. The radon-free air drawn into the soil from both the building and the atmosphere also dilutes the radon concentration in the soil adjacent to the building (43). This system has been successfully applied in a number of locations in Canada, Sweden (22–24), and the United States (25–27) to buildings with concrete block foundations as well as to those with poured concrete foundations.

The average natural pressure difference between the soil and building is only a few Pa, and even a small axial fan is able to produce suctions of 25–50 Pa in the pipe network. A passive vented stack extending into the low-pressure zone over the building roof produces a negative pressure of a few Pa, comparable to that existing between the building and the soil, for it is produced by the same wind and thermal forces. As the collection system has to compete with the building for soil gas, a passive system always needs a much larger collection network than a powered exhaust. For this reason, passive systems are rarely as cost-effective as powered ones.

Although soil ventilation is generally effective, it is not a panacea. The use of low permeability fill, local variations in soil permeability, or large building-to-soil connections, can prevent reversal of the soil-building pressure gradient over a portion of the foundation, particularly in retrofit situations. It is hard to predict the size of fan required; a 40-L/s (100-cfm) axial fan is often satisfactory, but more permeable soils or substructures with many openings can require large centrifugal fans to achieve the needed pressure drop. The fan noise can cause difficulties in fan location.

In areas where winter temperatures fall below freezing for considerable periods, the cold air drawn from the atmosphere may cause the frost line to penetrate deeper around the foundation than normal, which might cause structural damage. The soil gas discharged by the system is saturated with moisture, which can freeze in the exhaust portions of the system and may block the exhaust, or damage the fan. To prevent this, fans in colder areas are mounted on the end of long vertical risers (44). Condensation or freezing takes place in the riser, thus protecting the fan.

2.4.2 Collection Systems. The subsoil collection system must produce slightly subatmospheric pressures in the soil adjacent to each wall and the floor. This can be achieved by excavation around the building perimeter to install a perforated pipe and cutting the basement floor or slab, installing perforated pipes in the subfloor fill, and patching the floor. Installation of a system of this size is expensive and causes considerable disruption, but is needed if a passive vented stack is to be used.

If an exhaust fan is used, the extent of the collection system can be reduced, since a fan can generate much higher suctions than a passive stack. In many cases, the collection network can be dispensed with entirely, and the existing structure utilized to control the airflow. Three common systems used in low-cost mitigation work are discussed below.

2.4.2.1 Subfloor Exhaust. If the building has a concrete floor slab, "subfloor" ventilation can be used. This uses an exhaust pipe simply inserted through the floor into a cavity filled with crushed stone. The opening around the pipe is sealed, and a small suction fan is placed on the end of the pipe outside the house. The suction draws the soil gas to the cavity through the layer of coarse material present under most floor slabs and in turn draws air from the building atmosphere through every crack and opening in the floor slab and through the wall-floor joint, thereby preventing soil gas and radon from moving from the soil into the building through these openings. This is very effective if the basement walls are poured concrete, so that the entry routes are entirely cracks through the floor and wall-floor joint. If the walls are concrete block, this system is less effective, for it may not eliminate the flow of soil gas into the building through the block walls.

The effective suction radius is hard to predict, as it depends on the permeability of the subfloor fill, and on the size and distribution of openings, but it is usually 4–5 m with a fan that develops 50–100 Pa suction. Small houses of approximately square plan may require only a central exhaust location for satisfactory performance, but larger rectangular houses generally require two locations so that no portion of the floor is further than 4–5 m from the fan. To reduce costs both exhaust pipes can be joined together with a tee to use one fan.

2.4.2.2 Weeping-Tile Exhaust. The peripheral groundwater drain (weeping-tile) pipe can be used as a collection system by connecting an exhaust fan. Air is drawn from the atmosphere through the soil adjacent to the walls, and a smaller amount is also drawn from the basement through wall cracks and the wall/floor joint. This not only reduces the radon concentration in the soil adjacent to the walls, but also decreases or prevents the flow of soil gas into the building through wall openings. As a result, this reduces radon entry rates even in buildings with concrete block walls, provided that the floors do not have too many openings.

Not all weeping-tile installations are satisfactory as soil gas collection systems. For example, in some areas window wells are drained to the weeping tile either by coarse fill to the footing or by an open-ended pipe connected to the weeping tile. Both provide a low-resistance path for air to reach the tile. Up to a point this can be compensated for by increasing the fan size, but generally drains will have to be excavated and the open end partially closed so that the airflow is reduced but water can still enter.

There are two different practical methods to exhaust the weeping tile. The first is to dig down outside the building and attach an exhaust pipe via a tee piece. To prevent the fan from simply drawing air along the water discharge pipe, it must be closed by a water trap. The second method, applicable if the discharge is to an internal sump, is sump ventilation.

2.4.2.3 Sump Exhaust. Weeping tiles are often drained into a sump inside the building. In this case the weeping tile can be exhausted with minimum effort and cost by placing an airtight cover over the sump and exhausting it to the exterior by a fan. This provides a double benefit, for not only is the suction transmitted to the weeping tile via the drainpipe, but any openings between the edge of the sump crock and the floor slab (which would normally be a route for radon entry) allow the fan to draw soil gas from beneath the floor slab. This widespread pressure reduction is usually effective in reversing the soil gas flow over most of the basement area. For houses with sumps, it is probably the most cost-effective measure available and is the mitigative action of first choice.

2.4.2.4 Wall Cavity. The major radon entry routes in buildings with hollow concrete block foundation walls are the walls themselves and the wall/floor joint. If there is no weeping-tile system, both these routes can be attacked by using the wall cavities as the collector system, exhausted either by a small fan inserted into each wall or by a header collection system tapped into each wall. A fan is needed at each wall because the blocks at the corners are often filled with concrete for reinforcement, so there is no connection between walls. If the pressure in the block cavities is significantly lower than in the building, air will flow into the wall at all connections—including the wall/floor joint.

A problem with this approach is that the leakage area of the walls is large and predominantly on the building side of the wall. Some work is needed to reduce the size of the openings. This could be as little as gluing sheets of foam insulation to the inside face of the wall or painting the walls with waterproofing paint, but access to the walls is necessary to do this. If there is no cap block at the top of the wall, as is the case in some areas, the block cavities will have to be closed by filling them with mortar or an expanding foam. A high standard of closure is needed, for the walls will be filled with soil gas that is high in radon content, which may be forced into the house from the upwind walls when the wind blows.

2.4.2.5 Methods. The entry of soil gas from exposed soil in unpaved crawl spaces can be reduced by placing a perforated collection pipe network over the soil and then covering it with an air barrier. The barrier does not have to be completely airtight, as long as the openings are small enough to allow a small fan to produce the required suction. Barriers can be concrete, plastic sheet, or even a sprayed and formed-in-place membrane material. The advantages of this, over ventilation of the space itself, are that the amount of air withdrawn from the building is small, and the impact on energy costs is negligible.

Although the discussion above has been on the basis of exhaust systems, in some circumstances pressurized soil ventilation systems will perform as effectively and may be preferable. These systems work entirely by reducing the radon concentration adjacent to the building and are suspected to work best in areas of high soil permeability, where the relatively high air velocities in the soil directed away from the house will lead to low radon concentrations in the soil gas.

2.4.3 Costs. To provide an indication of the cost of these mitigation measures, the approximate costs of work in existing houses utilizing contractors' personnel having some prior experience are listed below:

Installation	Cost ($U.S.)
Passive subfloor system (floor trenched plus external excavation)	7000
Single-point subfloor system	700
Exhaust weeping tile via sump	250
Exhaust weeping tile externally	500–700
Exhaust concrete blockwall (each)	300
Crawl-space collection system	800

2.4.4 Performance. If the collection and exhaust system is large enough to reverse the house-to-soil pressure gradient over the entire foundation surface, these systems can be very effective. Examples from Pennsylvania (27) in houses with concrete block walls include active wall ventilation reducing average radon concentrations of 56 kBq/m^3 in a basement to 70–100 Bq/m^3, and active weeping-tile ventilation reducing 8.1 kBq/m^3 to 70–140 Bq/m^3. Even in a case where the weeping tile did not pass completely around the building, large concentration reductions were still achieved, e.g., 2.6 kBq/m^3 to 250 Bq/m^3.

3   DISCUSSION

When an area is identified as having elevated indoor radon levels, the housing resale and construction market is disrupted. Purchasers ask for a radon measurement before buying a home, and buildings with high concentrations become virtually unsalable. Given this situation, there are considerable financial incentives for homeowners to carry out mitigation work in their homes and for builders to produce houses with low radon levels.

3.1   Financing Mitigation Work

At the time of writing, there is a major paradox in North America in the funding of mitigation work against radon. In cases where the radon source is radium-rich materials that have been translocated, radon is perceived as a public-health problem. There is little difficulty in obtaining government funds to carry out immediate mitigation action in houses with high levels and to permanently reduce levels by source removal within a few years. In contrast, if the source is the local environment, radon is apparently perceived as a problem for the homeowners to deal with individually—as if it were comparable to a leaking roof. Immediate mitigation action has not been undertaken by state or federal agencies even in cases where the levels were well in excess of the action levels used in the other projects. For example, no immediate action was undertaken in Pennsylvania houses that routinely had potential alpha-energy concentrations due to radon progeny in the 1–3-WL (4–10 kBq/m^3) range.

This disparity in approach is not because the radon from translocated radium is more hazardous than the radon from in situ radium, but is the result of legislative gaps. The hazards of improper waste disposal were recognized many years ago, and money has been provided to "clean up" historical sites. When the legislation was framed, it was taken for granted that the environmental radon background in ordinary houses was low, and therefore the question of what to do about high natural levels never entered the discussion.

The recent discovery in Pennsylvania and New Jersey of houses with potential alpha-energy concentrations of up to 10 WL (40 kBq/m^3) has dramatically redefined our perception of the range of variability in the natural background. Evidence is accumulating to indicate that conditions there are not unique, and that there are many areas in the United States where the radon levels in some houses result in exposures that exceed 2 WLM/y, recently recommended as a remedial action level by the U.S. National Council on Radiation Protection and Measurements (45). In light of this, it seems likely that a more even-handed source-independent treatment of elevated radon levels in houses will emerge over the next few years.

The number of houses that would require mitigation depends on the action level adopted, but if it were in the region of the occupational exposure standard—equivalent to about 0.1 WL annual average—there could be 15,000 houses in the United States in excess of that figure if the NCRP estimate of the distribution is correct

(45)   It seems likely that a significant reduction in radon levels could be achieved in these houses for an expenditure of less than $5000 per house, so radon levels in all these houses could be mitigated for a cost of less than 75×10^6. This would be comparable in cost to some of the other major uranium processing cleanup projects, but due to the much higher radon levels encountered in these houses, and the large numbers of people involved, the cost effectiveness of environmental radon mitigation programs on a health-effect-averted basis could be up to 2 orders of magnitude higher than that of most other radon/radium cleanup programs to date.

In the meantime, it seems as if mitigative actions against environmental radon will remain the entire responsibility of the homeowner. The active soil ventilation methods are within the capability of a homeowner or small contractor to install and would provide a significant reduction in radon concentration at moderate cost, but it is a major task to disseminate the information to all interested parties. Very few individuals in the United States have experience in selecting mitigation methods, and in the absence of a determined effort to spread their knowledge and experience, the situation will not improve. Significant sums have been spent by some homeowners to achieve small reductions in radon concentrations, where better guidance would have enabled them to get larger reductions for less money.

3.2 New Housing

When an area is identified as having elevated radon levels in conventional housing, developers have three choices. They can stop development in a particular area; they can continue to build as usual in the hope and expectation that public concerns will die down once the newspapers stop writing about radon; or they can change their construction techniques to produce foundations that limit soil gas and radon entry. Some areas are so attractive for development, except for radon, that the added cost of producing radon-resistant foundations would be no deterrent to their adoption if the builders knew how to build them.

There are three basic designs for radon-resistant foundations:

1. Constructing the portions of the building in contact with the soil of poured concrete with sealed joints and sealed service entries.

2. Placing the building above grade with an insulated floor supported on piers or walls to provide natural ventilation between the soil and building.

3. Constructing a conventional foundation with added piping for a soil ventilation system.

Each of these designs can be effective. The choice between them depends largely

---

*According to more recent work by Nero et al., discussed in Chapter 1, and assuming a mean equilibrium factor of 0.4, the annual average potential alpha energy concentration exceeds 0.1 WL in an estimated 37,000 single-family houses.

on local construction practices, in areas where concrete foundations are the rule, the first design would be attractive. In areas where concrete blocks are the usual construction medium, only a ventilated subfloor space or a soil ventilation system will exclude soil gas and radon at a reasonable cost (44, 46, 47).

Sealing the openings or providing ventilation spaces beneath the building are obviously passive methods and, thus, do not require the homeowner to maintain any equipment. Soil ventilation requires that the air pressure in the soil adjacent to the foundation be less than the pressure in the house. This can be achieved "passively" by means of a large pipe network beneath and around the house connected to an uninsulated central stack that runs to near the roof peak. Suction is developed by the buoyancy of the warmer air in the stack and by the low-pressure area that develops over the roof when the wind blows.

If a fan is used to provide the suction, the installation cost can be considerably reduced, for it is expensive to run a stack up through a house. A fan can be mounted on a duct at ground level, and the capital cost savings over a stack installation alone will pay for the fan and its running costs over the life of the building (46).

The success of weeping-tile ventilation as a retrofit mitigative measure suggests that new housing in areas where radon levels may be elevated might have weeping tile installed with connections for ventilation as a low-cost precautionary measure. The added costs of water traps on the weeping tile and a riser for the fan would be insignificant at the time of construction. If subsequent measurements showed an elevated radon level, a fan could be attached to the riser at minimal cost, and would produce a major reduction in radon concentration.

If standard designs were developed for use in a particular area, the additional costs of building radon-resistant foundations by any method are estimated to be less than 1–2% of the final price of the building. The ventilated subfloor space method would be the most expensive, followed by a passive soil ventilation system. Depending on construction styles, sealing concrete structures or installing an active soil ventilation system could be similar in cost. A modified weeping-tile system would be the cheapest of all.

3.3 Obstacles

The technical problems involved in the production of radon-resistant foundations have been largely solved. The obstacles to their use are twofold. First, there is no general method at the moment to determine in advance of construction where radon-resistant foundations are needed. This will be less of a problem in the future, as house survey programs identify large areas as "radon prone" or "radon free" and present work on predictive methods (48, 49) bears fruit. Second, it is only within the past few years that the scientific community has realized the potential extent of radon problem areas, so there has not been time to disseminate information to the large number of firms that make up the building trade. In particular, there has not been a general demonstration to the trade that the routine construction of radon-resistant foundations by any method is feasible.

3.4 Summary

A variety of techniques are available for low-cost mitigation in existing houses. The costs and difficulties associated with them are largely those of obtaining access to parts of the building structure that are concealed by subsequent work and the numerous slight variations in construction methods that cause the physical layout of similar systems to differ from house to house. All systems are effective when properly installed, but the best performance/cost ratio is achieved by active soil ventilation systems. The same basic techniques can be used in new construction to produce radon-resistant foundations at minimal additional cost. The major obstacles to their implementation are the rate at which information can be disseminated to the building trades and the lack of a demonstration to the trade that the proposed methods are effective and economical.

REFERENCES

1. Kukacka, L. E. and Isler, R. J. (1978). *Cost Estimate for Remedial Action Program for Residences in the Grand Junction, Colorado Area*, report BNL 17433, Brookhaven National Laboratory, Upton, NY.
2. Tappan, J. T. (1978). Personal communication.
3. Schiager, K. J., and Olson, H. G. (1973). *Radon Progeny Exposure Control in Buildings*, Colorado State University, Fort Collins, CO.
4. Culot, M. V. J., Olson, H. G., and Schiager, K. J. (1973). Field applications of a radon barrier to reduce indoor radon progeny, *Health Phys.*, **34**, 498.
5. Tappan, J. T. (1974). *Operational Evaluation of the C.S.U. Sealant Demonstration Project*, Nelson, Haley, Pattern and Quirk, Inc., Grand Junction, CO.
6. Case, G., and Maruska, R. (1979). Site investigation techniques. In *Second Workshop on Radon and Radon Daughters in Urban Communities Associated with Uranium Mining and Processing*, report AECB-1164-2, Atomic Energy Control Board, Ottawa.
7. Case, G. (1980). A summary and historical review of the radioactive clean-up in Port Hope, Ontario. In *Third Workshop on Radon and Radon Daughters in Urban Communities Associated with Uranium Mining and Processing*, report AECB-1164-3, Atomic Energy Control Board, Ottawa.
8. Knight, G. B., and Makepeace, C. E. (1980). Modification of the natural radionuclide distribution by some human activities in Canada. In T. F. Gesell and W. M. Lowder (eds.), *Natural Radiation Environment III*, DOE symposium ser. 51, CONF-780422, Washington, DC.
9. Eaton, R. S. (1982). Radon and radon daughters in public, private and commercial buildings in communities associated with uranium mining and processing in Canada. In K. G. Vohra, U. C. Mishra, K. C. Pillai, and S. Sadasivan (eds.), *Natural Radiation Environment*, Wiley Eastern Ltd., New Delhi, India.
10. DSMA ATCON Ltd. and Acres Consulting Services Ltd. (1978). *Report on Investigation and Implementation of Remedial Measures for the Radiation Reduction and Radioactive Decontamination of Elliot Lake, Ontario*, Atomic Energy Control Board, Ottawa.

11. Scott, A. G. (1978). The source of radon at Elliot Lake. In *First Workshop on Radon and Radon Daughters in Urban Communities Associated with Uranium Mining and Processing*, report AECB-1164-1, Atomic Energy Control Board, Ottawa.

12. DSMA ATCON Ltd. and Acres Consulting Services Ltd. (1979). *Natural Radioactivity in Ontario Sands*, Toronto.

13. DSMA ATCON Ltd. and Acres Consulting Services Ltd. (1979). *Variation of Radon Concentration in Soil Gas*, Toronto.

14. DSMA ATCON Ltd. and Acres Consulting Services, Ltd. (1978). *Radon Diffusion Through Concrete*, Elliot Lake Technical Note Series, Toronto.

15. DSMA ATCON Ltd. and Acres Consulting Services Ltd. (1978). *Isolation Module Tests*, Toronto.

16. DSMA ATCON Ltd. and Acres Consulting Services Ltd. (1978). *Elliot Lake Remedial Program*, Elliot Lake Technical Note Series, Toronto.

17. DSMA ATCON Ltd. and Acres Consulting Services Ltd. (1978). *Elliot Lake Remedial Program Proposed Remedial Treatment*, Toronto.

18. DSMA ATCON Ltd. and Acres Consulting Services Ltd. (1982). *Final Report on Investigation and Implementation of Remedial Measures for the Radiation Reduction and Radioactive Decontamination of Elliot Lake, Ontario*, Atomic Energy Control Board, Toronto.

19. DSMA ATCON Ltd. and Acres Consulting Services Ltd. (1982). *Final Report on Investigation and Implementation of Remedial Measures for the Radiation Reduction and Radioactive Decontamination of Uranium City, Saskatchewan*, Atomic Energy Control Board, Ottawa.

20. James F. MacLaren Ltd. (1979). *Investigation and Implementation of Remedial Measures for the Reduction of Radioactivity Found in Bancroft, Ontario and Its Environs*, Atomic Energy Control Board, Ottawa.

21. Hildingson, O., Gustafsson, J., and Nilsson, I. (1984). Locating and limiting radon in dwellings, *Radiat. Prot. Dosim.*, **7**, 403.

22. Ehdwall, H. (1980). Tracing and dealing with dwellings with high radon and radon daughter concentrations. In *Third Workshop on Radon and Radon Daughters in Urban Communities Associated with Uranium Mining and Processing*, report AECB-1164-3, Atomic Energy Control Board, Ottawa.

23. Ericson, S-O. (1980). Some remarks about remedial actions and research program in Sweden. In *Third Workshop on Radon and Radon Daughters in Urban Communities Associated with Uranium Mining and Processing*, report AECB-1164-3, Atomic Energy Control Board, Ottawa.

24. Ericson, S-O., Schmied, H., and Clavensjo, B. (1984). Modified technology in new constructions, and cost effective remedial action in existing structures, to prevent infiltration of soil gas carrying radon, *Radiat. Prot. Dosim.*, **7**, 223.

25. Nitschke, I. A., W. S. Fleming and Associates, Syracuse, NY (1984). Personal communication.

26. Nitschke, I. A., Wadach, J. B., Clarke, W. A., Traynor, G. W., Adams, G. P., and Rizzuto, J. E. (1984). A detailed study of inexpensive radon control techniques in New York state houses. In B. Berglund, T. Lindvall, and J. Sundell (eds.), *Indoor Air*, Vol. 5: *Buildings, Ventilation and Thermal Climate*, Swedish Council for Building Research, Stockholm, p. 111.

27. Henschel, D. B., and Scott, A. G. (1986). The EPA program to demonstrate mitigation measures for indoor radon: Initial results. In *Indoor Radon* (Proc. of Specialty Conf., Philadelphia, February 1986), Air Pollution Control Association, Pittsburgh; Turk, B. H., Prill, R. J., Fisk, W. J., Grimsrud, D. T., Moed, B. A., and Sextro, R. G. (1986). Radon and remedial action in Spokane River Valley residences, report LBL-21399, Lawrence Berkeley Laboratory, Berkeley, CA.

28. DSMA ATCON Ltd. and Acres Consulting Services Ltd. (1979). *Concrete Block Basement Remedial Action Evaluation Program*, Elliot Lake Technical Note Series, Toronto.

29. Eaton, R. S., and Scott, A. G. (1984). Understanding radon transport into houses, *Radiat. Prot. Dosim.*, **7**, 251.

30. DSMA ATCON Ltd. and Acres Consulting Services Ltd. (1979). *Laboratory Tests of External Coatings*, Toronto.

31. DSMA ATCON Ltd. and Acres Consulting Services Ltd. (1980). *Tests on Roofing Cement as a Sealant*, internal report.

32. DSMA ATCON Ltd. and Acres Consulting Services Ltd. (1980). *Remedial Work Specification—Sealing*, internal report.

33. DSMA ATCON Ltd. and Acres Consulting Services Ltd. (1981). *Effect of Form Release Oil on the Performance of Two Rubber-Based Sealants*, Toronto.

34. Desrochers, D., and Scott, A. G. (1985). Residential ventilation rates and indoor radon daughter levels, presented at APCA Specialty Conference on Indoor Air Quality in Cold Climates, Ottawa, May 1985.

35. Desrochers, D., and Robertson, A. (1985). The effects of occupancy and furnace operation on residential indoor air quality, presented at APCA Specialty Conference on Indoor Air Quality in Cold Climates, Ottawa, May 1985.

36. Smith, D., and Scott, A. G. (1981). Ventilation as a means of radon control, presented at the Health Physics Society Annual Meeting, Louisville, KY.

37. American Atcon Inc. (1983). *Demonstration of Remedial Techniques Against Radon in Houses on Florida Phosphate Lands*, report EPA 520/5-83-009, US Environmental Protection Agency, Washington, DC.

38. Keith Consulting Ltd. (1980). Summary of Uranium City, Saskatchewan, remedial measures for radon reduction with special attention to vent fan theory. In *Third Workshop on Radon and Radon Daughters in Urban Communities Associated with Uranium Mining and Processing*, report AECB-1164-3, Atomic Energy Control Board, Ottawa.

39. Nazaroff, W. W., and Doyle, S. M. (1985). Radon entry into houses having a crawlspace, *Health Phys.*, **48**, 265.

40. Rundo, J., and Toohey, R. E. (1983). Radon in homes and other technologically enhanced radioactivity, presented at the Nineteenth Annual Meeting of the National Council on Radiation Protection and Measurements, Washington, DC.

41. Haubrich, E., and Leung, M. K. (1980). Further efforts at remedial measures for houses with block walls. In *Third Workshop on Radon and Radon Daughters in Urban Communities Associated with Uranium Mining and Processing*, report AECB-1164-3, Atomic Energy Control Board, Ottawa.

42. Leung, M. K. (1979). Further studies on remedial measures and radon infiltration routes for houses with block walls. In *Third Workshop on Radon and Radon Daughters in*

Urban Communities Associated with Uranium Mining and Processing, report AECB-1164-2, Atomic Energy Control Board, Ottawa.

43. Scott, A. G. (1979). Comments on subfloor ventilation. In *Second Workshop on Radon and Radon Daughters in Urban Communities Associated with Uranium Mining & Processing*, Report AECB-1164-2, Atomic Energy Control Board, Ottawa.

44. DSMA ATCON Ltd. and Acres Consulting Services Ltd. (1981). *Remedial Work Specification—Soil Ventilation Systems*, internal report.

45. *Exposures from the Uranium Series with Emphasis on Radon and Its Daughters* (1984). NCRP report no. 77, National Council on Radiation Protection and Measurements, Bethesda, MD.

46. DSMA ATCON Ltd. and Acres Consulting Services Ltd. (1981). *Evaluation of Existing Experience in Building Construction Relative to Indoor Radon Levels*, report to the Collaborative Design Program—Elliot Lake Housing, sponsored by the Ontario Ministry of Housing, Rio Algom Ltd., and Dension Mines Ltd.

47. DSMA ATCON Ltd. and Acres Consulting Services Ltd. (1980). *Comparative Costs Study of Building Low Radon Houses*, Toronto.

48. Wilson, C. (1984). Mapping the radon risk of our environment. In B. Berglund, T. Lindvall, and J. Sundell (eds.), *Indoor Air*, Vol. 2: *Radon, Passive Smoking, Particulates and Housing Epidemiology*, Swedish Council for Building Research, Stockholm, p. 85.

49. DSMA ATCON Ltd. (1985). *A Computer Study of Soil Gas Movement into Buildings*, report no. 1389/1333, Department of Health and Welfare, Ottawa.

▬ 11

Removal of Radon and Radon Progeny from Indoor Air

NIELS JONASSEN
Laboratory of Applied Physics I, Technical University of Denmark, 2800
Lyngby, Denmark

J. P. McLAUGHLIN
Physics Department, University College, Dublin, Ireland

1 INTRODUCTION

During the past 25 years considerable effort has taken place aimed at controlling
the levels of airborne radon progeny in the industrial workplace. This has been
true in particular in the case of the mining industry (1). It is only in the last decade
that any serious attention has been devoted to strategies aimed at the reduction of
radon progeny and associated PAEC* in the indoor air (2, 3). The development
of cost-effective and socially acceptable remedial strategies for this problem has
been a slow process. The reasons for this delay are both scientific and sociopolit-
ical and in many cases have interacted with each other.

In the scientific area there has until recently been a considerable lack of precise
experimental information on the behavior of radon progeny in the indoor air of
normal houses. In general, it is known that wide variations may be expected in
such important parameters as the indoor aerosol concentration and size distribution
and their temporal and spatial variations. The same is true of other important parameters such as indoor ventilation and energy conservation practices, human occupancy factors, and so forth. A number of studies principally in North America
and Europe, have, however, taken place in recent years which have helped considerably in quantifying the expected ranges of some of these parameters in indoor
environments in developed countries (4–8). Regulatory and control bodies, which
for decades have recognized the radiation hazard arising from the inhalation of
radon progeny, have been slow in coming to terms with the problem of enhanced
exposure of members of the general public in the indoor environment. The increas-

---

*Potential alpha-energy concentration, see Chapter 1, Section 8.1.

435

ing awareness of this problem is, however, reflected by the many national surveys that have taken place or are currently in progress, notably in Europe and Canada (9–13). A national survey in the United States is long overdue. As recommendations of the International Commission on Radiological Protection (ICRP) are generally treated with due consideration by national regulatory authorities, it is interesting to consider briefly what appears to be the stance of the ICRP in this indoor radon problem. ICRP recommendations have traditionally dealt with exposures from artificial radiation or, where natural radiation was involved, with occupational exposure from enhanced natural radiation (as in the case of uranium and other categories of mining). Recent ICRP publications have, however, referred specifically to exposure of the general public arising from indoor radon (14). In the case of ICRP publication 39, it is suggested (rather than the stronger term ''recommended'') that, for a simple remedial action, an action level of equilibrium equivalent radon concentration (EEC-Rn*) in the region of 200 Bq m^{-3} might be considered.

This publication does recommend that national authorities establish investigation levels to separate exposures that require investigation from those that do not. An EEC-Rn of 100 Bq m^{-3} as an investigation level would appear to correspond approximately to current ICRP thinking on this matter. It is to be expected that over the next decade a number of regulatory bodies will incorporate these suggestions and recommendations within their national regulations. It is reasonable to expect, therefore, that remedial actions or strategies should be capable of maintaining the indoor PAEC from radon progeny at a level corresponding to approximately 150 Bq m^{-3} or lower for future housing stock.

The direct transfer of existing radon progeny control methods from mining or other industries to the indoor environment is not possible for a variety of economic, social, and scientific reasons. In broad terms, of course, any successful indoor control strategy will have its counterpart in the industrial environment.

Controlling radon progeny in the air spaces of houses may be divided into three principal categories:

1. Prevention of radon entry into the indoor air space by the use of sealants, barriers, subfloor ventilation, choice of building materials, choice of house location, etc.
2. Dilution of the indoor air with outdoor air containing a low radon concentration (i.e., ventilation).
3. The use of various air treatments (filtration, electric field methods, radon adsorption, etc.) to directly remove radon progeny, or in some cases the radon gas itself.

*The equilibrium equivalent radon concentration (EEC-Rn) of a nonequilibrium mixture of short-lived radon progeny is defined as that concentration of radon for which the short-lived progeny in equilibrium would have the same potential alpha-energy concentration as the nonequilibrium mixture. See also the discussion of units in Chapter 1, Section 2.1 and 8.1.

[*Editors' note:* This chapter does not treat removal of radon gas, usually considered to be an impractical approach. However, the interested reader may wish to consult a recent paper on this topic: Bocanegra, R., and Hopke, P. K. (1987). The feasibility of using activated charcoal to control indoor radon. In P. K. Hopke (ed.), *Radon and Its Decay Products: Occurrence, Properties and Health Effects*, ACS Symposium Series 331, American Chemical Society, Washington, DC, p. 560.]

The present concern of the developed world with energy conservation has caused a significant reduction in the ventilation rates in some countries. Consequently, strategy (2) may need to be modified by the use of heat recovery devices. In this context it is obvious that houses—with a given radon entry—which are better sealed than heretofore will have higher indoor radon and progeny levels than in the days when inexpensive energy was available. However, as discussed in Chapters 2 and 10, sealing of penetrations in parts of the building shell can reduce both energy loss and the radon entry rate. In this chapter only strategies (2) and (3) will be described.

2 STEADY-STATE MODEL

As an aid in estimating the possible effectiveness of a remedial strategy, it is instructive to use a model that describes the principal features of the behavior of radon and its progeny in an enclosed space. Probably the best model available for this purpose is that originally presented by Jacobi (15) and extended by Porstendörfer et al. (8, 16). In Chapter 5 of this book, Knutson gives a detailed account of this model. It is, however, necessary in this chapter to consider some of the principal features of this model that are relevant to indoor remedial or control strategies.

Essentially an indoor environment may be considered an enclosure in which the activity concentrations of radon and its progeny in their various states occur as a result of the interplay between production and loss rates for these species. Here we shall consider only steady-state conditions in which

$$dA_j/dt = 0 \qquad (1)$$

where A_j is the airborne activity concentration of radon and its three short-lived decay products ^{218}Po, ^{214}Pb, and ^{214}Bi ($j = 0\text{--}3$).* It is a reasonable stance to consider only the steady-state case, both on the grounds of simplicity of treatment and also because in terms of human exposure we are generally concerned more with long-term mean exposures rather than with the effect of short-term variations.

---

*The alpha radiation from the fourth radon decay product, ^{214}Po, can be taken as coming from ^{214}Bi because of the extremely short half-life ($\sim 10^{-4}$ s) of ^{214}Po.

In the further interest of simplicity and clarity we will make the following reasonable assumptions:

1. The activity distributions within the air space and deposited on surfaces are uniform in each category.
2. The radon source term is constant (i.e., exhalation from walls and ingress from subsoil or water is constant).
3. Outside radon and progeny concentrations may be considered negligible compared to inside air (i.e., $(A_0)_{outdoor} \ll (A_0)_{indoor}$).

Using the above assumptions we can thus write the following expressions for radon and progeny activity concentrations in the indoor enclosure:

radon:

$$A_0 = \lambda_0 S_r / [V(\lambda_0 + \lambda_v)] \tag{2}$$

where S_r/V is the radon entry rate per unit volume;

unattached (free) airborne radon progeny:

$$A_1^u = \lambda_1 A_0 / (\lambda_1 + \lambda_v + \lambda_d^u + \lambda_a) \tag{3}$$

$$A_2^u = \lambda_2 (A_1^u + pA_1^a + p_1^* A_1^{s*}) / (\lambda_2 + \lambda_v + \lambda_d^u + \lambda_a) \tag{4}$$

$$A_3^u = \lambda_3 A_2^u / (\lambda_3 + \lambda_v + \lambda_d^u + \lambda_a) \tag{5}$$

attached airborne radon progeny:

$$A_1^a = A_1^u \lambda_a / (\lambda_1 + \lambda_v + \lambda_d^a) \tag{6}$$

$$A_2^a = ((1-p)\lambda_2 A_1^a + \lambda_a A_2^u) / (\lambda_2 + \lambda_v + \lambda_d^a) \tag{7}$$

$$A_3^a = (\lambda_3 A_2^a + \lambda_a A_3^u) / (\lambda_3 + \lambda_v + \lambda_d^a) \tag{8}$$

plateout (deposited) radon progeny:

$$A_1^{s*} = (\lambda_d^u A_1^u + \lambda_d^a A_1^a) / \lambda_1 \tag{9}$$

$$A_2^{s*} = ((1-p^*)\lambda_2 A_1^{s*} + \lambda_d^u A_2^u + \lambda_d^a A_2^a) / \lambda_2 \tag{10}$$

$$A_3^{s*} = (\lambda_3 A_2^{s*} + \lambda_d^u A_3^u + \lambda_d^a A_3^a) / \lambda_3 \tag{11}$$

From these formulae we further find the unattached fractions of airborne activity:

$$f_1 = A_1^u / (A_1^u + A_1^a) \tag{12}$$

(and correspondingly for f_2 and f_3) and the equilibrium factor with respect to the PAEC:

$$e_p = \left[0.1045 (A_1^u + A_1^a) + 0.516 (A_2^u + A_2^a) + 0.3795 (A_3^u + A_3^a) \right] / A_0 \quad (13)$$

In the equations above the symbols used have the following meaning: λ_v represents the aggregate effect of imposed removal processes, such as ventilation, filtration, or electrostatic deposition. The plateout rates are denoted λ_d^u and λ_d^a for unattached and attached progeny, respectively, and are assumed to have the same values for each nuclide. λ_j, $j = 0$–3, represents the radioactive decay rate constant for the jth species. λ_a is the aerosol attachment rate constant. The constant p^* refers to recoil into the airspace following alpha decay of plateout ^{218}Po activity. Although no measurements of p^* specific to indoor surfaces are reported in the literature, we may expect p^* to be ≤ 0.5 and probably closer to 0.25 (17). In the case of p, the recoil factor for alpha decay of attached airborne ^{218}Po activity, we may expect $0.8 \leq p \leq 1.0$ (18, 19). It should be noted in these equations that the plateout activity $A_j^s{}^*$ is expressed as an equivalent volumetric concentration. This can readily be converted into a surface activity density by multiplying it by the surface-to-volume ratio for a room or indoor space.

3 DOSIMETRIC MODELS

The equilibrium factor, e_p, is a measure of the potential alpha-energy concentration at a given radon level. The radiological impact of being exposed to a given atmosphere, however, is only partly determined by the potential alpha-energy concentration. The likelihood of deposition of the inhaled activity at specific sites of the respiratory tract is also important.

The unattached radon progeny, having relatively high diffusivity, preferentially deposit in the upper part of the respiratory tract, where most tumors seem to develop. Consequently, the radiological effect—the dose value—per unit potential alpha-energy concentration is expected to be higher for unattached than for attached radon progeny. This has been recognized in the development of several models for the dose received over a given time by a given part of the respiratory tract.

Commonly used models are (i) the James-Birchall, (ii) the Harley-Pasternack, and (iii) the Jacobi-Eisfeld model (20). See Chapter 7 for recent developments in lung dosimetry.

Generally the dose, D, can be expressed as

$$D = Lt(A'A_1^u + B'A_2^u + C'A_3^u + AA_1^a + BA_2^a + CA_3^a) \quad (14)$$

or

$$D = Lt\left[A'f_1A_1 + B'f_2A_2 + C'f_3A_3 + A(1 - f_1)A_1 \right.$$
$$\left. + B(1 - f_2)A_2 + C(1 - f_3)A_3 \right] \quad (15)$$

where A_1, A_2, and A_3 are the total (unattached + attached) airborne activity concentrations of the radon progeny, L is the breathing rate characteristic of the population group considered, t is the exposure time, and A, B, C, A', B', and C' are constants characteristic for the model, group of individuals, and aerosol distribution. The three models differ both in the absolute values of the constants A, B, C, A', B', and C' and, in particular, in the ratios between the dose values per unit of potential alpha-energy concentration ascribed to unattached and attached progeny, respectively. The James-Birchall and the Harley-Pasternack models ascribe much higher dose values per unit of potential alpha-energy concentration to the unattached than to the attached progeny, making these models very sensitive to changes in the partitioning of the progeny between the attached and unattached states. In the Jacobi-Eisfeld model, the ratio between the dose values of unattached and attached progeny is generally much smaller (in some cases less than 1). Unless the changes in unattached fractions are very dramatic, the variation in the dose predicted by this model will usually follow the change in the potential alpha-energy concentration, and thus—for constant radon concentration—the equilibrium factor.

4 VENTILATION, PLATEOUT, ATTACHMENT

It is useful at this stage to consider the effect on radon and its progeny due to the range of the rate constants (in particular λ_v and λ_a) likely to be encountered in normal dwellings. In the case of radon, assuming constant entry rate, its concentration, A_0, is controlled mainly by the effect of ventilation. Here ventilation refers to the replacement of indoor air with outdoor air, commonly of low radon content. If λ_v values in a normal dwelling might be considered to range from 0.3 to 2 h^{-1}, then $\lambda_v \gg \lambda_0$ ($= 7.6 \ 10^{-3}$ h^{-1}).

Thus, for A_0 we may write

$$A_0(\lambda_v) \simeq \lambda_0 S_r / V \lambda_v \tag{16}$$

It may be noted that

$$A_0(\lambda_v)/A_0(0) \simeq \lambda_0/\lambda_v \tag{17}$$

The latter equation shows that even for a low ventilation rate, say 0.3 h^{-1}, $A_0(0.3)$ $\simeq 2.5\%$ $A_0(0)$. At first sight this seems to indicate a very powerful effect of ventilation at reducing indoor radon concentrations and, as a consequence, the PAEC from its progeny. In practice, however, a house that has a radon problem already has a ventilation rate much greater than zero. If increased ventilation is to be considered as part of the remedial strategy, then its effect must be considered within an acceptable range of ventilation rates rather than with respect to the somewhat academic situation of $\lambda_v = 0$. If we take a tolerable λ_v range of 0.3–2 h^{-1}, we find that, when the ventilation rate is changed from a value λ_{v1} to a new, higher rate λ_{v2}, the radon concentration is, from Equation 16, reduced by the factor $\lambda_{v1}/\lambda_{v2}$. If one takes, as an example, a home with an initial ventilation rate of 0.3 h^{-1}, then increasing λ_v to 2 h^{-1} for remedial purposes reduces the radon concentration to approximately 15% of the initial value. If a dwelling has a severe radon problem, as found in the high-radon-level houses in Eastern Pennsylvania, Finland, or Sweden, such a reduction may be inadequate. In such high-radon-level houses the ventilation rates required to adequately reduce the PAEC may exceed those compatible with household comfort and energy budgeting. In using ventilation as a means of controlling radon progeny concentrations, energy requirements must be considered. Some work in recent years indicates that the conflicting requirements of energy conservation by means of making dwellings more airtight, and increased ventilation for radon reduction, may be made compatible by the use of heat recovery devices.

In the many cases in which soil is a significant source of indoor radon, the rate of radon entry may be influenced by the same pressure differences that determine the ventilation rate. Thus, depending on how it is achieved, a change in ventilation rate may also lead to a change in radon entry rate, and the corresponding change in indoor radon concentration may be greater or lesser than predicted by the ratio of ventilation rates. This interplay between radon entry and ventilation is discussed further in Chapters 2 and 10.

The case of direct control of radon progeny is quite complex. Because of uncertainties that exist concerning important aspects of the microphysics and chemistry of the progeny, it is difficult to predict with confidence the effect on the PAEC and lung dose of any action aimed directly at progeny control. Here it is again instructive to consider the range of rate constants likely to be encountered.

Of the two plateout rates λ_d^u and λ_d^a it is only possible to quote λ_d^a values with any degree of confidence. For a typical room λ_d^a values in the range of 0.2–0.8 h^{-1} may be expected, depending on the surface-to-volume ratio and the aerosol characteristics. The values of λ_d^u to be expected are less certain, and a review of the recent literature suggests that λ_d^u values as low as 3 h^{-1} and as high as 50 h^{-1} may be present in dwellings (4, 5, 7, 8, 20, 21). The wide range in λ_d^u values reflects both the variety of flow conditions that may exist indoors and the lack of knowledge that still exists concerning the nature of what is called the "unattached" or "free" fraction of airborne radon progeny. It is becoming more generally accepted that the division of airborne activity into unattached and attached fractions is at best an approximation and that the airborne species may exist in a size continuum from small cluster size (≈ 5 nm) up to the size of the indoor aerosol (22, 23). (See also Chapter 6.) In the present treatment, however, we shall adhere to the practice of discussing unattached and attached fractions of each decay product as separate species.

The attachment rate λ_a, which describes the attachment of the unattached progeny to the room aerosol, may be expected to show wide variations. A limited number of studies have taken place, principally in North America and Europe, in which the characteristics of the indoor aerosol and to a lesser extent the size distribution of airborne radon progeny have been studied (4–6, 24). For example, Knutson et al. (6), from measurements in U.S. houses, found a bimodal size distribution for the PAEC with the major mode centered at ≈ 100-nm diameter and a minor mode at 5–10 nm. The mean attachment rate at a particle number concentration of approximately 80,000 cm^{-3} was 146 h^{-1}. Other similar measurements in German houses by Reineking et al. (25) show that attachment rates may range from as low as 36 h^{-1} (clean air) to as high as 1700 h^{-1} where cigarette smoking has taken place. In rooms where intensive filtration is taking place, the λ_a value may even be as low as 4 h^{-1}

In summary, we therefore must consider that before any remedial action is to take place we may reasonably expect the rate constants to lie within the ranges shown in Table 11.1.*

The ranges quoted in Table 11.1 are somewhat wider than those to be found in the literature. The logic for this is that the number of determinations of rate constants is still rather small, and thus the relevant ranges are known only with a high degree of uncertainty. In order to better see the effect of variations in the rate constants, the ranges considered have therefore been chosen rather widely.

We shall not describe in detail the dependence of the various concentrations and derived quantities on the rate constants, but a few characteristic relations should be pointed out.

The maximum possible values of the relative concentrations of the airborne progeny products for a given value of the attached plateout rate λ_d^a are reached (theoretically) when $\lambda_a \gtrsim 400 \lambda_d^a$ and $\lambda_v = 0$ and are given by

$$e_{1,\text{max}} = \frac{1}{(1 + \lambda_d^a/\lambda_1)}$$

$$e_{2,\text{max}} = \frac{e_{1,\text{max}}}{(1 + \lambda_d^a/\lambda_2)}$$

$$e_{3,\text{max}} = \frac{e_{2,\text{max}}}{(1 + \lambda_d^a/\lambda_3)} \tag{18}$$

where $e_j = A_j/A_0$.

TABLE 11.1   Rate Constants for Radon Progeny in Indoor Environment

Parameter	Value (h^{-1})
λ_0, decay constant for ^{222}Rn	7.6×10^{-3}
λ_1, decay constant for ^{218}Po	13.37
λ_2, decay constant for ^{214}Pb	1.55
λ_3, decay constant for ^{214}Bi	2.10
	Likely range
Ventilation λ_v	0.3–2
Attached plateout λ_d^a	0.08–0.8
Unattached plateout λ_d^u	3–50
Aerosol attachment λ_a	4–2000

*An analogous table in Chapter 5 (Table 5.5) shows somewhat different ranges. The differences are small compared with the size of the ranges and reflect independent appraisals of a common body of literature.

For a likely lowest value $\lambda_d^a = 0.08 \text{ h}^{-1}$ we thus find

$$e_{1,\max} = 0.99$$

$$e_{2,\max} = 0.94$$

$$e_{3,\max} = 0.91$$

corresponding to an equilibrium factor $e_{p,\max} = 0.93$. For a likely highest value $\lambda_d^a = 0.8 \text{ h}^{-1}$

$$e_{1,\max} = 0.94$$

$$e_{2,\max} = 0.62$$

$$e_{3,\max} = 0.45$$

with an equilibrium factor $e_{p,\max} = 0.59$. In these two cases plateout of attached progeny alone causes the deviation from equilibrium. In general, however, as is seen in equations 3–11, ventilation and plateout of unattached progeny are also effective removal processes.

We shall consider a few characteristic examples, and for the sake of simplicity we choose $\lambda_d^a = 0.08 \text{ h}^{-1}$, $\lambda_d^u = 3 \text{ h}^{-1}$, $p = 0.8$, and $p^* = 0$. It should be mentioned that e_1 does not depend on p or on p^* and that the influence of p and p^* on the values of e_2 and e_3 is small. Table 11.2 shows the relative concentrations of the airborne radon progeny, their unattached fractions, and the equilibrium factor for the ventilation rates $\lambda_v = 0.3$ and $\lambda_v = 2.0 \text{ h}^{-1}$ and for $\lambda_a = 2000, 100,$ and 4 h^{-1}, corresponding to approximately 500,000, 25,000, and 1000 aerosol particles per cm^3, thus covering both extremes and an intermediate value of λ_a. The cases with $\lambda_v = 0.3 \text{ h}^{-1}$ correspond to a house with a low ventilation rate. We see that under these conditions the equilibrium factor may vary from 0.47 in the case of very clean air to 0.75 at very (unlikely) high aerosol loading of the atmosphere. With a ventilation rate of 2 h^{-1}, on the other hand, the equilibrium factor can be expected to fall in the range from 0.24 to 0.35.

TABLE 11.2   Airborne Radon Progeny Characteristics for Different Indoor Conditions[a]

λ_v (h^{-1})	λ_a (h^{-1})	Relative Concentrations $e_0 : e_1 : e_2 : e_3$	f_1	f_2	f_3	e_p
0.3	2000	1:0.97:0.78:0.66	0.01	0	0	0.75
0.3	100	1:0.95:0.74:0.63	0.12	0.02	0	0.72
0.3	4	1:0.84:0.47:0.37	0.77	0.30	0.09	0.47
2.0	2000	1:0.86:0.37:0.19	0.01	0	0	0.35
2.0	100	1:0.84:0.35:0.18	0.13	0.03	0	0.34
2.0	4	1:0.75:0.24:0.10	0.79	0.45	0.19	0.24

[a]Assumptions: $\lambda_d^a = 0.08 \text{ h}^{-1}$, $\lambda_d^u = 3 \text{ h}^{-1}$, $p = 0.8$, $p^* = 0$.

Considering human exposures it is not useful to simply compare the values of the equilibrium factor corresponding to the two ventilation rates, since the radon concentration, A_0, to which e_p refers will be different in the two cases. From Equation 2 we should expect A_0 to be inversely proportional to λ_v (for $\lambda_v \gtrsim 0.1$ h^{-1}), and consequently A_0 at $\lambda_v = 2$ h^{-1} should be about 7 times smaller than A_0 at λ_v

TABLE 11.3   **Radiological Doses from Exposures to Various Radioactive Atmospheres[a]**

λ_v (h^{-1})	λ_a (h^{-1})	e_p	Bronchial dose (10^{-4} Gy y^{-1} Bq^{-1} m^3) C6Y[b]	A3[c]
0.3	2000	0.75	0.62 (JB)[d]	0.47 (JB)
			0.40 (HP)[e]	0.33 (HP)
			0.80 (JE)[f]	0.52 (JE)
0.3	100	0.72	0.88 (JB)	0.73 (JB)
			0.47 (HP)	0.50 (HP)
			0.78 (JE)	0.57 (JE)
0.3	4	0.47	2.66 (JB)	2.61 (JB)
			0.94 (HP)	1.73 (HP)
			0.64 (JE)	0.72 (JE)
2.0	2000	0.35	0.30 (JB)	0.23 (JB)
			0.19 (HP)	0.16 (HP)
			0.37 (JE)	0.24 (JE)
2.0	100	0.34	0.54 (JB)	0.46 (JB)
			0.25 (HP)	0.31 (HP)
			0.38 (JE)	0.28 (JE)
2.0	4	0.24	2.08 (JB)	2.05 (JB)
			0.69 (HP)	1.35 (HP)
			0.38 (JE)	0.49 (JE)

The coefficients[g] obtained from the models and used in Equation 14 are:

(10^{-8} Gy / Bq)

	JB C6Y	JB A3	HP C6Y	HP A3	JE C6Y	JE A3
A'	5.67	1.64	1.82	1.11	1.00	0.45
B'	20.51	7.29	6.05	4.46	1.06	0.82
C'	20.48	6.40	8.31	5.11	3.65	2.27
A	0.28	0.06	0.15	0.04	0.31	0.06
B	1.20	0.29	0.79	0.20	1.69	0.35
C	0.93	0.22	0.65	0.17	1.15	0.24

[a] $\lambda_d^a = 0.08$ h^{-1}, $\lambda_d^y = 3$ h^{-1}, $p = 0.8$, $p^* = 0$.
[b] Children, 6 years of age.
[c] Adults, breathing rate $= 1.2$ m^3 h^{-1}.
[d] James-Birchall model.
[e] Harley-Pasternack model.
[f] Jacobi-Eisfeld model.
[g] The coefficients were supplied by A.C. James, whose help is gratefully acknowledged.

$= 0.3 \text{ h}^{-1}$. As a result, the potential alpha-energy concentration is expected to be reduced by a factor of about 7 times the ratio between the relevant values of the equilibrium factor, i.e., reduction by a factor of 14, when changing the ventilation rate from 0.3 to 2 h^{-1}. If the characteristics for the atmospheres considered in Table 11.2 are introduced into Equations 14 or 15, we obtain the results presented in Table 11.3 for the dose to the bronchial epithelium per unit of radon concentration, expressed in 10^{-4} Gy per year per Bq m^{-3} of radon concentration.

Table 11.3 shows that, although a decrease in the aerosol attachment rate from 2000 h^{-1} to 4 h^{-1} causes the equilibrium factor, and thus the potential alpha-energy concentration, to decrease by a factor from 1.5 to 1.6, the radiological doses are predicted to increase in two of the cases (JB and HP), by factors ranging from 2 to 9. In the case of the Jacobi-Eisfeld model, the change in dose varies from a decrease of 20% to an increase by a factor of 2. It also appears that the change in the rate of attachment to aerosols from $\lambda_a = 2000 \text{ h}^{-1}$ to $\lambda_a = 100 \text{ h}^{-1}$ produces a much smaller effect, both in equilibrium factor and in dose, than does the change from $\lambda_a = 100 \text{ h}^{-1}$ to $\lambda_a = 4 \text{ h}^{-1}$.

5 DIRECT REMOVAL OF RADON DECAY PRODUCTS

5.1 Filtration

When air is passed through a filter, be it electro- or mechanical, airborne particles, both inactive and radioactive, are removed with an efficiency that depends on the type of filter and the size distribution of the particles. In many ways filtration and ventilation are thus equivalent. However, it should be kept in mind that filtration on one hand does not involve the energy-consuming side effect of introducing cold air, but may, on the other hand, cause a change in the partitioning of the progeny between attached and unattached and thus partly counteract the direct removal of radioactive material. If we disregard this latter problem, Equations 3–12 can be used to predict the effect of filtration on the radon progeny by replacing λ_v with the filtration rate (or the sum of the ventilation and filtration rates). The results in Tables 11.2 and 11.3 can be used to estimate the effect of filtration, assuming that the filtration does not change the aerosol concentration and size distribution (which it often does). If λ_v is taken to mean the (effective) filtration rate of some filtering device, we see that a change in filtration rate from 0.3 h^{-1} to 2 h^{-1} is predicted to lower the equilibrium factor to about 50% of its original value and the dose to somewhere from 46 to 78% of the original value, depending on the attachment rate, dose model, and population group considered.

For filtration rates of about 2–3 h^{-1} the simple theory thus predicts that it is possible by filtering the air to lower the radiological exposure and the dose received by about 50%.

The possibility of using filtration as a means of removing radon progeny from indoor air has been recognized for several years, but the experimental results reported so far are few. The experiments show that it is possible by filtration to reduce the PAEC by up to 90% or more (26–35). The reduction depends primarily on the filtration rate, the surface-to-volume ratio of the room, and the aerosol condition.

Several investigations also demonstrate a substantial increase in the unattached fraction of the radon progeny. The degree of agreement between the experimental results and the predictions of the steady-state model was investigated in a series of experiments (31, 32) where the air in a virtually unventilated room was filtered by an electrofilter with rates from 0 to about 3 h^{-1} at different aerosol concentrations. The concentration and unattached fractions of individual radon progeny products were measured under steady-state conditions at various filtration rates. Table 11.4 shows some of the results of the measurements at intermediate aerosol concentrations, together with the model predictions from the same filtration rates, for an atmosphere characterized by $\lambda_d^a = 0.08$ h^{-1}, $\lambda_d^u = 3$ h^{-1}, $\lambda_a = 100$ h^{-1}, $p = 0.8$, and $p^* = 0$. It appears that for the particular atmosphere investigated, filtration is considerably more effective in lowering the potential alpha-energy concentration than predicted by the model. One possible reason is that the applicable value of λ_d^u is higher than the 3-h^{-1} value used in the model, since mechanically induced mixing may play a role in increasing the plateout (see below). Furthermore, the aerosol attachment rate is likely to be lowered as the filtration rate increases. Table 11.5 shows the radiological doses calculated from the experimental results in Table 11.4.

The results in Tables 11.4 and 11.5 show that, although filtration can be very effective in removing radioactive material from the air, as illustrated by the decrease in equilibrium factor, it may at the same time shift the partitioning of the remaining airborne radon progeny toward the unattached state with a higher predicted dose per unit of potential alpha energy, and thus, as far as the predicted doses are concerned, partly counteract the direct removal effect of filtration. It should be pointed out, however, that the results quoted here were obtained in an experimental room under circumstances (for example, a ventilation rate of about 0.01 h^{-1}) unlikely to be encountered in a normal living and working environment. The actual effect of filtration on the doses in practical circumstances can be determined accurately only by additional experiments.

[Editors' note: Recent work has directly addressed the effect on radon decay product concentrations of a range of commercially available air-cleaning devices based on panel filters, HEPA filters, electrostatic precipitators and negative-ion generators (Sextro, R. G., Offermann, F. J., Nazaroff, W. W., Nero, A. V., Revzan, K. L., and Yater, J. [1986]. Evaluation of indoor aerosol control devices and their effects on radon progeny concentrations, Environ. Int., **12**, 429). An earlier report described the effect of these devices on particles, with respect to both the total number concentration and the size distribution (Offermann, F. J., Sextro, R. G., Fisk, W. J., Grimsrud, D. T., Nazaroff, W. W., Nero, A. V., Revzan, K. L., and Yater, J. [1985]. Control of respirable particles in indoor air with portable air cleaners, Atmos. Environ., **19**, 1761).]

TABLE 11.4 Experimental and Theoretically Predicted Results of Filtration on Radon Progeny in an Atmosphere with Intermediate Aerosol Concentration

Filtration rate (h^{-1})	Experimental results					Model predictions				
	Relative concentrations $e_0:e_1:e_2:e_3$	f_1	f_2	f_3	e_p	Relative concentrations $e_0:e_1:e_2:e_3$	f_1	f_2	f_3	e_p
0	1:0.88:0.85:0.72	0.11	0.02	0.01	0.80	1:0.97:0.90:0.87	0.12	0.01	0	0.89
0.44	1:0.83:0.49:0.35	0.22	0.04	0.02	0.47	1:0.94:0.69:0.55	0.12	0.02	0	0.66
0.88	1:0.69:0.34:0.16	0.31	0.07	0.03	0.31	1:0.91:0.55:0.38	0.13	0.02	0	0.52
1.76	1:0.56:0.14:0.07	0.43	0.13	0.10	0.16	1:0.86:0.38:0.20	0.13	0.03	0	0.36
2.64	1:0.49:0.11:0.04	0.49	0.18	0.13	0.12	1:0.81:0.29:0.13	0.14	0.03	0	0.28

TABLE 11.5   Effect of Filtration on Equilibrium Factor and Radiological Dose; intermediate Aerosol Concentration

Filtration rate (h^{-1})	e_p	Bronchial dose (10^{-4} Gy y^{-1} Bq^{-1} m^3)	
		C6Y	A3
0	0.80	0.96 (JB)	0.80 (JB)
		0.52 (HP)	0.55 (HP)
		0.87 (JE)	0.61 (JE)
0.44	0.47	0.86 (JB)	0.76 (JB)
		0.39 (HP)	0.52 (HP)
		0.54 (JE)	0.41 (JE)
0.88	0.31	0.80 (JB)	0.73 (JB)
		0.33 (HP)	0.49 (HP)
		0.37 (JE)	0.31 (JE)
1.76	0.16	0.73 (JB)	0.68 (JB)
		0.26 (HP)	0.46 (HP)
		0.22 (JE)	0.23 (JE)
2.64	0.12	0.68 (JB)	0.64 (JB)
		0.24 (HP)	0.43 (HP)
		0.18 (JE)	0.20 (JE)

For abbreviations, see notes to Table 11.3.

5.2   Reduction of Radon Progeny by Mechanical Mixing

Sizable reductions in the PAEC of radon progeny by the use of air-circulating fans have been reported by Hinds et al. (36). In this and other similar reports it appears that deposition on fan surfaces as such is not a significant factor, but rather the increased circulation of the air causes a corresponding increase in the plateout rate constants throughout the room. Rudnick et al. (27) have reported an increase in the plateout rate constant for unattached progeny from about 8 h^{-1} when no fan is used to 30–50 h^{-1} when fans are used. The actual deposition of activity on the blades is reported to be about 7% of the total. The generally observed increase of plateout rates with the use of mechanical mixing by fans may be viewed in terms of the enhanced deposition velocity of radon progeny as a result of turbulent flow over room surfaces. The resulting increase in plateout or deposition velocity is more important for the unattached rather than the attached fraction of the radon progeny. The relationship between plateout velocity and air velocities in a room depends on the particle size distribution, surface roughness, and the friction velocity (8). Measurements in dwellings of plateout velocities of unattached progeny by Scott (5) have shown, even under conditions of free circulation, a five-to-one variation, depending on surface orientation and air velocity. It cannot be reasonably expected that this type of circulation-assisted deposition will ever be used alone as a remedial technique, but its presence in conjunction with the operation of other remedial methods, such as filtration, may be expected to give rise to an additional reduction in PAEC.

5.3 Electric Field Methods

Early studies of radon progeny usually involved exposure of a metal plate or wire to a radon atmosphere for a period of a few hours for collection of what was known as the induced or excited activity or, more commonly, the active deposit of radon. This method of collection, however, was not very effective, and it was soon found that the activity collected could be greatly increased if the collector was negatively charged, indicating that part of the radon progeny carry a positive charge (37).

Although the alpha decay of a radon atom involves emission of a doubly charged positive particle, the 0.11-MeV recoil energy of the residual ^{218}Po atom is sufficiently high to ensure that most of these atoms will be positively (singly) charged. This elementary ^{218}Po ion will rapidly cluster with a number of other molecules, probably mostly water, forming an unattached ^{218}Po (positive) ion, which in turn may pass through a series of charged and uncharged states (cf. Chapter 6):

1. The initially positively charged ^{218}Po ion may become neutralized by combination with an ordinary negative air ion, or by removing an electron from a colliding neutral molecule, thus forming a neutral unattached ^{218}Po;
2. It may combine with a neutral aerosol particle forming a positively charged attached ^{218}Po ion;
3. The neutralized unattached ^{218}Po may combine with a positive, negative, or neutral aerosol particle forming an attached positive, negative, or neutral ^{218}Po;
4. Attached ^{218}Po (neutral, positive, and negative) may combine with ordinary small ions and thus change their state of charge.

Other combination processes are possible but less likely. When ^{218}Po decays to ^{214}Pb and ^{214}Bi, these products will participate in similar processes, and we can therefore generally expect to find the airborne radon progeny in the unattached state as neutral and positive and in the attached state as neutral, positive, and negative.

The partitioning of the progeny between these various states is governed by equations similar to those used to describe the interaction between ordinary small and large ions and aerosol particles. If the radon and aerosol concentrations in a given atmosphere are known, together with the relevant attachment coefficients, it is thus possible, in principle, to estimate the concentrations of the various states—attached and unattached, charged and uncharged—of the progeny products.

The properties of the charged radon progeny products or, as they are also called, the radon daughter ions, have been studied by many researchers. The early investigations were mainly concerned with the behavior of the radon daughter ions in the free atmosphere, often as a tool for atmospheric or atmospheric electric research (38–46). In most of the investigations only positive radon progeny ions have been studied, although negative radon progeny ions have been shown to exist in measurable amounts under certain circumstances, e.g., in underground environments (40, 46).

5.3.1 Mobilities of Radon Progeny Ions.

A major problem in both these and more specialized investigations has been the determination of the mobility or mobility distribution of the radon progeny ions. Bricard and co-workers (47, 48) determined that the small radioactive ions in unfiltered, artificially radon-enriched air have mobilities in the range $(0.3–2.3) \times 10^{-4}$ m^2 V^{-1} s^{-1} with the major part occupying the range $(0.3–1.2) \times 10^{-4}$ m^2 V^{-1} s^{-1}. Wilkening et al. (41) found that most of the ions had mobilities greater than 0.67×10^{-4} m^2 V^{-1} s^{-1}, and Jonassen and Wilkening (43) found that in outdoor air the mobilities were less than 1.7×10^{-4} m^2 V^{-1} s^{-1}. Fontan et al. (49) found in unfiltered air a maximum mobility of 2.2×10^{-4} m^2 V^{-1} s^{-1}, which decreased as the age of the air examined increased. Thomas and LeClare (50), in their experiments on the determination of diffusion coefficients, deduced an ion mobility of 3.2×10^{-4} m^2 V^{-1} s^{-1}. In experiments with laboratory air Jonassen and Hayes (51) determined the mobility distribution for small radon progeny ions to have a mode of 0.51×10^{-4} m^2 V^{-1} s^{-1} and a mean value of 0.94×10^{-4} m^2 V^{-1} s^{-1}. The results refer to unattached radon progeny ions only and show that this species has mobilities in the same range as ordinary small ions. A further result from these studies is that these radioactive ions only appear positively charged.

Although attached radon progeny ions, or radioactive aerosols as they are often called, have also been studied (42, 48), very little is known about their electrical behavior. Recent studies, however, seem to show (52) that positively and negatively charged attached radon progeny ions appear in more or less equal concentrations and that the major part of both polarities have mobilities in the range 10^{-8}–10^{-7} m^2 V^{-1} s^{-1}, which is the range populated by ordinary large ions (charged aerosol particles).

5.3.2 Charged Fractions of Radon Progeny Products.

The electrical behavior of airborne radon progeny is often conveniently characterized by the fractions of each progeny product, attached and unattached, which are charged. This quantity may, at least for ^{218}Po, be deduced from a knowledge of the concentration of ordinary small and large ions, the aerosol concentration, and the attachment coefficients (18, 48, 53, 54). However, actual experimental determinations of charged fractions of radon progeny, in particular in indoor air of normal houses, are few (52, 55, 56). Busigin et al. (55) report values ranging from 0 to 27% for unattached radon progeny ions in two Canadian uranium mines. The charged fractions were determined by measuring the decrease in airborne activity when letting the air to be sampled pass through an electric field. It should be mentioned that no attempt was made to determine the polarity of the ions removed from the air. The results showed variations from 0 to the maximum value in less than 1 h and reflect a high degree of uncertainty, maybe both in definition of the quantity to be measured and in the measuring equipment (57).

Jonassen (52) reports, for filtered laboratory air with an aerosol number concentration of a few thousands per cm^3, fractions of positively charged unattached ions of about 10–20% for ^{218}Po and somewhat higher for ^{214}Pb. The concentration of ^{214}Bi was, because of the filtration, too low to allow a determination of the charged fraction with a reasonable degree of accuracy. Of the attached progeny a fraction of perhaps 60–70% of each decay product could be deflected by an electric field, rather independently of the direction of the field. This did not seem to be due to a polarization of the aerosol, and it was concluded that about 60–70% of the attached progeny products were charged, with a more or less even distribution between positive and negative charges. Naturally these values can only be taken to be valid for the special circumstances under which they were determined, and it can also not be completely ruled out that polarization effects contribute under certain circumstances to the motion of attached radon progeny products in an electric field.

5.3.3 Electrostatic Field Deposition.
Those airborne radon progeny products that are charged or can be polarized may be extracted from the air by being exposed to an electric field. This has been demonstrated experimentally by placing metal disks kept at a negative potential in a radon-rich atmosphere (33, 58, 59). Khan and Phillips (58) found that the alpha activity from the disks increased linearly with the collecting voltage up to -1750 V at constant potential alpha-energy concentration and with the ^{218}Po concentration at constant collection voltage. The distribution (between individual progeny products) of the collected activity was not analyzed. Jonassen (33, 59) expressed the collection properties of the disks by their cleaning rates defined as the activity collected per unit time of each progeny product divided by the concentration of that particular nuclide and showed that, for filtered air at low aerosol concentrations, the cleaning rates would saturate at collection voltages of about $-(10-15)$ kV and give the relative values $1:0.67:0.03$ for ^{218}Po, ^{214}Pb, and ^{214}Bi respectively. It was also demonstrated that only (positive) unattached progeny ions were collected to any significant degree by this method.

The effect of electrostatic deposition on the level of radon progeny activity has been investigated in several studies. Bigu et al. (60, 61) demonstrated that it is possible to lower the PAEC of both radon and thoron progeny (in a relatively small box, ~ 3 m^3) by operating a negative ion generator in the box. The effect on individual nuclide concentrations and on the dose was not examined, and no suggestion of the mechanisms involved was given. Maher, Rudnick, and Moeller (62) have shown that the operation of ion generators in a larger room (78 m^3) causes the concentrations of each of the progeny nuclides to decrease. The decrease appears to be larger when positive ions are used rather than negative ions. The effect on unattached fractions and on dose is not reported; the theory offered is rather opaque; and the experimental conditions are only vaguely described. The results, however, are interesting, and the experiments should be repeated with measurements of the electrical parameters as well as of the unattached fractions of the individual nuclides.

The direct effect of an electrical field on the radon progeny has been examined in a couple of preliminary studies by Jonassen (33, 63). It was shown that by placing a thin metal wire, maintained at a negative voltage, at a distance of approximately 1 m from the walls, it was possible to lower the concentrations of the radon progeny products in an atmosphere with low aerosol concentration from about 13% (^{218}Po) to about 60% (^{214}Bi) at a wire voltage of -5 kV. The resulting decrease in the potential alpha-energy concentration was about 50%. In a similar series of experiments (64) the reduction in potential alpha-energy concentration was again found to be about 50%. The corresponding reductions in the radiological doses to the basal cells in the bronchial epithelium for the three dose models and two age groups are shown in Table 11.6, both when the air was exposed only to a field and when the air was simultaneously filtered through an electrofilter.

The effect of electric fields on the level of airborne radon progeny activity depends on the fraction and the mobility distribution of the charged radon progeny. The (positively) charged unattached radon progeny, having mobilities about 10^{-4} m^2 V^{-1} s^{-1}, will, when exposed to even moderate electric fields (say 10^4 V m^{-1}), obtain such velocities (~ 1 m s^{-1} for this example) that it is possible to extract this species electrically from even relatively large volumes of air. This was confirmed in the series of experiments referred to above, where it was found that with a negative voltage (-5 kV) on the wire, no charged unattached radon progeny could be detected in the air. The charged attached progeny, on the other hand, having mobilities in the 10^{-8}–10^{-7} m^2 V^{-1} s^{-1} range, will obtain very low velocities (10^{-4}–10^{-3} m s^{-1}) in electric fields of moderate strengths (say 10^4 V m^{-1}), which means that the rate at which these species can be removed from the air is so slow that the charge equilibrium is not appreciably affected. This was also confirmed by the series of experiments mentioned. Although the field did reduce the concentration of attached radon progeny, the charged fractions stayed constant within the uncertainty of the measurements.

The effect of an electric field on the concentration of attached radon progeny is

TABLE 11.6 Reduction (%) in Radiological Dose Induced by an Electrical Field Alone and by an Electrical Field with Simultaneous Filtration

	Reduction in dose (%)	
Treatment	Children (6 years)	Adults (1.2 m³/h)
Electric field	25 (JB)	23 (JB)
(wire at -5 kV)	32 (HP)	24 (HP)
	46 (JE)	41 (JE)
Electric field	54 (JB)	53 (JB)
(wire at -5 kV)	65 (HP)	53 (HP)
+ electrofilter	85 (JE)	76 (JE)
(6–7 h^{-1})		

For abbreviations, see notes to Table 11.3.

determined not only by the fractions charged, but also by the half-lives of the individual progeny products. This can be seen by the following considerations: Let us consider a section of a wire, with radius r, kept at a voltage V with respect to grounded surroundings at a distance R. The field at a distance x from the wire has the magnitude

$$E = V/(x \ln (R/r)) \tag{19}$$

A charged particle with mobility k (and proper polarity) will travel, in a time T, from a distance X to the surface of the wire, where

$$X^2 = 2 \, V k \, T\left(\ln (R/r)\right)^{-1} + r^2 \tag{20}$$

If we put $V = 5$ kV, $R = 1$ m, $r = 1$ mm, $k = 10^{-7}$ m^2 V^{-1} s^{-1}, we find for ^{218}Po, with a mean life of 260 s, that an attached ^{218}Po ion has to start within 20 cm of the wire in order to be deposited on the surface of the wire before it is transformed to ^{214}Pb. For ^{214}Pb ions and ^{214}Bi ions, on the other hand, with respective mean lives of 2300 and 1700 s, the corresponding distances are about 60 and 50 cm, respectively. This means that on the average the volume from which the field is able to effectively extract charged attached radon progeny products is about 9 and 6 times greater for ^{214}Pb and ^{214}Bi than for ^{218}Po. This is also reflected in the changes in the relative concentrations of the progeny products when the air is exposed to an electric field. With field geometries other than the cylindrical one considered here, the relative influences on the individual progeny products may be different.

6 SUMMARY AND CONCLUSION

In the present context the ultimate objective of any remediation or preventive technique is to reduce lung doses to an acceptable level. Where this objective is being pursued by means of either preventing radon entry into a dwelling or by ventilation, it may, as a first approximation, be reasonably expected that any reduction achieved in the indoor radon concentration will lead to a corresponding reduction in lung dose. In the case of techniques like filtration (mechanical or electrical) aimed at removing radon progeny from the air, such an expectation is not realistic. On the basis of current lung dose models it can be shown that the relative reduction achieved in dose may be much less than the corresponding relative reduction in total PAEC (64). Model predictions of this type discourage the development of techniques aimed directly at removing radon progeny from the air. There are a number of reasons for this situation, the most important of which is the relative value of the dose-exposure conversion factors for inhaled unattached and attached radon progeny. Current radon dosimetry models are in broad agreement that the dose-exposure conversion factor for unattached progeny is substantially greater than that for attached progeny. Recently, for example, James (65) has estimated, in a reconsideration of cells at risk, that the dose conversion factor for unattached progeny is 130 mGy/WLM, which is a factor of 16 greater than that for the attached fraction at a typical indoor AMD of 0.12 μm (see also Chapter 7). It follows from this that any remediation technique, such as filtration, that has the effect of increasing the unattached fraction while at the same time reducing the absolute value of the total PAEC may prove to be somewhat inefficient.

Notwithstanding this, dose reductions may in fact be achieved by filtration. For example, if filtration reduces the total PAEC by a factor of 10 and at the same time causes an increase in the unattached fraction from 5% to 20%, then according to the new dose conversion factors of James, a substantial reduction of approximately a factor of 4 in dose will occur. In this regard it should be stressed that the very large dose-exposure conversion factor ascribed to the unattached fraction is a theoretical prediction and has not yet been experimentally verified. There are, for example, no experimental measurements showing that the size of either unattached or attached radon progeny remains unchanged after entering the lung airways, where the air is always close to saturation humidity (66). Any substantial growth in the inhaled unattached fraction, in particular, would considerably reduce its dose-exposure conversion factor. Similarly, there seems to be considerable uncertainty about the fraction of the unattached progeny that deposits in the airways before reaching the lung. It is usually assumed that with nose breathing this fraction is 50%, but it could very well be higher. It should also be noted that the critical cells at risk for cancer initiation in the lung have not yet been identified (67). The vogue held until recently by the basal cells of the bronchial epithelium has now somewhat declined and is shared by the secretory cells, which are now considered to be equally sensitive targets.

In light of these considerations and in anticipation of likely future developments in microdosimetry of the lung, the established ability of filtration to reduce the absolute levels of PAEC in air, possibly in combination with electric fields and/or ion production, should be considered a useful technique for radon progeny control in the indoor air environment.

REFERENCES

1. *Proceedings of the Specialist Meeting on Personal Dosimetry and Area Monitoring Suitable for Radon and Daughter Products* (1978). NEA/OECD, Paris, November 20–22, 1978.
2. Ericson, S-O. (1984). Cost benefit analysis of decreased ventilation rates and radon exhalation from building materials. In B. Berglund, T. Lindvall, and J. Sundell (eds.), *Indoor Air: Buildings, Ventilation and Thermal Climate*, vol. 5, Swedish Council for Building Research, Stockholm, Sweden, p. 271.
3. Hartley, J. N., Koehmstedt, P. L., Esterl, D. J., and Freeman, H. D. (1979). *Asphalt Emulsion Sealing of Uranium Mill Tailings*, 1979 Annual Report, PNL 3290, Battelle Northwest Lab, Richland, WA.
4. George, A. C., Knutson, E. O., and Tu, K. W. (1983). Radon daughter plateout—I. measurements, *Health Phys.*, **45**, 439.

5. Scott, A. G. (1983). Radon daughter deposition velocities estimated from field measurements, *Health Phys.*, **45**, 481.

6. Knutson, E. O., George, A. C., Knuth, R. H., and Koh, B. R. (1984). Measurements of radon daughter particle size, *Radiat. Prot. Dosim.*, **7**, 121.

7. McLaughlin, J. P., and O'Byrne, F. D. (1984). The role of daughter product plateout in passive radon detection, *Radiat. Prot. Dosim.* **7**, 115.

8. Porstendörfer, J. (1984). Behaviour of radon daughter products in indoor air, *Radiat. Prot. Dosim.*, **7**, 107.

9. Letourneau, E. G., McGregor, R. G., and Walker, W. B. (1984). Design and interpretation of large surveys for indoor exposure to radon daughters, *Radiat. Prot. Dosim.*, **7**, 303.

10. Mjönes, L., Burén, A., and Swedjemark, G. A. (1984). Radonhalter i svenska bostäder, report a84-23, Statens Stralskyddsinstitut, Stockholm.

11. Schmier, H., and Wicke, A. (1985). Results from a survey of indoor radon exposures in the Federal Republic of Germany, *Sci. Total Environ.*, **45**, 307.

12. McLaughlin, J. P. (1987). Population doses in Ireland. In P. K. Hopke (ed.), *Radon and Its Decay Products: Occurrence, Properties, and Health Effects*, ACS Symposium Series 331, American Chemical Society, Washington, DC, p. 113.

13. Stranden, E. (1987). Radon-222 in Norwegian dwellings. In P. K. Hopke (ed.), *Radon and Its Decay Products: Occurrence, Properties, and Health Effects,* ACS Symposium Series 331, American Chemical Society, Washington, DC, p. 70.

14. International Commission on Radiological Protection (1984). Publication no. 39, Principles of limiting exposure of the public to natural sources of radiation, *Ann. ICRP*, **14**, 1.

15. Jacobi, W. (1972). Activity and potential alpha energy of Rn-222 and Rn-220 daughters in different air atmospheres, *Health Phys.*, **22**, 441.

16. Porstendörfer, J., Wicke, A., and Schraub, A. (1978). The influence of exhalation, ventilation and deposition processes upon the concentration of radon, thoron and their decay products in room air, *Health Phys.*, **24**, 465.

17. Jonassen, N., and McLaughlin, J. P. (1976). On the recoil of RaB from membrane filters, *J. Aerosol Sci.*, **7**, 141.

18. McLaughlin, J. P. (1972). The attachment of radon daughter products to condensation nuclei, *Proc. Roy. Irish Acad.*, Sect. A, **72**, 51.

19. Mercer, T. T. (1976). The effect of particle size on the escape of recoiling RaB atoms from particulate surfaces, *Health Phys.*, **31**, 173.

20. Dosimetry aspects of exposure to radon and thoron daughter products (1983). NEA/OECD, Paris.

21. Knutson, E. O., George, A. C., Frey, J. J., and Koh, B. R. (1983). Radon daughter plateout—II. Prediction model, *Health Phys.*, **45**, 444.

22. Busigin, A., van der Vooren, A., Babcock, J. C., and Phillips, C. R. (1981). The nature of unattached RaA (Po-218) particles, *Health Phys.*, **40**, 333.

23. Frey, G., Hopke, P. K., and Stukel, J. J. (1981). Effects of trace gases and water vapor on the diffusion coefficient of polonium-218, *Science*, **211**, 480.

24. Johansson, G. I., Samuelsson, C., and Pettersson, H. (1984). Characterisation of the aerosol and the activity size distribution of radon daughters in indoor air, *Radiat. Prot. Dosim.*, **7**, 133.

25. Reineking, A., Becker, K. H., and Porstendörfer, J. (1985). Measurements of the unattached fractions of radon daughters in houses, *Sci. Total Environ.*, **45**, 261.

26. Miles, J. C. H., Davies, B. L., Algar, R. A., and Cliff, K. D. (1980). The effect of domestic air treatment equipment on the concentration of radon-222 daughters in a sealed room, *Roy. Soc. Health. J.*, **100**, 82.

27. Rudnick, S. N., Hinds, W. C., Maher, E. F., Price, J. M., Fujimoto, K., Gu Fang, and First, M. W. (1982). *Effect of Indoor Air Circulation Systems on Radon Decay Product Concentrations*, final report on research supported by EPA Contract 68-0106029, Harvard School of Public Health, Boston, MA.

28. Jonassen, N., and McLaughlin, J. P. (1982). Air filtration and radon daughter levels, *Environ. Int.*, **8**, 71.

29. Jonassen, N., and McLaughlin, J. P. (1984). Airborne radon daughters, behavior and removal. In B. Berglund, T. Lindvall, and J. Sundell (eds.), *Indoor Air: Radon, Passive Smoking, Particulates and Housing Epidemiology*, Vol. 2, Swedish Council for Building Research, Stockholm, Sweden, p. 21.

30. Jonassen, N., and McLaughlin, J. P. (1985). The reduction of indoor air concentrations of radon daughters without the use of ventilation, *Sci. Total Environ.*, **45**, 485.

31. Jonassen, N. (1983). *Radon Daughter Levels in Indoor Air, Effects of Filtration and Circulation*, progress rep. III, Laboratory of Applied Physics I, Tech. Univ. Denmark, Lyngby.

32. Jonassen, N. (1984). *Radon Daughter Levels in Indoor Air, Effects of Filtration and Circulation*, progress rep. VI, Laboratory of Applied Physics I, Tech. Univ. Denmark, Lyngby.

33. Jonassen, N. (1985). Electrical properties of radon daughters. In H. Stocker (ed.), *Occupational Radiation Safety in Mining, Proc. Int. Conf.*, Vol. 2, Canadian Nuclear Association, Toronto, p. 561.

34. Jonassen, N. (1986). Removal of radon daughters from indoor air, *ASHRAE Transactions*, **91**, 1980.

35. Rajala, M., Janka., K., Lehtimäki, M., Kulmala, V., and Graeffe, G. (1986). The influence of an electrostatic precipitator and a mechanical filter on Rn decay products, *Health Phys*, **50**, 447.

36. Hinds, W. C., Rudnick, S. N., Maher, E. F., and First, M. W. (1982). Control of indoor radon decay products by air treatment devices, *J. Air Pollut. Contr. Assoc.*, **33**, 134.

37. Briggs, G. H. (1921). Distribution of the active deposits of radium, thorium and actinium in electric fields, *Phil. Mag.*, **41**, 357.

38. Burke, P. T., and Nolan, J. J. (1950). Observations on the radium A content of the atmosphere, *Proc. Roy. Irish Acad.*, Sect A, **53A**, 145.

39. Wilkening, M. H. (1964). Radon daughter ions in the atmosphere. In J. A. S. Adams and W. M. Lowder (eds.), *The Natural Radiation Environment*, Univ. Chicago Press, Chicago, p. 359.

40. Stanley, R. D. (1964). Mobility distribution of radon-daughter ions, M.Sc. thesis, New Mexico Inst. Mining and Technology, Socorro, NM.

41. Wilkening, M. H., Kawano, M., and Lane, C. (1966). Radon daughter ions and their relations to some electrical properties of the atmosphere, *Tellus*, **18**, 679.

42. Kawano, M., Ikebe, Y., Nakayama, T., and Shimizu, K. (1970). The interaction between radioactive ions and condensation nuclei, *J. Meteorol. Soc. Japan*, **48**, 69.

43. Jonassen, N., and Wilkening, M. H. (1970). Airborne measurements of radon 222 daughter ions in the atmosphere, *J. Geophys. Res.*, **75,** 1745.

44. Roffman, A. (1971). Radon 222 daughter ions in fair weather and thunderstorm environments, Ph.D. thesis, New Mexico Inst. Mining and Technology, Socorro, NM.

45. Jonassen, N., and Hayes, E. I. (1972). Relative concentrations of radon-222 daughter ions in air, *J. Geophys. Res.*, **77,** 2648.

46. Romero, V. (1979). Atmospheric electric parameters in the Carlsbad Caverns, M.Sc. thesis, New Mexico Inst. Mining and Technology, Socorro, NM.

47. Bricard, J., Girod, P., and Pradel, J. (1965). Spectre de mobilité des petits ions radioactifs de l'air, *C.R. Acad. Sci.*, **260,** 6587.

48. Bricard, J., and Pradel, J. (1966). Electric charge and radioactivity of naturally occurring aerosols. In C. N. Davies (ed.), *Aerosol Science*, Academic Press, London.

49. Fontan, J. D., Blanc, M., Huertas, and Marty, M. L. (1969). Mesure de la mobilité et du coefficient de diffusion des particles radioactives. In S. Coroniti and J. Hughes (eds.), *Planetary Electrodynamics*, vol. 1, Gordon and Breach, New York, p. 257.

50. Thomas, J. W., and LeClare, P. C. (1970). A study of the two-filter method for radon 222, *Health Phys.*, **18,** 113.

51. Jonassen, N., and Hayes, E. I. (1972). Mobility distribution of radon 222 daughter small ions in laboratory air, *J. Geophys. Res.*, **77,** 5876.

52. Jonassen, N. (1985). *Radon Daughter Levels in Indoor Air, Effects of Filtration and Circulation*, progress rep. VIII, Laboratory Applied Physics I, Tech. Univ. Denmark, Lyngby.

53. Raabe, O. G. (1969). Concerning the interactions that occur between radon decay products and aerosols, *Health Phys.*, **17,** 177.

54. Chu, K-D., and Hopke, P. K. (1985). Continuous monitoring method of the neutralization phenomena of polonium-218, presented at 78th Annual Meeting of the Air Pollut. Contr. Assoc., Detroit, MI, June 1985.

55. Busigin, C. J., Busigin, A., and Phillips, C. R. (1983). Measurements of charged and unattached fractions of radon and thoron daughters in two Canadian uranium mines, *Health Phys.*, **44,** 165.

56. Dua, S. K., Kotrappa, P., and Gupta, P. C. (1983). Influence of humidity on the charged fraction of decay products of radon and thoron, *Health Phys.*, **45,** 152.

57. Scott, A. G. (1984). Comment on "Measurement of unattached and charged fractions of radon and thoron daughters in two Canadian uranium mines," *Health Phys.*, **46,** 480.

58. Khan, A., and Phillips, C. R. (1984). Electrets for passive radon daughter dosimetry, *Health Phys.*, **46,** 141.

59. Jonassen, N. (1984). Removal of radon daughters by filtration and electric fields, *Radiat. Prot. Dosim.*, **7,** 407.

60. Bigu, J. (1983). On the effect of a negative ion-generator and a mixing fan on the plate-out of radon decay products in a radon box, *Health Phys.*, **44,** 259.

61. Bigu, J., and Greiner, M. (1984). On the effect of a negative ion-generator and a mixing fan on the attachment of thoron-decay products in a thoron box, *Health Phys.*, **46,** 933.

62. Maher, E. F., Rudnick, S. N., and Moeller, D. W. (1984). Removal of radon decay products with ion generators—Comparison of experimental results with theory. In *Proc.*

18th DOE Nucl. Airborne Waste Managem. and Air Clean. Conf., Baltimore, MD August 1984.

63. Jonassen, N. (1983). The effect of electric fields on ^{222}Rn daughter products in indoor air, *Health Phys.*, **45**, 487.

64. Jonassen, N. (1984). *Radon Daughter Levels in Indoor Air, Effects of Filtration and Circulation*, progress rep. VII, Laboratory Applied Physics I, Tech. Univ. Denmark, Lyngby.

65. James, A. C. (1987). A reconsideration of cells at risk and other key factors in radon daughter dosimetry. In P. K. Hopke (ed.), *Radon and Its Decay Products: Occurrence, Properties, and Health Effects*, ACS Symposium Series 331, American Chemical Society, Washington, DC, p. 400.

66. Blanchard, J. D., and Wielleke, K. (1985). Total deposition of ultrafine sodium chloride particles in human lungs, *J. Appl. Physiol.*, **57**, 1850.

67. Hofmann, W. (1984). Lung cancer induction by inhaled radon daughters—What is the relevant dose? *Radiat. Prot. Dosim.*, **7**, 367.

▬ 12

Elements of a Strategy for Control of Indoor Radon

ANTHONY V. NERO, Jr.

Indoor Environment Program, Lawrence Berkeley Laboratory, University of California, Berkeley, California

1 INTRODUCTION

During the last decade or so, efforts to characterize the levels of ^{222}Rn decay products in homes have demonstrated that even average indoor concentrations are high enough to entail an unusually large estimated risk compared with other identifiable environmental insults. Furthermore, the higher concentrations found are unacceptable by virtually any standard. During the same time period—and, indeed, as early as the late 1960s in Sweden—public and political awareness of the radon problem has risen substantially, at least in areas tending to have high levels. A notable example recently is the United States, where concern among policy makers and the general public has grown sharply during the last few years, partly as a result of the discovery of unusually high concentrations in the ''Reading Prong'' geological structure in Pennsylvania. The result has been substantial, sometimes frantic, efforts to identify and control excessive concentrations in a few of the areas where these are known to occur.

These recent efforts, and indeed much of the research of the last decade, have demonstrated a number of difficulties in formulating a program to control the indoor radon problem. One is that of identifying areas or types of buildings where high concentrations tend to occur: it has become apparent that the various possible approaches, including monitoring in small numbers of houses or examining fundamental geological or structural parameters affecting radon entry rates, do not as yet yield consistently reliable results. And even when a high-concentration area is identified, finding individual houses with excessive concentrations involves difficult choices in monitoring protocol and interpretation. Even more fundamental is the difficulty of determining what constitutes an acceptable level: existing regulatory structures and building codes give little guidance on the control of pollutants in private environments, as a result of which past and current control efforts have had to rely on makeshift, often arbitrary, guidelines. And even when a house is judged to need remedial action, difficulty of deciding what measure(s) might be appropriate is compounded by the sparse and inconsistent experience, to date, with various control techniques. Finally, all these difficulties are amplified by a single important point, that homes are essentially private environments: the entire process of setting standards or guidelines, finding houses with high levels, and deciding on what control techniques—if any—are to be employed entails deciding who is responsible for what part and, indeed, how necessary information is to be communicated to homeowners and occupants.

The purpose of this chapter is to examine briefly these essential questions as a basis for formulating a control strategy that takes proper account of important technical and social requirements. The major elements of a control strategy (and the underlying scientific understanding or technical capabilities) are indicated in Figure 12.1. The present examination of these elements is intentionally a rather detached view of what might be seen as an urgent problem. But, however important and urgent, indoor radon has been with us since we began to live in enclosed spaces. And, except perhaps in Sweden, only a few percent of the houses that ought to be considered for remedial action have so far been identified. Careful consideration of basic issues can substantially increase the effectiveness and efficiency of a control strategy that may involve—even within the United States—a million homes, millions of individuals, and billions of dollars.

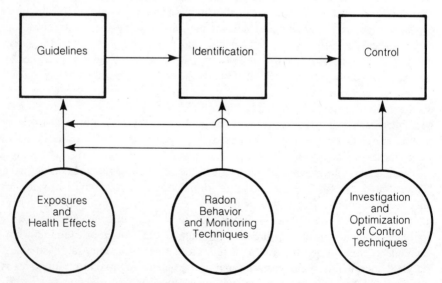

Figure 12.1. The main elements of a control strategy are a system of guidelines, means for identifying the portion of the building stock requiring action, and a framework for choosing appropriate control actions. Formulation of the guidelines and implementation of the control strategy in general depend on scientific understanding of the health risks of indoor exposures, of the behavior of radon and its decay products, and of the principles by which excessive concentrations can be controlled. (Courtesy of Lawrence Berkeley Laboratory.)

2 STANDARDS FOR INDOOR RADON?

One of the main elements of a control program is a system of standards or guidelines embodying an agreed-upon judgment of what exposures are acceptable or unacceptable. As suggested in Figure 12.1, this system must be developed considering the risks involved, current concentrations in the building stock, and the practical possibilities for identification and control. It might be thought that the only consideration is that of risk, which should be reduced as much as *possible*. But, in virtually any real situation, the risk is only controlled as much as is *practical*, a descriptor that takes into account not only the risk, but also the difficulties (and costs) of implementing controls and the value or importance of the activity or entity involved.

Before treating standards for radon per se, we look briefly at the use of health risk as a basis for control of indoor air quality and at the applicability of current standards to indoor radon. Some aspects of these questions have been explored previously (1, 2). I note that the word standard has two potential interpretations in the present context: a regulatory standard with compliance generally assured by governmental action, and an advisory standard with conformance either voluntary or assured by other than governmental means. Examples of both types will be given below.

I also note that virtually the entire discussion below is couched in terms of decay-product concentrations. For practical purposes, one can usually use a nominal equilibrium factor of 0.5, in which case the given (equilibrium-equivalent) decay-product concentrations (given in Bq/m^3) can merely be multiplied by 2 to yield the corresponding ^{222}Rn concentrations, also in Bq/m^3 (or can be divided by 18.5 to yield ^{222}Rn concentrations in the traditional units, pCi/L).

2.1 Estimated Health Risk as a Basis for Action on Indoor Air

One of the principal bases for environmental standards in general is the potential for the pollutants in question to cause human disease or death. Even for a given setting, it is usually difficult to formulate a consistent set of standards for different pollutants, not only for practical reasons having to do with their origin and cost of control, but also because it is difficult to assess the risk on a uniform basis. Pollutants have different types of risks, often not comparable, and the quality of the information base used for assessing risk differs from one pollutant to another. This inescapable difficulty is usually compounded by the fact that, from one situation to another, the level of risk that is considered acceptable can change. The result is that the indoor environment cannot sensibly be treated on the same basis as either the outdoor environment or occupational environments, which also have rationales that differ from one another.

To illustrate this point, consider one risk measure—i.e., an individual's lifetime risk of early death—associated with the following situations or exposures. Mortality is not, of course, the only risk criterion that could be used. (And, indeed, such risk might better be measured in terms of estimated loss of life, rather than chance of early death.)

1. Personal criteria for risk aversion tend to cause avoidance of lifetime risks exceeding levels of 10^{-1}–10^{-2} if the risks in question are under individual control. The larger number (10% or more) is associated with cigarette smoking and the smaller (1–2%) with automobile accidents. One to a few percent lifetime risk may be the approximate level at which people begin to worry about chronic risk over which they have some control, and—as is clear—even at this level many people will deem the risk acceptable because of some perceived benefit.

2. Occupational criteria for exposures that are specifically related to the type of work, such as a substance arising from an industrial process, and over which the worker has limited control tend to lie in the range of 10^{-2}–10^{-3}. These exposures must be distinguished from incidental ones, such as those that occur merely because a worker is in an indoor space (e.g., an office). It is interesting to note that, except possibly for the recently lowered benzene standard, the lifetime risk associated with ^{222}Rn decay product exposures in mines may be the highest occupational risk from pollutant exposure, several percent according to current risk estimates.

3. Finally, environmental criteria for risks that arise externally to the people exposed, over which they have no control, and that are not directly related to a benefit to them, are typically less than 10^{-3} and often in the vicinity of 10^{-5}, or even 10^{-6}, a range that the U.S. Environmental Protection Agency (EPA) appears to use commonly as a criterion for examining and regulating environmental risks.

Environmental risks are to be distinguished from the risks that individuals suffer in connection with situations of direct benefit to themselves, specifically in their own homes and places of work. It is clear that we choose to live indoors because of a wide range of benefits, including comfort, convenience, and health. One might therefore anticipate that risk criteria for this environment, hitherto largely uncontrolled with respect to pollutants, should be in the range between environmental criteria and either occupational or personal criteria. An exception might be cases of industrial contamination of living spaces, for which a more stringent standard might be thought appropriate because of the externality of the insult.

Pollutant exposures also cause risks other than that of early death. In the indoor environment, emissions from unvented (or improperly operating) combustion appliances, organic chemicals from a variety of materials and products, and cigarette smoke are often found to cause larger exposures to a variety of substances than occur in the outdoor environment. These may lead not only to early death, but to a significant risk of acute irritant or allergic response or to chronic respiratory illness. It is difficult to compare such risks with that of lung cancer, in terms of either frequency or detriment. Given better knowledge of the full range of risks, either indoors or in other settings, one approach might be to express all risks in terms of estimated days of life lost or ill, then to assign weighting factors that

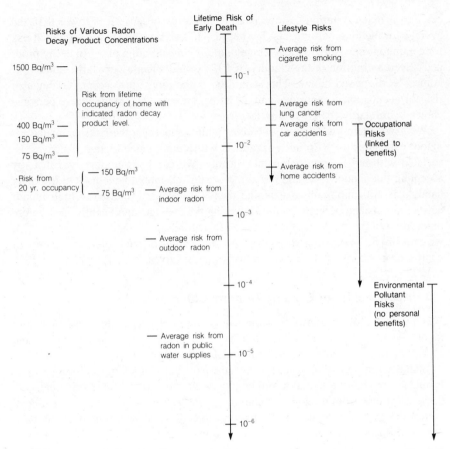

Figure 12.2. Comparison of risk of early death for various exposures and settings. The risks associated with indoor radon exposures, including those that are somewhat higher than average, are comparable to risks that the public assumes as part of their normal life-style, often exceed those from occupational exposures in industrial settings, and exceed by large factors the risks associated with regulated pollutant exposures in the general environment. (Courtesy of Lawrence Berkeley Laboratory.)

depend on the severity of illness. This contrasts with Figure 12.2, where the risk of early death is indicated independently of the associated *amount* of life lost.

Simply considering the risk of early death estimated to arise from ^{222}Rn-decay-product exposures, the level of risk associated with the average U.S. single-family home—having a ^{222}Rn concentration of about 55 Bq/m^3 (1.5 pCi/L) (3)—appears to be about 0.3×10^{-2} (0.3%). And—as indicated in Chapter 1—although some homes have lower concentrations, implying risks in the range of 10^{-3}–10^{-4}, a significant number have risks exceeding 10^{-2} (i.e., 1%) and even 10^{-1} (10%) for lifetime occupancy. It is apparent that a risk criterion in the vicinity of 10^{-5} or even 10^{-4} is impractical for indoor environments. In fact, it is difficult to conceive of a radon criterion as low as 10^{-3}, not only because it is lower than the average for indoor environments, but because it is comparable to the estimated risk for continuous exposure to the average *outdoor* concentration of ^{222}Rn decay products. Even a criterion in the vicinity of 10^{-2} would affect a very large number of homes, as discussed below. This would be at the top of the acceptable range of risk for occupational exposures and at the beginning of the range where personal choice is ordinarily the governing factor.

We must, therefore, content ourselves with the fact that the risks estimated for indoor exposures to ^{222}Rn decay products will remain much higher than risks associated with most "environmental" insults. We can console ourselves that, by accepting this indoor risk (and others), we gain substantial benefits. On the other hand, it is still important to examine means of avoiding unusually high indoor concentrations and perhaps even of lowering the average significantly. But before proceeding to the question of a corresponding structure of standards (Section 2.3), we turn briefly to existing structures. An illustration of the costs and benefits of control programs, with various concentration objectives, is given in Section 2.4.

2.2 Applicability of Existing General Standards

Several classes of standards may offer us some guidance for the case of indoor radon. Among these are existing radiation standards, general occupational and environmental standards, and building-related standards.

Standards for radiation have, for the most part, been based on recommendations formulated within the radiation protection community, represented principally by the International Commission on Radiological Protection (ICRP) and, in the United States, the National Council on Radiation Protection and Measurements (NCRP), organizations with official standing internationally and nationally. Although properly describing the potentially applicable standards is confused significantly by various special radiation units (as are many papers and meetings on indoor radon), the general standard for protection of the public in the United States has been that no individual should suffer radiation doses of more than 0.5 rem per year from man-made radioactivity (4). Furthermore, the average exposure rate to large groups of people, i.e., to the population as a whole, should not exceed one-third of this rate, 0.17 rem per year.

These numerical standards, or their present reformulation in terms of sieverts, can be seen not to apply to indoor radon, which exists completely naturally. To put it another way, no agent is *subjecting* anyone to indoor radon. It is done, albeit inadvertently, by all of us to ourselves by choosing to live indoors. But what is disconcerting is that, uncertainties in conversion factors aside, a *typical* indoor concentration of ^{222}Rn decay products, i.e., an equilibrium-equivalent decay-product concentration (EEDC) of about 20 Bq/m^3 (equal to 0.005 WL—see Chapter 1, Section 8.1), corresponds to an exposure rate that is as significant as 0.17 rem/y, and very large numbers of homes cause exposures much more significant than 0.5 rem/y.

Occupational standards, in particular for radiation, may prove slightly more useful as guidance. The basic limit for radiation has been 5 rem/y, 10 times the value noted above for members of the general public (4), or—for exposures to ^{222}Rn decay products—4 WLM/y*, an exposure rate, expressed in traditional units, that is approximately equivalent to continuous exposure to an EEDC of 300 Bq/m^3 (0.08 WL). There is significant pressure, in the United States at least, to lower this occupational standard by a factor of 2 or more. This is ironic since, to the extent that standards for environmental radon exposures have been developed by international or national bodies, they tend to be in the range of 2–4 WLM/y or the equivalent, prompted partly by the fact that so many homes (e.g., about a million in the U.S.) have exposure rates of 2 WLM/y or more.

Before turning to the guidance being developed for environmental or indoor radon, it is worth mentioning other classes of standards that directly or indirectly limit human exposures to pollutants in air and other media. The most general pollutant-specific class includes environmental and occupational standards for a wide range of substances. These standards typically have philosophies and structures similar to those just described for radiation. For example, the limit for the public is often a factor of 10 lower than that for occupational exposures. In other cases, the environmental standards are based on explicit risk considerations, often seeking to limit risk to less than 10^{-5} or even 10^{-6}, much lower than is possible for indoor radon. In some cases, such as certain outdoor air quality standards, other effects than human health are considered. And for a variety of pollutants, indoor exposures often exceed outdoor, and even occupational, limits.

Another important class of standards apply particularly to the indoor environment, but not to indoor radon alone, i.e., various standards for new construction. A principal example is ASHRAE Standard 62-1981 on "Ventilation for Acceptable Indoor Air Quality," formulated by the American Society of Heating, Refrigerating, and Air-Conditioning Engineers (ASHRAE) (5). The main orientation of this standard is provision of a sufficiently high ventilation rate to assure adequately low levels of human-related pollutants, e.g., CO_2 and odors.

Nonetheless, the basic ventilation rates recommended—approximately 0.5 air changes per hour for homes—also provide adequate assurance of general indoor air quality, assuming that no unusually large pollutant sources are present. Ironically, the current version of this standard—now undergoing revision—also permits an alternative approach to assuring adequate air quality, i.e., not by prescribing ventilation rates, but by checking that concentrations of certain airborne pollutants are below specified levels. As pointed out in Ref. 2, this alternative—as set forth in Ref. 5—does not appear adequate to the purpose and might even be counterproductive. Nonetheless, it does indicate the interest in and need for complementing specified ventilation requirements with guidance on important identified indoor pollutants, including radon. Ultimately, specification of radon-related con-

---

*One working level month (WLM) is an exposure of 173 WL-h, e.g., 1 WL (3740 Bq/m^3) for 173 hours (approximately one month's work).

struction measures for new housing in radon-prone areas might have the broadest effect on public exposures, affecting houses that would otherwise have concentrations below 200 Bq/m³ (0.05 WL) more than would remedial programs. Improvements can be implemented more efficiently in new homes, in the same way that improved specifications on electrical wiring can have a wide effect at low cost in new homes.

2.3   Present Standards for Radon in Homes

Significant steps have been taken in recent years toward development of standards for radon in homes. This guidance has been developed primarily for two situations that must be distinguished: (i) remedial action in buildings whose indoor concentrations are (or appear to be) elevated due to industrial activities or contamination and (ii) remedial measures in ordinary homes, where the radon comes from sources in their natural state or, at least, without elevation due to special types of industrial processing. A final class of standard is that for new homes, exemplified—as indicated above—by the ASHRAE standard for ventilation.

2.3.1   Industrial Contamination. The three major examples of elevated indoor radon concentrations associated with industrial activities are buildings that have been affected by uranium mill tailings, phosphate lands, and refined radium residues. Each of these cases has a long and complex history, so that I mention only the essential points and give a key reference for each. Although these examples are taken only from the United States and Canada, other countries also have some degree of experience with such problems.

A seemingly severe problem with residential contamination by uranium mill tailings was discovered in Grand Junction Colorado during the 1960s. Radon decay product concentrations up to approximately 4000 Bq/m³ (1 WL) were discovered in a variety of structures, including homes and schools. The resulting remedial action program used as guidance recommendations of the U.S. Surgeon General that remedial action was "indicated" for levels exceeding 0.05 WL (185 Bq/m³) and "suggested" above 0.01 WL (37 Bq/m³) (6). In recent years, continued and even increased efforts have been devoted to the disposal of existing uranium tailings, either dispersed in otherwise normal environments or still in major piles. The major environmental impact of these tailings piles appears to be from the release of radon. Although very few people are exposed to concentrations exceeding 0.05 WL (or even 0.01 WL) as a result, it is anticipated that billions of dollars will be spent in isolating these piles. In Canada, remedial programs have been instituted in four communities with prior radium or uranium processing operations. The criterion used for these communities has been to take action to reduce levels below 74 Bq/m³ (0.02 WL). In subsequent consideration of the general housing stock, Canadian authorities have decided not to apply so stringent a standard (7).

"Elevated" decay product concentrations were found during the 1970s in structures built on or with materials from the phosphate mining industry, primarily in Florida. For example, in 133 structures on reclaimed land, one-third were found to have concentrations exceeding 37 Bq/m^3 (0.01 WL), with a few exceeding 185 Bq/m^3 (0.05 WL) (8). In response to a request from the governor of Florida, the EPA recommended that remedial action be taken in residences with concentrations exceeding 0.02 WL (74 Bq/m^3). The EPA also recommended that remedial action be evaluated, on a structure-by-structure basis, for lower levels, but noted that they would be unlikely to be justified for concentrations less than 0.005 WL (18 Bq/m^3) above normal indoor background (9). Ironically, the levels found in these houses are not far above the distribution that appears to be typical of U.S. single-family houses (see Chapter 1).

During this century, numerous industrial facilities that used radium-bearing materials for commercial or military purposes have left a residue of radioactive material. Although natural, the radium has been concentrated so that it can pose an elevated risk for those exposed to the penetrating radiation or to the elevated air-borne concentrations of radon and its decay products. A recent example of such local contamination came to view during 1984, when elevated indoor radon concentrations were found in several New Jersey communities, including Montclair, Glen Ridge, and Orange (10). The U.S. EPA and Centers for Disease Control (CDC) subsequently recommended that remedial action be taken in houses with decay product concentrations exceeding 74 Bq/m^3 (0.02 WL). New Jersey and federal agencies have since implemented remedial actions in a portion of the homes affected, resulting in the problem of disposing of the radium-contaminated soil excavated from around some of these houses.

As is evident from the manner in which these situations have been handled, regulatory agencies have felt a special responsibility for intervening in situations where industrial activities have resulted in elevated radon exposures in people's homes. Analogous as this is to the "environmental" regulatory situation, where an external nonbeneficial agent is the cause of the exposure, the action in these cases has been unusually quick, severe, and costly, as compared with the cases where comparable concentrations are found in ordinary homes, where no external agent is culpable. Indeed, in many cases the cost per unit exposure reduction has been truly extraordinary.

2.3.2 Ordinary (Uncontaminated) Homes.
The history of standards for radon in ordinary homes is somewhat shorter than for cases of contamination. However, considering the experience in Sweden and the growing evidence of a significant incidence of high concentrations in many countries, the radiation protection community has made substantial progress in formulating guidance for ordinary homes. This class of homes is much larger than those with contamination, and the number of people exposed to high concentrations from undisturbed natural sources of radon is much larger than the number seriously affected by industrial residues.

The ICRP and the NCRP have made explicit, although slightly different, recommendations for radon in buildings. In 1983, the ICRP made recommendations both for remedial action and for new housing, suggesting that, for the first, "if the remedial action considered is fairly simple, an action level in the region of 200 Bq/m^3 (0.055 WL) might be considered," but that "for severe and disrupting remedial action, a value several times larger might be more appropriate'' (11). The NCRP, on the other hand, recommended that remedial action be taken, when necessary, to limit individuals' total exposure to 2 WLM/y (12). This is equivalent to an average concentration of about 0.04 WL or, assuming as much as 80% occupancy, an indoor concentration of 0.05 WL (185 Bq/m^3). Although the NCRP said nothing about new construction, the ICRP did, stating the belief that ''a reasonable upper bound . . . is of the order of 100 Bq/m^3 (0.027 WL) and that, in many countries, a value of this magnitude would prevent radon from becoming a dominating source of risk in dwellings.'' Although neither of these reports thoroughly considered the causes of and influences on high radon concentrations, both showed substantial sophistication in the formulation of guidance for existing and (in the case of the ICRP) future housing.

More recently, the World Health Organization, in draft recommendations for indoor and outdoor pollutants, dealt with radon and formaldehyde in the indoor environment. The basic recommendation for radon was that remedial actions in buildings with concentrations higher than 400 Bq/m^3 (0.11 WL) be considered in all cases and that the total dose before remedial action should not exceed 2000 Bq m^{-3} y (e.g., that a home with 400 Bq/m^3 should be modified within 5 years). It also recommended that, where simple measures are possible, action be considered for concentrations higher than 100 Bq/m^3 (0.027 WL). Finally, it recommended that building codes be formulated to avoid levels higher than 100 Bq/m^3 (0.027 WL) in new structures. This framework of recommendations is similar to the guidance now employed in Sweden, where the relatively high remedial action limit of 400 Bq/m^3 was chosen largely for practical reasons.

During 1986, the EPA issued guidance for U.S. householders, recommending that houses with decay-product concentrations greater than 74 Bq/m^3 be altered to reduce levels (13). The suggested urgency of the action depends on how high the concentration is, with the speediest action recommended for houses having levels above 3740 Bq/m^3 (1 WL). The guidelines are also stated in terms of radon concentration (assuming a 50% equilibrium factor). This is a sensible provision considering that the preferred monitoring techniques measure the radon concentration, as discussed below, and that this appears to be a more reliable indicator of risk than the decay product concentration (cf. Chapter 7). However, as indicated in Table 12.1, the recommended remedial action level is lower than that suggested by others, thereby affecting a much larger number of homes.

2.4 Objectives and Implications of Radon Standards

Based on current risk estimates, a radon standard that results in reduction of indoor concentrations will presumably lead to a decrease in the incidence of lung cancer. It will also entail the expenditure of substantial effort or funds to modify buildings as needed. Depending on the choice and design of the standard, these efforts will be more or less efficient in accomplishing the desired exposure (and risk) reduction.

TABLE 12.1   Recommended Limits on ^{222}Rn Decay Product Concentrations in Buildings

	Existing buildings		Future buildings	Ref.
	Ordinary	Contaminated		
Professional Organizations				
ICRP	200 Bq/m³ (0.054 WL) (higher level for more difficult remedial actions)		100 Bq/m³ (0.027 WL)	11
NCRP	185 Bq/m³ (0.050 WL)[a]			12
WHO	400 Bq/m³ (0.11 WL)[b] (100 Bq/m³ if simple measures)		100 Bq/m³ (0.027 WL)	17
ASHRAE			37 Bq/m³ (0.01 WL)[c]	5
Countries				
United States	74 Bq/m³ (0.02 WL)	37–185 Bq/m³ (0.01–0.05 WL)		9, 13
Canada		74 Bq/m³ (0.02 WL)		7
Nordic countries[d]	400 Bq/m³ (0.11 WL) (consider action above 100 Bq/m³)		100 Bq/m³ (0.027 WL)	18

[a]Recommended limit is 340 WL-h per year, equivalent to 0.050 WL for 80% occupancy.
[b]Remedial action to be performed before added exposure exceeds 2000 Bq m^{-3}y (27 WLM).
[c]Likely to be raised in 1987 revision.
[d]These countries are Denmark, Finland, Iceland, Norway, and Sweden. In earlier recommendations (19), Sweden had specified a 70 Bq/m³ limit for new buildings and had not specifically recommended consideration of action, in existing buildings, for levels in the range 100–400 Bq/m³.

Effects of a standard on risk of lung cancer will manifest themselves in two ways, either in reducing the total population risk or in reducing the risk of the highly exposed fraction of the population. The relative importance of these two potential objectives affects the form of the standard (and associated control strategy) adopted.

Under any scheme, individuals at high risk due to living in very high concentrations will experience a substantial reduction in exposures and risk. A strategy aimed primarily at high-concentration houses, a small fraction of the housing stock, will—not surprisingly—substantially affect the fraction of the population at highest risk, but will have only a modest effect on the average population exposure and therefore on the total rate of lung cancer attributable to indoor radon. On the other hand, a strategy that also aims at the relatively large number of houses with concentrations within a factor of 5 or so of the average will also substantially reduce the average population exposure and risk. The cost of this exposure reduction will depend greatly on whether it is effected in existing houses or primarily in new construction.

Attaching specific estimates to these generalizations depends critically on (i) the assumed distribution of exposures, (ii) the assumed risk per unit exposure, and (iii) the costs of exposure reduction, either as remedial action or as construction techniques for new buildings. To illustrate this, let us presume the U.S. distribution discussed in Chapter 1, and a dose–response factor similar to that of the NCRP (14) or ICRP (see Chapter 7). The U.S. Environmental Protection Agency has tended to use higher dose-response factors (cf. upper limit cited in Ref. 13), which would significantly influence the calculation of cost effectiveness given below.

We can estimate, from the lognormal distribution discussed in Chapter 1, that about 7% of U.S. single-family homes have annual-average *radon* concentrations exceeding 150 Bq/m^3 (4 pCi/L), which—for an equilibrium factor of 0.5—corresponds to decay product concentrations of 75 Bq/m^3 (0.02 WL). For a lifetime risk factor of $2 \times 10^{-6}/(\text{Bq m}^{-3}\text{y})$ (i.e., $1.4 \times 10^{-4}/\text{WLM}$), lifetime occupancy of a house with 75 Bq/m^3 of decay products entails an added risk of about 0.8%, assuming 80% of one's time is spent at home. Furthermore, the roughly 7% of houses exceeding this level contribute about 35% of the total population exposure. The corresponding fraction of houses having at least *twice* this concentration, i.e., 300 Bq/m^3 (8 pCi/L) of radon (or about 150 Bq/m^3—0.04 WL—of decay products), is about 2%. The added risk for lifetime occupancy of a house at 150 Bq/m^3 of decay products is 2%; about 15% of the total population risk is incurred within the small percentage of houses exceeding this level. Finally, the individual risk for lifetime occupancy of a house with a decay product concentration of 400 Bq/m^3 (0.1 WL) is about 5%, somewhat more than twice the risk of death from automobile accidents and approximately the same in terms of years of life lost. Approximately 0.1% of U.S. houses are expected to have decay product concentrations exceeding this level, based on extrapolation of the frequency distribution found in Ref. 3.

Aiming remedial measures at this 0.1% of the population would focus efforts toward assisting those at significant risk, but would have little effect on the *average* exposure. On the other hand, these efforts would be extremely effective in terms of reduction in risk per dollar. Assume, for illustrative purposes, that installation of remedial features costs about $2000 per house, with only a modest dependence on the concentration. Then action in the higher-level houses, i.e., those over 400 Bq/m^3 (0.1 WL), would result in reduction of estimated risk to lifetime occupants by several percent. Assuming a reduction of risk by 4% per 70 years of occupancy and 3.5 occupants per house, this would imply a cost of about $50,000 per life saved, if the measure is effective over a house's remaining life—taken here to be about 30 years—and if maintenance costs over this period total half of the initial installation cost. On the other hand, application of the same measures—at roughly the same cost—in lower-level houses would achieve less reduction in risk. In contrast, adoption of measures for new buildings would entail costs, we can now guess, of only hundreds of dollars per dwelling, implying a cost effectiveness comparable to remedial measures among the higher-level houses.

(The estimate for remedial action's cost effectiveness does not include the cost of finding houses with high concentrations, which may cost as much as the remedial actions themselves. The amount of these costs may also depend on the concentration chosen as a remedial action level. The net cost will reflect two contrasting tendencies. At one extreme, if a high fraction of houses are thought to require action, so that virtually every house is monitored, the cost per "high" house found may be less than $2000 for a national program. At the other extreme, if the remedial limit is set at a high level, the houses requiring remediation will occur in clusters in a small fraction of a country's area, so that—once such areas are located—the cost per house identified may be similar to the more broad-scale program.)

Compared with *public* expenditures for reduction of risks from pollution caused by government or industry, the cost of remedial measures may appear modest even for houses at lower levels. However, we are here considering *private* environments and efforts. A rough analogy may be made with installation of smoke detectors, which can be estimated to save one life per $30,000, roughly consistent with the cost effectiveness of remedial action for the higher-level houses. Yet these are not required in private homes. Drawing the analogy with automobile accidents, virtually no effort is required of passengers to use seat belts and thereby reduce a risk of early death that is comparable to that from the "high" decay product concentration of 400 Bq/m^3. On the other hand, an investment of about $200 per car in passive restraints could save lives at a cost of about $100,000 each, comparable to the cost effectiveness of implementing remedial measures above 200 Bq/m^3. Expenditures for cleaning up *contaminated* houses and sites are typically far less cost effective than this (by factors of many thousand in the case of cleaning up the uranium tailings piles), a situation that often occurs when there is public or industrial culpability, explicit or implied. These comparisons are sensitive to the assumptions made about costs and risks, so that they should be regarded as illustrative only.

Finally, as will be seen below, the design of any radon standard interacts significantly, in the context of an overall control strategy, with measures for identification and with decisions on remedial measures.

3   INTERRELATIONSHIP OF GUIDELINES, IDENTIFICATION, AND CONTROL

The foregoing discussion has illustrated the important connections between choosing standards for indoor radon and the means for identifying high concentrations and controlling them. As noted before, an overall control strategy consists of three main elements: a system of standards, methodologies for identification, and a framework for control. These components are based on an underlying scientific and technical understanding, and—once framed—interact with one another directly.

Before proceeding to a discussion of identification and control, it is useful to

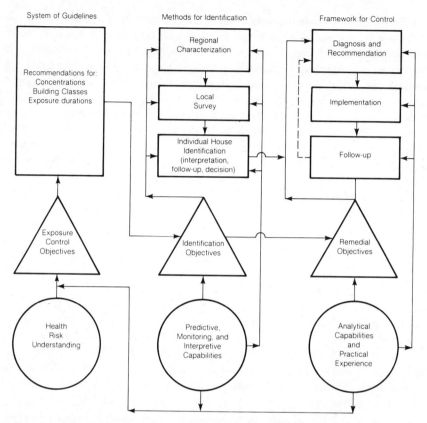

Figure 12.3. Structure of the main elements of a radon control strategy. Each of the elements of a control strategy is actually a moderately complex system or framework in itself. In addition, the main elements are joined by a linked set of objectives for exposure control, for identification, and for selection of control measures. The underlying scientific understanding provides direct support for essential parts of each of the main elements. (Courtesy of Lawrence Berkeley Laboratory.)

indicate these interrelationships somewhat more explicitly, as is done in Figure 12.3. Several important observations can be made at this point:

1. Each of the "elements" discussed here is really a system or framework. The system of guidelines would specify several kinds of standards applying to various classes of buildings (e.g., existing or future) and indicating objectives or limits for concentrations, ventilation rates, etc., as well as time frames for implementation, either for the control program as a whole or for measures in individual houses, once identified. Similarly, the methodology for identification includes (sub)strategies for locating or identifying high-radon areas or housing classes, for surveying these areas or classes, and for measuring and interpreting concentrations in individual houses. Finally, the framework for control includes a methodology

for analyzing the situation in individual houses and choosing appropriate technical measures, for implementing the measures chosen, and for subsequently determining their effectiveness.

2. Each major element in the strategy is driven by a set of objectives or goals. In the case of the system of guidelines, the goals are set by the kinds of risk, cost, and benefit considerations set forth in the last section. In turn, the guidance system, once determined, helps to specify the objectives for identification and control. This interrelationship will become evident in the discussion below.

3. The underlying scientific understanding, including that from prior experience with control techniques, affects the overall control strategy in two important ways. First, it directly or indirectly determines the objectives for each area. The objectives for the system of guidelines, especially, are affected directly by a consideration of radon risks and behavior in general—including not only exposures and health risks, but also the scientific understanding of radon and decay product behavior and the corresponding design and effectiveness of methods for identification and control (which also directly affect the objectives specified for these two areas). Second, the actual manner in which the identification methodology and control techniques are implemented is guided directly by the general scientific understanding of radon behavior, as well as information pertaining to the area or situation at hand. (An example discussed below is how knowledge of the variability in radon concentrations affects the interpretation of monitoring results.)

The overall framework shown in Figure 12.3 can be interpreted at two levels. First, it indicates the basic elements needed in formulating and implementing an overall national strategy for control of indoor radon. Second, some of the key operative elements apply directly to individual structures, i.e., the utilization and interpretation of monitoring results and the choice and implementation of appropriate control techniques. It will be noted that the perspective shifts as the discussion proceeds.

Furthermore, the discussion of identification and control emphasizes the problem of finding and alleviating high concentrations in the existing housing stock, with particular attention to the case of single-family houses. However, the overall framework presented here can also be applied to other aspects of the indoor radon question, including future housing, multifamily structures, or buildings devoted to other purposes.

4 IDENTIFYING AREAS, HOUSING CLASSES, OR INDIVIDUAL HOMES WITH HIGH LEVELS

Although an overall strategy for controlling exposures to radon decay products indoors will include attention to the total population exposure, a major focus in the near term can be expected to be on existing homes that have higher-than-average concentrations. An essential element of a control strategy is therefore to identify this portion of the housing stock. Two key considerations in formulating a strategy for identification are (i) the number of houses thought to be involved and (ii) the manner in which they are distributed, by location or other characteristics, within the full housing stock. The question of preventing high radon concentrations in future housing or of controlling the average radon concentration by means of building codes is considered briefly in Section 6.

In view of the apparent frequency distribution of concentrations, the number of houses requiring identification depends critically on the concentration above which remedial action is desired. As indicated in the example discussed above, a change of a factor of 2 in the remedial action level may cause a change of a factor of 5–10 in the total number of houses involved. If a small fraction of the housing stock is sought, then identification efforts can be staged, focusing the most intensive monitoring efforts on areas (or classes of housing) that are found to have higher-than-average mean concentrations and that therefore contain most of the high-concentration houses.

That there is substantial clustering of such houses by area is clear from very practical experience and also from the systematic examination of the U.S. monitoring data described in Ref. 3. This is illustrated in Figure 12.4, which shows the cumulative distribution of mean concentrations from the 22 data sets that formed the principal basis of that examination. These means range over more than a factor of 10, even within this small number of areas. (A comparable result was reported in Ref. 15.) For any remedial action criterion, the individual data sets show that the houses with excessive concentrations tend to be clustered in the areas with

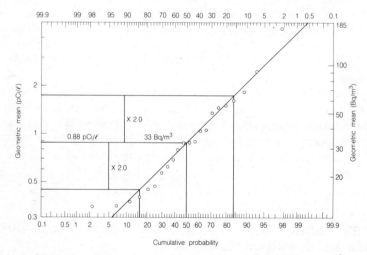

Figure 12.4. Distribution of annual-average geometric means for U.S. data. The geometric means (GMs) from 22 sets of data from around the United States (analyzed in Ref. 3) are plotted versus the probability that the mean is less than the given value. On this scale, if the GMs are distributed lognormally, they should lie along a straight line. The geometric standard deviation of the indicated line is 2.0, providing a measure of the variability of GMs for these various areas. (Courtesy of Lawrence Berkeley Laboratory.)

mean concentrations that are above the average. Conversely, a significant portion of the country will be found to have virtually no houses above the remedial action level, provided that it is selected to be well above typical levels.

Nonetheless, even for areas with low mean concentrations, a very small fraction of houses will have concentrations above any remedial action level selected. Attention to the area-mean concentration may thus be regarded to be a way of prioritizing the effort, causing the earliest and most substantial attention to be focused on areas that have the bulk of the houses needing remedial action or that have houses with genuinely high concentrations. Furthermore, a substantial portion of the country might be expected to have such a low probability of high-concentration houses that no action is taken.

A strategy for identifying the housing having high concentrations can thus be divided practically into two stages: characterization of concentration by area or housing class, and intensive efforts in the areas or classes thought to have the highest probability of high concentrations. The first stage can be carried out by a combination of prediction and monitoring. Because of the variability of concentration, even in a high-concentration area or class, the final identification of houses for which remedial action should be considered requires actual monitoring. A key element in monitoring individual houses will be a framework for interpreting monitoring results as a basis for deciding whether action is needed, what kind, and how fast.

4.1 Methodologies for Identifying High-Concentration Areas or Classes

The most direct way to find areas (or types of houses) with unusually high radon concentrations is to conduct broad-scale surveys that measure levels in a sample of homes over a large region. The efficacy of this approach depends to some extent, but not substantially, on the detailed design of the survey. Virtually any scheme of selecting participants and any measurement technique will yield a useful representation of area-mean concentrations. The only important details of survey design and analysis for this purpose are the fraction of homes selected for the survey and the manner in which the data are interpreted in view of the particular monitoring technique and protocol employed.

To date, the identification of high-concentration areas has not resulted from such a systematic approach. Rather, in the course of local monitoring conducted for a variety of reasons, a number of areas have been identified, almost incidentally, as having high levels. In only one case in the United States, that of Pennsylvania's Reading Prong, has other information—i.e., the basic geological characteristics of this particular formation—*then* been used as an indicator of the potential for high levels in other areas; in particular, monitoring has been conducted elsewhere in this formation to locate other areas with high concentrations, e.g., in New Jersey. This is suggestive of the other, essentially complementary, approach to locating high-concentration areas, i.e., attention to the factors affecting indoor concentrations.

As is clear from the previous chapters of this book, the basic characteristics determining indoor radon concentrations begin with the source material and end with the physical behavior of the indoor atmosphere. For radon entering from the ground, the essential elements affecting indoor concentrations are (i) the radium content of local soil and rock, as well as the fraction of radon generated that enters the pore spaces of these materials, (ii) the transport characteristics of the ground, especially its permeability to airflow, (iii) the house characteristics, especially its understructure, overall leakiness, and mode of operation, and (iv) meteorological conditions. Consideration of these factors—the first two affecting the availability of radon and the second two determining the actual movement into and out of the house—can provide a basis for predicting the indoor radon potential by area or housing class. One difficulty so far is that what appears to be the most influential single factor—the permeability of the soil to flow of radon-bearing air—is the one about which we have the least information on a broad scale.

At present, the relative importance of these factors, and their dependence on more accessible underlying characteristics, have been established only in a very general way. However, as more complete experimental investigations are being undertaken, such as those in connection with practical mitigation efforts, work is continuing on the formulation of a theoretical framework for predicting the dependence of the average indoor radon potential on the factors mentioned above. Such a framework could form the basis of a predictive methodology that substantially increases the efficiency of finding high-radon areas. Such a methodology would be validated and refined by surveys that measure indoor radon concentrations in areas where the factors affecting radon entry (and removal) are also determined. Subsequently, a combination of prediction and monitoring would provide a more efficient basis for locating areas where radon concentrations are a significant concern.

As noted above, there is substantial latitude in design of surveys to locate high-radon areas. The main considerations are that enough homes be selected to provide information on a useful physical scale and that the resulting data be utilized properly. As a crude example, in urban or suburban areas where the density of housing is of the order of 500 units/km², the sampling frequency necessary to provide adequate area-means on a physical scale of 5 km × 5 km is only about one residence in 500: this would provide 25 indoor readings (per 25 km²), determining the mean with a (standard) uncertainty of about 20%, more than adequate for the purpose. For sampling in rural areas or in areas where geological information suggests a finer physical grid seems appopriate, a higher proportion of homes should be sampled.

As another key element, care must be taken to interpret data consistently with the monitoring procedure used. For example, the sampling period has a significant effect on interpretation of results in terms of annual-average concentrations, as does the time of year during which the measurements are performed. Often a particular sampling technique and protocol may require auxiliary measurements in a subset of houses and additional information (such as meteorological) as a basis for interpretation.

These two examples—sample density and data interpretation—are given only to illustrate the types of considerations and features to be included in design and conduct of surveys to find high-radon areas or classes. As indicated above, the efficiency of such surveys can be substantially enhanced by a theoretical framework relating indoor concentrations to the factors affecting them.

4.2 Techniques and Strategies for Identifying High-Radon Homes

Once houses in an area or class are known to have a high probability of excessive concentrations, it is necessary to monitor each house of concern to determine actual levels. The objective of such monitoring is to obtain a useful estimate of the annual-average concentration in the living space. Achieving this simply stated objective is complicated by two factors: first, measurement techniques differ substantially in their suitability for determining this quantity; and, second, the annual-average has an intrinsic variability because of its dependence on a variety of factors, including such obvious ones as the local meteorology and the pattern of use of the home being examined. As a result, any measurement outcome must be utilized within an interpretive framework associated with the concentration guidelines being applied.

Three simple techniques are presently available for measuring the radon concentration. Grab sampling typically uses alpha scintillation or comparable principles for on-site analysis of a sample of air drawn at a particular time. Charcoal sampling collects radon over a period of a day to a week for later laboratory analysis using gamma detection. Etched-track detection exposes a piece of plastic material for up to a year, followed by laboratory etching and counting of alpha-induced tracks in the material. These techniques are discussed briefly here and in more detail in the appendix to this book.

Because it can be left in place for a year, the etched-track technique is most directly suited to measuring the desired quantity. However, even for this technique, the resulting value is not unambiguous. A single detector measures the concentration in one location, so it may not accurately reflect the average living-space concentration, even if placed in the most heavily occupied room. Thus, even aside from the intrinsic variability in the concentration due to meteorology and use patterns, every technique has limitations associated with protocol, as well as analytical uncertainties intrinsic to the technique itself. The resulting concentration therefore has an uncertainty that must be considered in any use to which it is put. However, not too much concern should be associated with uncertainties on the order of 20 or 30%: the risk associated with radon exposures is assumed to be a smooth function with no threshold, so that the guidelines should not have sudden thresholds, nor should occupants' decisions ordinarily be affected by modest uncertainties in measurement results.

Utilization of the charcoal techniques requires attention to the issues of variability over medium to long times, e.g., from week to week and from one season to another. This can introduce substantial uncertainties, which, however, can be reduced significantly with knowledge of meteorological conditions at the time of measurement, coupled with a theoretical or experiential framework within which to make necessary adjustments. Nonetheless, there are significant limitations. For example, in an area with moderate summertime conditions, it is unlikely that a low reading from summer monitoring is a useful indicator of the annual-average concentration.

Finally, grab sampling—because it does not even average over the very large *daily* variation known to occur—gives little basis for any kind of decision, not even about whether or not to monitor further, unless performed a number of times, as indicated below. Ironically, single grab samples can be used—with proper interpretation—to indicate area-means (and even distributions) in a regional survey. But there is at present no adequate measurement methodology or interpretive framework for determining that, in a single house, one low reading indicates a low annual average or that a high reading indicates the need for remediation. In any area where high concentrations occur, every grab-sample measurement would have to be followed by an integrated measurement, which is to say that the grab-sample measurement has provided no usable information. An alternative is to perform a *number* of grab samples in a house, effectively simulating an integrated sample. (However, it is important to recognize the importance of grab sampling or real-time measurements for following the concentration during attempts to implement control measures in a specific house.)

As indicated, even if a useful measurement technique is employed, some interpretation has to be applied and uncertainties considered in utilizing the result within a system of guidelines. This extends even to the consideration of temporal variability from year to year. But the most difficult variability to consider is that arising from different patterns of occupancy and operation of homes, as well as different personal habits (such as cigarette smoking). Creating a control strategy that copes explicitly with all such matters is probably not practical. In fact, considering that houses typically have a sequence of occupants, it may be best that the concentration estimate sought from any monitoring approach and interpretive framework be that characteristic of some "normal" use pattern and not be linked to personal habits, but only to key operational questions.

Perhaps the dominant operational question is the amount of controllable ventilation, either through open windows or because of mechanical (heating, ventilating, or air-conditioning) systems. As an example of the kind of criterion that might be used, in many areas windows are normally kept closed during the heating season, and this is the period during which the higher indoor concentrations occur. If current occupants leave windows open during the heating season, the concentration estimation should probably adjust monitoring results to the "normal" condition in some way, at least for subsequent occupants. Formulating a consistent approach for handling such complexities, although sometimes perplexing, is a necessary part of a long-term radon control strategy.

4.3   Framework for Interpreting and Utilizing Monitoring Results

Just as the results of a regional survey must be interpreted in light of design and objectives of the survey, the results of monitoring in an individual house must be used intelligently. First, using the result to estimate an annual-average concentration in the living space ordinarily requires some degree of interpretation. Second, the manner in which this estimate is used depends on how it fits into the applicable guidance structure and on what means might be appropriate for achieving a reduction in concentration. For this reason, the main elements of a control strategy as indicated in Figure 12.3 have an inherent structure whose implementation depends on an effective scientific understanding of the behavior of radon and its decay products.

Obtaining an estimate of the annual-average concentration and its uncertainty requires consideration of the various factors just discussed in connection with monitoring techniques. Some of these arise directly from the measurement technique itself, so that their effect may be evaluated by contractors or individuals performing measurements. Others require more sophistication, e.g., an analytical approach and sufficient local information to convert a reading from, say, charcoal collection over several days to an estimated annual average. It is likely that this capability could only be maintained by a central (although, perhaps, local) authority or contractor. To some extent, such complications can be minimized by careful design of the framework for utilizing the resulting estimate.

This interpretive framework is an essential functional element in any local con-

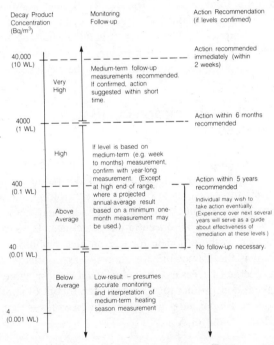

Figure 12.5. Possible responses to initial monitoring results: follow-up monitoring and remedial action. Concentrations found in single-family homes vary over a very wide range. An important part of a control strategy as it applies to individual houses is indication of appropriate courses of action as a response to various possible monitoring results. These recommendations should take into account the monitoring protocol, the resulting estimated concentration as it compares with recommended limits, and the appropriate time scale for action. (Courtesy of Lawrence Berkeley Laboratory.)

trol program. Specifically, it must match a specific measurement result to the structure of guidelines and yield a course of action, if any. The guidelines presumably would have a series of concentration ranges with differing recommendations. As suggested in Figure 12.5, these might be ranked as follows: a below-average range in which no consideration of action is suggested, an above-average (but not high) range for which it is suggested only that individuals may wish to consider remedial action, a high range in which action is recommended at some time, a very high range in which action is recommended soon (e.g., within a year), and an extreme range in which action is recommended essentially immediately (e.g., within weeks). Depending on where a measurement result fits into this scheme, a decision either for or against remedial action might be appropriate or subsequent monitoring might be indicated. For example, a charcoal sample result that falls into the lowest range or into the very high range would probably be reliable enough to make a decision, specifically to decline action in the first case and to investigate the choice of remedial measure(s) in the second. On the other hand, a charcoal sample result in the above-average or high ranges would probably warrant further monitoring (i.e., a year-long measurement or a sequence of charcoal measurements) to determine the annual-average concentration with more assurance, after which a decision could be made on a sounder basis. The details of such a structure for decision require careful consideration. But it is clear that such a structure must be adopted, either explicitly or implicitly. The default structure, where no such consideration is given, is simply the one where all measurement results are utilized as though they yield the annual-average concentration with the same degree of assurance.

5 A FRAMEWORK FOR CHOOSING REMEDIAL MEASURES IN INDIVIDUAL HOMES

As suggested by the discussion to this point and illustrated in Figure 12.3, the essential elements of a strategy for control of indoor radon are three frameworks providing the basis for decisions to be made in controlling indoor concentrations both on a strategic level and, ultimately, in individual homes. One of these ''frameworks'' is a structure of concentration guidelines. The second, as it applies to individual houses, is the rationale for interpreting monitoring results, just discussed. The third is the framework for choosing appropriate remedial measures where they are deemed necessary. In point of fact, these three frameworks are inextricably linked, constituting together the overall control strategy as it applies to individual houses. Properly designing these frameworks is therefore essential to designing an effective control strategy.

5.1 Major Features of a Framework for Choosing Remedial Measures

The presumed situation for choosing remedial measures is one where the results of monitoring, interpreted in light of some set of guidelines, have prompted a decision to seek a reduction in the concentration in a particular house. Along with this specific decision will have come some sense of the importance of the action (reflected indirectly in the degree of concentration reduction sought) and of its urgency (manifested in terms of a recommended time during which action should be implemented). These two factors or objectives are determined in view of monitoring results and the remedial action guidelines, possibly after some diagnosis of potential causes of the high levels, and constitute the broad premises for choosing the course of action and specific measures suited to the house in question. Thus, the overall framework for remedial action utilizes objectives designated (at least tentatively) for the house being considered and includes (i) choice of appropriate control measures, (ii) a capability for implementing this plan of action, and (iii) any necessary follow-up.

Choosing specific remedial measures in individual homes is the most difficult aspect of operating a remedial action program. The indoor concentration depends in a very complex way on many factors. In particular, the pathways and forces accounting for radon entry in a given house are often extremely complicated and heterogeneous. Owing in part to this complexity, as well as to limited experience, procedures for characterizing the specific entry process in a given house are tentative at best. At present, one can—on the basis of limited examination and measurements—formulate a hypothesis (i.e., a diagnosis), but this can only be tested in a very practical way, i.e., by implementing an associated control measure or set of measures. Should this attempt not work, a different approach—based on a somewhat different hypothesis—can be attempted. After one or more attempts, something approximating the desired reduction will be achieved.

Even then, the apparent success of remedial measures should be confirmed by a follow-up measurement that provides a basis for estimating the new annual-average concentration associated with the house. An apparent change in concentration during the course of remediation cannot be considered sufficient of itself. It is possible, for example, that the apparent success depends on the specific meteorological or operational conditions of the moment. Hence it is still often appropriate to perform long-term monitoring as a follow-up. Moreover, even if the efficacy of the control approach that has been implemented is confirmed by such monitoring, future changes in characteristics of the house structure (e.g., continued settling in the understructure) might cause a later problem. The probability of such difficulties will depend on features of the house being considered and on the type of remedial measures that have been implemented. The confirmation and follow-up procedures should handle this possibility.

5.2 Diagnosis and Selection

It is useful to illustrate crudely the process of selecting appropriate remedial measures by indicating two of the primary possibilities to be examined and choices to be made. Specifically, one class of choices has to do with the seriousness and urgency of the problem and another has to do with the type of house.

Considering the first, if the concentration falls into the extreme range, something should be done in a short time. The only measures immediately available to most occupants are temporary evacuation, increased ventilation, or the immediate attention of a contractor. None of the options is extremely attractive. Evacuation is inconvenient and expensive. Sufficient ventilation to effect a large reduction in concentration is ordinarily uncomfortable and costly. And securing the rapid attention of a contractor is likely to increase the cost substantially and, perhaps, decrease the quality of the alterations made. Fortunately, very few houses fall into the range where action is recommended so rapidly. In such cases the optimal choice will often be to provide substantial temporary ventilation to reduce the concentration to one of the lower ranges until a reasonable attempt at remedial action can be arranged.

The more usual situation, i.e., where action is recommended "sometime" or "soon," or where the owner decides to do something even though action is not specifically recommended, will occur with much higher frequency and should be the main focus of a structure for choosing measures. In that case, decisions can be made in the light of the relative priority of the factors that affect indoor concentrations. Ordinarily, the ventilation rate in a high-radon house is in the normal range, so that the main focus of potential control efforts will be on radon entry. (Should this not be true, i.e., if the house is one in which the infiltration rate is unusually low because of special construction practices, then some consideration should be given to increasing the ventilation rate, as discussed below.)

Because the main mechanism for radon entry is ordinarily movement of air from the ground into the house, associated control techniques seek either to reduce this flow or to reduce the radon concentration in the nearby soil air, or both (cf. Chapter 10). The technique appropriate to a specific house depends on the type of structure, details of the substructure and underlying ground, and the reduction factor sought. The most effective means have often been found to involve specialized (but basically simple) systems for altering the pressure balance between the lower part of the house and the ground or specifically for venting radon from underlying soil directly to the outdoors. The effectiveness of these systems can be increased by sealing the understructure, even though such sealing of itself is often ineffective.

Thus, in considering the seriousness of the problem and focusing on the case of moderately high levels, we have turned already to the usual case in terms of house type, i.e., where the overall difficulty is an excessive entry rate and the most likely solution is to be found in reducing flow from the ground. However, there is a smaller probability of situations where other means are appropriate, either where ventilation is used on a temporary basis to alleviate truly extreme concentrations, or—somewhat more frequently—where the house has much lower-than-average ventilation rates owing to unusual construction practices.

Houses with unusual features designed to lower infiltration rates substantially in order to save energy can be expected to have higher-than-average concentrations of radon and other indoor pollutants. Such levels can be reduced by using mechanical systems to increase the overall ventilation rate of the house to a normal level, say 0.5 air changes per hour. The simplest such system is some form of exhaust ventilation. However, because exhaust fans increase the pressure across the building shell, they may also increase the rate of radon entry, thus changing the concentration little or even increasing it. For this reason, systems to increase the house ventilation rate ordinarily should be balanced, incorporating both an air intake and air exhaust. (As a general rule, such systems can also include heat exchange between the incoming and outgoing airstreams, thus avoiding most of the energy loss associated with increased ventilation rates (16). Similarly, exhaust ventilation, utilized for reasons other than radon, can include heat recovery.)

A comprehensive scheme for diagnosis and selection must be more detailed than suggested by this overall consideration of urgency, house type, and control approach. It must also be tailored to the type of houses and radon entry modes characteristic of a locale or region. Indeed, even the system of guidelines and the methodologies for survey, monitoring, and interpretation can be expected to depend on the characteristics of the region and the frequency and severity of radon problems in the local building stock.

6 RELATED ISSUES

The foregoing examination of basic elements in radon control strategies suggests a number of important issues whose detailed examination is beyond the scope of this summary, but which ought to be considered as part of a complete strategy. Among these are local or regional variability, strategies for future housing, allocation of responsibilities, and communication of the nature of the problem and probable solutions among responsible entities and to the general public and contractors.

6.1 Local and Regional Variability

Variability in conditions from one area to another affects indoor concentrations, the factors determining them, and the response appropriate to the situation. The design of investigatory efforts in an area depends on the frequency of high levels expected, and the interpretation of monitoring results to yield annual-average concentrations requires an understanding of factors affecting concentrations locally. Such an understanding also underlies diagnosis of the problem in an individual house and selection of control techniques.

The local situation can also substantially affect the system of guidelines for control. This applies both to guidance formulated in terms of concentration limits and to building codes aimed specifically at controlling radon concentrations (as opposed to more general measures setting ventilation objectives). It can be expected that areas tending to have a high frequency of homes with excessive radon concentrations might alter code requirements to include specific control measures or to facilitate their implementation on a remedial basis. Conversely, in an area tending to have high levels, the concentrations thought to be acceptable might be higher than in other areas. This arises from practical considerations that reflect (i) the fundamental presumption that any concentration goal is based on a tradeoff between benefits (e.g., risk reduction) and costs (e.g., implementation of control measures) and (ii) the fact that the cost to reduce the concentration to a given level will tend to be higher in high-radon areas. It is inevitable that the average concentration will continue to vary from one area to another.

6.2 Future Buildings

Although many of the considerations treated here can be applied generally, they are most specifically oriented toward the problem of excessive radon concentrations in existing houses. Much of what is said can be adapted to the problem of future housing, provided two practical considerations are kept in mind: (i) lower concentrations should be sought in future housing because the cost of doing so is less than for implementation of control techniques in existing housing, and (ii) a major component in a strategy for future housing can be expected to be incorporation of radon-specific provisions in building codes and practices.

These practical considerations also interact with fundamental issues. First, the balance of strategic objectives between reducing the total population risk and limiting individual risk in new housing may be altered substantially from the balance adopted for existing housing. Second, the time scale for change may be considerably longer when accomplished in new buildings because the housing stock only turns over at a rate of about 2% per year. On the other hand, virtually the entire stock can be altered over a long period of time.

6.3 Responsibilities

Those inevitably involved in addressing the problem of excessive indoor radon concentrations range from the national government to the individual homeowner or occupant and include local authorities and contractors. A complete radon strategy encompasses not only the specific elements of a control strategy indicated here, but the research underlying it (as suggested in Fig. 12.1). The question of who is responsible for which aspect of an overall radon strategy is, in principle, open. At one extreme, all responsibility could be assigned to federal entities, and at the other, the general population could be left to fend for itself.

An effective approach would appear to involve an intermediate distribution of responsibilities. Thus, development of the most general understanding and of the basic strategic elements is most efficiently relegated to federal agencies and the scientists whose research they support. States and local entities are in the best position to implement a radon strategy locally. And individuals and their immediate agents—private contractors—are ultimately responsible for action in their own homes, at least in a country such as the United States. The boundaries between these areas of responsibility might be crossed in certain respects, e.g., to increase efficiency or cope with financing difficulties. But ultimately the allocation of responsibility ought to align reasonably well with capabilities and immediacy of interest.

6.4   Communication

A critical element in a control strategy involving a diversity of responsibilities and actors is effective communication. This is particularly important when members of the public are those whose effective action is sought and, in this case, whose health is threatened. But, in fact, difficulties exist at every link in the chain of responsibility, including those where scientific results must be utilized properly by agencies having to formulate programs, those where federal pronouncements require interpretation by state and local officials, and—of course—those where information has to be interpreted and utilized by the public.

Perhaps the largest failure in communication has to do with acting before examining carefully the premises for action and the probable results of proposed actions. This is particularly important in the case of indoor pollutants, where the risks are much higher than most "environmental" risks (but not higher than other real-life risks), and where governmental agencies ordinarily do not have jurisdiction—but still have a responsibility. The ambiguities in this situation require more than normal care in examining the premises for action, in formulating criteria appropriate to the indoor setting, and in communicating effectively the elements of a control strategy suggested on the basis of these criteria.

7   CONCLUSIONS

Although identification of the elements needed for a control strategy is straightforward, development of them to an effective form is not. Thus, all agree that guidelines based on clear objectives for exposure reduction are needed, but few agree on what these objectives should be, let alone how they should be framed in terms of standards for ventilation rates, other building characteristics, or concentrations. Similarly, an approach for identifying areas and houses with high concentrations is needed, but development of such an approach is not very advanced, nor is there adequate appreciation of how it connects with a complex system of guidelines or set of control measures. Finally, the basis for selecting a strategy for control in an individual house needs improvement.

An important contributor to the difficulties in developing a control strategy is that, although there is a significant amount of information in each of the required areas, there is not yet enough to provide a sound basis for decision. The current understanding of health effects, although useful, is incomplete and uncertain. The development of predictive capabilities for assisting in the search for high-radon areas or in the interpretation of radon measurements is only at a preliminary stage. And our scientific understanding of radon entry, and experience with methods for reducing it, are not yet adequate for efficient diagnosis and remedy. It is important that substantial efforts be devoted to improving our basic understanding of radon health effects and behavior.

Equally important as improving the scientific understanding is more careful examination of the strategic structure for control. Specifically, the kind of analysis that is indicated in this chapter needs to be developed more systematically and completely. Most decisions and recommendations—whether by radiological protection organizations or national authorities—have not been based on such an analysis, the main possible exception being in Sweden. What is called for—development of a "criteria document," examining the premises for action and defining the associated criteria for a control strategy—has not occurred. Such a document would set forth a systematic analysis and subject it to the scrutiny of the scientific and policy community, laying the basis for a strategy whose objectives and components are understood, optimized, and agreed upon.

Perhaps the most important element in such an analysis would be examination of premises. It is unfortunate, but probably unavoidable, that there is significant disagreement on estimates of risk due to indoor radon. Furthermore, there is no agreement on a general approach to dealing with pollutant exposures in the home environment. In the absence of careful consideration of these matters, proceeding with programs that can affect a large portion of the housing stock is likely to cause confusion and misplaced effort. Conversely, careful consideration of these matters, and of the spectrum of indoor exposures characteristic of the housing stock, will lay the basis for an effective program for reducing excessive radon concentrations. In this context, we will also understand better the scientific needs of this program.

As is evident from the different approaches already taken in the matter of indoor radon, there is some controversy over the premises for action and the objectives to be sought. For example, should significant reduction in the average exposure be sought by remedial actions in existing houses? Or should the main goal of remedial action be reduction of concentrations in the houses with much higher-than-average levels, leaving reduction in the average exposure to alterations in the construction of new buildings?

As a practical matter, no change in the average concentration is likely to occur in the near future, simply because of the effort and time required for such a change. The near-term objective should therefore be fairly clear, i.e., to focus efforts relatively rapidly on houses with unusually high concentrations, in the meantime evaluating whether or how to reduce intermediate concentrations. There is considerable disagreement about whether the latter levels need substantial attention. But even those who believe so would agree that those at higher levels deserve attention first. In the United States, we will be fortunate indeed to have provided remedies for most of the houses exceeding 400 Bq/m^3 EEDC—or about 20 pCi/L of radon—within a decade. In the interim, we will gain substantial experience with identification and control, thereby permitting more efficient future action in the intermediate-level houses. At the same time, we can seek substantial improvement in our understanding of health risks and of the behavior of radon and its decay products in the indoor environment.

REFERENCES

1. Nero, A. V. (1983). Indoor radiation exposures from ^{222}Rn and its daughters: A view of the issue, *Health Phys.*, **45**, 277.
2. Nero, A. V., and Grimsrud, D. T. (1984). Air quality issues in ventilation standards.

In *Proc. 5th AIC Conference*, held Reno, Nevada, Oct. 1–4, 1984, Air Infiltration Centre, Bracknell, England, p 8.1.

3. Nero, A. V., Schwehr, M. B., Nazaroff, W. W., and Revzan, K. L. (1986). Distribution of airborne radon 222 concentrations in U.S. homes, *Science*, **234**, 992.

4. National Council on Radiation Protection and Measurements (1971). *Basic Radiation Protection Criteria*, rep. no. 39, NCRP, Bethesda, MD.

5. American Society of Heating, Refrigerating, and Air-Conditioning Engineers (1981). *Ventilation for Acceptable Indoor Air Quality*, ASHRAE Standard 62-1981, ASHRAE, Atlanta, GA.

6. US Atomic Energy Commission (1972). Grand Junction remedial action: Proposed criteria, *Fed. Register*, **37**, 203.

7. Létourneau, E. G. (1986). Radon standard for Canada. In D. S. Walkinshaw (ed.), *Indoor Air Quality in Cold Climates: Hazards and Abatement Measures*, Air Pollution Control Association, Pittsburgh, PA.

8. Guimond, R. J., Ellett, W. H., Fitzgerald, Jr., J. E., Windham, S. T., and Cuny, P. A. (1979). *Indoor Radiation Exposure Due to Radium-226 in Florida Phosphate Lands*, report EPA-520/4-78-031, US Environmental Protection Agency, Washington, DC.

9. Costle, D. M. (1979). Recommendations for radiation protection of persons residing on phosphate lands, contained in letter from U.S. EPA Administrator Costle to the Governor of Florida, May 30, 1979.

10. Feldman, J., Johnson, D. W., Stoddard, K. M., and Czapor, J. V. (1986). Evaluation of radon levels in residential properties contaminated with radium processing residues. In *Indoor Radon*, Proc. of ACPA Int. Specialty Conf., Philadelphia, PA, Feb. 1986, Air Pollution Control Association, Pittsburgh, PA, p. 78.

11. International Commission on Radiological Protection (1984). *Principles for Limiting Exposure of the Public to Natural Sources of Radiation*, ICRP publication 39, Annals of the ICRP 14, No. 1.

12. National Council on Radiation Protection and Measurements (1984). *Exposures from the Uranium Series with Emphasis on Radon and Its Daughters*, report no. 77, NCRP, Bethesda, MD.

13. US Environmental Protection Agency (1986). *A Citizen's Guide to Radon*, report OPA-86-004, Washington, DC.

14. National Council on Radiation Protection and Measurements (1984). *Evaluation of Occupational Exposures to Radon and Radon Daughters in the United States*, report no. 78, NCRP, Bethesda, MD.

15. Cohen, B. L. (1986). A national survey of ^{222}Rn in U.S. homes and correlating factors, *Health Phys.*, **51**, 175.

16. Fisk, W. J., and Turiel, I. (1983). Residential air-to-air heat exchangers: Performance, energy savings, and economics, *Energy Buildings*, **5**, 197.

17. World Health Organization (1986). *Indoor Air Quality: Radon and Formaldehyde*, Environmental Health Series no. 13, WHO Regional Office for Europe, Copenhagen.

18. The Radiation Protection Institutes in Denmark, Finland, Iceland, Norway, and Sweden (1986). *Naturally Occurring Radiation in the Nordic Countries—Recommendations*, published by the named Radiation Protection Institutes.

19. Swedjemark, G. A. (1986). Swedish limitation schemes to decrease Rn daughters in indoor air, *Health Phys.*, **51**, 569.

APPENDIX

Measurement Techniques

WILLIAM W. NAZAROFF

Environmental Engineering Science, California Institute of Technology, Pasadena, California
Indoor Environment Program, Lawrence Berkeley Laboratory, University of California, Berkeley, California

1 INTRODUCTION

Many techniques have been established for measuring the concentrations of radon and its decay products in air; many of these are suitable for measurements in indoor environments. The objectives of this appendix are to describe briefly the major techniques in current use and to provide a window into the scientific literature on this topic. Further information can be found in several reviews (1–4).

All of the techniques for measuring radon and its decay products are based on the detection of emissions from radioactive decay. Most methods rely on detection of alpha particles; some are based on detection of gamma emissions; only a few utilize beta decays.

In addition to the type of radiation that is detected, several other characteristics distinguish the measurement techniques. An important one is whether the technique measures radon or its decay products, and, if the latter, whether the individual decay product concentrations or the potential alpha-energy concentration is measured. A second major characteristic, for which there are three broad classes, is time resolution. In *grab-sample* techniques, the radioactive content of discrete samples of air—usually collected over a short time at a single point—is analyzed. *Continuous* techniques are designed to provide information on the time dependence of concentrations. *Integrating* techniques provide a single concentration determination, generally averaged over a period of a few days to a year. This classification is useful, even though the boundaries are indistinct. Integrating techniques are most commonly used for survey work or to determine, for example, the annual-average radon concentration of a specific building. Continuous monitors are useful in research applications and in testing remedial techniques. One may, of course, obtain an integrated result from a continuous record; however, this approach is generally more expensive than making a direct integrated measurement. Grab sampling has some application in each of the cases indicated above, particularly for tracking the radon concentration as a remedial measure is being installed; however, it is most useful for the associated analytical techniques which may constitute a secondary calibration standard against which to test integrating and continuous instruments.

Because environmental concentrations of radon and its decay products are often low, the precision and accuracy of the measurement techniques are important issues. Measurement uncertainty arises from several sources, such as the random nature of radioactive decay, variations in detector response, interference by unmeasured species, and unfulfilled assumptions concerning the atmosphere being sampled (e.g., that concentrations are constant over the sampling interval). At the lower end of the range of concentrations of interest to investigators of indoor radon, uncertainty due to the randomness of radioactive decay becomes prominent. For most techniques, one can improve precision of low-level measurements by increasing the volume of air sampled, or by lengthening the sampling or analysis time. The other sources of error can be maintained, with moderate care, at less than about 15%.

2   TECHNIQUES FOR MEASURING RADON

2.1   Analytical Techniques and Grab-Sampling Methods

In this category, the most useful device is the scintillation flask, which was introduced in the 1950s (5, 6). In one of its more common forms, it has become known as the Lucas cell, in recognition of the contributions of H. F. Lucas to its development (7).

The device consists of a vessel, whose inside is at least partially coated with $ZnS(Ag)$ phosphor, and which has one transparent surface, usually flat, that constitutes a viewing window. The vessel has one or two sampling ports, each fitted with a valve. An alpha particle that is produced within the vessel may strike the phosphor, generating a flash of light that is sensed by a photomultiplier tube— which is optically coupled to the vessel window—and associated electronics.

For analysis, a sample of air is admitted into the vessel. In the most precise method, a delay of at least 3 h permits the in-growth to radioactive equilibrium of ^{218}Po and ^{214}Po, after which alpha decays are counted over a period of time. For given delay and counting intervals, the amount of radon contained in the vessel is proportional to the net number of decays observed above the background count rate. In faster, less precise field-sampling methods, counting can begin immediately.

The flask designed by Lucas has the shape of a right circular cylinder with a hemispherical cap. Its diameter and volume are 5 cm and 100 cm^3, respectively. Typically, the detection efficiency is 75–80%, and, with care, a background count rate of about 0.1 counts/min is achieved. Under these conditions, the uncertainty in measuring a sample containing 10 Bq m^{-3}, using 3-h sample-count and background-count intervals, is about 30%. Improved efficiency may be achieved by extracting radon from a larger volume of air and transferring it to the flask (7, 8). Other flask designs have been proposed (9–14), generally to reduce the cost of fabrication or, by using a larger volume, to increase the sensitivity without using a concentration step.

Among other techniques for grab-sample measurement of indoor radon are the two-filter method (15), a method for electrostatic collection of newly formed radon decay products in a chamber (16), and a solvent-extraction technique (17).

2.2 Continuous Monitors

In contrast to the case of grab-sampling methods, no consensus has evolved in favor of a single approach for continuous radon monitoring. Several techniques have merit and these are described below.

One major class of instruments in this category is based on the electrostatic collection of ^{218}Po. The first such instrument, reported by Wrenn et al. (18), has a hemispherical detection chamber with a volume of several liters. Centrally located in the flat bottom surface is a light pipe coupled to a photomultiplier tube. The light pipe is covered with a phosphor, which in turn is covered by a thin layer of aluminized mylar. The upper portion of the chamber is formed by a wire screen covered by foam. A high-voltage electric field is established between the screen ($+$) and the mylar ($-$). The instrument is placed in the room to be monitored, and radon, but not its decay products, diffuses into the detection chamber. Positively charged ^{218}Po, formed from the decay of ^{222}Rn in the chamber, is drawn to the mylar by the electric field. (See Chapters 6 and 11.) Alpha particles from the decays of ^{218}Po and ^{214}Po may strike the phosphor, producing a light pulse which is detected. ^{220}Rn is not detected because it may not diffuse through the foam during its short half-life. The instrument is suitable for measuring concentrations down to about 10 Bq m^{-3}. One limitation of this device is that it is sensitive to humidity, apparently owing to the effects of water vapor on the rate of ^{218}Po neutralization. This problem is solved by placing desiccant in the detection chamber.

A second limitation of this technique is time resolution. Because of the relatively long half-lives of ^{214}Pb and ^{214}Bi, the measurement integration interval cannot be less than a few hours, regardless of the concentration. Although this is acceptable in many situations, there are circumstances in which more rapid response is needed. This constraint has been removed in one variation by replacing the detection apparatus with a solid-state detector (19). In this configuration, alpha spectroscopy is used, and only the counts from ^{218}Po, which has a half-life of 3 min, are registered. In this way, the time resolution is improved to the order of 10 min. Porstendörfer et al. devised a similar instrument that used active sampling by means of a pump rather than passive sampling by means of diffusion (20). With this system, measurement of both ^{222}Rn and ^{220}Rn is possible. Another device using the same approach was recently developed (21).

A second major class of devices in this category uses a two-port scintillation flask with continuous flow (22). As with the device of Wrenn et al., this instrument suffers time-resolution problems: alpha decays of ^{218}Po and ^{214}Po deposited on the walls of the cell contribute to the count rate. Busigin et al. developed a calibration procedure for improving the time response by determining the detection efficiency of ^{222}Rn separately from that of the decay products (23). With this procedure, the scintillation flask monitor may be used with integration intervals as short as 30 min.

Chittaporn et al. devised a promising instrument that combines the scintillation flask with electrostatic collection of ^{218}Po by means of an electret (24). However, in contrast to the instruments described previously, electrostatic collection is used to prevent the decay products from being detected. With this device, measurement of 10 Bq m^{-3} of ^{222}Rn over a 15-min interval is achieved with 30% uncertainty.

The two-filter method (15) has been adapted for continuous monitoring of low concentrations of ^{222}Rn in outdoor air (25–27). Although these specific instruments are too large for use in indoor environments, the technique could be applied to this purpose.

2.3   Integrating Monitors

The most widely used integrating radon monitor is based on materials alternatively known as solid-state nuclear track detectors or as etched-track detectors. The technique is simple to use and relatively inexpensive. It provides a single measure that indicates the integrated exposure. For measurement of environmental levels, exposures of a few weeks to a year are necessary to obtain adequate precision at low analysis cost. This technique is well suited to determining annual-average concentrations, but is less useful for rapidly obtaining information on indoor concentrations.

Several detector materials have been developed. The most suitable for indoor radon measurements appears to be CR-39, a polymer derived from the monomer oxydi-2, 1-ethanediyl di-2-propenyl diester of carbonic acid (28, 29). Alpha particles penetrating the material cause damage to the chemical bonds. Upon etching, the damaged regions become visible, with each alpha particle producing a distinguishable track. By counting the tracks in a given area, the exposure of the detector to alpha-producing nuclides may be determined.

Several configurations have been developed for using etched-track detectors to measure indoor radon concentrations (30). In the most useful one, the detector is taped to the bottom of a plastic cup. The cup is covered either with a filter, to prevent radon decay products from entering, or with a membrane, which also prevents the entry of ^{220}Rn. By diffusion, then, the radon concentration in the cup is equal, on average, to that in the surrounding air. Alpha particles from radon that has diffused into the cup, and from the polonium isotopes that have been produced therein, may strike the detector and be registered. Some concern has been expressed that static charge on the cup may affect the response of the device by altering the deposition pattern of the decay products. This may account in part for the approximately 20% variation in response that is observed beyond the uncertainty owing to the random nature of radioactive decay (30, 31). In addition to its use as a survey device, the etched-track detectors have proven useful for certain research applications (32, 33).

A more recent development in integrated measurements of indoor radon concentration is the use of activated charcoal (34–37). The most useful configuration has a diffusion barrier to separate the charcoal from the air being sampled. In a manner similar to the operation of other passive samplers for indoor air pollutants, a linear concentration gradient is established along the barrier and the rate of pollutant collection is proportional to the airborne concentration (38, 39). Following exposure, the quantity of radon adsorbed by the charcoal is analyzed, most commonly by gamma spectrometry, although desorption followed by scintillation counting is possible.

The charcoal adsorption technique is suitable for measuring concentrations less than 40 Bq m^{-3} with an integration time of a few days. The primary limitations on this technique arise from the fact that the charcoal only *collects* the radon, it does not *detect* it. Because the half-life of ^{222}Rn is only 3.8 days, the exposure period cannot usefully be longer than a week, and the sampler must be returned to the laboratory for prompt analysis following exposure. For the same reason, this technique does not provide a true time average, but rather averages with a weighting factor that varies exponentially with a time-constant equal to the radon half-life. The measurement is sensitive to humidity and temperature, but to a relatively small degree (37). Despite its limitations, this technique is a useful complement to the etched-track detector, particularly for survey work.

Other instruments for integrated radon measurement have been developed but are not now in wide use (40–43).

3 TECHNIQUES FOR MEASURING RADON DECAY PRODUCTS

3.1 Grab-Sampling Methods

Almost all methods for measuring radon decay products entail drawing a specified volume of air through a filter capable of retaining the decay products at or near its surface. Radioactive decays on the filter are detected and the data used to determine the concentration(s) in the sampled air.

To pass beyond this cursory level of understanding and delve into the details of the measurement techniques, one needs knowledge of the behavior of the radioactive chain of radon decay products. A useful description has been written by Evans (44).

Consider for the moment an atmosphere that contains ^{222}Rn and its decay products, but not ^{220}Rn or its products. As the half-life of ^{214}Po is too short for the number concentration of this species to be of consequence (see Fig. 1.2), there are three radioisotopes of interest: ^{218}Po, ^{214}Pb, and ^{214}Bi. The concentrations of the three species represent three independent variables. An approximate measure of a parameter, such as EEDC (or PAEC), may be obtained by measuring only one or two parameters and making reasonable assumptions about the state of equilibrium, as discussed below. However, to determine the three concentrations without prior assumption, measurement of at least three independent parameters is required.

Tsivoglou et al. (45) were the first to devise a measurement technique that recognized this principle. It was developed for use in mines and is not sensitive enough for measurements in most indoor environments; however, the method remains an archetype for many of the techniques in current use. Their procedure is to sample air through a filter for 5 min, collecting radon decay products on the filter. A ratemeter is then used to obtain the alpha decay rate as a function of time for the next 45 min. Alpha activity at 5, 15, and 30 min following sampling is determined, satisfying the requirement for three independent measurements. The concentrations of ^{218}Po, ^{214}Pb, and ^{214}Bi are computed as linear combinations of the three net count rates.

Following the work of Tsivoglou et al. there have been numerous developments to make this technique more suitable for indoor measurements. Thomas suggested replacing rate measurements with integrated counts over the intervals 2–5, 6–20, and 21–30 min following sampling (46, 47). Cliff devised an approach in which the first counting interval coincided with sampling (48). Busigin and Phillips (49) and Nazaroff (50) proposed different counting intervals to improve precision. Scott proposed an alternative set of counting intervals to facilitate field measurements (51). Khan et al. developed a five-count technique for simultaneously measuring the concentrations of the decay products of ^{220}Rn: ^{212}Pb and ^{212}Bi (52).

The precision of the these variants of the three-count total-alpha technique for determining concentrations of individual decay products is adequate for measurements in many indoor environments. Precision is poorest for ^{218}Po, particularly if sequential sampling and counting intervals are used. The equilibrium-equivalent decay product concentration (EEDC) is measured with good precision by these methods. For example, assuming a total measurement time of 60 min, and a product of detector efficiency and sampling flow rate of 5 L min^{-1}, an EEDC of 1 Bq m^{-3} (0.0003 WL) can be measured with 20% uncertainty using sequential sampling and counting intervals (50). With overlapping intervals, an EEDC of 0.3 Bq m^{-3} can be measured with equivalent precision.

A further development along this line (even though it predated much of the work mentioned above) is the technique of Raabe and Wrenn, in which more count intervals than unknowns are used (53). A least-squares fit to the count rate versus time provides somewhat more precise determinations of ^{222}Rn and ^{220}Rn decay products than is possible with the "exact" techniques. The cost is a somewhat greater computational effort.

In addition to these developments in analysis, the ratemeter of Tsivoglou et al.'s day has been supplanted by a ZnS (Ag) phosphor plus photomultiplier tube and associated electronics, or by a solid-state diffused-junction or surface-barrier detector.

One is not restricted to total alpha decays as a measurement parameter, and much work has been devoted to techniques using other decay information. The most prevalent alternative is the use of alpha spectroscopy, whereby the decays of

^{218}Po and ^{214}Po, and, in some cases, ^{212}Po, are distinguished according to their energy. This cannot be done with a phosphor, but is readily accomplished with a solid-state detector. The first use of alpha spectroscopy for this purpose was reported by Martz et al. (54). In analogy to Tsivoglou et al., they proposed the determination of decay rates at two distinct times. Jonassen and Hayes reported an alpha-spectroscopic technique using two counting intervals (55). Optimization of the count-interval timing was studied by Tremblay et al. (56) for the case in which the counting and sampling intervals overlap, and by Nazaroff (57) for the case in which the intervals are distinct. Aprilesi et al. (58) have reported on a technique based on alpha spectroscopy for which counting occurs during sampling and a least-squares fit to the growth and decay curves is used to determine concentrations. An interesting aspect of their instrument is that decay products are collected by electrostatic precipitation, rather than by filtration.

Overall, the alpha-spectroscopic techniques with sequential sampling and counting intervals are capable of measuring indoor ^{222}Rn decay product concentrations of less than 20 Bq m^{-3} within an hour with a precision of better than 20% (e.g., Ref. 57). Compared with the total-alpha techniques, measurement precision for ^{218}Po is greatly improved.

The instrument with possibly the greatest potential for rapid, high-precision measurements was developed by Groer and co-workers (59, 60). In this case a single postsampling counting interval is used with a total $\beta + \gamma$ determination supplementing alpha-spectroscopic measurement.

Irfan and Fagan reported on a technique analogous to the modified Tsivoglou method in which detection of gamma emissions from ^{214}Bi was substituted for the total alpha detection (61). However, this technique does not appear to offer any advantages over the total-alpha methods for indoor measurements.

In addition to the techniques that obtain enough information to determine separately the concentrations of the decay products, much effort has been devoted to the development of simpler techniques to measure EEDC (62–75). These developments are broadly analogous to those for the "exact" methods described above. In comparison with the "exact" methods, the approximate techniques have the advantage of being simpler to execute and analyze. In addition to having less information, the main disadvantage is the introduction of a procedural error that arises because the relationship between EEDC in air and decays on a filter depends on the relative activity concentrations of the decay products. The "exact" and approximate methods require the same types of equipment and offer similar measurement precision for determining EEDC.

3.2 Continuous Monitors

The "continuous" monitors for radon decay products are based on the grab-sample methods described above, with modifications to permit automatic sampling, counting, and, in some cases, analysis. In most cases they are not truly continuous, but rather collect and analyze discrete samples at intervals from several minutes to an hour. Three instruments based on the alpha-spectroscopic technique have been reported: filter collection (57) and electrostatic collection (76) with sequential sampling and counting intervals; and filter collection with overlapped sampling and counting intervals (77). The procedure of Groer et al. has also been automated (60).

3.3 Integrating Monitors

Only one approach to integrated measurement of radon decay products indoors has been widely used (78, 79). In one form it is commonly known as the radon progeny integrated sampling unit (RPISU). The essential elements of the device are a sampling head and a constant-flow-rate pump. The sampling head has a thermoluminescent dosimeter (TLD), commonly a thin crystal of LiF, mounted in a holder facing the upstream side of a filter. The pump draws air at a low rate (typically $100 \text{ cm}^3 \text{ min}^{-1}$) through the filter, collecting radon decay products.

Some of the alpha particles from subsequent decay strike the TLD, creating electron-hole pairs which may enter a metastable state above the ground state. The analysis procedure involves heating the detector through a prescribed temperature cycle and observing, by means of a photomultiplier tube, the light emitted as the electrons and holes recombine. The amount of light observed is related to the average EEDC sampled.

This same configuration may be used with other detectors, such as etched-track detectors (80, 81) or solid-state diffused-junction detectors. One concern with this approach that has not been resolved is the potential loss of decay products on the sampling head in advance of the filter. This is a particular concern for the unattached decay products, which have a high mobility. It has also been proposed that to save weight and expense the pump and filter may be replaced with an electret (82). The latter approach would seem to be very sensitive to environmental conditions, such as the degree of air motion and the relative humidity.

An effort has been made to develop a technique for measuring integrated EEDC based entirely on etched-track detectors. One approach uses an array of detectors covered by absorbers of varying thicknesses and mounted in a diffusion box (83, 84). Interpretation of the data is based on a simplified model of decay product behavior within the box. Results of a test of the technique indicate that, although the approach may have some value, further work is needed before it can be considered reliable in routine application.

There are no techniques for integrated measurement of individual decay product concentrations.

4 CALIBRATION

The calibration of instruments for measuring ^{222}Rn is traced to solutions of ^{226}Ra, such as the standard-reference-method (SRM) solutions available from the U.S. National Bureau of Standards. Research groups that maintain independent calibration facilities usually have a set of devices, such as scintillation flasks, that are directly calibrated against the SRM solution. Procedures for transferring ^{222}Rn from the solution to scintillation flasks have been reported (e.g., Refs. 7 and 8).

Calibration of continuous and integrating instruments for measuring radon is seldom done directly with an SRM solution. Instead, an atmosphere whose radon concentration is determined with a calibrated device is simultaneously sampled with the uncalibrated instrument. The sampling is often done in a chamber established specifically for such a purpose.

To provide further quality assurance, calibration intercomparisons between laboratories that routinely make airborne radon measurements have been initiated (85, 86).

For the case of radon decay products, the basis for absolute assurance in the results is not so well established. Ideally, one seeks a procedure by which an atmosphere may be established to contain known concentrations of radon decay products. Other important characteristics, such as particle concentration and size distribution, should be independently variable so that the typical range of indoor conditions can be simulated. The calibration procedure would then be to determine the efficiency of the entire measurement system by sampling and analyzing the known decay product concentrations.

Although limited attempts have been made in this direction, such an ideal has not been achieved (87). Instead, calibration of decay product measurement techniques is limited to components of the measurement system. Sampling pumps and flowmeters are routinely calibrated against absolute displacement devices. Detector efficiency may be determined using an electrodeposited radioactive source, such as ^{241}Am for alpha-measurement techniques, having the same geometry as the sampled decay products. It is commonly assumed that filters collect decay products with perfect efficiency. This appears reasonable for membrane filters with submicron pore size, and, possibly for glass fiber filters (88–91). One also generally assumes that, once collected, decay products are retained on the filter. However, Jonassen and McLaughlin have shown that, in a vacuum, the recoil loss of ^{214}Pb from membrane filters may be large (92). Under typical conditions this may cause an underestimate by about 10% in the determination of ^{214}Pb, with smaller errors for the other two radioisotopes (93).

It appears, then, that with modest care satisfactory calibration may be attained for instruments that are important in survey and other field applications. This situation also holds for instruments used for radon measurements and some kinds of decay product measurements in laboratory experiments. The problem of developing and calibrating specialized measurement techniques is more difficult, a prime example being instruments aimed at elucidating the behavior of radon decay products with respect to indoor aerosols (see Chapter 6).

REFERENCES

1. Nuclear Energy Agency Group of Experts (1985). *Metrology and Monitoring of Radon, Thoron and Their Daughter Products*, OECD, Paris.

2. Budnitz, R. J., Nero, A. V., Murphy, D. J., and Graven, R. (1983). *Instrumentation for Environmental Monitoring*, 2nd ed., Vol. 1, *Radiation*, Wiley, New York, p. 395.

3. George, A. C., and Breslin, A. J. (1977). Measurements of environmental radon with integrating instruments. In *Proc. Workshop on Methods for Measuring Radiation in and Around Uranium Mines*, Albuquerque, NM.

4. Budnitz, R. J. (1974). Radon-222 and its daughters: A review of instrumentation for occupational and environmental monitoring, *Health Phys.*, **26**, 145.

5. Damon, P. E., and Hyde, H. I. (1952). Scintillation tube for the measurement of radioactive gases, *Rev. Sci. Instrum.*, **23**, 766.

6. Van Dilla, M. A., and Taysum, D. H. (1955). Scintillation counter for assay of radon gas, *Nucleonics*, **13**(2), 68.

7. Lucas, H. F. (1957). Improved low-level alpha-scintillation counter for radon, *Rev. Sci. Instrum.*, **28**, 680.

8. Ingersoll, J. G., Stitt, B. D., and Zapalac, G. H. (1983). A fast and accurate method for measuring radon exhalation rates from building materials, *Health Phys.*, **45**, 550.

9. Collinson, A. J. L., and Haque, A. K. M. M. (1963). A scintillation counter for the measurement of radon concentration in air, *J. Sci. Instrum.*, **40**, 521.

10. Kraner, H. W., Schroeder, G. L., Lewis, A. R., and Evans, R. D. (1964). Large volume scintillation chamber for radon counting, *Rev. Sci. Instrum.*, **35**, 1259.

11. Kristan, J., and Kobal, I. (1973). A modified scintillation cell for the determination of radon in uranium mine atmosphere, *Health Phys.*, **24**, 103.

12. Scheibel, H. G., Porstendörfer, J., and Wicke, A. (1979). A device for the determination of low natural ^{222}Rn and ^{226}Ra concentrations, *Nucl. Instrum. Methods*, **165**, 345.

13. Cohen, B. L., El Ganayni, M., and Cohen, E. S. (1983). Large scintillation cells for high sensitivity radon monitoring, *Nucl. Instrum. Methods*, **212**, 403.

14. Barton, T. P., and Ziemer, P. L. (1984). A simple, inexpensive scintillation cell, *Health Phys.*, **47**, 93.

15. Thomas, J. W., and LeClare, P. C. (1970). A study of the two-filter method for radon-222, *Health Phys.*, **18**, 113.

16. Srivastava, G. K., Raghavayya, M., Khan, A. H., and Kotrappa, P. (1984). A low-level radon detection system, *Health Phys.*, **46**, 225.

17. Prichard, H. M. (1983). A solvent extraction technique for the measurement of ^{222}Rn at ambient air concentrations, *Health Phys.*, **45**, 493.

18. Wrenn, M. E., Spitz, H., and Cohen, N. (1975). Design of a continuous digital-output environmental radon monitor, *IEEE Trans. Nucl. Sci.*, **NS-22**, 645.

19. Negro, V. C., and Watnick, S. (1978). FUNGI: A radon measuring instrument with fast response, *IEEE Trans. Nucl. Sci.*, **NS-25**, 757.

20. Porstendörfer, J., Wicke, A., and Schraub, A. (1980). Methods for continuous registration of radon, thoron and their decay products indoors and outdoors. In T. F. Gesell and W. M. Lowder (eds.), *Natural Radiation Environment III*, CONF-780422, US Dept. of Commerce, National Technical Information Service, Springfield, VA, p. 1293.

21. Watnick, S., Latner, N., and Graveson, R. T. (1986). A ^{222}Rn monitor using α spectroscopy, *Health Phys.*, **50**, 645.

22. Thomas, J. W., and Countess, R. J. (1979). Continuous radon monitor, *Health Phys.*, **36**, 734.

23. Busigin, A., van der Vooren, A. W., and Phillips, C. R. (1979). Interpretation of the response of continuous radon monitors to transient radon concentrations, *Health Phys.*, **37**, 659.

24. Chittaporn, P., Eisenbud, M., and Harley, N. H. (1981). A continuous monitor for the measurement of environmental radon, *Health Phys.*, **41**, 405.

25. Newstein, H., Cohen, L. D., and Krablin, R. (1971). An automated atmospheric radon sampling system, *Atmos. Environ.*, **5**, 823.

26. Thomas, J. W. (1972). An automated atmospheric radon sampling system, *Atmos. Environ.*, **6**, 285.

27. Schery, S. D., Gaeddert, D. H., and Wilkening, M. H. (1980). Two-filter monitor for atmospheric ^{222}Rn, *Rev. Sci. Instrum.*, **51**, 338.

28. Cartwright, B. G., Shirk, E. K., and Price, P. B. (1978). A nuclear-track-recording polymer of unique sensitivity and resolution, *Nucl. Instrum. Methods*, **153**, 457.

29. Cassou, R. M., and Benton, E. V. (1978). Properties and applications of CR-39 polymeric nuclear track detector, *Nucl. Track Detection*, **2**, 173.

30. Alter, H. W., and Oswald, R. A. (1983). Results of indoor radon measurements using the track etch method, *Health Phys.*, **45**, 425.

31. Cohen, B. L. (1986). Comparison of nuclear track and diffusion barrier charcoal adsorption methods for measurement of ^{222}Rn levels in indoor air, *Health Phys.*, **50**, 828.

32. Abu-Jarad, F., Wilson, C. K., and Fremlin, J. H. (1981). The registration of the alpha-particles from polonium isotopes plated-out on the surface of the plastic detectors LR-115 and CR-39, *Nucl. Tracks*, **5**, 285.

33. Abu-Jarad, F., Fremlin, J. H., and Bull, R. (1980). A study of radon emitted from building materials using plastic alpha-track detectors, *Phys. Med. Biol.*, **25**, 683.

34. Cohen, B. L., and Cohen, E. S. (1983). Theory and practice of radon monitoring with charcoal adsorption, *Health Phys.*, **45**, 501.

35. George, A. C. (1984). Passive, integrated measurement of indoor radon using activated charcoal, *Health Phys.*, **46**, 867.

36. Prichard, H. M., and Mariën, K. (1985). A passive diffusion ^{222}Rn sampler based on activated carbon adsorption, *Health Phys.*, **48**, 797.

37. Cohen, B. L., and Nason, R. (1986). A diffusion barrier charcoal adsorption collector for measuring Rn concentrations in indoor air, *Health Phys.*, **50**, 457.

38. Palmes, E. D., Gunnison, A. F., DiMattio, J., and Tomczyk, C. (1976). Personal sampler for nitrogen dioxide, *Am. Ind. Hyg. Assoc. J.*, **37**, 570.

39. Geisling, K. L., Tashima, M. K., Girman, J. R., Miksch, R. R., and Rappaport, S. M. (1982). A passive sampling device for determining formaldehyde in indoor air, *Environ. Int.*, **8**, 153.

40. Sill, C. W. (1969). An integrating air sampler for determination of radon-222, *Health Phys.*, **16**, 371.

41. Bedrosian, P. H. (1969). Photographic technique for monitoring radon-222 and daughter products, *Health Phys.*, **16**, 800.

42. George, A. C. (1977). A passive environmental radon monitor. In *Proc. Radon Workshop*, February 1977, report HASL-325, Health and Safety Laboratory, New York.

43. Kotrappa, P., Dua, S. K., Pimpale, N. S., Gupta, P. C., Nambi, K. S. V., Bhagwat, A. M., and Soman, S. D. (1982). Passive measurement of radon and thoron using TLD or SSNTD on electrets, *Health Phys.*, **43**, 399.

44. Evans, R. D. (1969). Engineers' guide to the elementary behavior of radon daughters, *Health Phys.*, **17**, 229.

45. Tsivoglou, E. C., Ayer, H. E., and Holaday, D. A. (1953). Occurrence of nonequilibrium atmospheric mixtures of radon and its daughters, *Nucleonics*, **11**(9), 40.

46. Thomas, J. W. (1970). Modification of the Tsivoglou method for radon daughters in air, *Health Phys.*, **19**, 691.

47. Thomas, J. W. (1972). Measurement of radon daughters in air, *Health Phys.*, **23**, 783.

48. Cliff, K. D. (1978). The measurement of low concentrations of radon-222 daughters in air, with emphasis on RaA assessment, *Phys. Med. Biol.*, **23**, 55.

49. Busigin, A., and Phillips, C. R. (1980). Uncertainties in the measurement of airborne radon concentrations, *Health Phys.*, **39**, 943.

50. Nazaroff, W. W. (1983). Optimizing the total-alpha three-count technique for measuring concentrations of radon progeny in residences, *Health Phys.*, **46**, 395.

51. Scott, A. G. (1981). A field method for measurement of radon daughters in air, *Health Phys.*, **41**, 403.

52. Khan, A., Busigin, A., and Phillips, C. R. (1982). An optimized scheme for measurement of the concentrations of the decay products of radon and thoron, *Health Phys.*, **42**, 809.

53. Raabe, O. G., and Wrenn, M. E. (1969). Analysis of the activity of radon daughter samples by weighted least squares, *Health Phys.*, **17**, 593.

54. Martz, D. E., Holleman, D. F., McCurdy, D. E., and Schiager, K. J. (1969). Analysis of atmospheric concentrations of RaA, RaB, and RaC by alpha spectroscopy, *Health Phys.*, **17**, 131.

55. Jonassen, N., and Hayes, E. I. (1974). The measurement of low concentrations of the short-lived radon-222 daughters in the air by alpha spectroscopy, *Health Phys.*, **26**, 104.

56. Tremblay, R. J., Leclerc, A., Townsend, M. G., Mathieu, C., and Pepin, R. (1979). Measurement of radon progeny concentration in air by alpha-particle spectrometric counting during and after air sampling, *Health Phys.*, **36**, 401.

57. Nazaroff, W. W. (1983). Radon daughter carousel: An automated instrument for measuring indoor concentrations of ^{218}Po, ^{214}Pb, and ^{214}Bi, *Rev. Sci. Instrum.*, **54**, 1227.

58. Aprilesi, G., Loria, A., Magnoni, G., Marseguerra, M., Morelli, S., and Rivasi, M. R. (1978). Absolute estimation of radon daughter concentrations in air by alpha-spectroscopy, *Nucl. Instrum. Methods*, **148**, 187.

59. Groer, P. G., Evans, R., and Gordon, D. A. (1973). An instant working level meter for uranium mines, *Health Phys.*, **24**, 387.

60. Keefe, D. J., McDowell, W. P., and Groer, P. G. (1983). The EWLM-II, a measurement and data acquisition system for radon daughters. In *International Meeting on Radon-Radon Progeny Measurements: Proceedings*, report EPA 520/5-83/021, US Environmental Protection Agency Office of Radiation Programs, Washington, DC, p. 5.

61. Irfan, M., and Fagan, A. J. (1979). Measurement of radon daughters in air using gamma spectroscopy, *Nuclear Instrum. Methods*, **166**, 567.

62. Kusnetz, H. L. (1956). Radon daughters in mine atmospheres: A field method for determining concentrations, *Am. Ind. Hyg. Assoc. Q.*, **17**, 85.

63. Markov, K. P., Ryabov, N. V., and Stas', K. N. (1962). A rapid method for estimating

the radiation hazard associated with the presence of radon daughter products in air, *Soviet J. Atomic Energy*, **12**, 333.

64. Harley, N. H., and Pasternack, B. S. (1969). The rapid estimation of radon daughter working levels when daughter equilibrium is unknown, *Health Phys.*, **17**, 109.

65. Rolle, R. (1969). Improved radon daughter monitoring procedure, *Am. Ind. Hyg. Assoc. J.*, **30**, 153.

66. Rolle, R. (1972). Rapid working level monitoring, *Health Phys.*, **22**, 233.

67. Groer, P. G. (1972). The accuracy and precision of the Kusnetz method for the determination of the working level in uranium mines, *Health Phys.*, **23**, 106.

68. Hill, A. (1975). Rapid measurement of radon, decay products, unattached fractions, and working level values of mine atmospheres, *Health Phys.*, **28**, 472.

69. Schiager, K. J. (1977). The 3R-WL working level survey meter, *Health Phys.*, **33**, 595.

70. Stranden, E. (1980). A two-count filter method for measurement of Rn-220 and Rn-222 daughters in air, *Health Phys.*, **38**, 73.

71. Holub, R. F. (1980). Evaluation and modification of working level measurement methods, *Health Phys.*, **39**, 425.

72. Nazaroff, W. W. (1980). Improved technique for measuring working levels of radon daughters in residences, *Health Phys.*, **39**, 683.

73. Borak, T. B., Franco, E. D., and Holub, R. F. (1982). An evaluation of working level measurements using a generalized Kusnetz method, *Health Phys.*, **42**, 459.

74. Revzan, K. L., and Nazaroff, W. W. (1983). A rapid spectroscopic technique for determining the potential alpha energy concentration of radon decay products, *Health Phys.*, **45**, 509.

75. Bigu, J., and Grenier, M. (1984). Thoron daughter working level measurements by one and two gross alpha-count methods, *Nucl. Instrum. Methods*, **255**, 385.

76. Andrews, L. L., Schery, S. D., and Wilkening, M. H. (1984). An electrostatic precipitator for the study of airborne radioactivity, *Health Phys.*, **46**, 801.

77. Bigu, J., Raz, R., Golden, K., and Dominguez, P. (1984). Design and development of a computer-based continuous monitor for the determination of the short-lived decay products of radon and thoron, *Nucl. Instrum. Methods*, **225**, 399.

78. Schiager, K. J. (1974). Integrating radon progeny air sampler, *Am. Ind. Hyg. Assoc. J.*, **35**, 165.

79. Guggenheim, S. F., George, A. C., Graveson, R. T., and Breslin, A. J. (1979). A time-integrating environmental radon daughter monitor, *Health Phys.*, **36**, 452.

80. Auxier, J. A., Becker, K., Robinson, E. M., Johnson, D. R., Boyett, R. H., and Abner, C. H. (1971). A new radon progeny personnel dosimeter, *Health Phys.* **21**, 126.

81. Johnson, D. R., Boyett, R. H., and Becker, K. (1970). Sensitive automatic counting of alpha particle tracks in polymers and its applications in dosimetry, *Health Phys.*, **18**, 424.

82. Khan, A., and Phillips, C. R. (1984). Electrets for passive radon daughter dosimetry, *Health Phys.*, **46**, 141.

83. Fleischer, R. L., Turner, L. G., and George, A. C. (1984). Passive measurement of working levels and effective diffusion constants of radon daughters by the nuclear track technique, *Health Phys.*, **47**, 9.

84. Fleischer, R. L. (1984). Theory of passive measurement of radon daughters and working levels by the nuclear track technique, *Health Phys.*, **47**, 263.

85. Fisenne, I. M., George, A. C., and McGahan, M. (1983). Radon measurement intercomparisons, *Health Phys.*, **45**, 553.

86. Miles, J. C., Stares, E. J., Cliff, K. D., and Sinnaeve, J. (1984). Results from an international intercomparison of techniques for measuring radon and radon decay products, *Radiat. Prot. Dosim.*, **7**, 169.

87. McLaughlin, J. P., and Jonassen, N. (1983). The intercalibration of a radon daughter detection system with a radon detection system, *Health Phys.*, **45**, 556.

88. Anderson, D. E. (1960). Efficiencies of filter papers for collecting radon daughters, *Am. Ind. Hyg. Assoc. J.*, **21**, 428.

89. Lindeken, C. L. (1961). Use of natural airborne radioactivity to evaluate filters for alpha air sampling, *Am. Ind. Hyg. Assoc. J.*, **22**, 232.

90. Holmgren, R. M., Wagner, W. W., Lloyd, R. D., and Pendleton, R. C. (1977). Relative filter efficiencies for sampling radon daughters in air, *Health Phys.*, **32**, 297.

91. Busigin, A., van der Vooren, A. W., and Phillips, C. R. (1980). Collection of radon daughters on filter media, *Environ. Sci. Technol.*, **14**, 531.

92. Jonassen, N., and McLaughlin, J. P. (1976). On the recoil of RaB from membrane filters, *J. Aerosol Sci.*, **7**, 141.

93. Jonassen, N., and McLaughlin, J. P. (1976). The effect of RaB recoil losses on radon daughter measurements, *Health Phys.*, **30**, 234.